Infectious Disease Emergencies

Infectious Disease Emergencies
Preparedness & Response

Chief Editor
Dale Fisher

Editorial Advisors
David Heymann, Soumya Swaminathan,
Myriam Henkens, Ali S. Khan, Paul Effler,
Carlos Navarro Colorado, Pat Drury

Associate Editors
Joycelyn Soo, Sai Arathi Parepalli, Archith Kamath, Chen Xiaoyu

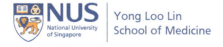

© 2025 The authors

Published by:
NUS Press
National University of Singapore
AS3-01-02
3 Arts Link
Singapore 117569

Fax: (65) 6774-0652
E-mail: nusbooks@nus.edu.sg
Website: http://nuspress.nus.edu.sg

ISBN: 978-981-325-247-9 (case)
ePDF ISBN: 978-981-325-248-6

All rights reserved. This book, or parts thereof, may not be reproduced in any form or by any means, electronic or mechanical, including photocopying, recording or any information storage and retrieval system now known or to be invented, without written permission from the Publisher.

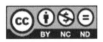 Creative Commons Attribution-NonCommercial-NoDerivatives 4.0 International License (CC-BY-NC-ND 4.0)

National Library Board, Singapore Cataloguing in Publication Data
Name(s): Fisher, Dale, editor. | NUS Press, publisher.
Title: Infectious disease emergencies : preparedness & response / chief editor, Dale Fisher.
Description: Singapore : NUS Press, National University of Singapore, 2025.
Identifier(s): ISBN 978-981-325-247-9 (case) | 978-981-325-248-6 (ePDF)
Subject(s): LCSH: Communicable diseases--Transmission--Prevention. | Pandemics--Prevention. | Epidemics--Prevention. | Medical emergencies. | Health services administration.
Classification: DDC 616.9045 --dc23

Cover image: Naoki Ichiryu

Typeset by: Ogma Solutions Pvt. Ltd.
Printed by: Integrated Books International

Contents

Preface *Dale Fisher*		ix
Foreword *David L. Heymann*		xi
List of Abbreviations		xiii
List of Contributors		xvii
1.	Infectious Disease Emergencies: Introduction *Dale Fisher*, National University of Singapore	1
2.	What Causes Outbreaks? *Joycelyn Soo*, SingHealth *Catherine Moore*, University of Oxford *George Gao*, Director, Chinese Center for Disease Control and Prevention *David L. Heymann*, London School of Hygiene and Tropical Medicine	9
3.	Leading and Partnering in a Crisis *Iris Hunger*, Robert Koch Institute *Johanna Hanefeld*, Robert Koch Institute *Carolin Meinus*, Robert Koch Institute *Lothar H. Wieler*, Hasso Plattner Institute *David Nabarro*, WHO	20
4.	Legal Frameworks for Outbreak Response *Elyssa Liu*, UNICEF *Dena Kirpalani*, Geneva Graduate Institute *Ayelet Berman*, National University of Singapore	29
5.	Ethics to Inform Decision-making *Sarah J.L. Edwards*, University College London *Caitlin Gordon*, National Health Service, U.K. *Blessing Silaigwana*, University of Cape Town *Roli Mathur*, Indian Council of Medical Research	45
6.	Teamwork and Decision-making *Nikita Devnarain*, CAPRISA *Salim S. Abdool Karim*, Columbia University	62
7.	Operational Logistics Support and Supply Chains *Matthew Y.S. Lai*, University of Oxford *Pierre Boulet-Desbareau*, Médecins Sans Frontières *J.C. Azé*, WHO *Robert Blanchard*, WHO	71
8.	Border Controls and Public Health Emergencies of International Concern *Vivianne Ihekweazu*, Nigeria Health Watch *Sarin K.C.*, Ministry of Public Health, Thailand *David L. Heymann*, London School of Hygiene and Tropical Medicine	86

9. Surveillance, Outbreak Detection, and Early Warning — 98
   Rachel Peh, London School of Hygiene and Tropical Medicine
   Geoffrey Namara, WHO
   Oyeronke Oyebanji, Coalition for Epidemic Preparedness Innovations
   Chikwe Ihekweazu, Nigeria Centre for Disease Control and Prevention

10. Field Epidemiology and Outbreak Investigation — 111
    Alexander Spina, Applied Epi
    Erika Valeska Rossetto, ProEpi, the Brazilian Field Epidemiology Network
    Neale Batra, Executive Director, Applied Epi

11. The Evolution of Contact Tracing — 130
    Zheng Jie Marc Ho, Ministry of Health, Singapore
    Vernon Lee, Ministry of Health, Singapore
    Yang Luo, National Healthcare Group, Singapore

12. Non-pharmaceutical Interventions — 139
    Caitriona Murphy, The University of Hong Kong
    Benjamin J. Cowling, The University of Hong Kong

13. One Health: the Animal-Human Interface — 155
    Sai Arathi Parepalli, University of Oxford
    Archith Kamath, NHS Lothian, U.K.
    John S. Mackenzie, Curtin University
    Mahmudur Rahman, Bangladesh Global Health Development/EMPHNET

14. Healthy Populations and Strong Health Systems for Outbreak Resilience — 168
    Thomas Bentley, North Bristol NHS Trust
    Anders Nordström, Stockholm School of Economics
    Helena Legido-Quigley, NUS Saw Swee Hock School of Public Health, Singapore

15. Complicating Humanitarian Emergencies — 179
    Kate McNeil, University of Cambridge
    Joycelyn Soo, SingHealth
    Myriam Henkens, Médecins Sans Frontières

16. Modelling to Inform Strategy — 193
    Louisa Sun, Alexandra Hospital, Singapore
    Gabriel Leung, The University of Hong Kong
    Alex R. Cook, National University of Singapore

17. Integrated Outbreak Analytics (IOA) — 211
    Simone E. Carter, UNICEF
    Pascale Lissouba, Epicentre–MSF

18. Research to Inform Practice — 222
    Thomas A.J. Rowland, University of Oxford
    David Paterson, National University of Singapore
    Mo Yin, National University Hospital, Singapore

19. Establishing Laboratory Capacity — 237
    Rosanna W. Peeling, London School of Hygiene and Tropical Medicine
    Noah Takah Fongwen, London School of Hygiene and Tropical Medicine
    Amadou Sall, Institut Pasteur Dakar

20. Evaluating and Implementing New Diagnostics — 252
   Devy Emperador, FIND
   Camille Escadafal, FIND
   Daniel G. Bausch, FIND

21. Pathogen Genomics for Surveillance and Outbreak Investigations — 270
   Tze-Minn Mak, Bioinformatics Institute, Singapore
   Marc Stegger, Statens Serum Institut, Denmark
   Kåre Mølbak, Statens Serum Institut, Denmark
   Sebastian Maurer-Stroh, Bioinformatics Institute, Singapore

22. Clinical Care in Challenging Settings — 289
   Sean Wu Jiawei, National University Hospital, Singapore
   Lubaba Shahrin, icddr,b, Bangladesh
   Robert Fowler, University of Toronto

23. Maintaining Essential Health and Social Services — 300
   Zheng Huan Javier Thng, Medical Corps, Singapore Armed Forces
   Simone E. Carter, UNICEF
   William Fischer, University of North Carolina

24. Critical Care in Outbreaks — 314
   Ziwei Liu, University of Cambridge
   Richard Kojan, Kinshasa Teaching Hospital, The Alliance for International Medical Action (ALIMA)
   William Fischer, University of North Carolina

25. Healthcare Facilities and Infrastructure — 331
   Shreya Dwarakacherla, University of Cambridge
   Moi Lin Ling, Singapore General Hospital
   Craig Kenzie, Médecins Sans Frontières

26. Strengthening Infection Prevention and Control Systems — 353
   Amy R. Kolwaite, U.S. Centers for Disease Control and Prevention
   S. Kushlani Jayatilleke, Sri Lanka College of Microbiologists
   Folasade T. Ogunsola, University of Lagos, Nigeria
   Benjamin Park, U.S. Centers for Disease Control and Prevention

27. Enabling Research for Therapeutics — 365
   Xin Hui Sam, National Centre for Infectious Diseases, Singapore
   Marissa Alejandria, University of the Philippines
   John Amuasi, Kwame Nkrumah University of Science and Technology
   Barnaby Young, National Centre for Infectious Diseases, Singapore

28. Pandemic Vaccine Development — 379
   Qi Rou Yap, National University of Singapore
   Wei Chuen Tan-Koi, Centre of Regulatory Excellence, Singapore
   John C.W. Lim, Centre of Regulatory Excellence, Singapore
   Eng Eong Ooi, SingHealth Duke-NUS Global Health Institute

29. Vaccine Implementation Strategies: Equity and Hesitancy — 396
   Jolyn Koh, University of Cambridge
   Leesa Lin, London School of Hygiene and Tropical Medicine
   Heidi J. Larson, London School of Hygiene and Tropical Medicine

30. Managing Risk in Mass Gatherings	408
Jacob Lewis, University of Cambridge	
Ziad Memish, Mass Gatherings Research & Innovation Center, King Saudi Medical City, Alfaisal University, Saudi Arabia	
Brian McCloskey, Public Health England	
31. Mental Health and Psychosocial Support	420
Heather Boagey, University of Oxford	
Maha Barakat, Mubadala, Abu Dhabi	
Cristina Carreño Glaría, Médecins Sans Frontières	
32. Protecting the Vulnerable	434
Elyssa Liu, UNICEF	
Louisa Sun, Alexandra Hospital, Singapore	
33. Successful Risk Communication and Community Engagement	450
Wai Jia Tam, National University of Singapore (NUS)	
Rachel Peh, London School of Hygiene and Tropical Medicine	
34. Infodemics and Information Management	465
Sarah Hess, WHO	
Sylvie Briand, WHO	
Tim Nguyen, WHO	
Elisabeth Wilhelm, UNICEF	
Tina D. Purnat, Harvard University	
35. Working with Communities and Volunteers	474
Sylvia Phua, Ministry of Health Holdings, Singapore	
Gwendolen Eamer, Red Cross Red Crescent	
36. Learning the Lessons: Recovery and Review	489
Jen O. Lim, University of Cambridge	
Ebere Okereke, Public Health England	
Magda Robalo, The Institute for Global Health and Development	
Renu Bindra, U.K. Health Security Agency	
37. Capacity Building through Stakeholder Training	501
Renée Christensen, The Global Outbreak Alert and Response Network	
Paul Effler, Western Australian Department of Health	
Ashley Greiner, U.S. Centers for Disease Control and Prevention	
Sharon Salmon, WHO	
38. Till the Next Pandemic: National Preparedness	517
Danielle A. Thies, University of Nebraska	
Carlos Navarro Colorado, UNICEF	
Ali S. Khan, University of Nebraska	
39. Moving Forward Globally to Improve Health Outcomes	540
Thomas Frieden, Resolve to Save Lives	
Amanda McClelland, Resolve to Save Lives	
Precious Matsoso, Resolve to Save Lives	
List of Reviewers	550
Index	551

Preface

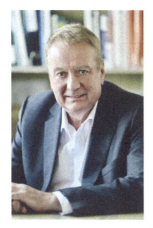

This book represents the knowledge and experience of some of the greatest in the field of outbreak preparedness and response. We have paired around 100 esteemed experts with early career professionals to provide readers with unprecedented insights into how to prepare for and respond to outbreaks and pandemics. The project began in 2021 after being inspired by a group of medical students from the National University of Singapore (NUS), the University of Oxford, and the University of Cambridge. These (now) doctors have been on the journey throughout and became our associate editors, assisting in the writing and other later refinements.

I believe the book will appeal to many, including early career professionals developing skills in outbreak response as well as seasoned experts in a particular discipline who seek to gain a more holistic understanding of outbreak preparedness and response by better appreciating the efforts undertaken in other disciplines. While it is quite technical, we expect that many key partners in outbreak response—political and community leaders and the media—would get value from the book, particularly on confronting an outbreak.

With the generous support of the Yong Loo Lin School of Medicine, National University of Singapore, this book will be a valuable resource for those involved in training in outbreak preparedness and response. Access is supported by its free availability online. Further, we intend for this book to be available in many key languages.

I thank the many authors who have given generously of their time. I'm particularly pleased to acknowledge the junior authors, students, and early career practitioners who worked with their senior colleagues on many of the chapters. The publishing team at NUS, led by Peter Schoppert, has gone above and beyond the typical role of a publisher. While acknowledging the authors and publishers, one cannot forget that behind each author is a supportive network: family, friends, and employers who are the true enablers of this book which has emerged successfully for the benefit of so many.

Dale Fisher, FRACP

Foreword

The COVID-19 pandemic revealed weaknesses in preparedness for such an event globally. While some health systems struggle to provide adequate services in the best of times, even apparently strong, well-resourced systems were often found wanting in areas such as leadership, coordination, and community engagement.

No country can be completely satisfied with its response with a diversity of lessons to be learned and improvements to be made. If the pillars of outbreak response are not coordinated and adapted within the context of the emergency, then the outcome is destined to be suboptimal.

This book, *Infectious Disease Emergencies: Preparedness & Response*, arrives at a pivotal juncture, offering a useful tool for strengthening global health security. Over 100 world renowned authorities in outbreak preparedness and response have contributed thereby providing a sound mix of evidence-based knowledge and practical application relevant to high-, middle-, and low-income countries across all continents.

The 39 chapters leave no gaps in describing how to prepare for and respond to infectious disease emergencies. It can be read from cover to cover for those studying the field or wishing to understand the breadth of issues, from how outbreaks start to vaccine development and mental health issues to hospital infrastructure. Alternatively, it can be used as a reference for those who may have a question on managing misinformation or mass gatherings in a pandemic.

Everyone will find something for themselves in this book. Some will be stimulated by the ethics chapter and others will enjoy understanding the legal frameworks or why some individuals can be particularly vulnerable during the emergency.

I would also like to highlight the clever use of "boxed stories" which add to the readability of each chapter with specific real-world examples that illustrate points in the main text. There are also great graphics and tables readers will find useful in their own presentations.

I'd like to congratulate the editor-in-chief, Dale Fisher, who tenaciously spearheaded the project for over four years. To my knowledge, there is no such book as this with such esteemed authors sharing their knowledge and having it compiled in one place.

This book is not merely a theoretical treatise. It can be seen as a practical toolkit, informed by real-world experiences in infectious disease emergencies, to guide policymakers, public health officials, healthcare providers, and community leaders in their efforts to build more resilient health systems and strengthen our collective defence against future pandemics.

David L. Heymann, MD

List of Abbreviations

3 Rs	renaissance in public health, robust primary care, resilience
4S's	staff, stuff, system, space
ACTT-1	Adaptive COVID-19 Treatment Trial
Africa CDC	Africa Centres for Disease Control and Prevention
Africa PGI	Africa Pathogen Genomics Initiative
AMCs	advance market commitments
AMRH	African Medicines Regulatory Harmonization
APAs	advance purchase agreements
ART	antigen rapid test
AU	African Union
AVAREF	African Vaccine Regulatory Forum
BIPAP	bilevel positive airway pressure
C-TAP	COVID-19 Technology Access Pool
CAM-ICU	Confusion Assessment Method for ICU patients
CDC	Centers for Disease Control and Prevention
CEPI	Coalition for Epidemic Preparedness Innovations
CGIN	Coalition for Ghana's Independence Now
CIDT	culture-independent diagnostic tests
vCJD	Creutzfeldt-Jakob disease
CMA	Conditional Marketing Authorisation
COHRED	Council on Health Research for Development
CTAP	Coronavirus Treatment Acceleration Program
DRC	Democratic Republic of the Congo
DTP3	diphtheria-tetanus-pertussis vaccine
ECMO	extra-corporeal membrane oxygenation
EDCARN	Emerging Diseases Clinical Assessment and Response Network
EDCTP	European & Developing Countries Clinical Trials Partnership
EIOS	Epidemic Intelligence from Open Sources initiative
EMA	European Medicines Agency
EPHF	essential public health function
EPREP	emergency preparedness and response plan
ETAT	Emergency Triage Assessment and Treatment
EUA	emergency use authorisation
EUL	Emergency Use Listing Procedure

FIF PPR	World Bank Financial Intermediary Fund for Pandemic Prevention, Preparedness and Response
Gavi	Gavi, the Vaccine Alliance
GDP	gross domestic product
GHSA	Global Health Security Agenda
GHSI	Global Health Security Index
GHSI	Global Health Security Initiative
GISRS	Global Influenza Surveillance and Response System
GLP	Good Laboratory Practices
GMP	Good Manufacturing Practices
GOARN	Global Outbreak Alert and Response Network
GPHIN	Global Public Health Intelligence Network
GPS	Global Positioning System
GVAP	Global Vaccine Action Plan
HAI	hospital-acquired infections
HCW	healthcare worker(s)
HIS	health information system(s)
IA2030	Immunization Agenda 2030
IBS	indicator-based surveillance
ICMRA	International Coalition of Medicines Regulatory Authorities
IDCC	Infectious Diseases Control Centre
IFRC	International Federation of Red Cross and Red Crescent Societies
IHR	International Health Regulations
IMS	incident management system
IOA	integrated outbreak analytics
IPC	infection prevention and control
IPC-WASH	Infection Prevention and Control-Water, Sanitation, and Hygiene
IRBs	institutional review boards
ISARIC	International Severe Acute Respiratory and emerging Infection Consortium
ISID	International Society for Infectious Diseases
JEE	Joint External Evaluation(s)
JRC	Joint Research Centre of the European Commission
LAMP	loop-mediated isothermal amplification
MERS	Middle East respiratory syndrome
MERS-CoV	Middle East respiratory syndrome coronavirus
MHPSS	mental health and psychosocial support
ML	Maturity Level
MLT	mobile laboratory truck
MSF	Médecins Sans Frontières

List of Abbreviations

NFPs	national focal points
NGS	next-generation sequencing
NHSPI	National Health Security Preparedness Index
NiV	Nipah virus
NPI	non-pharmaceutical intervention
NRAs	national regulatory authorities
ORE	Open Research Europe
OWS	Operation Warp Speed
PCR	polymerase chain reaction
PEF	Pandemic Emergency Financing Facility
PHEIC	public health emergency of international concern
PHSMs	public health and social measures
PIP	Pandemic Influenza Preparedness Framework
PPE	personal protective equipment
PREVAIL 1	Partnership for Research on the Ebola Virus in Liberia
PTSD	post-traumatic stress disorder
R&D	research and development
RAT	rapid antigen testing
RCCE	risk communication and community engagement
RCT	randomised controlled trial
RDT	rapid diagnostic test
REMAP-CAP	Randomized Embedded Multifactorial Adaptive Platform for Community-acquired Pneumonia
RI	routine immunisation
RPA	recombinase polymerase amplification
RRMLs	rapid response mobile laboratories
RT-PCR	reverse transcription-polymerase chain reaction
RVFV	Rift Valley fever virus
SARS	severe acute respiratory syndrome
SARS-CoV-1	severe acute respiratory syndrome coronavirus 1
SDOH	social determinants of health
SLIPTA	Stepwise Laboratory Improvement Process Towards Accreditation
SLMTA	Strengthening Laboratory Management Toward Accreditation
SNPs	single nucleotide polymorphisms
SPRN	Special Pathogens Research Network
TDR	Special Programme for Research and Training in Tropical Diseases
TPP	Target Product Profile
UHC	universal health coverage
UHDR	United Nations Universal Declaration of Human Rights
UHPR	Universal Health and Preparedness Review

List of Abbreviations

UNMEER	United Nations Mission for Ebola Emergency Response
U.S. FDA	U.S. Food and Drug Administration
U.S. HHS	U.S. Department of Health and Human Services
U.S. NIAID	U.S. National Institute of Allergy and Infectious Diseases
VAERS	Vaccine Adverse Event Reporting System

List of Contributors

Alphabetised by surname

Marissa Alejandria is Professor of Clinical Epidemiology and Infectious Diseases at the University of the Philippines College of Medicine and the Philippine General Hospital. During the COVID-19 pandemic, she served as the National Coordinator for the World Health Organization (WHO) Solidarity Trials in the Philippines. She also led the development of the Philippine COVID-19 Living Clinical Practice Guidelines and served as a member of the Department of Health Technical Advisory Group for COVID-19. Her research interests are TB, HIV, sepsis, antimicrobial resistance, and COVID-19, particularly epidemiological and clinical studies, as well as health systems and quality improvement projects.

John Amuasi heads the Global Health Department at the Kwame Nkrumah University of Science and Technology in Ghana. He holds a W2 Professorship and is Group Leader of the Global One Health Research Group at the Bernhard Nocht Institute of Tropical Medicine in Hamburg, Germany, and at the Kumasi Centre for Collaborative Research in Tropical Medicine in Ghana. Dr. Amuasi's research involves both field epidemiologic and clinical studies (including trials) across Africa on emerging and re-emerging infectious diseases, neglected tropical diseases, and antimicrobial resistance. Dr. Amuasi also co-chairs the Lancet One Health Commission and is an Honorary Visiting Research Fellow at the Nuffield Department of Medicine at the University of Oxford.

J.C. Azé started humanitarian work in 1990 in Mozambique as a logistician and administrator in a number of non-governmental organisations (NGOs). He spent twelve years in Médecins Sans Frontières (MSF) (1992–2004) as country coordinator and HQ Projects Manager, mainly dealing with contexts of complex crisis and conflict. In 2005, he joined the World Health Organization (WHO) as a logistics officer in the Boxing Day tsunami response, moving on to Syria in 2006 and Palestine in 2007 to coordinate an important medicine supply project. That same year, he was appointed the head of WHO's outbreak response logistics unit with the mission to develop and strengthen the global logistics capacity of the organisation (Operation Support and Logistics). This unit had the opportunity to demonstrate its pertinence and efficiency in all the numerous epidemic responses in which the WHO was involved around the world including major ones: H1N1 pandemic response (2009), the West Africa Ebola response (2014/2015), the Ebola outbreak in East Democratic Republic of the Congo (DRC) (2018), and more recently, the response to the COVID-19 pandemic. J.C. Azé is now retired.

Maha Barakat, a U.K.-trained consultant endocrinologist, is Assistant Minister for Health and Life Sciences at the UAE Ministry of Foreign Affairs, the Director-General of the Frontline Heroes Office, and a Senior Advisor at Mubadala. In addition to being a Board Member of Mubadala Health, she is the Board Chair of the RBM Partnership to End Malaria, and Board Member of the Global Institute for Disease Elimination (GLIDE), the Cleveland Clinic Abu Dhabi, the Abu Dhabi Quality Conformity Council, and the Family Development Foundation. She was previously the Director-General of the Health Authority Abu Dhabi from 2013 to 2018. Prior to this, she co-founded the Imperial College London Diabetes Centre in Abu Dhabi and was its Medical and Research Director.

Neale Batra is an applied epidemiologist and the Executive Director of Applied Epi, a non-profit organisation that provides training, support, and tools for applied epidemiologists worldwide. He previously worked in emergency response and communicable disease control for local health departments in the U.S. and other countries with the U.S. Agency for International Development (USAID), the World Health Organization, and Médecins Sans Frontières.

Daniel Bausch, MPH&TM, FASTMH, is the Senior Advisor for Global Health Security at FIND, contributing to efforts on pandemic preparedness and response, surveillance, humanitarian emergencies, and antimicrobial resistance. He specialises in the research and control of emerging tropical viruses, with over 25 years' experience in sub-Saharan Africa, Latin America, and Asia combating viruses such as Ebola, Lassa, hantavirus, and SARS coronaviruses. Previously, he held posts at the U.K. Public Health Rapid Support Team (London, U.K.), the World Health Organization (Geneva, Switzerland), the U.S. Naval Medical Research Unit No. 6 (Lima, Peru), the Tulane School of Public Health and Tropical Medicine (New Orleans, U.S.), and the U.S. Centers for Disease Control and Prevention (Atlanta, U.S.). Daniel holds an appointment as a Professor of Tropical Medicine at the London School of Hygiene & Tropical Medicine and is the 2021–2023 President of the American Society of Tropical Medicine and Hygiene.

Thomas Bentley is an academic foundation doctor with a strong interest in evidence-based humanitarian response and global public goods. He has published on a range of topics including vaccinology, antimicrobial resistance, well-being, and ethnic inequality in health.

Ayelet Berman is Visiting Associate Professor at the National University of Singapore (NUS) Saw Swee Hock School of Public Health, the Lead of the Law & Governance Program at the Asia Centre for Health Security, and the Lead of the Global Health Law & Governance Program at the NUS Centre for International Law (CIL). Her work focuses on the law, policy, and governance aspects of global health and biosecurity. Her expertise also covers international law, global governance, and international investment law. Before academia, she practised international trade law and regulatory/commercial law in Big Law. Among her many professional leadership roles, she is on the editorial board of *BMJ Public Health*, and was Co-Chair of the American Society of International Law International Organizations Interest Group.

Renu Bindra is Deputy Director Public Health Clinical Response at the U.K. Health Security Agency. She is an experienced public health physician with significant expertise in all hazards incident management and in policy, strategy, and service development. She has extensive infectious disease outbreak management experience and was the Head of COVID Advice and Guidance for Public Health England at the height of the pandemic, leading across government on the coordination of evidence and advice to inform policy on all aspects of testing, tracing, and isolation. She previously established and chaired a regional TB Control Board, overseeing a comprehensive programme of regional TB control activities, as well as leading national work on multidrug-resistant (MDR)-TB. Renu has a strong interest in healthcare leadership and has received the National Health Service (NHS) Leadership Academy Award in Executive Healthcare Leadership.

Robert Blanchard heads the World Health Organization's Global Logistics Hub, responsible for rapidly responding to acute health emergencies driven by outbreaks of infectious diseases, natural disasters, and conflicts around the world. He was previously a health scientist with the U.S. Agency for International Development's Emerging Pandemic Threats programme, specialising in preparedness and control measures to counter the threat posed by the highly pathogenic avian influenza H5N1 virus. He has over a decade of experience responding to health emergencies including COVID-19, Ebola, cholera, yellow fever, mpox, and avian and pandemic influenza. He holds a Master's degree in public health from George Washington University and is a former Health and Child Survival Fellow with the Johns Hopkins University Bloomberg School of Public Health.

Heather Boagey completed her medical training at the University of Oxford. She is an Honorary Clinical Fellow at the University of Glasgow and currently works in psychiatric intensive care.

For the past 25 years, **Pierre Boulet-Desbareau** has developed extensive expertise in designing, conducting, and improving health emergency preparedness and response to sudden-onset disasters and protracted crises induced by major epidemics, food crises, natural hazards, armed conflicts, NRBC threats, and mass displacement of populations. Following his wide-ranging professional experience as a logistician in more than 50 countries, including ten years as Director of Logistics for Médecins Sans Frontières (MSF) Headquarters and founder of the International Committee of the Red Cross (ICRC) Regional Humanitarian Procurement Centre in Abidjan, Pierre specialised in negotiating, opening, and leading emergency health programmes in complex and hostile operating environments, including urban and sea SAR operations. During the COVID-19 crisis, Pierre was detached as Special Advisor of the Health Minister in Brussels to guide and model the strategic and operational response of the Belgium government to the pandemic and the asylum crisis. He was also to advise the European Union (EU) Emergency Response Coordination Centre (ERCC).

Sylvie Briand is currently leading the Global Preparedness Monitoring Board (GPMB) secretariat which is co-convened by the World Health Organization (WHO) and the World Bank. She was previously the Director of the Epidemic and Pandemic Preparedness and Prevention department at the WHO Headquarters. She has been at the forefront of managing epidemic and pandemic preparedness and response for more than 20 years including COVID-19, Middle East respiratory syndrome (MERS), avian and pandemic influenza, Ebola, Zika, yellow fever, plague, Nipah, cholera, smallpox, mpox, and many other public health emergencies of international concern. She holds a Medical Doctor degree with a specialisation in infectious diseases, a PhD in Health Systems' Analysis, a Master's degree in Sociology and Anthropology, and a Master's degree in Public Health.

Cristina Carreño Glaría is a Mental Health Advisor and leader of the Médecins Sans Frontières Mental Health and Psychosocial Support International Working Group. She is a psychiatrist, has a Master's Degree in Psychotherapy, and another Master's Degree in International Health. She has worked in humanitarian settings for 15 years.

Simone E. Carter is currently working in the Democratic Republic of the Congo (DRC), leading UNICEF's Social Science Analytics Cell (CASS) for outbreaks. She is also UNICEF's lead on Integrated Multidisciplinary Outbreak Analytics for the Public Health Emergencies team in Geneva, where she provides support to countries in their use of evidence in outbreak response. Simone joined the Eastern DRC Ebola outbreak response in September 2018, where she, under the strategic coordination of the Ministry of Health (MOH), developed, set up, and managed the CASS, which is now operational for Ebola, COVID-19, and cholera. Simone has a Master's of Science in Epidemiology from the University of British Columbia's Faculty of Medicine. Following her field research, she has spent the last ten years working across Latin America, sub-Saharan Africa, and the Middle East in humanitarian response and interventions, of which she spent six years working for Oxfam's rapid response team leading the humanitarian and public health emergency response. Since 2014, in the West Africa Ebola outbreak, she has specifically supported operational research to inform programme response, aiming to improve accountability to communities through evidence.

Renée Christensen leads the Capacity Strengthening and Training portfolio for the Global Outbreak Alert and Response Network (GOARN) based at the World Health Organization in Geneva. She is responsible for the strategic design, development, and implementation of the multifaceted and layered GOARN Capacity Building and Training Programme, leading a collaboration with over 40 of the world's leading public health and emergency response institutions to collectively enhance global outbreak response capacity. Renée has over 15 years' experience with the United Nations (UN) across Africa, Asia, and Europe in building capacity for post-conflict, humanitarian, and infectious disease emergency response. She holds a Master's of Education, a Graduate Diploma in Teaching, a Graduate Diploma in Experimental Particle Physics, and a Bachelor of Science (Physics) from the University of Melbourne (Australia). She is a published author in global education.

Alex R. Cook is Professor and Vice Dean (Research) at the National University of Singapore (NUS) Saw Swee Hock School of Public Health. He works on infectious disease modelling and statistics, including for COVID-19, dengue, influenza, and other respiratory pathogens, and on population modelling to assess the effects of evolving demographics on non-communicable diseases such as diabetes.

Benjamin Cowling is currently Chair Professor of Epidemiology and head of the Division of Epidemiology and Biostatistics at the School of Public Health at The University of Hong Kong, and Co-Director of the World Health Organization Collaborating Centre for Infectious Disease Epidemiology and Control. He conducts research into the epidemiology of respiratory virus infections, with a focus on transmission dynamics and the effectiveness of control measures, including vaccination. Since early 2020, he has conducted research on the epidemiology and control of COVID-19 including highly cited publications in *NEJM, Science,* and *Nature Medicine.* He holds major research grants to study how individual measures of immunity translate to population immunity, and to estimate the impact of public health measures for influenza and COVID-19. He has authored more than 750 peer-reviewed journal publications to date. He is Editor-in-Chief of *Influenza and Other Respiratory Viruses,* and an Associate Editor of the journal *Emerging Infectious Diseases.* In June 2021, he was awarded an MBE by Her Majesty Queen Elizabeth II for services to public health and COVID-19 research.

Nikita Devnarain is a Research Associate at the Centre for the AIDS Programme of Research in South Africa (CAPRISA), an Honorary Senior Lecturer at the University of KwaZulu-Natal, and Manager of the DSI-NRF Centre of Excellence in HIV Prevention. She has a research background in medical and pharmaceutical sciences, with a strong interest in investigating potential anticancer, antibacterial, and antiviral therapies.

Shreya Dwarakacherla, a medical student at the University of Cambridge, has a keen interest in public health. She is eager to contribute to initiatives that promote preventative care, health equity, and evidence-based interventions that can improve health outcomes, especially in underserved populations.

Gwendolen Eamer holds a dual role at the International Federation of Red Cross and Red Crescent Societies, as Head of Emergency Operations and Public Health in Emergencies. In this role, she provides operational and strategic leadership in red-level emergencies and works to continually improve emergency response systems and tools. She has worked in emergency response for 18 years, in epidemics, natural disasters, population movements, and both outbreak response and long-term health programming in complex and conflict-affected contexts. Most of this experience has focused on supporting communities, volunteers, and local health workers to provide adapted, localised, and relevant public health services to populations in need. Her academic background includes an MSc in Global Health, with a focus on innovation and health service delivery in times of crisis.

Sarah Edwards is Professor of Bioethics at University College London (UCL). Her body of work has helped inform the academic and policy agendas in the field of research ethics and law, particularly within a health context. Her main achievements have often come from identifying new issues in the ethics of health research and forecasting changing circumstances, then studying these issues from different disciplinary perspectives in philosophy and social sciences. Her academic research has been widely adopted by policymakers locally, nationally, and internationally. Her work has been consistently cited as examples of high-impact research in the U.K. She is the current Chair of the UCL Research Ethics Committee and is a member of several international working groups on the ethics of research, especially in low-income settings.

Paul Effler received a Doctorate in Medicine from the University of California and a Master's of Public Health degree from the University of Hawaii. After completing a residency in Public Health and Preventive Medicine, he served as an Officer in the Epidemic Intelligence Service at the U.S. Centers for Disease Control and Prevention (U.S. CDC). For more than a decade, he served as the State Epidemiologist for Hawaii, where he oversaw disease surveillance activities, bioterrorism, and pandemic preparedness efforts, and directed the public health response to outbreaks. In 2008, he moved to Western Australia where he is currently a Senior Medical Advisor in communicable disease control. Dr. Effler has been actively involved in the Global Outbreak Alert and Response Network (GOARN) since 2009 and is the current partner lead for the GOARN Capacity Building and Training Programme. He has an appointment as a Clinical Professor with the School of Medicine at the University of Western Australia and is an Associate Editor for the U.S. CDC's *Emerging Infectious Diseases* journal.

Devy Emperador joined FIND in 2017 and is currently a Senior Scientist in the Pandemic Threats Programme, supporting diagnostic development for outbreak-prone and emerging diseases for low- and middle-income countries. With over ten years of experience in both private and public sectors and a focus on global health and infectious diseases research, she believes that fostering partnerships and relying on local knowledge improve health outcomes. Her interests lie in laboratory capacity strengthening and outbreak preparedness, specifically through the evaluation and implementation of appropriate diagnostic tools for outbreak-prone diseases such as Ebola, Lassa, mpox, Zika, and COVID-19. Devy completed her BSc in Biochemistry and Molecular Biology and her MPH with a concentration in infectious diseases and vaccinology. She is currently a doctoral student in global health at the University of Geneva, Switzerland.

Camille Escadafal joined FIND–the global alliance for diagnostics in 2017, holding posts as Scientific Officer in the Malaria & Fever programme, and currently as Senior Scientist in the Pandemic Threats programme. She trained as a biochemistry engineer at the Institut National des Sciences Appliquées in Toulouse, France, and worked for three years as a research engineer at the Pasteur Institute in Senegal, where she oversaw the development and standardisation of diagnostic techniques for arboviral infections. Camille completed her PhD with a focus on quality assessment and the development of diagnostic methods for vector-borne viruses, particularly yellow fever. She later joined the Institut Pasteur's Laboratory for Urgent Biological Threats as coordinator of their human virology activities, focusing on creating a laboratory network for emerging viruses in the Mediterranean region. She also coordinated a project on point-of-care tests for epidemic-prone viruses and took part in international field missions during the Ebola and Zika virus outbreaks in Guinea and Brazil, respectively.

William Fischer is a pulmonary and critical care trained physician-scientist and full-time faculty member at the University of North Carolina. He has specific expertise in severe emerging viral pathogens including Ebola Virus Disease, Lassa fever, and SARS-CoV-2. He has hands-on experience in providing care to patients with Ebola Virus Disease and Lassa fever, is a member of the World Health Organization (WHO) Health Emergencies Clinical Team, served as a content-matter expert on call with the U.S. Centers for Disease Control and Prevention Ebola Response Team, and has served as the lead consultant to the WHO for the last two Ebola outbreaks in the Democratic Republic of the Congo and the most recent Ebola Sudan outbreak in Uganda. He is an experienced clinical researcher with expertise in designing and implementing clinical research studies, including therapeutic trials and observational studies.

Dale Fisher is an Australian infectious diseases physician who first moved to the National University Hospital, Singapore, in March 2003 during the SARS outbreak. He is Professor of Medicine at the National University of Singapore (NUS) and Group Chief of Medicine at National University Health Systems. He became involved in international outbreak response in 2009, being deployed for H1N1 outbreaks to Asian countries through the Global Outbreak Alert and Response Network (GOARN). He attended Liberia during its Ebola crisis, providing expertise in case management and infection prevention and control. In 2010, he was part of the writing team for the heralded GOARN scenario training and helped in delivery on numerous occasions in Africa, Central America, Asia, and the Middle East. He was selected to the GOARN Steering Committee in 2013 and was Chair from 2018 to 2022, during which time he addressed the World Health Assembly on matters including the safety of international deployees and capacity building for outbreak response. In addition, he was one of 12 international technical experts who visited China in February 2020 to investigate the COVID-19 outbreak and subsequently became part of the World Health Organization (WHO) Director-General's global advisory panel. In 2022, he founded the Centre for Outbreak Preparedness and Response based at NUS with the intention of creating a regional educational hub for infectious disease emergency preparedness.

List of Contributors

Noah Takah Fongwen is the coordinator for diagnostic access at the Africa Centres for Disease Control and Prevention (Africa CDC). He is a clinician and global health expert with an interest in diagnostics. At Africa CDC, he leads continental efforts towards diagnostic development, evaluation, regulatory harmonisation, policy development, and uptake.

Robert Fowler is critical care physician and H. Barrie Fairley Professor of Medicine at the University of Toronto. He is Chief of the Trauma-Critical Care programme at the Sunnybrook Health Sciences Centre and the past Chair of the Canadian Critical Care Trials Group. Rob's clinical and academic focus includes access and outcomes of care for critically ill patients and infection-related critical illness. He has assisted or worked with the World Health Organization during the SARS, pandemic and avian influenza, Middle East respiratory syndrome, COVID-19, and Ebola outbreaks in Guinea, Liberia, Sierra Leone, and the Democratic Republic of the Congo.

Thomas Frieden, a physician with training in internal medicine, infectious diseases, public health, and epidemiology, served as Commissioner of the New York City Health Department and Director of the U.S. Centers for Disease Control and Prevention (U.S. CDC). His work has improved the care of TB patients and control of TB outbreaks. Dr. Frieden led the U.S. CDC's work to control Ebola, Zika, and other health threats, and created global initiatives to reduce tobacco use and prevent cardiovascular diseases. He is the founder and CEO of Resolve to Save Lives, a global non-governmental organisation.

George Gao, or Gao Fu, served as Director of the Chinese Center for Disease Control and Prevention from August 2017 to July 2022, and has been Dean of the Savaid Medical School of the University of Chinese Academy of Sciences since 2015. Educated at Shanxi Agricultural University, Beijing Agricultural University, and the University of Oxford, where he also later taught, Gao returned to China in 2004 to serve as Professor and Director of the Institute of Microbiology, Chinese Academy of Sciences. Gao was appointed Deputy Director of the Chinese Center for Disease Control and Prevention in 2011. Gao also serves as Vice-President of the National Natural Science Foundation of China.

Caitlin Gordon is a Clinical Research Fellow (Infectious Diseases) at the University Hospitals Sussex NHS Foundation Trust. She received her MBBS from the Queen Mary University of London.

Ashley Greiner is a board-certified emergency medicine physician with over 15 years of emergency public health experience. She is currently leading the U.S. Centers for Disease Control and Prevention's (U.S. CDC's) Emergency Response Capacity Team which aims to strengthen emergency operations and surge workforce capacity globally, working with foreign governments, international partners, and within the U.S. CDC's global response structure. In addition, Dr. Greiner focuses on operational research to enhance the resiliency of health systems responding to public health emergencies.

Johanna Hanefeld is the Head of the Centre for International Health Protection (ZIG) at the Robert Koch Institute. She is also Associate Professor of Health Policy and Systems at the London School of Hygiene & Tropical Medicine and the head of its Berlin office. A policy analyst by training, she researches and works on global health protection, health systems, governance, and migration issues in global health. She uses innovative social science techniques to understand these issues.

Myriam Henkens, MD, MPH, is formerly International Medical Coordinator, now Senior Advisor, for Médecins Sans Frontières (MSF). From 1982 till 1988, Myriam worked in positions with MSF in Africa and Asia. After completing an MPH at Johns Hopkins University, she became the Director of the Medical Department at MSF in Brussels and then created the MSF's international medical coordination function. Besides coordinating the medical departments of all MSF sections, Myriam was involved in several medical topics such as meningitis, cholera, and vaccination, focusing on outbreak responses as well as the availability of and access to necessary tools for diagnosis, treatment, and prevention. Till 2021, she represented MSF at interagency platforms such as the International Coordination Group for meningitis, yellow fever, and cholera. She has acted as an expert to several platforms on cholera vaccines, meningitis, and yellow fever. She coordinated the MSF inputs to the World Health Organization's Essential Medicines list and Essential Diagnostics list. Myriam was the leader of the MSF intersection team for the quality assurance of medicines, medical devices including diagnostic tests, and therapeutic food. She was a member of the Global Outbreak Alert and Response Network steering committee. Now retired, she continues to act as a senior advisor for the MSF International Medical Team.

Sarah Hess is a public health expert skilled in global public health policy, health emergency preparedness, infectious diseases, community engagement, and communication. She currently serves as a World Health Organization technical officer with the Health Emergencies Programme on High Impact Events Preparedness. Sarah also works in the "Infodemic Management" pillar of the COVID-19 response, leading work on partnerships and community empowerment.

David Heymann is currently Professor of Infectious Disease Epidemiology at the London School of Hygiene & Tropical Medicine and a Distinguished Fellow at the Centre on Universal Health at Chatham House, London. He served as the Chief of Research of the Global Programme on AIDS and Founding Director of the Programme on Emerging and Other Communicable Diseases at the World Health Organization. When Prof. Heymann served as the Executive Director of the Communicable Diseases Cluster, he headed the global response to SARS, and subsequently named the Assistant Director for Health Security and the Director-General's Representative for Polio Eradication.

Zheng Jie Marc Ho is Group Director for Policy and Systems at the interim Communicable Diseases Agency under the Ministry of Health, Singapore. A public health physician by training, he oversees policy development, pandemic preparedness, disease intelligence, surveillance systems, technology, and analytics. He is also Lead for Pandemic Preparedness at the Asia Centre for Health Security and Adjunct Associate Professor at the Saw Swee Hock School of Public Health, National University of Singapore. Marc was previously the technical lead for urban health emergency preparedness and health systems for health security at the World Health Organization Headquarters. During the COVID-19 pandemic, he was Director of the Contact Tracing and Epidemiology Centre in Singapore.

Iris Hunger co-heads the Centre for International Health Protection (ZIG) of the Robert Koch Institute (RKI) in Berlin, Germany, where she focuses on strategic programme development, partnership support, and networking. Iris moved to ZIG from RKI's Information Centre for Biological Threats and Special Pathogens, where she focused on national public health emergency preparedness and response. From 2006 to 2011, Iris headed the Hamburg Research Group for Biological Arms Control at the University of Hamburg, Germany, where her work concentrated on biological arms control and security aspects of the life sciences. She also held positions at the Office for Disarmament Affairs at the United Nations in Geneva and the Planning Staff of the Germany Federal Foreign Office. Iris has a Master's in Biochemistry and a PhD in International Relations.

Chikwe Ihekweazu is a medical doctor and Assistant Director-General and Deputy Executive Director of the Health Emergencies Programme at the World Health Organization. Before this, he was the first Director-General of the Nigeria Centre for Disease Control (NCDC). He has held leadership positions in several national public health agencies including the South African National Institute for Communicable Diseases, the U.K. Health Protection Agency, and the Robert Koch Institute, Germany. Dr. Ihekweazu has a further specialisation in infectious disease epidemiology and public health, holding a Master's in Public Health, a Fellowship of the European Programme for Intervention Epidemiology Training, and a Fellowship of the U.K.'s Faculty of Public Health. He has 200 publications in medical peer review journals mostly focused on the epidemiology of infectious diseases. He is the recipient of an Honorary Doctor of Science, awarded by the Liverpool School of Tropical Medicine, U.K., and the Officer of the Order of the Niger (OON), awarded by the President of the Federal Republic of Nigeria, for his service.

Vivianne Ihekweazu is the Managing Director of Nigeria Health Watch, a health communication and advocacy organisation advocating for improved health and access to services in Nigeria. She leads the strategic direction and designs health communication and advocacy strategies for governments, non-profits, and development partners. With over 20 years of experience, her work focuses on nutrition, maternal and child health, routine immunisation, sexual and reproductive health and rights, and health security. She played a leading role in COVID-19 crisis communications, supporting the Nigeria Centre for Disease Control. Vivianne holds an MSc in Global Health Policy from the London School of Hygiene & Tropical Medicine and is an African Public Health Leaders Fellow at Chatham House's Centre for Universal Health.

Kushlani Jayatilleke is the Consultant Microbiologist at Sri Jayewardenepura Hospital and an Honorary Senior Lecturer, Faculty of Medicine, University of Sri Jayewardenepura, Sri Lanka. She has worked in the Lancashire Teaching Hospital and Leeds Teaching Hospital NHS Trust, U.K. She has won many awards, including the President's Award for Scientific Publications from Sri Lanka's National Research Council. She was also a member of the expert committee for revision of the list of critically important antimicrobials for human medicine, World Health Organization, Geneva. She is currently the Liaison Officer for the Asian Network for Surveillance of Resistant Pathogens. She was the President of the Sri Lanka College of Microbiologists, an Assistant Secretary of the Sri Lanka Medical Association, and a member of the National Advisory Committee for Combating Antimicrobial Resistance, Sri Lanka. She holds an MBBS, a Diploma in Medical Microbiology, and an MD in Medical Microbiology.

Archith Kamath is an ophthalmology registrar (resident) in Edinburgh, and a Fellow of the Higher Education Academy. He read Medicine and Medical Sciences at the University of Oxford, and has a research interest in global health and surgery. He served as one of the assistant editors of this book.

Craig Kenzie is a medical doctor, project coordinator, and Hospital Logistics/Water and Sanitation manager with Médecins Sans Frontières.

Ali S. Khan, MD, is the Richard Holland Presidential Chair and Dean of the College of Public Health at the University of Nebraska Medical Center. He is a former Assistant Surgeon General with the U.S. Public Health Service. His career has focused on health security, global health, climate change, and emerging infections. He completed a 23-year career as a senior director at the U.S. Centers for Disease Control and Prevention (U.S. CDC), where he led and responded to numerous high-profile domestic and international public health responses. Dr. Khan was one of the main architects of the U.S. CDC's national health security programme and serves as an executive member of the World Health Organization's Global Outbreak Alert and Response Network. He is the author of *The Next Pandemic: On the Front Lines Against Humankind's Gravest Dangers*.

Dena Kirpalani is an emerging scholar in the field of global health law. She holds a Master of Law in Global Health Law & International Institutions from the Geneva Graduate Institute and Georgetown Law. She is pursuing a PhD in International Law (with a minor in Anthropology and Sociology) from the Geneva Graduate Institute. Her research investigates the transformation of the global health landscape through the financing of the global health agenda. Dena is an English-qualified solicitor, and was a consultant with the Health Law & Ethics team at the World Health Organization Western Pacific Regional Office.

Jolyn Koh is a geographer and urban planner, and graduated from the University of Cambridge in 2024. She has an interest in social inequalities and the phenomenology of everyday life.

Richard Kojan is a clinician who has been practising emergency medicine and intensive and critical care in low- and middle-income countries for the last 20 years. He has contributed to clinical work on emerging infectious diseases including filovirus diseases (Ebola and Marburg), Lassa fever, COVID-19, and mpox. His team helped develop the Portable Biosecurity Emergency Care Unit (CUBE) which optimises the standard of care for patients in low-resource settings, and so enables the better implementation of clinical trials during outbreaks. He is currently working in collaboration with different teaching hospitals and international research societies around the world. He is currently a member of the scientific committee for the Inter-universities Hemorrhagic Fever programme from Ouagadougou University, Burkina Faso. Richard is President of the Alliance for International Medical Action (www.alima.ngo).

Amy Kolwaite is a nurse epidemiologist and Chief of the Health Systems Strengthening, Resilience, and Training Branch in the U.S. Centers for Disease Control and Prevention Division of Healthcare Quality Promotion. She leads a multidisciplinary group of clinicians, epidemiologists, and health scientists to develop and deliver targeted resources to help health systems successfully train all healthcare personnel to implement infection prevention and control (IPC) measures for routine and emerging pathogens, and measure and target factors that can put health systems and their patients at risk for IPC lapses. She has been a public health clinician for more than ten years and has worked in domestic and international settings, including expertise in policy, programme development, and public health outbreak response. She is an acute and primary care-certified paediatric nurse practitioner with more than twenty years of experience in paediatric intensive care units and emergency departments.

List of Contributors

Matthew Yunshen Lai is a resident doctor working in the University Hospitals Bristol and Weston NHS Trust. He graduated with first-class honours in medical sciences and a BM BCh from the University of Oxford in 2023 and has worked in a digital health company where he developed preventative approaches for non-communicable diseases in his role as Vice-President of Research and Development.

Heidi J. Larson is Professor of Anthropology, Risk and Decision Science, and Director of the Vaccine Confidence Project, the London School of Hygiene & Tropical Medicine, U.K., and Clinical Professor, Institute for Health Metrics & Evaluation, University of Washington, Seattle, U.S. Her research focuses on managing risk and building trust. In 2021, Prof. Larson founded the Global Listening Project to investigate public experiences and trust relations during the COVID-19 pandemic to inform societal preparedness for future crises. Prof. Larson previously led vaccine strategy and communication at UNICEF and served on the World Health Organization SAGE Working Group on vaccine hesitancy. She is the author of *STUCK: How Vaccine Rumors Start – and Why They Don't Go Away*. In 2021, she was awarded the 2021 Edinburgh Medal for Science.

Vernon Lee is the Executive Director of the National Centre for Infectious Diseases, Senior Director of the Communicable Diseases Division at Singapore's Ministry of Health, and Adjunct Professor at the Saw Swee Hock School of Public Health. He is an avid educator and researcher and has published about 200 scientific papers, many in top journals such as *NEJM*, *JAMA*, and *The Lancet*. Formerly an Advisor to the Assistant Director-General for Health, Security, and Environment at the World Health Organization (WHO) Headquarters, Medical Epidemiologist in the WHO Office in Indonesia, and the Head of the Biodefence Centre in the Singapore Armed Forces, Prof. Lee has been involved in major global health security collaborations, and has developed pandemic preparedness plans, risk assessments, and disease management programmes at the global and national levels. Prof. Lee completed his medical education at the National University of Singapore, and also holds Master of Public Health and Master of Business Administration degrees from Johns Hopkins University, as well as a PhD in infectious diseases epidemiology from the Australian National University.

Helena Legido-Quigley joined The George Institute for Global Health, U.K., and the School of Public Health, Imperial College London, in 2023 as Chair in Health Systems Science. Prof. Legido-Quigley also holds an Associate Professorship in Health Systems at the Saw Swee Hock School of Public Health, National University of Singapore, is an Associate Fellow of Chatham House, a member of the Council of the World Economic Forum, and is Editor-in-Chief of Elsevier's *Journal of Migration and Health*. She is also a member of Women in Global Health, Spain, a role reflective of her commitment to redistributing power in global health and of her broader emphasis on championing the next generation of global health researchers through mentorship and teaching.

Gabriel Leung is the Executive Director (Charities and Community) of The Hong Kong Jockey Club, overseeing its Charities Trust. He is one of Asia's most respected higher education, health, and philanthropic leaders, and is known for his commitment to improving human capabilities, nurturing impactful innovation, and building strong institutions. His career has straddled academia, public service, and philanthropy. From 2013 to 2022, he was the longest serving Dean of Medicine and inaugural Helen and Francis Zimmern Professor in Population Health at The University of Hong Kong (HKU). Formerly, he was Hong Kong's first Under Secretary for Food and Health and fifth Director of the Chief Executive's Office in government. Dr. Leung's research defined the epidemiology of three novel viral epidemics, namely SARS in 2003, H7N9 influenza in 2013, and most recently, COVID-19. In government, he led Hong Kong's response against the 2009 influenza pandemic. He was the founding Co-Director of HKU's World Health Organization Collaborating Centre for Infectious Disease Epidemiology and Control and established the Laboratory of Data Discovery for Health (D24H) at the Hong Kong Science and Technology Park.

Jacob M. Lewis is a medical student at the University of Cambridge. His interests range from public health initiatives to general psychiatry and pseudoscientific misinformation.

Jen Lim is a medical student at the University of Cambridge with a special interest in eye conditions and genetic diseases. He is the recipient of several academic awards and has been involved in widening access and cancer awareness efforts at his university.

John C.W. Lim is Professor and founding Executive Director of the Duke-NUS Centre of Regulatory Excellence, inaugural Chairman of the Consortium for Clinical Research & Innovation, Singapore, Senior Advisor at Singapore's Ministry of Health (MOH), and Policy Core Lead at the SingHealth Duke-NUS Global Health Institute. He was formerly Chief Executive Officer of Singapore's Health Sciences Authority and Deputy Director of Medical Services at MOH. A medical graduate from the National University of Singapore (NUS), he has postgraduate degrees in public health from NUS and health policy and management from Harvard University, and holds joint appointments at Duke-NUS and the NUS Saw Swee Hock School of Public Health. He sits on the Singapore Food Agency Board, Singapore Medical Council, and U.S. Pharmacopeia Council of the Convention as Asia-Pacific Regional Chapter Chair, among others. Prof. Lim has been awarded the DIA Global Connector Inspire Award and the Regulatory Affairs Professional Society's Founder's Award for leadership in promoting global collaboration and shaping regulatory practice and policy throughout his career.

Leesa Lin, Assistant Professor at the London School of Hygiene & Tropical Medicine, serves as Co-Director of the Vaccine Confidence Project and the head of the AI/Digital Health programme, with a special focus on the Asia-Pacific region. She leads a multidisciplinary team that leverages AI, big data analytics, machine learning, social and behavioural sciences, and statistical modelling to predict and mitigate public health risks. Her research tackles critical issues and evaluates system responses during large-scale emergencies including pandemics, climate disasters, antimicrobial resistance, vaccine hesitancy, infodemics, misinformation, and public trust. Dr. Lin has contributed to the World Health Organization's Coronavirus R&D Preparedness and has translated her research into practical tools, training programmes, and digital products, including chatbots and other innovative technologies.

Moi Lin Ling received her medical education at the National University of Singapore, postgraduate training in microbiology at the Victoria University of Manchester, is a member of the Royal College of Pathologists of Australasia, and a certified professional in healthcare quality (CPHQ). She is currently the Director of Infection Prevention & Epidemiology at the Singapore General Hospital, Director of Infection Prevention, SingHealth, and Lead, Infection Prevention, Regional Health System, SingHealth. She is the President of the Asia Pacific Society of Infection Control (APSIC),

President of the Infection Control Association (Singapore), and President of the Healthcare Quality Society of Singapore. She is an active member of the World Health Organization (WHO) Global Infection Prevention and Control Network and the WHO COVID-19 IPC Guidance Development Group of experts. She is also an active member of the National Infection Prevention Committee at the Ministry of Health, Singapore.

Pascale Lissouba joined Médecins Sans Frontières in 2014 and Epicentre in 2016. A field epidemiologist on various missions in Africa and South East Asia in stable and emergency contexts, she is currently the focal point of the mixed methods research technical support group. Previously, she was a social scientist at the French National Institute for Health and Medical Research (INSERM).

Ziwei Liu is a specialty registrar in Public Health, training in the East of England. She obtained her medical degree and an MPhil in population health sciences from the University of Cambridge, and has a strong interest in global health and health policy.

Elyssa Liu is an international health lawyer who leads the Legal Frameworks team at the Centre for Outbreak Preparedness in Singapore, where she focuses on strengthening legal systems to enhance health outcomes, particularly in emergency preparedness. Her career spans global, regional, and local levels, with expertise in global health, law, and bioethics. Elyssa has held roles at the World Health Organization Headquarters and Western Pacific Region (WPRO), specialising in health law, ethics, human rights, and ageing. At UNICEF, she worked on health in emergencies and humanitarian settings, community health, and antimicrobial resistance. She also brings experience from her work with non-profits such as HelpAge and Women in Global Health. Elyssa holds an LLM in Global Health Law, an LLB (Honours), and is currently pursuing an MPH.

Yang Luo began his medical career at the height of the COVID-19 pandemic. A recipient of the National University of Singapore (NUS) Merit Scholarship, Dr. Luo completed his medical studies at NUS. With a deep passion for primary care and community health, he is now pursuing a Master of Medicine in Family Medicine through the residency programme.

John S. Mackenzie retired as Professor from Curtin University in 2008 where he had been one of the inaugural WA Premier's Fellows, and a deputy CEO of the Australian Biosecurity Cooperative Research Centre. Prior to that, he held the Chair of Microbiology at The University of Queensland from 1995 to 2004, and senior academic appointments at the University of Western Australia. His research interests have been concerned with mosquito-borne viral diseases, and more recently with the concept of One Health. He has been involved with a number of World Health Organization committees including the Global Outbreak Alert and Response Network, and has been a member of various emergency committees under the International Health Regulations.

Sandy **Tze-Minn Mak** is a researcher at the A*STAR Bioinformatics Institute (BII), with prior experience in laboratory public health, where she led the incorporation of next-generation sequencing workflows for virological surveillance and outbreak investigations. During the COVID-19 pandemic, she developed diagnostic tools and conducted genomic epidemiological investigations in Singapore. Sandy also contributed to drafting the World Health Organization's technical guide for genomic sequencing of SARS-CoV-2. Since joining A*STAR's BII, she has been involved in tracking viral phylogenies and curating reports for the ASEAN region. She is also actively involved in regional capacity development efforts though collaboration with GISAID as well as the Asia Pathogen Genomics Initiative.

Roli Mathur has worked over the years, developing national policies and guidelines and building capacity for research ethics in India. She heads the Bioethics Unit at the Indian Council of Medical Research (ICMR), Ministry of Health and Family Welfare, Government of India, and is the Scientific Advisor to the National Ethics Committee Registry. She is a Professor, Faculty of Medical Research at the Academy of Scientific & Innovative Research. Her department is recognised as a World Health Organization (WHO) Collaborating Centre for Strengthening Ethics, the very first one in the WHO South East Asia Region. She is a member of several WHO expert groups, including Ethics and Governance, Ethics of Artificial Intelligence in Health, Benchmarking Indicators for Ethics Oversight, Global Clinical Trial Ecosystem, and Clinical Care and Ethics. She is also a member of the Forum for Ethics Committees in Asia and Western Pacific (FERCAP) and Executive Committee Member of the Council for International Organizations of Medical Sciences (CIOMS). Recently, she was elected to serve as the Chairperson for the Global Network of WHO Collaborating Centres in Bioethics for a two-year term. She is also presently appointed to serve as an External Evaluator of the functioning of the WHO Headquarters Ethics Review Committee.

Precious Matsoso was appointed to the RTSL Board of Directors for a term of 26 January 2023 to 7 November 2025. She is Co-Chair of the World Health Organization (WHO) Intergovernmental Negotiating Body and Director of the Health Regulatory Science Platform, a division of the Wits Health Consortium. Previously, she served as Director-General of the South African National Department of Health and WHO's Director of Public Health Innovation and Intellectual Property and Department of Technical Cooperation for Essential Drugs and Traditional Medicines. Additionally, she was the Registrar of the Medicines Control Council in South Africa for six years and has served on various advisory bodies both nationally and internationally.

Coming from Vienna and Brussels to Singapore, **Sebastian Maurer-Stroh** has led the sequence analytics portfolio at the A*STAR Bioinformatics Institute (BII) since 2007 and has served as Executive Director of BII since January 2021. His computational team is well known for successes at the public–private interface in Singapore, from precision medicine to consumer products and food safety, and of course, for his critical contributions to national and global viral pathogen surveillance through the GISAID Data Science Initiative—the single most important source for virus outbreak data sharing and analysis in this pandemic—powering public health responses globally. He also transformed BII into a hub connecting biomedical data in A*STAR and Singapore.

Amanda McClelland has more than 15 years of experience in international public health management. Amanda previously served as Global Emergency Health Advisor for the International Federation of Red Cross and Red Crescent Societies (IFRC) where she focused on emergency health, epidemic control, mass casualty in low-resource settings, disease prevention, and response operations. Amanda earned her Master's of Public Health and Tropical Medicine from James Cook University in Queensland, Australia, and her Bachelor of Nursing from the Queensland University of Technology. In her capacity as Senior Vice-President of the Prevent Epidemics (PE) team, Amanda will lead the prioritisation and planning of interventions/support in identified countries and regions to strengthen the action packages in prevention, detection, and response to epidemics.

Brian McCloskey has worked in public health at local, national, and international levels, focusing on emergency planning and the response to major emergencies. He was an advisor on health security to the World Health Organization (WHO), Co-Chair of the WHO COVID-19 Mass Gatherings Expert Group, and a member of the WHO's Emergency Committees for COVID-19 and Ebola. Dr. McCloskey worked with the WHO's Mass Gatherings Advisory Group from 2008, heading up the U.K. Collaborating Centre on Mass Gatherings and Global Health Security. He acted as the U.K. National Incident Director for Ebola in 2014 and was seconded to work with the United Nations Special Envoy on Ebola in Geneva. He was subsequently a member of the post-Ebola International Health Regulations Review Committee. Between 2015 and 2017, Dr. McCloskey was responsible for establishing the U.K.'s Public Health Rapid Support Team developed to deploy in serious outbreaks globally. He is the public health advisor to the International Olympic Committee's Medical and Scientific Commission and was responsible for developing the COVID-19 countermeasures for the Tokyo 2020 and Beijing 2022 Olympics.

Kate McNeil is a doctoral student in the Department of Politics and International Studies at the University of Cambridge, where she researches the science–policy interface during health emergencies.

Carolin Meinus, MD, is a paediatrician and project leader at the Robert Koch Institute, Germany.

Ziad A. Memish is Senior Infectious Diseases Consultant at the College of Medicine, Alfaisal University, Riyadh, Saudi Arabia, and Adjunct Professor at the Hubert Department of Global Health, Rollins School of Public Health, Emory University, Georgia, U.S. Widely recognised as a pioneer in Mass Gathering Medicine and Infection Control, Dr. Memish established the World Health Organization (WHO) Collaborating Centre for Mass Gathering Medicine in the Ministry of Health and WHO Collaborating Centre for Infection Prevention and Control in the Saudi Ministry of National Guard (Health Affairs). He is the Editor-in-Chief of three medical journals and has published more than 850 papers and book chapters.

Mo Yin is an infectious diseases physician and a clinician scientist based at the National University Hospital, Singapore. She is driven by the ideal of using quality clinical research to influence patient care and propel health policies. She has been active in clinical research, medical education, and hospital administration. She has received numerous awards for her achievements in clinical care, research, and teaching. Dr. Mo Yin's career goal is to serve her community, focusing on translational research to influence regional and global policies.

Kåre Mølbak is a medical doctor with an interest in infectious diseases epidemiology and control. He served as state epidemiologist of Denmark and Vice-President of Statens Serum Institut (SSI). He has extensive international research experience and has authored some 400 publications. He had a key role in the Danish response to the COVID-19 pandemic, serving on the COVID-19 Advisory Panel and providing advice to the President of the European Commission. He has now retired from the position at SSI but continues as part-time consultant and Professor at the University of Copenhagen.

Catherine Moore is a junior doctor in the U.K. She read Medicine at the University of Oxford, then completed her foundation training in the NHS during the COVID-19 pandemic.

Caitriona Murphy is a PhD student at the School of Public Health at The University of Hong Kong. She was previously trained as a microbiologist at The University of Galway, Ireland, and then spent two years researching the burden of respiratory syncytial virus in infants in Zambia. She later graduated with an MPH from The University of Hong Kong and has since continued her research on the epidemiology of respiratory viruses, including influenza and COVID-19. Her primary research focus is on the effectiveness of control measures including non-pharmaceutical interventions and vaccination.

David Nabarro is currently Co-Director (since mid-2019) and Chair of Global Health at the Institute of Global Health Innovation, Imperial College London. After beginning his career as an academic, he joined the U.K. Government Foreign Office as Senior Health Advisor for East Africa (1989–1990) and Chief Health and Population Advisor (1990–1997). He then became Director for Human Development in the U.K. Department for International Development (DFID; 1997–1999). In 1999, David moved into the United Nations (UN) system, starting as an Executive Director at the World Health Organization (WHO), responsible for the Roll Back Malaria Project and the Office of the Director-General. He was Special Representative of the WHO Director-General for Health Action in Crises (2002–2005). He was then appointed as UN System Senior Coordinator for Avian and Pandemic Influenza (2005–2014), the UN Secretary-General's Special Representative for Food Security and Nutrition (2008–2014), Coordinator of the Movement for Scaling Up Nutrition (2011–2014, as Assistant Secretary-General), the UN Secretary-General's Special Envoy for the West Africa Ebola Outbreak Response (2014–2015), and the UN Secretary-General's Special Advisor for the 2030 Agenda for Sustainable Development and Climate Change (2016–2017, as Under-Secretary-General). He was appointed, by the Director-General of the WHO, as Chair of the expert group on the reform of WHO's work on outbreaks and emergencies in 2015. In October 2018, David received the World Food Prize, together with Lawrence Haddad, for leadership on nutrition.

Geoffrey Namara is an accomplished public health professional with over two decades of experience in statistics and epidemiology, public health monitoring and evaluation (M&E), and health emergency response. He currently serves as the Country Support Officer at the World Health Organization (WHO) Hub for Pandemic & Epidemic Intelligence in Berlin, Germany. In this role, he leads efforts to support countries in strengthening their surveillance, detection, and early warning systems. Throughout his career, Geoffrey has engaged extensively with country officials and development partners to strengthen public health systems. His experience in implementing routine monitoring and surveillance systems for facility and community-based health programmes, as well as his capacity building and mentorship in research and M&E, reflect his commitment to advancing public health initiatives. Previously, Geoffrey served as the WHO's Team Lead for the Health Emergency Information Management and Risk Assessment team at the Nigeria Country Office and as the Africa Head of M&E for the Malaria Consortium. A Ugandan national, Geoffrey holds a Master of Science in Epidemiology from the London School of Hygiene & Tropical Medicine, and a Bachelor of Statistics from Makerere University, Kampala.

Carlos Navarro Colorado is currently an independent consultant for climate change and public health emergencies with the World Bank. Carlos was most recently the Principal Advisor for Public Health Emergencies for UNICEF. He has previously worked at the U.S. Centers for Disease Control and Prevention as an emergency epidemiologist (2010–2017), as an independent consultant on health and nutrition in emergencies (2005–2010), and in a number of field assignments and coordination positions for Action Contre la Faim (ACF) and Médecins Sans Frontières (1994–2004). He has completed dozens of field emergency and outbreak assignments in field and leadership positions. Carlos's research work in emergency response has focused on outbreak response and the treatment and prevention of acute malnutrition. He started the research department of ACF in 2000, and has been involved in the design and implementation of operational research in emergency settings since 1997, obtaining an MSc from the London School of Hygiene & Tropical Medicine and a PhD from Aberdeen University.

Tim Nguyen is the Head of Unit for High Impact Events in the Epidemic and Pandemic Preparedness and Prevention Department of the World Health Organization (WHO) Health Emergencies Programme. His unit develops innovative approaches to community co-creation and decision-making tools. He joined the WHO in 2006, working as a Technical Officer in the Yellow Fever Programme which coordinated an initiative funded by Gavi, the Vaccine Alliance to provide 40 million doses of vaccine to the most at-risk populations. In 2008, he joined the WHO's Global Influenza Programme and took part in the global response work to the first influenza pandemic of the 21st century. From 2014 to 2017, he was the Unit Leader for Knowledge Management, Evidence, and Research for Policymaking at the WHO Regional Office for Europe based in Copenhagen, Denmark. There, he established the scientific journal *Public Health Panorama* and developed the WHO/Europe resolution and action plan for evidence-informed policymaking.

Anders Nordström is a medical doctor and advisor at the Stockholm School of Economics and the Karolinska Institute where he leads the Health Diplomacy Initiative. He was Ambassador for Global Health at the Swedish Ministry for Foreign Affairs for 13 years. In 2020/21, Dr. Nordström served as Head of Secretariat for The Independent Panel for Pandemic Preparedness and Response. He was instrumental in establishing the Global Fund to Fight AIDS, Tuberculosis and Malaria, and served at the World Health Organization for many years, including as Acting Director-General in 2006–2007.

Folasade Ogunsola is the Vice-Chancellor of the University of Lagos. She is a medical doctor and has been a professor of clinical microbiology since 2008. Her research interest has centred around the diagnosis and prevention of infectious diseases as well as antibiotic resistance. She has worked extensively on understanding the epidemiology and ecology of resistant organisms in the hospital environment and preventing their transmission to patients and staff. She has also worked extensively in the community, providing HIV and TB treatment and prevention services to slum dwellers. She has consulted on infection prevention and control at various times since 2003 for the World Health Organization (WHO) and was a member of the Africa Centres for Disease Control and Prevention Taskforce for COVID-19 and the Lagos State Think-Tank for COVID-19. She currently serves as a member of the WHO Strategic and Advisory Group on Infectious Hazards with epidemic and pandemic potential (Stag-IH) and is on the Expert Review Committee on polio eradication and routine immunisation in Nigeria.

Ebere Okereke is recognised for her expertise shaping public health policy, designing strategic frameworks, and executing complex health programmes. Her work primarily focuses on global health security, health system strengthening, and the cultivation of effective leadership in the field. Most recently, Ebere was the CEO of the Africa Public Health Foundation. Her previous roles include Lead Consultant in Public Health England's International Health Regulations Strengthening Programme, Senior Advisor to the Tony Blair Institute for Global Change, Honorary Senior Advisor to the Director of the Africa Centres for Disease Control and Prevention, and co-lead for the African Union's Partnerships for African Vaccines Manufacturing. She is a Fellow of the U.K. Faculty of Public Health and an Associate Fellow at Chatham House. A graduate of the University of Nigeria College of Medicine, she holds a Master's of Science degree from Newcastle University and an honorary Doctor of Science degree from the Liverpool School of Tropical Medicine.

Eng Eong Ooi trained in medicine at the University of Nottingham and then completed his PhD studies at the Department of Microbiology, National University of Singapore (NUS). He is a professor in the Emerging Infectious Diseases programme and Associate Dean (Early Research Career Development) in the Office of Academic Medicine, Duke-NUS Medical School. He holds a joint Professorship at the Saw Swee Hock School of Public Health, NUS. He received the Clinician-Scientist (Senior Investigator) Award from the National Medical Research Council of Singapore in 2010, 2014, and 2019, and the Singapore Translational Research (STaR) Award in 2023. He was one of six to be named the *Straits Times* Asians of the Year and a member of the team that was named the *Straits Times* Singaporean of the Year, both in 2020. He is a member of the Scientific Advisory Board of *Science Translational Medicine* and an editorial board member of *PLoS Biology*.

Oyeronke Oyebanji is a public health professional, currently leading country and regional engagement for Lassa vaccine development at the Coalition for Epidemic Preparedness Innovations (CEPI). With nearly ten years of experience in global health, Oyeronke has demonstrated strong leadership skills by leading successful projects and providing strategic support to public health leaders, working at national, regional, and global levels. Oyeronke worked at the Nigeria Centre for Disease Control (NCDC) from 2016 to 2020 where she played a critical role in developing policies, managing partnerships, implementing International Health Regulations projects and activities, and executing NCDC's Strengthening States for Health Security strategy. In 2021, Oyeronke was part of the COVAX Strategic Coordination Office, where she managed projects that contributed to the delivery of nearly two billion COVID-19 vaccines worldwide. Oyeronke holds a Bachelor of Science in Public Health from Babcock University, Nigeria, and a Master's in Global Health Policy from the London School of Hygiene & Tropical Medicine (LSHTM). She is also a doctoral candidate at LSHTM. Additionally, Oyeronke is a Senior Fellow at the Aspen Institute.

Sai Arathi Parepalli is a medical doctor and clinical researcher with a strong interest in global/population health. She read Medicine at the University of Oxford prior to starting clinical training with the NHS U.K., and is now working as a researcher with the University of Edinburgh. She served as one of the assistant editors of this book.

Benjamin Park is a senior scientist with the U.S. Centers for Disease Control and Prevention (U.S. CDC), currently seconded to the Global Fund in Geneva, Switzerland, where he works to improve Global Fund investments in antimicrobial resistance, infection prevention and control, and waste management. He is the formal Chief of the International Infection Control Program in the U.S. CDC Division of Healthcare Quality Promotion, where he leads a multidisciplinary group of clinicians, epidemiologists, and health scientists to improve healthcare delivery in international settings. He has been a public health official for more than 20 years and has worked in domestic and international settings, has expertise in outbreak investigations, public health responses, and programme delivery, and has authored or co-authored 100 publications.

David Paterson is an infectious diseases physician who directs ADVANCE-ID (ADVANcing Clinical Evidence in Infectious Diseases), a clinical research network based in Asia, and is currently focused on antimicrobial resistance. Prof. Paterson is a tenured professor at the National University of Singapore and was formerly Director at the University of Queensland Centre for Clinical Research. He has featured in the Clarivate Highly Cited Researchers list regularly since 2015.

Rosanna W. Peeling is Professor Emeritus, Diagnostics Research, at the London School of Hygiene & Tropical Medicine, Professor, Department of Medical Microbiology, University of Manitoba, Canada, and the founding Director of the International Diagnostic Centre (IDC) Network. Trained as a medical microbiologist, she previously held positions as the Chief of the Canadian National Laboratory for Sexually Transmitted Diseases, and Research Coordinator and Head of Diagnostics Research at the UNICEF/United Nations Development Programme/World Bank/World Health Organization (WHO) Special Programme for Research and Training in Tropical Diseases in Geneva. Her research focuses on defining unmet diagnostic needs and facilitating test development, evaluation, and implementation. Prof. Peeling has served on WHO guideline development groups for HIV, hepatitis, and dengue, and as a member of many expert advisory committees, including the WHO Strategic Advisory Group of Experts on In Vitro Diagnostics (SAGE IVD), the Global Validation Advisory Committee for the Elimination of Mother-to-Child Transmission of HIV, Syphilis, and Hepatitis B, the WHO STI POC Test Initiative, and the Africa Centres for Disease Control and Prevention Laboratory Working Group, among others. Prof. Peeling was awarded the Royal Society of Tropical Medicine and Hygiene's George MacDonald Medal for outstanding contribution to tropical medicine in 2014 and was made an Honorary Fellow of the Society in 2021.

Rachel Wei Chun Peh is a researcher at SingHealth Polyclinics, focusing on health programme evaluation and implementation science in primary care settings. She holds a Bachelor's degree in Life Sciences from the National University of Singapore and a Master's degree in Epidemiology from the London School of Hygiene & Tropical Medicine.

Sylvia Phua is a Family Medicine resident with the National University Health System. She is passionate about community service and promoting preventative care in Singapore. She aspires to collaborate with like-minded professionals to provide holistic patient care and make meaningful contributions to public health initiatives.

Tina D. Purnat is a Doctor of Public Health (DrPH) student and Prajna Leadership Fellow at the Harvard T.H. Chan School of Public Health. Her work focuses on enhancing services for vulnerable and at-risk communities facing social, economic, and health information disparities. With over two decades of global experience in health informatics, Tina has worked across academia, the World Health Organization, and public health organisations, advancing digital public health, AI technologies, and health information systems, and addressing health misinformation. She is passionate about modernising public health through the integration of cutting-edge technology and human-centred solutions. Tina is a recognised conference speaker and academic lecturer, particularly in the areas of health misinformation and AI for health.

Mahmudur Rahman served as Director of the Institute of Epidemiology, Disease Control and Research (IEDCR) and National Influenza Centre in Bangladesh for 12 years, capping a 33-year career in epidemiological and public health research. Retiring from government service in June

2016, he continued to work as a consultant and is currently the Global Health Development (GHD)/ EMPHNET Country Representative in Bangladesh. Rahman contributed significantly to establishing the National Influenza Centre, BSL3, Nipah laboratory, and web-based disease surveillance in Bangladesh. He founded several epidemiology courses at IEDCR with U.S. Centers for Disease Control and Prevention support and led the national 2009 H1N1 pandemic response. Rahman has chaired numerous panels on epidemiology and public health policies, including for the World Health Organization, and served on various international committees. Currently, he chairs the South-East Asia Regional Commission for Certification of Polio Eradication (SEARCCPE) and is a member of multiple global health advisory groups. He has conducted extensive research in communicable and non-communicable diseases, authoring 153 studies and publications. Rahman holds a Master's in Primary Health Care Management from Mahidol University and a PhD in Epidemiology from the University of Cambridge.

Magda Robalo is the President and co-founder of The Institute for Global Health and Development (IGHD). She is a public health physician and infectious diseases expert whose career spans over 30 years in the global health ecosystem. She held senior leadership positions at the domestic and international levels in various professional settings, working with government, multilateral, and civil society organisations. She has a track record in promoting gender equality and equitable access to quality health care, social justice, ethics, and accountability. She has worked on a broad range of public health issues, and actively works on gender equality, ethics, and governance. She spearheaded successful initiatives as former Minister of Health, High Commissioner for the COVID-19 response in Guinea-Bissau, World Health Organization (WHO) Representative and WHO Director of Communicable Diseases, and the Global Managing Director of Women in Global Health. She serves on several boards and councils. Dr. Robalo is a medical doctor (Universidade do Porto, Portugal) with a Postgraduate Certificate in Public Health and Tropical Medicine (Universidade Nova, Portugal) and a Master of Sciences degree in Epidemiology (Université Laval, Canada).

Thomas Rowland is a medical doctor working in Oxford. He has an MSc in Control of Infectious Diseases from the London School of Hygiene & Tropical Medicine and, alongside his clinical duties, has spent the last four years working part time for the U.K. Health Security Agency on COVID-19, avian influenza, and polio.

Salim Abdool Karim is a South African clinical infectious diseases epidemiologist widely recognised for scientific and leadership contributions in AIDS and COVID-19. He is Director of the Centre for the AIDS Programme of Research in South Africa (CAPRISA), Durban, and CAPRISA Professor of Global Health at Columbia University, New York. He is a Special Advisor (on pandemics) to the Director-General of the World Health Organization (WHO). He is Adjunct Professor of Immunology and Infectious Diseases at Harvard University, Boston, Adjunct Professor of Medicine at Cornell University, New York, and Pro Vice-Chancellor (Research) at the University of KwaZulu-Natal, Durban. He served as President of the South African Medical Research Council and is a Vice-President and Fellow of the International Science Council. He is a member of the WHO's Science Council, a Commissioner of the African Union Commission on COVID-19 and the Lancet Commission on COVID-19, and a Fellow of the Royal Society.

Amadou Sall is the CEO of Institut Pasteur de Dakar in Senegal and Director of the World Health Organization (WHO) Collaborating Centre for Arboviruses and Viral Haemorrhagic Fever. Dr. Sall has been Chairman of the Global Outbreak Alert and Response Network (GOARN) and a member of the Coalition for Epidemic Preparedness and Innovation Scientific Advisory Board. He is a virologist with a PhD in public health, and an expert in epidemic response and control, more specifically for arboviruses, viral haemorrhagic fevers, and high consequence pathogens. Dr. Sall is a member of several expert committees for WHO (GOARN, TDR, SAGE, STAG-IH) and OIE. Dr. Sall is the Co-Chair of the COVID-19 laboratory technical working group for the Africa Centres for Disease Control and Prevention and a member of the African Union AFTCOR Steering Committee, as well as the Senegalese Committee for COVID-19. He is Chairman of the Pasteur Network.

Sarin K.C. is Head of the Environmental Economics Unit at HITAP, Ministry of Public Health, Thailand. Previously, he worked as a research analyst at the LSE and the Ministry of Health in Nepal. As a health economist, he has helped institutionalise processes for health technology assessment in countries like Bhutan, Ghana, and India. During the COVID-19 pandemic, he was part of the COVID-19 Multi-Model Comparison Collaboration (CMCC) which provided guidance on adapting high-income models for low-income settings. He co-led a study on vaccination certificates, influencing Thailand's risk-based border policies, including the Phuket sandbox and bilateral agreements with Singapore. Currently, Sarin is the lead Secretariat for the Lancet Commission on Strengthening the Use of Epidemiological Modelling of Emerging and Pandemic Infectious Diseases. His work in the Environmental Economics Unit aims to make the Thai health system climate and carbon resilient, exploring cost-effective, environmentally-friendly health interventions and advancing methodology to integrate environmental impacts into health technology assessment.

Sharon Salmon is the Technical Officer, Global Outbreak Alert and Response Network (GOARN), Emergency Operations, the World Health Organization (WHO) Health Emergencies Programme, WHO Regional Office for the Western Pacific. Sharon is an experienced WHO Incident Manager dealing with emerging and re-emerging outbreak alert and response, acute emergencies, and crises, with public health experience at national and international levels, including WHO country, regional, and global levels. Sharon leads operational partnerships and has been part of GOARN since 2008, helping to shape the training programme, and has deployed numerous times to Liberia for Ebola Virus Disease and during COVID-19 to Papua New Guinea and the Philippines. Sharon coordinated the deployment of 72 experts on 89 missions to 14 countries in the WHO Western Pacific Region for the COVID-19 response. Sharon holds a Bachelor of Nursing and Master's of Public Health from the University of Sydney and a PhD from the University of New South Wales, Australia.

Xin Hui Sam is a former Research Fellow at the National Centre for Infectious Diseases. She holds a BSc in Biotechnology and a Master of Science in Molecular Biotechnology. She has years of working experience in research laboratories and different healthcare settings in Singapore for various biomedical studies and clinical trials. Her current role at the Lee Kong Chian School of Medicine, Nanyang Technological University, focuses on engagement with general practitioners and family physicians for research in primary care.

Lubaba Shahrin, MBBS, FCPS, is a paediatrician at the Dhaka Hospital of the icddr,b where she has been working since 2006. She currently holds a scientist position. Her research focuses on emerging infectious diseases, diarrhoeal illnesses, malnutrition, child TB, sepsis, and acute respiratory infections. In 2014, she was awarded an HIV/ID clinical observership programme at New York-Presbyterian Hospital—Weill Cornell Medical College, U.S. In 2017, she was deployed to Ethiopia for three weeks. She has authored more than 30 journal publications and more than 10 conference proceedings in her research career, including clinical trials on severe pneumonia. Currently, she is conducting a U.S. Agency for International Development (USAID)-funded multicentre clinical, genomic, and immunopathological study on the dengue outbreak in Bangladesh.

Blessing Silaigwana is a Senior Manager in Research Ethics at the University of Cape Town's Faculty of Health Sciences. He completed his PhD with the South African Research Ethics Training Initiative (SARETI) at the University of KwaZulu-Natal and pursued postdoctoral fellowships in bioethics in the U.K. He is interested in the ethical governance of biomedical research, operations of research ethics committees, and health research ethics systems in Africa. He is a member of the Ethics Working Group on Africanising ethical frameworks for research in outbreak emergencies.

Joycelyn Soo was a medical student at the National University of Singapore (NUS); she graduated in 2024. She has an interest in public health and policy and this project was sparked off with her observation to the Dean of the NUS Yong Loo Lin School of Medicine that there was no single textbook covering preparedness for infectious disease emergencies, and incorporating the lessons learned from the COVID-19 pandemic. She served as one of the assistant editors of this book.

Alexander Spina is an infectious disease epidemiologist and doctor. He has consulted for a variety of emergency response organisations at national and international levels. He is the Co-Founder and current President of Applied Epi alongside his work in the National Health Service of Scotland.

Marc Stegger has a strong interest in genomics and bioinformatics to aid in understanding microbial evolution, selection, and dissemination. This applies specifically to dynamics in microbial communities, antimicrobial usage in humans and livestock, nosocomial infections by coagulase-negative staphylococci, and in later years, to SARS-CoV-2. Here, genomic data has been crucial to his work regarding microbial resistance and human pathogens. He heads the Department of Bioinformatics at the Statens Serum Institut in Copenhagen, Denmark, and is an Adjunct Professor at Murdoch University, Perth, Australia.

Louisa Sun is an Infectious Diseases and Infection Control physician at Alexandra Hospital, National University Health System, Singapore. She also serves as Deputy Director of the Centre for Infectious Disease Emergency Response at the National University of Singapore. As a junior infectious diseases consultant, Dr. Sun played a key role in various COVID-19 outbreak response operations. Through her clinical practice, research, and policy work, she continues to develop her expertise in emerging infectious diseases and outbreak preparedness and response.

Wai Jia Tam is Senior Adjunct Lecturer at the National University of Singapore (NUS) Centre for Infectious Disease Emergency Response (CIDER). She is a risk communication and community engagement (RCCE) specialist with an interest in vulnerable communities, and experience in field deployment globally with the World Health Organization, Global Outbreak Alert Response Network, and UNICEF during outbreaks. She catalysed, coordinated, and led nationwide health communication efforts among low-wage migrant workers in Singapore during the COVID-19 outbreak, raising up to a million dollars in funding over four years. Her efforts were recognised with the Public Service Medal from Singapore's Prime Minister's Office. She leads the curricula design and teaching of the RCCE module in the MSc in Infectious Disease Emergencies (MSc IDE) at NUS CIDER to train leaders and build response capacity to outbreaks in the region. She is in the midst of moving to Tanzania, Africa, to serve as a public health specialist at the Kilimanjaro Christian Medical Centre.

Wei Chuen Tan-Koi is Assistant Professor and Lead of Regulatory Systems Strengthening at the Duke-NUS Centre of Regulatory Excellence (CoRE). Asst. Prof. Tan-Koi's work focuses on health policy research and capacity building in biomedical innovation and regulatory science. She is a consultant for the Asian Development Bank–CoRE Vaccine Regulation Project and a faculty member in international capacity building programmes, including the Asia-Pacific Economic Cooperation Pharmacovigilance Centre of Excellence Pilot Programme and the ASEAN Vaccine Security and Self-Reliance Vaccine Human Resource Development Programme for Enhancing Vaccine Development and Deployment Capacities. Prior to joining the Duke-NUS Medical School, Asst. Prof. Tan-Koi was Regulatory Consultant and Team Lead of the Regulatory Research and Risk Communication teams at Singapore's Health Sciences Authority. A pharmacist by training, Asst. Prof. Tan-Koi was awarded the Singapore Health Manpower Development Plan Fellowship for Graduate Research Programme in Public Health and received her doctoral degree from the NUS Saw Swee Hock School of Public Health.

Danielle A. Thies, MPH, MA, currently works at the University of Nebraska Medical Center (UNMC) in the College of Public Health (COPH) for the Center of Global Health and Development (CGHAD). She is developing global health opportunities for COPH students and faculty through coursework development, international travel courses, engagements, partnerships, scholarships, and communications.

Zheng Huan Javier Thng is a Medical Officer in the Healthcare Policy Centre of the Singapore Armed Forces. He has a keen interest in health economics and healthcare systems. As a student, during the height of the pandemic in early 2021, he worked with the National University of Singapore Saw Swee Hock School of Public Health to write weekly COVID-19 science reports to support the national response.

Erika Valeska Rossetto is an epidemiologist and graduate of the Field Epidemiology Training Program (Brazil FETP, 2008), with Master's and Doctorate degrees in Tropical Medicine and International Health. She has local, national, and international experience with demonstrated success in field epidemiology, emergency response, international health regulations, and global health. Her professional work experience includes assignments in Angola, Bangladesh, Chile, Colombia, India, Mozambique, and Paraguay, and regional support in South America and Portuguese-speaking countries in Africa. She received additional training in outbreak response (México, 2017) through the Global Outbreak Alert and Response Network in partnership with the World Health Organization. She served as President of the Brazilian Field Epidemiology Professionals Network.

Lothar H. Wieler, a veterinarian by training, is a microbiologist and global public health expert. Initially focusing on the molecular pathogenesis, genomic surveillance, and evolution of infectious agents, particularly zoonotic pathogens and antibiotic-resistant bacterial agents, he extended his research to public and global health, concentrating on disease prevention and the containment of pathogens with epidemic and pandemic potential. He currently extends his research to the prevention of non-communicable diseases, conducting studies in the field of digital health, with a particular focus on global public health issues. His goal is to reduce health inequalities by promoting digital public health at local, national, and international levels, with a particular focus on low- and middle-income countries.

Elisabeth Wilhelm is an award-winning global health expert in social behaviour change, infodemic management, and public health communication and strategy, with broad experience across immunisation, maternal and child health, and infectious diseases. She has worked at the U.S. Centers for Disease Control and Prevention, UNICEF, and the U.S. Agency for International Development, among other global health organisations. She has advised and led teams on domestic and global emergency and outbreak responses, served as principal investigator on implementation science research projects in multiple countries, and trained thousands of U.S. and global communicators and public health professionals. Elisabeth has a keen research and practice interest in infodemiology and infodemic management to address the uniquely 21st century challenges to health of misinformation, information overload, and information disorder, and how it affects communities, health systems, and society.

Sean Wu is an infectious diseases physician and the Deputy Director of the Infection Prevention and Control programme at the National University Hospital, Singapore. His academic interests include the role of the built environment in pathogen transmission, inclusive care in infectious diseases, and hospital preparedness in outbreaks.

Yap Qi Rou is a medical officer rotating through Singapore's public healthcare sector at Khoo Teck Puat Hospital. She is a medical alumnus of the National University of Singapore, and a member of the Singapore Medical Association.

Barnaby Young is an infectious diseases senior consultant at the National Centre for Infectious Diseases (NCID) and Tan Tock Seng Hospital (TTSH) and is jointly appointed Associate Professor (Clinical Practice) at the Lee Kong Chian School of Medicine. He is Head of the Singapore Infectious Disease Clinical Research Network (SCRN) at NCID and the database core lead for the Programme for Research in Epidemic Preparedness and Response (PREPARE), Ministry of Health. His research interests are in respiratory viral infections including SARS-CoV-2 and influenza. In 2023, he received a Clinician Scientist Award from the National Medical Research Council (NMRC) with the aim of conducting a SARS-CoV-2 controlled human infection study in Singapore.

CHAPTER 1

INFECTIOUS DISEASE EMERGENCIES: INTRODUCTION

by Dale Fisher

What is an infectious disease emergency? When does an outbreak start and end, and when does it become an epidemic or a pandemic? What is the emergency response cycle? Who are the actors involved in preventing, preparing for, responding to, and then recovering from an emergency? And what are the main pillars of the response process? This introduction provides the readers with an overview of the management of infectious disease emergencies, and an orientation to the different chapters of this book which take up all the topics in greater detail.

INTRODUCTION

An outbreak is generally defined as a significant increase in the number of cases of a disease over a short period of time. This may be due to more cases of an endemic condition or even just one case of a disease not previously present in that area. Outbreaks can last for just days or can go on for years. The outbreak is ended when there is a return to the baseline level of endemicity or the disease has been eradicated (with no new cases for two incubation periods). In the case of a novel pathogen that becomes endemic, the outbreak can be declared over when a baseline level of transmission has been established and all major countermeasures have been withdrawn.

A pandemic differs from an outbreak or epidemic in that a larger geographical area is involved, often worldwide. This is most likely to happen when there is little or no immunity and there is high community-level transmission. A novel agent most infective early in the disease, when symptoms are mild, is most likely to lead to a pandemic. The COVID-19 pandemic represents this scenario perfectly. The measured viral load of SARS-CoV-2 is highest at presentation and in the first few days of symptoms. In contrast, SARS-CoV-1 (responsible for the severe acute respiratory syndrome [SARS] outbreak in 2003) is most infective late in the disease when people are hospitalised; therefore, hospital outbreaks were responsible for a high proportion of cases. That is why good infection prevention and control (IPC) practices in hospitals (and laboratories) were responsible for its eradication, with community-level interventions unnecessary.

With its high levels of community transmission, SARS-CoV-2 could only be slowed, but usually slowed enough to prevent health systems from being overwhelmed. While some countries could eradicate it with draconian measures, this was not possible globally and therefore, no country could remain disease-free. It is not possible to declare a date of the end of the COVID-19 pandemic. While disease rates eventually reached a steady level (notwithstanding periodic fluctuations), each country reached its baseline on its own calendar and with varying approaches to the removal of social restrictions.

A universal and consistent anomaly in the delivery of healthcare is that the resources put into acute management dwarf those put into prevention. The patient with heart disease or cancer is very visible and their needs overt. There is much less public pressure to control the risk factors that would prevent disease. The same is true of outbreaks. Preparing for and preventing outbreaks rarely captures the imagination of leadership or the public yet the resources that have gone into or been lost during outbreak responses cannot be overstated.

The cost of COVID-19 to governments around the world is estimated at US$ 11 trillion. Even in 2018, epidemics cost the world US$ 60 billion (1). The impact goes well beyond the financial, with considerable morbidity, mortality, loss of livelihood, and social impact. Therefore, it is not difficult to pitch for greater efforts to prevent and respond better through strategic preparation.

THE EMERGENCY CYCLE

Preparing for an infectious disease emergency sets the scene for the response. While many external observers may feel response is an isolated event, it is indeed part of a cycle (**Figure 1.1**). After a **response**, it is critical to understand where improvements can be made while communities **recover** and the health system catches up on deferred work. After-action **reviews** feed into preparedness where all pillars of response can be reformed and improved. When there is an alert or early warning (this was late December 2019 during COVID-19), Readiness activities should begin. The World Health Organization (WHO) Health Emergencies Programme defines Readiness as the stage that links effective Preparedness to efficient Response through a specific communicable disease threat, with an outbreak anticipated to occur within 6 months. The emergency cycle can be described in a number of ways, some regarding readiness as synonymous with preparedness, but the consensus now is that it represents its own important "pre-response phase".

Communities with healthy individuals and good health systems, including primary care and universal healthcare coverage, are most able to be prepared. There are tools to assist countries (2–3) and by now, some basic principles have become well established, whether for low-, middle-, or high-income countries.

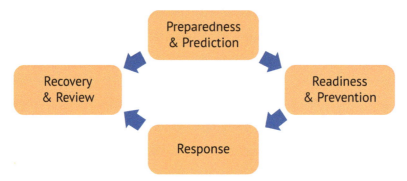

Figure 1.1: The emergency cycle as per the World Health Organization (WHO)
The emergency cycle starts with the imperatives to prevent, followed by prepare, respond, and recover. This version, with its focus on action verbs and process, leaves readiness as to be built up via prevention and preparation phases (https://www.who.int/europe/emergencies/emergency-cycle).

Table 1.1 provides examples of preparedness activities. The time to build hospitals, recruit and train staff, debate and make public health laws, establish strong systems, and stockpile essential items is not during a response. This is much better undertaken outside of an outbreak, rationally and in the fullness of time. Such efforts are almost always a routine benefit to the community, but also enable a much stronger response when an infectious disease (or other health) emergency arises.

Item	Consideration
Infrastructure	• adequate capacity for case management, isolation, quarantine • capacity for the underprivileged to be protected including the homeless, foreign workers, prisoners, refugees, and the elderly • consider risk in workplaces and other settings such as markets, cruise ships, transportation, and food processing plants
Human resources	• adequate numbers of staff with adequate training and experience
Legal framework	• public health laws relating to borders, business closures • ability to support a population suffering financial impact • relationship between national and subnational leadership
Public health governance and systems	• role of and relationship with public health institutions • surveillance • research • scenarios and frameworks for roles and interfaces
Pillars of response	• examine capacities in risk communication and community engagement, laboratories, case management, IPC security, epidemiology, contact tracing, and data management
Stockpile management	• therapeutics • personal protective equipment • supportive therapy, fluids, oxygen, ventilators, etc.

Table 1.1: Examples of preparedness activities

The Global Health Security Index (www.ghsindex.org) is an assessment of capabilities in 195 states and is a transparent ranking or comparison designed to drive improvement in six categories—prevention, detection and reporting, rapid response, health system readiness (*sic*), compliance with international norms, and risk environment. Many of the countries ranked highly in 2019 (including the U.S. and U.K., ranked first and second, respectively) had suboptimal responses to the pandemic in 2020 and 2021. This illustrates how difficult it is to use a score to predict performance when the static assessment of capacities does not necessarily translate to a well-executed multisectoral and coordinated response.

Readiness activities can begin at the first alert. The best health systems will use this period wisely to take advantage of preparedness efforts and gear towards what could happen (**Table 1.2**). This preparation should start before any cases arrive or while numbers are low and do not yet have an impact. Countries that addressed their capabilities well in January and February 2020 were able to respond robustly when cases of COVID-19 increased later in the year. Readiness efforts cannot be done in the preparedness phase, but they do build on the preparation undertaken. Preparedness and readiness, while being exercised in the response phase, should still be evolving during the outbreak. Public health laws can be adjusted, stockpiles developed, scenarios tested, and infrastructure needs addressed.

Item	Consideration
Health sector	• review pandemic plans and current surge capacities
Non-medical sectors	• establish a system engaging whole of government, whole of society
Early identification	• confirm sharing of what is known to the public and healthcare workers (HCWs), where patients should present, and that triage screening will facilitate prompt isolation • test availability, laboratory capacity, turnaround time, reporting
Community engagement	• establish communication conduits, roles of spokespeople for the public and HCWs
Scenario planning	• healthcare facilities, businesses, government departments
Knowledge	• establish what is known and gear toward new incoming information

Table 1.2: Examples of readiness activities

SIGNALS, EVENTS, AND RISK ASSESSMENTS

The WHO emergencies programme uses its surveillance systems to detect events (**See Chapter 9, Surveillance**). Through collaborative efforts between its regional and country offices, health ministries, and other available teams and partners, it will verify any signals and trigger a risk assessment. This involves an analysis of data and other contextual information to understand the risk and provide recommendations. The risk assessment considers the national, regional, and global threat to human health and the risk of spread, as well as the disease control capacities with available resources. The assessments will be graded along with the level of confidence. A low-risk event will be monitored with local support provided. If the event is assessed as high or very high risk, it is classified as an emergency and will be graded as 1, 2, or 3, which will correspond to the degree of support needed for the response. An incident management system will be established (**See Chapter 3, Leading and partnering**). Risk assessments require a "no regrets" approach but this may lead to perceived "overcalling".

OUTBREAK RESPONSE STRATEGIES

The natural history of an outbreak generally follows a normal bell curve pattern in infections, especially when the spread is human to human. Cases occur from a novel or re-emerging pathogen or from an endemic organism that for some reason has seen case numbers increase significantly. As people become infected, they develop immunity, and eventually when enough people are immune, case numbers will fall, and "herd immunity" is reached. After this, the pathogen may die out if there is no vulnerable host remaining and no source that can sustain it in the environment (e.g., in animal hosts). A novel pathogen that is sustainable will obtain a baseline rate of infection and the previously endemic organism will return to its pre-outbreak baseline. Of course, we do not allow an outbreak to follow its natural history if it has a significant health impact. We intervene. Non-pharmaceutical interventions (NPIs) **(See Chapter 12, NPIs)** work to reduce transmission so the peak of the curve never reaches its potential height; however, this means that "herd immunity" will be delayed. This is called "flattening the curve" and there are many reasons to do this. An infectious disease emergency that is capable of causing serious illness and death will impact health systems. The overwhelming of hospitals is less likely to occur if fewer people are sick at the same time. An overwhelmed hospital means that outcomes are much worse, and patients will not be able to receive adequate care for the outbreak disease or for any condition **(See Chapter 23, Essential services)**. Another reason to intervene and keep numbers down is to allow time for research to be undertaken so that we better understand what is needed **(See Chapter 27, Research for therapeutics)** and to enable the development of treatments and vaccines **(See Chapter 28, Vaccine development)**.

Early in the outbreak, when there are few cases, the strict implementation of countermeasures with quarantine of contacts, and identification, testing, and isolation of cases, means a much lower impact on society and lesser demand on resources. If such implementation is not undertaken until there are large numbers of cases, the resource needs rise considerably. Indeed, if numbers are so high that contact tracing (be it manual or technological) cannot keep up **(See Chapter 11, Contact tracing)**, then it may be necessary to assume much of the population is a contact. This was seen during the COVID-19 pandemic, which prompted lockdowns, the most severe of countermeasures. A lockdown is a response to uncontrolled transmission and confines households until eventually, control is regained. Unfortunately, it comes with the well-documented impact on mental health and livelihoods.

Another epidemiologic pattern is seen when there is apparent control of transmission either due to the countermeasures or to immunity (either a vaccine or past infection). As immunity wanes or countermeasures are eased, a resurgence of cases may occur, another so-called "wave". As the outbreak continues, fewer people are fully immunologically naïve, and it is likely that reinfections are less severe. In this stage of an outbreak, there is an uncoupling; earlier in the outbreak, transmission is associated with a greater impact, so countermeasures are crucial. After the acute phase when the health impact is less, countermeasures are not required.

THE ACTORS IN OUTBREAK PREPAREDNESS AND RESPONSE

Any outbreak response must be led by national (or subnational) authorities so ideally, the multidisciplinary, multisector effort will be undertaken by local players. In health, it will be those skilled in case management, epidemiologists, logisticians, laboratory and IPC experts, data managers, and so on. Coordination and strategies within each pillar will require leadership at national, subnational, and institutional or facility levels. Major outbreaks will impact all sectors and therefore, a whole-of-government approach will bring in those who manage security, education, tourism, transportation, pipelines of supplies, trade and industry, finance, and communications, among others. All players need to be involved in all phases of the emergency cycle described above. Some organisations also have a permanent presence across multiple countries, including the WHO, The International Federation of Red Cross and Red Crescent Societies (IFRC), Médecins Sans Frontières (MSF), and the U.S. Centers for Disease Control and Prevention (U.S. CDC).

The community is central, and their engagement will vastly improve the effectiveness of both prevention and response. Engagement and coordination with volunteers are an important resource.

The WHO is the world leader and through its emergencies programme, monitors dozens of events at any one time. The International Health Regulations form the framework for the prevention of spread of an infectious disease outbreak and under these regulations, the WHO—as an extreme measure—can declare a public health emergency of international concern (PHEIC) (**See Chapter 8, Border controls**).

When the needs of a response exceed national capacity, a country can seek external support. This could be for emergency medical teams or for small numbers of defined technical experts. National authorities have two key mechanisms to garner additional support. They may approach other countries bilaterally (e.g., via government-to-government arrangements) or they may work with the WHO and other international organisations and country and regional (and ultimately global) offices to establish the needs, and if required, decide where responders may come from, typically their own staff or sourced through partner networks with deployable staff.

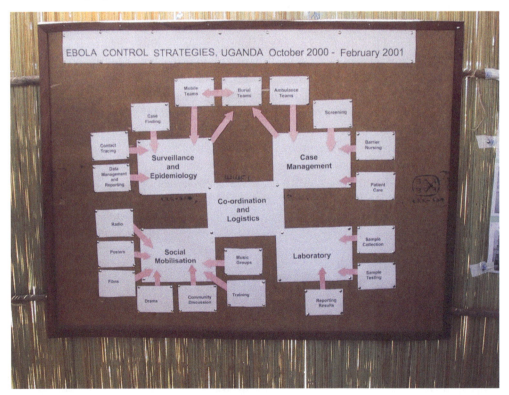

Figure 1.2: Pillars of the Ebola response, 2000–2001
(Credit: Dr Yoti Zabulon)

THE PILLARS OF OUTBREAK RESPONSE

For more than 20 years, outbreak response has been considered as requiring a series of coordinated pillars (**Figure 1.2**), each equally important. The number of pillars has grown accordingly with the complexity of responses today. There are many variations, but one important reference is the WHO's 2021 Strategic Preparedness and Response Plan for COVID-19, which outlines 10 pillars (4). My working version is similar, with 11 pillars (**Figure 1.3**).

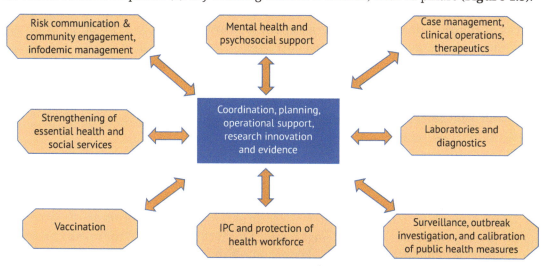

Figure 1.3: Pillars of infectious disease emergency response
(adapted from the WHO's COVID-19 Strategic Preparedness and Response Plan [SPRP] 2021) (4)

Each pillar requires attention during each of the four phases of the response cycle, beginning with effective **surveillance** to give responders as much time as possible when new cases emerge. **Case management, clinical operations, and therapeutics** will reflect on pre-existing systems and their capacity to respond to a surge in cases. This requires the consideration of infrastructure, trained human resources, and adequate supplies. Effective case management requires a high standard of **IPC systems**, again with trained staff, adequate supplies of personal protective equipment (PPE), and an enabling infrastructure. All staff need special consideration of their **mental health and well-being**, given the excessive strain over a long period of time (**See Chapter 31, Mental health**). However, efforts to promote mental health and well-being are, in their own right, a pillar because of the impact on all members of the community, as are efforts to **maintain essential services** in the midst of emergency response. **Risk communication and community engagement** (previously known as social mobilisation) is arguably one of the most complex pillars and starts with the establishment and maintenance of trust between political leaders, health leaders, scientists, and the community. Trust takes years to build and cannot be created during an emergency. The community and its concerns must be understood with two-way communication enabled. All members of society must be reached, the elderly and young, the vulnerable, the disabled, and those with possible language barriers. This requires the utilisation of all modes of communication. More recently, information monitoring and misinformation have risen to warrant specific attention within this pillar.

Vaccines are now such a crucial part of response—as seen in the COVID-19 pandemic and recent Ebola virus disease (EBOD) outbreaks—that they merit a pillar. The utilisation of vaccines illustrates just how the pillars are not silos. Vaccinations require **laboratory** research and advanced diagnostics for their production, **logistic supply chains** for their distribution, and community engagement to ensure uptake when useful vaccines are produced and distributed.

Effective **leadership** that balances clear lines of responsibility with flexibility and systems of **coordination** that also work to build networks of trust are two of the organisational pillars of effective emergency response.

While this discussion naturally leads to the consideration of major outbreaks which lead to PHEICs or at least a national-level crisis, the principles of outbreak preparedness and response actually apply to all outbreaks and contexts. The pillars of the response and emergency cycle equally apply to a small hospital outbreak or illnesses caused by contaminated food from a restaurant.

CONCLUSION

Led by the WHO emergencies programme, outbreak preparedness and response is becoming increasingly sophisticated, with an increasing number of pillars and an increased use of technology to detect, communicate, and manage an outbreak. The pillars need to be well coordinated and the community must be engaged for an effective response. Outbreaks are also a time for learning and integrating those lessons into better preparedness so as to reduce the health, social, and economic impacts of an outbreak in the future. This century has already seen countless outbreaks at a national level and a number of international outbreaks including SARS, Influenza A/H5N1, Middle East respiratory syndrome (MERS), EBOD, COVID-19, and mpox. Future outbreaks are inevitable. The question is whether we are making sufficient effort to improve at global, national, community, and institutional levels.

The discussion in this chapter, and indeed every chapter of the book, needs to come with a caveat that there is no perfect response. It is safe to say that perfection is not a term used in outbreak response.

"Perfect is the enemy of good" is a phrase commonly heard in the field and is the mantra one lives with. There are many interacting moving parts, with many stakeholders and priorities. The context and epidemiology are constantly changing and need to be addressed by balancing the need for swift and decisive actions against accuracy and risk assessments. The theory is clear but the reality in practice is tense and complex.

REFERENCES:

1. Wellcome. The cost of not preparing for infectious diseases. https://wellcome.org/news/cost-of-not-preparing-for-infectious-diseases.
2. The International Federation of Red Cross and Red Crescent Societies. Epidemic preparedness tools and resources. https://www.ifrc.org/our-work/health-and-care/emergency-health/epidemic-and-pandemic-preparedness/epidemic-preparedness.
3. World Health Organization. WHO guidelines for epidemic preparedness and response to measles outbreaks. https://www.who.int/publications/i/item/who-guidelines-for-epidemic-preparedness-and-response-to-measles-outbreaks.
4. World Health Organization. COVID-19 Strategic Preparedness and Response Plan (SPRP 2021). https://www.who.int/publications/i/item/WHO-WHE-2021.02.

CHAPTER 2

WHAT CAUSES OUTBREAKS?

by Joycelyn Soo, Catherine Moore, George Gao, and David L. Heymann

The circumstances that result in sources of transmission and the spread of pathogens are important to understanding disease outbreak. This chapter introduces the biological, environmental, and human factors contributing to infectious disease outbreaks. The concept of pathogen-host-environment interplay is explored in relation to biological drivers as well as environmental factors such as urbanisation and globalisation, and their impact on infection transmission. The steps needed to understand outbreaks will be outlined, covering both immediate tasks and measures for purposes of containment. System weaknesses that allow the propagation of disease will be discussed at the local, national, and global level with concluding statements describing the future of pandemic prevention.

INTRODUCTION

An infectious disease outbreak is defined as an incidence of cases that is increased beyond what is expected in a given population, geographic area, or season. Outbreaks, through history to the present day, can have rippling effects on wider health, social cohesion, economics, and geopolitics. In the past, civilisations have fallen as a result of epidemics. Many historians cite the "Antonine plague" as the trigger for the slow and eventual decline of the Roman empire in the West. Originating in Mesopotamia, where Roman warriors campaigned against the Parthians, successive epidemics significantly decreased the Roman population (1). The 1258 destruction of Abbasid Baghdad by the Mongols facilitated transmission of plague (2), establishing it in the Mongol Empire.

These examples illustrate the potential of disease outbreaks, especially when combined with other factors, to destabilise socioeconomic conditions and disrupt societal structure and functions. In order to mitigate the detrimental effects of disease outbreaks, international public health organisations have proposed, tested, and endorsed strategic approaches for outbreak investigation, response, and preparedness. The emergence of novel diseases and the re-emergence of known diseases occur through an interplay of numerous factors. Consequently, pinpointing and influencing these factors can assist in predicting and preventing future outbreaks.

Infectious disease emergence can be seen as a two-step process with the first phase being exposure of a new host population to a pathogen. The second phase is when the pathogen is established and disseminates within a community (3).

There is a spectrum of infectious disease outbreaks in a defined population ranging from sporadic occurrences to epidemics and pandemics (4). An outbreak that rapidly spreads to affect susceptible populations over much of the world is termed a pandemic. A disease that becomes established in a population or region is said to be endemic (5). Viruses are associated with large scale outbreaks, with the recent SARS-CoV-2 virus causing the COVID-19 pandemic, while bacteria, fungi, and parasites are sometimes neglected in discussions of potential outbreak-causing pathogens. This chapter will discuss the causes of outbreaks, detailing sources of transmission, pathogen-environment interplay, outbreak investigations, and system weaknesses allowing disease propagation, and will conclude with thoughts on the future of pandemic prevention.

SOURCES OF TRANSMISSION

Infectious disease outbreaks result from successful human pathogen transmission, originating from one of many potential sources. Human pathogen transmission occurs via different mechanisms. **Table 2.1** summarises the various sources of transmission, defining each route, mode, factors affecting transmission, and the common pathogens involved. With many factors in play, a "Convergence Model" is proposed to describe how the convergence of factors affects microbial-host interactions and hence, the emergence of infection. Factors are categorised under four domains namely (6):
- genetic and biological factors
- physical environmental factors
- ecological factors
- social, political, and economic factors

PATHOGEN-HOST-ENVIRONMENT INTERPLAY

Pathogens may be viruses, bacteria, or uni- or multicellular eukaryotes that cause disease in the host. Classically, pathogens comprise facultative and obligate pathogens, where the former can usually reproduce independently, and the latter requires one or multiple hosts to complete its life cycle. Facultative pathogens may be present in the environment and cause infections on a sporadic basis, as is the case with hospital-acquired microorganisms. All viruses, and certain bacteria and parasites, are obligate pathogens, and these are more often the cause of outbreaks (16).

Infection does not necessarily mean disease, as many infections are subclinical. This notion is best illustrated by the iceberg concept of infection in **Figure 2.1**. Post infection, the quantitative or relative measure of pathogenicity, or the severity of damage and symptoms caused, is termed virulence. The terms pathogenicity and virulence are not to be confused with contagiousness, transmissibility, or infectivity.

All pathogens have a specific obligatory pathogenesis pathway and methods of evasion from and preventing clearance by the immune system. The mechanisms by which viruses and bacteria cause disease will be briefly described in this section.

Viruses

Viruses (17) are normally inert particles that need to latch on to a body surface using specific proteins. They must bind to a cellular receptor molecule in order to gain entry into a cell. Upon successful attachment, three mechanisms of entry are generally observed:
- translocation of the virus across the cytoplasmic membrane
- viral endocytosis via vacuoles (where the virus is absorbed into small pockets within the cell)
- fusion of the viral envelope with the cell membrane itself

Route of transmission	Definition	Modes	Factors affecting transmission
Airborne and droplet (7–8)	Transmission of disease caused by the dissemination of droplet nuclei that remains infectious when suspended in air over long distance and time, and dissemination of droplets over relatively shorter distance and time	Airborne: Via a fine mist, dust, liquids, or aerosols (<100 microns) Droplets: >100 microns	• Distance from source • Weather (e.g., temperature, sunshine/UV rays, humidity, wind, extreme weather event) • Socioeconomic and living conditions (ventilation and air-conditioning) • Rural vs urban
Foodborne (9)	Contamination of food can occur at any stage of the food production, delivery, and consumption chain	During food consumption and infection of the gastrointestinal tract	• Freshness • Degree of contamination (including intentional contamination) • Food storage, preparation, and processes
Water related (10)	Water-related infectious disease includes waterborne, water-washed	• Waterborne • Water-washed (skin and eyes, diarrhoeal disease) • Water-based (penetrating skin, ingested) • Water-related insect vectors (biting near water, breeding near water)	Different points of the drinking water system: • Source water (surface or groundwater) • Treatment system • Distribution system • Storage system • Building distribution system • Point-of-use system Other potential sources: • Swimming pools (11)
Vector borne (12–13)	Diseases caused by parasites, viruses, and bacteria that are transmitted by vectors	• Mosquitoes • Aquatic snails • Blackflies, sandflies, Tsetse flies • Fleas, ticks, lice • Triatome bugs	Factors affecting vector-borne transmission: • Demographic • Environment • Social factors such as global travel, trade, unplanned urbanisation
Bloodborne (14–15)	Chronic infectious diseases caused by viruses and bacteria transmitted by contact with blood or other body fluids	• Direct blood contact on injured skin or mucosa • Iatrogenic procedures (e.g., transfusion, non-sterilised needles) • Intravenous drug abuse • Sexual contact	• Percutaneous injury • Accidental puncture • Human bites • Cuts • Abrasions

Table 2.1: Sources of infectious disease transmission in outbreaks

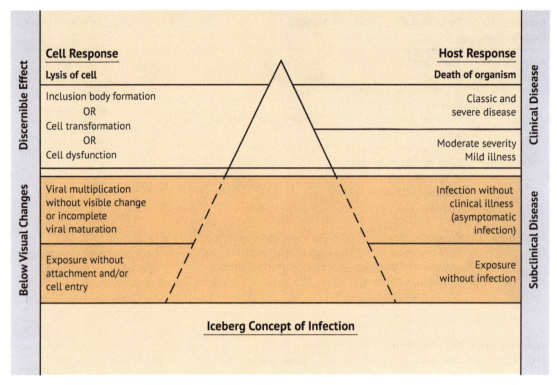

Figure 2.1: Iceberg concept of infection
(adapted from https://phil.cdc.gov/Details.aspx?pid=14928)

After this, uncoating, genome transcription, and replication occur via the host cellular mechanisms. Primary replication with subsequent maturation and release, and secondary viral replication can take place. Viral infections can either be localised or spread throughout the body, with different obstacles for the virus to overcome. The spread from a local to a systemic infection depends on the ability of the virus to enter skin cells, dodge the body's innate inflammatory and immune responses, reproduce, and spread via the bloodstream. This can lead to cytopathic effects in various organs.

Bacteria

While viruses are usually considered the most likely cause of future pandemics, bacterial infections (18) should not be overlooked. The increasing occurrence of bacteria that are resistant to drugs is a significant concern. Bacteria utilise virulence factors to evade clearance at infectious sites. For instance, they can have protective coatings of polysaccharides, cell walls which contain toxic components, and can release endotoxins, harmful proteinaceous or non-proteinaceous molecules that can cause cell damage. Much like viruses, adherence to cell surfaces is key to bacterial infection, and this is achieved via adhesin for cellular adhesion. Invasion mechanisms are extracellular or intracellular. In the former, lytic enzymes cause membrane breakdown while the bacteria remain outside the host cell. Alternatively, the bacteria can enter the host cell. With the evolution of virulence factors, antibiotic resistant bacteria pose a significant health threat. This is particularly the case as we have an insufficient process for developing or discovering new antibiotics (19).

FACTOR INTERPLAY AND OUTBREAKS

A shift in biological and ecological factors can create an opportunity for pathogens that may result in an emerging infection, one that is identified and confirmed for the first time in humans. Such emerging infections can be described based on their pathogens, their ecology, and their transmission dynamics (20):

- Novel host: this can happen when a pathogen jumps from one species to another, for instance during a spillover event.
- Mutant pathogen with a novel trait in an old host: this is when an existing pathogen develops a new characteristic in a familiar host, often due to evolutionary selection. An example would be an organism that becomes resistant to multiple drugs.
- New geographical location: pathogens can be introduced to new settings due to natural events or human actions. For example, mpox was exported from Africa in 2022.

Biological drivers

Most novel infectious diseases affecting humans are RNA viruses originating from animals. They make up 65 per cent of new pathogens discovered since 1980 (21). Pathogens which affect humans but come from non-human animals are known as zoonoses and they make up an estimated 61 per cent of all human pathogens (22). Worldwide, there are one billion cases of zoonotic disease annually, with a significant health and economic burden. Zoonotic viruses may spread to humans in domestic, agricultural, or most commonly, wild settings. Wild animals are the source of 91 per cent of zoonotic viruses, with 58 per cent from wild rodents.

The smaller the phylogenetic distance between animal host and human host, the more likely it is for viral adaptations to be applicable to the new host and for host barriers to be overcome. The likelihood of transmission from chimpanzees to humans is increased by their phylogenetic proximity, whereas transmission from rodents to humans is increased by the high frequency of interactions. Some pathogens, such as SARS coronavirus and Nipah virus, are found in a primary reservoir of bats spreading to humans via intermediate animal hosts that have closer frequent encounters with humans, such as animals in live food markets or domestic pigs.

The likelihood of a given virus to be transmissible from animals to humans is known as its zoonotic potential. This is affected by both natural and man-made factors and in turn, determines interventions under the One Health approach **(See Chapter 13, One Health)**.

Environmental and human drivers

Globalisation, which encompasses migration, tourism, and international trade, can directly amplify infection transmission. The density and scale of human settlements, and ease of movement, can spread a pathogen rapidly and internationally. A single case may be sufficient to spark an outbreak, as in MERS-CoV 2015 in South Korea (23).

Changes in the pattern of human activity in the last 50 years have greatly increased the risk of zoonotic transmission, principally by changes to the animal environment and human population (24). These changes include destruction of natural habitats, a growing animal produce trade, antimicrobial use, international travel, and human population growth. In particular, the loss of natural habitats with increased urbanisation can increase the contact between wild animals and humans.

Previous pandemics have been associated with the movement of people, such as the Black Death, spread in Europe along the Silk Road trade routes, and the 1918 Spanish flu, spread by the movements of military forces (25). In our globalised world, disease is only one flight away. Early data in the COVID-19 pandemic demonstrated that more globalised countries were among the first affected (26).

There are advantages, however, to living in a globalised world. Globalised countries are wealthier and more able to invest in research and in healthcare. The ease and rapidity of global information sharing can facilitate alerts and a coordinated response to an infectious disease threat.

Climate change is already having a multifaceted impact on global health and will continue to do so. Carrying capacities of ecosystems are affected by climate change and resultant fluctuations in the host or vector populations influence disease transmission. For instance, increased rainfall increases mosquito-transmitted Rift Valley fever, dengue, and malaria, while dry periods see a reduction in these diseases (27–28). Temperature changes also have profound effects on pathogen replication and therefore the load in a vector (29). Anthropogenic factors, including migration in response to climate change and various cultural and behavioural effects (30), and efforts to diminish the extent and effects of climate change further shape the development and progress of outbreaks (29).

Emergent human factors will further increase the likelihood of outbreaks, including increased numbers of potential human hosts in more tropical climates where changes in vector ecology are occurring (31). There is increased susceptibility to disease where malnutrition and other comorbid conditions are prevalent **(See Chapter 14, Outbreak resilience)**. Furthermore, more extreme weather is just one of the causes of humanitarian crises which will see increasing human displacement. Displacement combined with poor access to clean water and sanitation facilitates the spread of disease **(See Chapter 15, Humanitarian emergencies)**.

It is important to note that these risks disproportionately impact vulnerable populations, including migrants, poorer communities, women, and children.

OUTBREAK INVESTIGATION

The "Swiss cheese model" or Emmental cheese model (32), which typically explains accident causation, can be applied to disease outbreaks where various risk factors fall in line, resulting in an outbreak.

Steps of outbreak investigation can be divided into immediate measures and containment measures **(See Chapter 10, Field epidemiology for an 8-step version)**.

SYSTEM WEAKNESSES IN PROPAGATING OUTBREAKS

Strategies for suppression of disease should target factors that are associated with transmission, ideally until a vaccine is available. Infection prevention and control (IPC) measures with masks and social distancing, with quarantines and 'lockdowns' in extremis, have been shown to effectively reduce human-to-human transmission. However, the lack of IPC and risky human practices and behaviours can increase disease transmission.

Human activity plays a significant role in disease transmission. Globalisation amplifies the spread of disease geographically, but weaknesses in local, national, and international systems can exacerbate the situation.

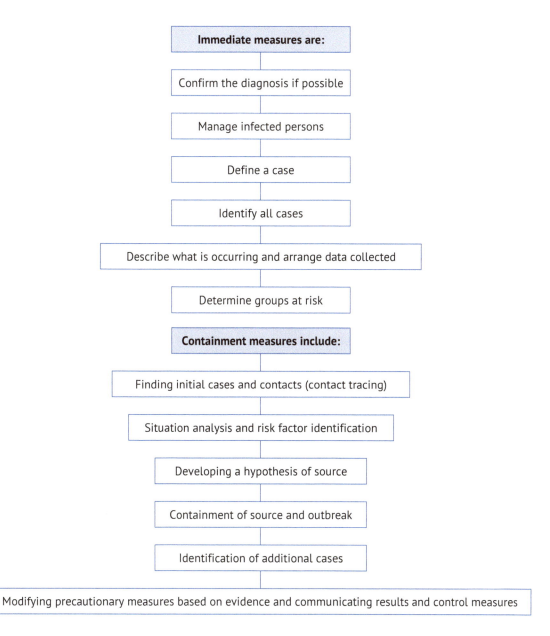

Person-to-person transmission of disease can be reduced by simple IPC measures. Healthcare workers (HCWs) are a particularly important group to target given their volume of interaction with patients. They can be both a source of infection and be themselves at higher risk of being infected. SARS-CoV-2 transmission between HCWs was well documented via respiratory droplets, including from asymptomatic individuals (34). The greatest risk to HCWs is from failure to identify infective patients, failure to put on and remove personal protective equipment (PPE) correctly, and inadequate supplies of PPE (34). Removing PPE is particularly high risk in viral haemorrhagic fever IPC, where cross-contamination poses a significant risk. Given these high-risk interactions, hospitals are a potential site of disease amplification, and indeed HCW infections are often how an outbreak is first identified.

Swiss cheese model in outbreak investigation

An outbreak of *Bacillus cereus* at a Singapore tertiary hospital illustrates the process of outbreak investigation (33). This outbreak was first identified when rates of *B. cereus* in inpatient clinical cultures exceeded two standard deviations above the mean of the preceding two years. Investigation was conducted by an outbreak team with environmental sampling carried out at wards most affected by the outbreak, including oncology wards. Plates containing bacterial growth media placed in linen trolleys revealed heavy growths of *B. cereus*. Laundry processes had recently changed. Samples from towels were cultured and found to be significantly more contaminated than sheets and other linen. Towel pieces cultured after laundering were still positive for *B. cereus* and more so when stored in a new non-porous wrapping, compared with looser porous bags. Infection rates were highest amongst immunocompromised patients in the oncology wards. The hypothesis was that aerosolised *Bacillus* from an adjacent excavation for construction works was entering the ventilation system and contaminating towels. The towels were trapping the pathogen and the load of bacteria was amplified by storage in warm areas with non-porous plastic wrapping. A smoke test demonstrated poor ventilation with air trapping in the patient rooms.

Measures implemented for outbreak control targeted laundry procedures, with the use of autoclaved towels, increasing the concentration of bleach to achieve a sporicidal effect during laundry, and a change of linen storage methods from plastic to canvas bags. Other interventions included a hospital-wide disinfectant change and the installation of additional filters in the ventilation system. During this time, cases dropped to pre-outbreak levels and interventions were relaxed. There was a consequent spike in *B. cereus* infection soon after, which further confirmed the hypothesis. The IPC team continued to work with laundry partners, maintaining measures until the construction was complete. **Figure 2.2** illustrates how identifying potential causative factors and utilising a Swiss cheese model (32) can assist in outbreak investigation.

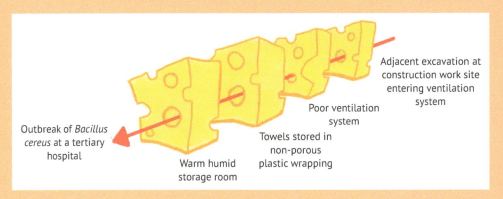

Figure 2.2: Reason's Swiss cheese model in outbreak investigation
(adapted from BMJ 2000;320(7237):768-770)

Local and national deficiencies in logistic supply chains often impact lower socioeconomic areas first, exacerbating health inequalities. Internationally, there is asymmetry in information sharing, differences in contact tracing protocols, challenges in diagnosis and treatment, and other discrepancies. Even if vaccines are available, poor immunisation programmes can make populations susceptible to infection. Increasingly, outbreaks are seen in insecure areas affected by conflict and civil disruption. This compromises the ability to implement effective control measures and end the outbreak at an earlier stage.

In the modern world, there are many additional emergent opportunities for transmission of disease including blood transfusion, the bushmeat trade, industrial food production, international travel, intravenous drug use, and immunosuppression (31). The technologies that facilitate these opportunities may hold benefits to humans; however, in many places they are not matched with sufficient IPC measures.

Additionally, misinformation and disregard for messages from public health authorities during pandemics can exacerbate system weaknesses. Dealing with human behaviours in such cases will require an active shift from epidemiological and virological modelling to a more holistic response (35), involving behavioural, psychosocial, and emotional factors **(See Chapter 34, Infodemics)**.

CONCLUSION

Understanding the causes of outbreaks is fundamental to outbreak preparedness and response. During the preparedness phase, state parties should strengthen prevention, detection, and response capacities targeting areas of highest risk. Coordination is needed at all levels, domestic to international. Concurrently, identifying areas requiring research and development will support these preparedness efforts. For example, in the field of Ebola Virus Disease there is the integrated outbreak analytics (IOA) system to produce data-based strategies and strengthen capacities **(See Chapter 17, Integrated outbreak analytics)**. Disease surveillance systems are also in place using a combination of indicator- and disease-based surveillance and procedures to confirm outbreak existence **(See Chapter 9, Surveillance; See Chapter 10, Field epidemiology)**. Teams preparing for and responding to outbreaks must work with communities as primary partners, establishing modes and functional systems of engagement. During outbreak response, there needs to be coordinated action in an accountable global effort and an ability to pivot quickly as required. Healthcare leaders need to recognise that healthcare needs persist beyond the outbreak and should take steps to enable health systems to address longer term medical complications and cope with pressures in the aftermath. A paradigm shift is needed in the way society prevents outbreaks and detects them early.

Infectious disease outbreaks have regularly featured in human history. Understanding the causative pathogens, modes of transmission, environment, and factors impacting outbreak amplification is essential to preventing and containing future outbreaks. Each of these components of an emergent or re-emergent disease presents an opportunity for intervention. The greater our understanding of the underlying causes of disease outbreaks, the greater our ability to predict and prevent disease emergence. In our globalised world, being several steps ahead of the pathogen and curtailing outbreaks before they have started must be the modern-day aim.

REFERENCES:

1. Benedictow OJ. Plague, Historical. In: International Encyclopedia of Public Health [Internet]. Elsevier; 2017. p. 473–88. http://dx.doi.org/10.1016/B978-0-12-803678-5.00332-5.
2. Fancy N, Green MH. Plague and the Fall of Baghdad (1258). Med Hist [Internet]. 2021 Mar 30;65(2):157–77. http://dx.doi.org/10.1017/mdh.2021.3.
3. Morse SS. Factors in the emergence of infectious diseases. Emerg Infect Dis [Internet]. 1995 Mar; 1(1):7–15. http://dx.doi.org/10.3201/eid0101.950102. PMID:8903148.
4. Brachman PS. Chapter 9: Epidemiology. In: Baron S, editor. Medical Microbiology. 4th ed. Galveston (TX): University of Texas Medical Branch at Galveston; 1996. https://www.ncbi.nlm.nih.gov/books/NBK7993/.
5. Heymann DL. Control of Communicable Diseases manual: An Official Report of the American Public Health Association. APHA Press; 2022.
6. Microbial Threats to Health [Internet]. National Academies Press; 2003. http://dx.doi.org/10.17226/10636.
7. Ather B, Mirza TM, Edemekong PF. Airborne Precautions [Updated 2023 Mar 13] StatPearls [Internet] Treasure Island (FL): StatPearls Publishing; 2023 Jan. https://www.ncbi.nlm.nih.gov/books/NBK531468/.
8. Wang CC, Prather KA, Sznitman J, Jimenez JL, Lakdawala SS, Tufekci Z, et al. Airborne transmission of respiratory viruses. Science [Internet]. 2021 Aug 27;373(6558). http://dx.doi.org/10.1126/science.abd9149. PMID:34446582.
9. Hussain MA. Food contamination: major challenges of the future. 2016 Mar;5(2):21. https://doi.org/10.3390/foods5020021. PMID:28231116.
10. World Health Organization. Surveillance and outbreak management of water-related infectious diseases associated with water-supply systems [Internet]. 2019. https://apps.who.int/iris/bitstream/handle/10665/329403/9789289054454-eng.pdf.
11. Ryan U, Lawler S, Reid S. Limiting swimming pool outbreaks of cryptosporidiosis – the roles of regulations, staff, patrons and research. J Water Health. 2017 Feb;15(1):1–16. https://doi.org/10.2166/wh.2016.160. PMID:28151435.
12. World Health Organization. Vector-borne diseases [Internet]. 2020. https://www.who.int/news-room/fact-sheets/detail/vector-borne-diseases.
13. Chala B, Hamde F. Emerging and re-emerging vector-borne infectious diseases and the challenges for control: a review. Front Public Health. 2021 Oct;9:715759. https://doi.org/10.3389/fpubh.2021.715759. PMID:34676194.
14. Pirozzolo JJ, LeMay DC. Blood-borne infections. Clin Sports Med. 2007 Jul;26(3):425–31. https://doi.org/10.1016/j.csm.2007.04.010. PMID:17826193.
15. Denault D, Gardner H. OSHA Bloodborne Pathogen Standards [Updated 2023 Jul 20] StatPearls [Internet]Treasure Island (FL): StatPearls Publishing; 2023 Jan. https://www.ncbi.nlm.nih.gov/books/NBK570561/.
16. Balloux F, van Dorp L. Q&A: what are pathogens, and what have they done to and for us? BMC Biol. 2017 Oct;15(1):91. https://doi.org/10.1186/s12915-017-0433-z. PMID:29052511.
17. Cann AJ. (2008). Replication of Viruses. Encyclopedia of Virology, 406–12. https://doi.org/10.1016/B978-012374410-4.00486-6.
18. Wilson JW, Schurr MJ, LeBlanc CL, Ramamurthy R, Buchanan KL, Nickerson CA. Mechanisms of bacterial pathogenicity. Postgrad Med J. 2002 Apr;78(918):216–24. https://doi.org/10.1136/pmj.78.918.216. PMID:11930024.
19. Salazar CB, Spencer P, Mohamad K, Jabeen A, Abdulmonem WA, Fernández N. Future pandemics might be caused by bacteria and not viruses: recent advances in medical preventive practice. Int J Health Sci (Qassim). 2022;16(3):1–3. PMID:35599938.
20. Engering A, Hogerwerf L, Slingenbergh J. Pathogen-host-environment interplay and disease emergence. Emerg Microbes Infect. 2013 Feb;2(2):e5. https://doi.org/10.1038/emi.2013.5. PMID:26038452.
21. Woolhouse M, Gaunt E. Ecological origins of novel human pathogens. Crit Rev Microbiol. 2007;33(4):231–42. https://doi.org/10.1080/10408410701647560. PMID:18033594.
22. Taylor LH, Latham SM, Woolhouse ME. Risk factors for human disease emergence. Philos Trans R Soc Lond B Biol Sci. 2001 Jul;356(1411):983–9. https://doi.org/10.1098/rstb.2001.0888. PMID:11516376.
23. Kim KH, Tandi TE, Choi JW, Moon JM, Kim MS. Middle East respiratory syndrome coronavirus (MERS-CoV) outbreak in South Korea, 2015: epidemiology, characteristics and public health implications. J Hosp Infect. 2017 Feb;95(2):207–13. https://doi.org/10.1016/j.jhin.2016.10.008. PMID:28153558.

24. Karesh WB, Dobson A, Lloyd-Smith JO, Lubroth J, Dixon MA, Bennett M, et al. Ecology of zoonoses: natural and unnatural histories. Lancet. 2012 Dec;380(9857):1936–45. https://doi.org/10.1016/S0140-6736(12)61678-X. PMID:23200502.

25. Tognotti E. Lessons from the history of quarantine, from plague to influenza A. Emerg Infect Dis. 2013 Feb;19(2):254–9. https://doi.org/10.3201/eid1902.120312. PMID:23343512.

26. Zimmermann KF, Karabulut G, Bilgin MH, Doker AC. Inter-country distancing, globalisation and the coronavirus pandemic. World Econ. 2020 Jun;43(6):1484–98. https://doi.org/10.1111/twec.12969. PMID:32836720.

27. Anyamba A, Linthicum KJ, Tucker CJ. Climate-disease connections: Rift Valley fever in Kenya. Cad Saude Publica. 2001;17 Suppl:133–40. https://doi.org/10.1590/S0102-311X2001000700022. PMID:11426274.

28. Julvez J, Mouchet J, Michault A, Fouta A, Hamidine M. Evolution du paludisme dans l'est sahélien du Niger. Une zone écologiquement sinistrée [The progress of malaria in ahelian eastern Niger. An ecological disaster zone]. Bull Soc Pathol Exot. 1997;90(2):101–4. French. PMID: 9289244.

29. Mills JN, Gage KL, Khan AS. Potential influence of climate change on vector-borne and zoonotic diseases: a review and proposed research plan. Environ Health Perspect. 2010 Nov;118(11):1507–14. https://doi.org/10.1289/ehp.0901389. PMID:20576580.

30. Reiter P, Lathrop S, Bunning M, Biggerstaff B, Singer D, Tiwari T, et al. Texas lifestyle limits transmission of dengue virus. Emerg Infect Dis. 2003 Jan;9(1):86–9. https://doi.org/10.3201/eid0901.020220. PMID:12533286.

31. Wolfe ND, Dunavan CP, Diamond J. Origins of major human infectious diseases. Nature. 2007 May;447(7142):279–83. https://doi.org/10.1038/nature05775. PMID:17507975.

32. Reason J. Human error: models and management. BMJ. 2000 Mar;320(7237):768–70. https://doi.org/10.1136/bmj.320.7237.768. PMID:10720363.

33. Balm MN, Jureen R, Teo C, Yeoh AE, Lin RT, Dancer SJ, et al. Hot and steamy: outbreak of Bacillus cereus in Singapore associated with construction work and laundry practices. J Hosp Infect. 2012 Aug;81(4):224–30. https://doi.org/10.1016/j.jhin.2012.04.022. PMID:22704635.

34. Shenoy ES, Weber DJ. Routine surveillance of asymptomatic healthcare personnel for severe acute respiratory coronavirus virus 2 (SARS-CoV-2): not a prevention strategy. Infect Control Hosp Epidemiol. 2021 May;42(5):592–7. https://doi.org/10.1017/ice.2020.1428. PMID:33427148.

35. Moeti M, Gao GF, Herrman H. Global pandemic perspectives: public health, mental health, and lessons for the future. Lancet. 2022 Aug;400(10353):e3–7. https://doi.org/10.1016/S0140-6736(22)01328-9. PMID:35934013.

CHAPTER 3

LEADING AND PARTNERING IN A CRISIS

by Iris Hunger, Johanna Hanefeld, Carolin Meinus, Lothar H. Wieler, and David Nabarro

International health emergencies are growing ever more complex. An interdisciplinary, well-coordinated response is needed to limit the impact of such events. The networks of health crisis responders are becoming more diverse and require new models of leadership. Recent events have shown that established incident management systems with their hierarchical structures need to be supplemented with well-managed networks to allow a more agile, context-aware crisis response.

Trusted leadership is a key element in functional networks which arise from careful trust-building efforts amongst network partners and the active promotion of ongoing meaningful communication and interaction. Preparing for the next health emergency requires investment in such functional networks of health crisis responders, including the building up of a sufficiently large and resourced healthcare and public health workforce at all levels. Strategic preparation enables a well-coordinated response.

All actors involved in the health emergency response require clear strategic direction. A shared vision, a consensus on goals, and clarity on how to reach those goals are central for actors at all levels to work collaboratively using their respective capacities and capabilities. A shared narrative, based on respected good-quality evidence, enables all actors to best use their respective strengths, expertise, and resources. The creation of such a narrative is a key leadership skill.

Effective coordination of actors and activities prevents duplication, interference, and gaps in emergency response. While always challenging in practice, effective coordination can create synergies and allows an agile, needs-based, community-centred, and broad health emergency response.

INTRODUCTION

The nature of infectious disease emergencies is hard to predict. Outbreaks are caused by a variety of agents, novel or known, each with its own source, transmission route, speed of spread, and geography. The health impact, mortality, and long-term effects are often influenced by the age and underlying health of the people affected, and by the availability and effectiveness of pharmaceutical as well as non-pharmaceutical countermeasures.

Health crises directly impact individuals' physical health. They also lead to a complex interaction between social, economic, and ecological effects on individual and public health. Overwhelmed health systems may cause a delay in treatment for acute and chronic conditions. This same pressure can compromise maternity and child health services, potentially leading to further fatalities. Social restrictions and business closures can disrupt trade and cause loss of income. These disruptions may result in a reduced availability of medical countermeasures and food. Mental health effects should also be expected due to the health crisis response and restrictions on movement and interaction (**See Chapter 31, Mental health**) (1).

Both direct and indirect effects are context-specific, and are dependent on population demographics (2), society-wide availability, and access to health services, as well as the strength of the public health system. They often reveal and reinforce, and can considerably deepen, pre-existing power structures and inequities (3). Robust social welfare systems may mitigate health and social effects.

THE LIMITS OF CENTRALISED MANAGEMENT STRUCTURES

The management of health emergencies is an "essential public health function" (EPHF) of every public health system (4). The first step in management is preparedness. It has always been difficult to create enough investment in emergency preparedness, even after the lessons from health crises such as HIV/AIDS and Ebola virus disease (EBOD).

Equally, our measures of preparedness may require adjustment. Many countries that had been expected to perform well during a health emergency did not meet expectations during the COVID-19 pandemic. Their preparedness as measured by different parameters—including the self-assessment tool under the International Health Regulations (IHR) or the Global Health Security Index—was not matched by performance (5–6). It is widely agreed that this has been at least in part due to "[i]nadequate compliance of states with obligations under the IHR [International Health Regulations], particularly on preparedness" (7). Such obligations include the establishment of core capacities to detect, assess, notify, and report events, and respond to public health risks and emergencies. A lack of integration and functionality in health emergency management capacities has also been cited (8). Additional explanations look to broader social factors that condition the acceptance of public health recommendations (9).

When health emergencies escalate, shortages of personnel and material cannot always be compensated through cross-district, cross-border, or international solidarity. Necessary healthcare and public health capacities may become unavailable and leadership on the ground is confronted with additional challenges, such as the need to prioritise the use of medical countermeasures on particular population groups, the lowering of standards of care, or an increasing reliance on volunteers (**See Chapter 35, Volunteers**) (10). As illustrated by the COVID-19 pandemic, severe crises can challenge international rules and partnerships. Restrictions on exports and prioritisation of national demand resulted in materials such as masks, gloves, diagnostics, and vaccines being inequitably distributed. International travel bans resulted in the economic isolation of countries and the hindrance of humanitarian support.

The management of health emergencies needs to take account of the complexity of disease outbreaks and the diversity of responders. Responders are placed at community, national, and international levels, and include government officials, United Nations (UN) agencies, non-governmental organisations (NGOs), communities, academia and research institutions, and the private sector. Types of activities include healthcare and public health, social services including food security, basic and higher education, emergency-related research and development, private sector support, political stability, and national security (11). Coordination is key to an effective response, but it has posed challenges in the past. While health emergency leadership is built on the protocols and clear lines of responsibility of incident management systems, the diversity of actors and types of activities involved in responding to health emergencies means that hierarchical leadership is sometimes hard to establish because responders come with different motives, mandates, and operational structures, and may just refuse to be aligned under an incident management system.

The solutions for coordination challenges will vary in different settings. While international approaches to the coordination of humanitarian aid, including the cluster approach, are well established, these have been implemented with varying success (12). National and local approaches to coordination have also had differing effectiveness (13).

The EBOD outbreak in West Africa in 2014–2015 is instructive. It was unprecedented in duration, severity, complexity of response, and loss of life. By June 2016, when the outbreak was over, it had caused 11,325 deaths and more than 28,600 infections (14). The outbreak had been declared a public health emergency of international concern (PHEIC) by the World Health Organization (WHO) on 8 August 2014. On 18 September 2014, the UN Security Council adopted Resolution 2177, calling the outbreak "a threat to international peace and stability", and one day later, the UN General Assembly adopted Resolution 69/1 establishing the UN Mission for Ebola Emergency Response (UNMEER), the first ever emergency health mission, modelled loosely on peacekeeping missions. This setting up of various coordination bodies at the highest levels was part of an explicit effort to "do better" to address coordination challenges that had been identified during earlier health emergency responses.

However, as seen in the number of infections and the long duration of the outbreak, the new approach did not work as well as hoped. Several reviews were conducted in the wake of the shortcomings of the international response to the 2014–2015 EBOD health emergency (15). A common thread across evaluation reports was the identified need for better leadership. For instance, the High-Level Panel on the Global Response to Health Crises stated in 2016 that "the absence of a strong WHO response capacity and the lack of clarity over the inter-agency leadership and coordination arrangements for health crises delayed an effective response" (16). At the same time, the central role of the WHO was reaffirmed by all reviews. There was strong agreement "that WHO should be the lead health emergency response agency" (17), requiring WHO Member States to provide the WHO Secretariat with appropriate authority and resources (18).

The WHO responded to the criticism and various recommendations by setting in train a reform process of its health emergencies work, guided by the Advisory Group on Reform of WHO's Work in Outbreaks and Emergencies. With its new Health Emergencies Programme, it brought all emergency-related activities into one programme "with one workforce, one budget, one set of rules and processes, and above all, one clear line of authority" (19).

While the High-Level Panel felt the WHO needed more clarity on lines of authority, the design of UNMEER, with its single unified command and control, proved to be unsuitable. The Ebola Interim Assessment Panel "… strongly recommended against the establishment of a [UN] mission for future emergencies with health consequences" (17). Part of the reason for rejecting UN missions for health emergency response was their "centralised command structure … viewed as inimical to many in the humanitarian community accustomed to a more horizontal management style", which also "led to the exclusion of many stakeholders from initial consultations" (20).

THE NEED FOR COLLABORATIVE LEADERSHIP IN NETWORKS OF PUBLIC HEALTH ACTORS

There are frequent challenges to unified management systems, where all groups of responders are managed in an integrated manner, particularly when there are big differences in the perceptions and motives of the political leaders who have authority and financial control over the different groups that interact at local levels. In such cases, a blend of centralised and network approaches will be the better leadership option.

Different layers of response—local, national, and international—are interconnected. The many response-related sectors of government and society are highly interdependent. Managing such complexity requires network management alongside centralised governance structures (21–23). In network management, we must recognise and consider the independent positions, strategies, and sometimes conflicting interests of all players (24–25). It is important to spark and guide discussions and explore new approaches cooperatively. This process calls for building relationships and a team spirit, understanding each other's abilities and skills, and engaging in participatory consensus reaching. Effective information exchange between partners is crucial. Trust underpins all these activities and is simultaneously the end product of such collaborative efforts (26).

The blending of unified incident response with a collaborative leadership of networks is required of the full range of actors from global to local. Accordingly, response coordination needs to be decentralised to a sufficient degree, using regional (as well as international) and local (as well as national) coordination structures to make health emergency response work. In the case of the EBOD outbreak in West Africa in 2014–2015, the response worked best once incident managers were established not just at the international and national, but also at the district and local levels (27). A study in Nigeria showed that moving the coordination of the COVID-19 pandemic response from the state to the local level improved coordination outcomes, resulting in, among other things, increased testing rates (28).

Africa Centres for Disease Control and Prevention (Africa CDC) provides regional leadership

Leaders of the African Union (AU) elevated public health to political significance during the COVID-19 pandemic. Africa CDC received greater recognition and resources. Within the continent, such public health and political leadership became a potent tool. AU at the level of Heads of State trusted "our Africa CDC". Nearly every month, Heads of State received a situation briefing from the heads of Africa CDC. These included the current needs to support the work of Africa CDC. Capital in the form of trust was established with Member States through the provision of diagnostics, personal protective equipment, and close to 20,000 community healthcare workers.

Africa CDC led with science-informed independent views, examples of which include their recommendations on the differentiated use of the AstraZeneca vaccine in the face of the emerging Beta variant of the virus in South Africa. Africa CDC and public health institutions in general provide the evidence for politicians to make decisions; they need to remain scientists. Most often, if the evidence and scientific argument are clear, the political leadership will follow. Close interaction of Africa CDC with the AU made it very effective during the COVID-19 crisis in terms of advising on policy for the continent.

As well as top-down direction, we need to empower and enable collaboration at the regional and local levels (29–30). This shift is especially necessary for effective community engagement.

Network governance research has shown not only that "resourceful and committed local partners" are essential for network effectiveness, but also that "good quality of collaborative processes characterise[d by] high level of resource sharing and trust among partners" is necessary (31). Therefore, for collaborative networks to work well during a crisis, they need to be established and functioning *before* the crisis (26). Strong collaborative networks consist of pre-established strong formal and informal partnerships and relationships, which in turn support awareness of interdependency, conflict resolution capacity, and in particular, trust. For networks to function well, continuous investment in partnership and governance is required.

EVIDENCE-BASED STRATEGIC DIRECTION AND TECHNICAL GUIDANCE

Whatever the mix of network and unified management structures, all actors involved require clear strategic direction. A shared vision, a consensus on the goals, and clarity on how to reach those goals are central for actors at all levels to work collaboratively towards the goals using their respective capacities and capabilities in their particular contexts (32). Network management experts have described the importance of "goal consensus" for network effectiveness (33). Finding the means to create and disseminate that vision is a key challenge for leadership in health crisis response. Solutions will vary in different contexts, but their necessity cannot be ignored.

A consensus on goals, and arguably on the ways to reach them, needs to be based on evidence. Evidence needs to be identified or, if found missing, be generated through research, including research during ongoing health emergencies. The WHO summarises the important aspects of evidence-based global health policy as follows (34–35):

- mobilising evidence
- institutionalising evidence-informed decision-making
- collaborating across the evidence ecosystem
- strengthening legitimacy and trust

During the COVID-19 pandemic, scientific exchange occurred internationally and was most effective at informing national policy when part of frank, open discussion and driven by an open-minded understanding of the needs of countries and different communities within them.

While strategies need to reflect the current state of the evidence, interventions need to take into account the different local contexts in which they are to be implemented. Outbreak response interventions need to be informed, not dictated by evidence, especially if the production of knowledge took place elsewhere or in a different population and is potentially not translatable to one's local context (36). Ideally, knowledge is co-produced and interventions co-created with all relevant sectors of society and together with communities to be tailored to their specific context. Community engagement and the specificity to the local context are particularly important to ensure an equitable and sustainable response (37–39).

The COVID-19 pandemic reinforced the importance of reliable data-driven technical guidance. Engaging in open dialogue with all stakeholders for joint decision-making was essential in this time of heightened social, economic, and political anxiety. This was especially the case when there was a lack of information, and when public health and treatment guidelines were changing rapidly. Evidence was limited or non-existent when the outbreak started in late 2019. As such, it had to be produced jointly, necessitating robust collaboration (35). This may be the case with other novel pathogens. Emerging evidence drove changes in recommendations through the course of the pandemic, creating unprecedented communication challenges. Also coming into sharp focus during the COVID-19 pandemic was the importance of evidence to policy pathways, the role of scientists as communicators, and the role of journalists, influencers, and social media, among others, in communicating science.

Legitimacy of evidence

During the pandemic, most countries and relevant international organisations either established or adapted pre-existing scientific advisory boards. These were often high profile and had important roles in advising on key aspects of national and international policy. Scientific expertise and legitimate authority for setting technical direction regarding health issues in many countries lie with health authorities such as national public health institutes. Such institutions are respected sources of evidence, if populations experience them as consistent, trustworthy, transparent, reliable, and learning actors. Professional societies and national science academies may also fulfil the role of trusted science advisors. The level of public trust in these bodies varies from country to country and is usually based on past performance.

In addition, at the international level, the WHO and specialised regional institutions such as Africa CDC and European CDC, and entities such as the International Association of National Public Health Institutes (IANPHI), provide scientific and technical leadership. For many countries, the WHO or regional public health institutions are the main source of scientific evidence and technical guidance. Established in 2018 following the aftermath of the 2014–2015 EBOD emergency in West Africa, the WHO's Strategic and Technical Advisory Group on Infectious Hazards with Pandemic and Epidemic Potential (STAG-IH) provides independent advice to the WHO and analysis on the infectious hazards that may pose a potential threat to global health. During COVID-19, this scientific advisory group met weekly to discuss the emerging evidence and develop recommendations. Well-established, transparent evidence to policy pathways do not only support policymakers at all levels in the rapid science-based development of policy decisions, but also inform scientists where evidence for informed policymaking is still missing.

More so than in previous health emergencies, individual scientists took on leadership roles in communicating and explaining government policy and interventions. This did not always go well. Not every scientist has the scientific expertise or skills to guide policy and the public in a crisis. Leading national and international public health actors, such as national public health institutes or scientific societies, often represented through their presidents, are the ideal champions for public health action and fair and equal access to healthcare. Their legitimacy is partly based on legal mandates awarded to such actors through legislation in their respective countries. More importantly, their legitimacy rests on their scientific excellence, independence, quality of data produced and used, and transparency. Individual scientists need to know the boundaries of their scientific expertise and stay outside the political spheres as much as possible.

CONCLUSION

We have observed recent health emergencies, learned from theories of network management and effectiveness, and reviewed the role of evidence in decision-making. We conclude that managing the complexity of health emergency response requires supplementing unified management structures with collaborative leadership by groups of responders, which in turn necessitates investment in functional networks of health actors at all levels *before* a health emergency occurs. A functional network arises with trusted leadership, the active promotion of meaningful frequent communication and interaction, and careful trust-building efforts amongst actors involved in outbreak response networks. Building-up of a sufficiently large and resourced public health and healthcare workforce, both at the national and local levels, is a must.

We also conclude that a shared narrative and goal consensus, based on good quality evidence (i.e., provided by trusted institutions), is needed for effective response, especially when relying on network management approaches. It is helpful if actors understand what they can contribute if they work effectively and collaboratively in the network of outbreak responders.

Strong collaborative networks can support readiness, response, and recovery across multiple levels through a high degree of resource sharing and trust among the partners. The mobilisation of networks can result in constant strategic renewal, as a cornerstone for an evidence-based adaptive response. The challenge for leadership is to mobilise such networks while getting the blend of centralised and networked approaches just right. The blend should be adapted to the distribution and impacts of the pathogen, the fabric of the society within which it is spreading, and the manner in which responses are organised and are being implemented. The scope for adapting the blend will depend on both political and institutional contexts.

Health emergencies require the engagement of the whole public health community and actors in other sectors, brought together by a shared narrative that is guided by technical expertise. National public health institutes, regional public health institutions, and the WHO are called on to play demanding leadership roles as champions of a health-for-all focused response. National authorities recognise that to be prepared for the next crisis, they need to invest in leadership structures and skills. National public health institutions need to be resourced sufficiently to fulfil their leadership functions. Individual crisis response leaders need to be versed in the art of collaborative leadership, the effective guidance of networks, and the recognition and use of high-quality evidence for decision-making.

REFERENCES:

1. Aknin LB, De Neve JE, Dunn EW, Fancourt DE, Goldberg E, Helliwell JF, et al. Mental health during the first year of the COVID-19 pandemic: a review and recommendations for moving forward. Perspect Psychol Sci. 2022 Jul;17(4):915–36. https://doi.org/10.1177/17456916211029964 PMID:35044275.
2. Gaertner B, Fuchs J, Möhler R, Meyer G, Scheidt-Nave C. Older people at the beginning of the COVID-19 pandemic: a scoping review. J Health Monit. 2021 Apr;6 Suppl 4:2–37. PMID:35586562.
3. Shadmi E, Chen Y, Dourado I, Faran-Perach I, Furler J, Hangoma P, et al. Health equity and COVID-19: global perspectives. Int J Equity Health. 2020 Jun;19(1):104. https://doi.org/10.1186/s12939-020-01218-z PMID:32586388.
4. World Health Organization. 21st century health challenges: can the essential public health functions make a difference?: discussion paper. 2022. https://www.who.int/publications/i/item/9789240038929.

5. Lal A, Erondu NA, Heymann DL, Gitahi G, Yates R. Fragmented health systems in COVID-19: rectifying the misalignment between global health security and universal health coverage. Lancet. 2021 Jan;397(10268):61–7. https://doi.org/10.1016/S0140-6736(20)32228-5 PMID:33275906.

6. Haider N, Yavlinsky A, Chang YM, Hasan MN, Benfield C, Osman AY, et al. The Global Health Security Index and Joint External Evaluation score for health preparedness are not correlated with countries' COVID-19 detection response time and mortality outcome. Epidemiol Infect. 2020 Sep;148:e210. https://doi.org/10.1017/S0950268820002046 PMID:32892793.

7. Aavitsland P, Aguilera X, Al-Abri SS, Amani V, Aramburu CC, Attia TA, et al. Functioning of the International Health Regulations during the COVID-19 pandemic. Lancet. 2021 Oct;398(10308):1283–7. https://doi.org/10.1016/S0140-6736(21)01911-5 PMID:34570995.

8. World Health Organization. Report of the review committee on the functioning of the International Health Regulations (2005) during the COVID-19 response. 2021. https://www.who.int/publications/m/item/a74-9-who-s-work-in-health-emergencies.

9. Badman RP, Wang AX, Skrodzki M, Cho HC, Aguilar-Lleyda D, Shiono N, et al. Trust in institutions, not in political leaders, determines compliance in COVID-19 prevention measures within societies across the globe. Behav Sci (Basel). 2022 May;12(6):170. https://api.semanticscholar.org/CorpusID:249216633 https://doi.org/10.3390/bs12060170 PMID:35735380.

10. Kaji A, Koenig KL, Bey T. Surge capacity for healthcare systems: a conceptual framework. Acad Emerg Med. 2006 Nov;13(11):1157–9. https://doi.org/10.1197/j.aem.2006.06.032 PMID:16968688.

11. Berman P, Cameron MA, Gaurav S, Gotsadze G, Hasan MZ, Jenei K, et al. Improving the response to future pandemics requires an improved understanding of the role played by institutions, politics, organization, and governance. PLOS Glob Public Health. 2023 Jan;3(1):e0001501. https://doi.org/10.1371/journal.pgph.0001501 PMID:36963068.

12. Durrance-Bagale A, Salman OM, Omar M, Alhaffar M, Ferdaus M, Newaz S, et al. Lessons from humanitarian clusters to strengthen health system responses to mass displacement in low and middle-income countries: a scoping review. J Migr Health. 2020;1-2:100028. https://doi.org/10.1016/j.jmh.2020.100028 PMID:33458716.

13. Yee D, Craig C, Earle-Richardson G. Lessons learned from 2014–2016 Ebola outbreak in Guinea, a review of RCCE related publications. Centers of Disease Control and Prevention. 2021. http://www.socialscienceinaction.org/wp-content/uploads/2021/04/21_323506-A_Yee_Ebola-Review_1.pdf.

14. World Health Organization. Ebola outbreak 2014-2016 - West Africa 2016. https://www.who.int/emergencies/situations/ebola-outbreak-2014-2016-West-Africa.

15. Gostin LO, Tomori O, Wibulpolprasert S, Jha AK, Frenk J, Moon S, et al. Toward a common secure future: four global commissions in the wake of Ebola. PLoS Med. 2016 May;13(5):e1002042. https://doi.org/10.1371/journal.pmed.1002042 PMID:27195954.

16. United Nations. High-Level Panel on the Global Response to Health Crises. Protecting humanity from future health crises : report of the High-Level Panel on the Global Response to Health Crises. 2016. https://digitallibrary.un.org/record/822489.

17. World Health Organization. Report of the Ebola Interim Assessment Panel - July 2015. 2015. https://www.who.int/publications/m/item/report-of-the-ebola-interim-assessment-panel---july-2015.

18. Moon S, Sridhar D, Pate MA, Jha AK, Clinton C, Delaunay S, et al. Will Ebola change the game? Ten essential reforms before the next pandemic. The report of the Harvard-LSHTM Independent Panel on the Global Response to Ebola. Lancet. 2015 Nov;386(10009):2204–21. https://doi.org/10.1016/S0140-6736(15)00946-0 PMID:26615326.

19. World Health Organization. Global Policy Group Statement on reforms of WHO work in outbreaks and emergencies. 2016. https://idwho.se/entity/dg/speeches/2016/reform-statement/en/index.html.

20. Snyder MR, Lupel A. Reimagining Crisis Response: Lessons from the UN's Ebola Mission 2017. https://theglobalobservatory.org/2017/02/ebola-unmeer-united-nations-sierra-leone-liberia/.

21. Sirleaf EJ, Clark H. Report of the Independent Panel for Pandemic Preparedness and Response: making COVID-19 the last pandemic. Lancet. 2021 Jul;398(10295):101–3. https://doi.org/10.1016/S0140-6736(21)01095-3 PMID:33991477.

22. World Health Organization. WHO's work in health emergencies. Strengthening WHO's global emergency preparedness and response. Report by the Director-General 2021. https://apps.who.int/gb/ebwha/pdf_files/EB148/B148_18-en.pdf.

23. Scottand R, Nowell B. Networks and Crisis Management. Oxford Research Encyclopedia. Oxford University Press. 2020.

24. Koppenjan, J., & Klijn, E.-H. Managing Uncertainties in Networks: Public Private Controversies (1st ed.). Routledge. 2004. https://doi.org/10.4324/9780203643457.
25. Nohrstedt, D. Networking and crisis management capacity: a nested analysis of local-level collaboration in Sweden. Am Rev Public Adm. 2018;48(3):232–44. https://doi.org/10.1177/0275074016684585.
26. Kapucu N. Collaborative emergency management: better community organising, better public preparedness and response. Disasters. 2008 Jun;32(2):239–62. https://doi.org/10.1111/j.1467-7717.2008.01037.x PMID:18380853.
27. Olu OO, Lamunu M, Chimbaru A, Adegboyega A, Conteh I, Nsenga N, et al. Incident management systems are essential for effective coordination of large disease outbreaks: perspectives from the coordination of the Ebola outbreak response in Sierra Leone. Front Public Health. 2016 Nov;4:254. https://doi.org/10.3389/fpubh.2016.00254 PMID:27917377.
28. Adejugbagbe AM, Adejugbagbe EA, Fatiregun AA, Dosumu MO, Itse O, Akanbiemu FA, et al. Lessons learnt from decentralization of COVID-19 response in a southwest state of Nigeria. Global Biosecurity; 2022. https://doi.org/10.31646/gbio.158.
29. Nabarro D, Atkinson J. Dealing with covid-19 means looking beyond immediate crisis response. BMJ Opinion. 2020. https://blogs.bmj.com/bmj/2020/07/03/david-nabarro-and-john-atkinson-dealing-with-covid-19-means-looking-beyond-immediate-crisis-response/.
30. Wilkinson A, Parker M, Martineau F, Leach M. Engaging 'communities': anthropological insights from the West African Ebola epidemic. Philos Trans R Soc Lond B Biol Sci. 2017 May;372(1721):372. https://doi.org/10.1098/rstb.2016.0305 PMID:28396476.
31. Han S, Kang M. Combinations of conditions for network effectiveness: a fuzzy-set qualitative comparative analysis of 37 international development intervention cases. Voluntas. 2021;32(4):731–49. https://doi.org/10.1007/s11266-021-00358-2 PMID:34092933.
32. Nabarro D, Atkinson J. Better, smarter, local response systems are the only way to avoid further lockdowns. The Guardian. 2020. https://www.theguardian.com/commentisfree/2020/nov/15/better-smarter-local-response-systems-are-the-only-way-to-avoid-further-lockdowns.
33. Keith G, Provan PK. Modes of network governance: structure, management, and effectiveness. J Public Adm Res Theory. 2008;18(2):229–52. http://dx.doi.org/10.1093/jopart/mum015.
34. World Health Organization. Evidence, policy, impact: WHO guide for evidence-informed decision-making. 2022. https://www.who.int/publications/i/item/9789240039872.
35. World Health Organization. Evidence as a catalyst for policy and societal change: towards more equitable, resilient and sustainable global health 2022. https://www.who.int/publications/i/item/9789240052130.
36. Turk E, Durrance-Bagale A, Han E, Bell S, Rajan S, Lota MM, et al. International experiences with co-production and people centredness offer lessons for covid-19 responses. BMJ. 2021 Feb;372:m4752. https://doi.org/10.1136/bmj.m4752 PMID:33593813.
37. Bedford J, Enria D, Giesecke J, Heymann DL, Ihekweazu C, Kobinger G, et al.; WHO Strategic and Technical Advisory Group for Infectious Hazards. Living with the COVID-19 pandemic: act now with the tools we have. Lancet. 2020 Oct;396(10259):1314–6. https://doi.org/10.1016/S0140-6736(20)32117-6 PMID:33038947.
38. World Health Organization. Integrated people-centred care. https://www.who.int/health-topics/integrated-people-centered-care#tab=tab_1.
39. Marten R, El-Jardali F, Hafeez A, Hanefeld J, Leung GM, Ghaffar A. Co-producing the COVID-19 response in Germany, Hong Kong, Lebanon, and Pakistan. BMJ. 2021 Feb;372(243):n243. https://doi.org/10.1136/bmj.n243 PMID:33593791.

CHAPTER 4

LEGAL FRAMEWORKS FOR OUTBREAK RESPONSE

by Elyssa Liu, Dena Kirpalani, and Ayelet Berman

The main international legal instruments that govern infectious disease outbreaks are the International Health Regulations (IHR), the Trade-Related Aspects of Intellectual Property Rights (TRIPS) Agreement, the Convention on Biological Diversity (CBD) and its Nagoya Protocol, the Pandemic Influenza Preparedness (PIP) Framework, and human rights treaties. These frameworks are pivotal in facilitating international collaboration, sharing scientific data, early outbreak reporting, and ensuring equitable access to medical countermeasures. National legal frameworks have a separate role in enabling preparedness and response at country and community levels via infectious disease acts and other laws.

In the wake of the global community's inadequate response to the COVID-19 pandemic, the deficiencies in national, regional, and international law have come to the forefront, prompting demands for reforms that address the identified shortcomings. Against this background, negotiations began at the World Health Organization (WHO), culminating in some revisions to the IHR and ongoing talks regarding a pandemic accord.

INTRODUCTION

This chapter explores the role of national, regional, and international legal frameworks in strengthening prevention, preparedness, and response to infectious disease outbreaks. It explains the importance of law for the fair, effective, and rapid management of outbreaks.

Laws enabling efforts to respond to infectious disease emergencies date back centuries. Quarantine, from the Italian *quaranta* meaning 40, was the cornerstone of disease control in Europe from the 14th century. Over 40 days, humans, animals, and goods deemed at risk would be segregated while their ships were fumigated and disinfected. During plague epidemics, some city states cordoned themselves off, with armed guards. The application of these laws was inequitable, inciting discrimination against merchants and minority groups.

During cholera outbreaks, compulsory quarantine and isolation measures (for those with symptoms) were adapted, as was the case with plague. Movement orders were placed disproportionately on marginalised groups such as beggars and prostitutes. In the 19th century, with the increase of travel and trade and the growing concern by imperial powers regarding the spread of infectious diseases across their empires, many countries and colonial administrations began enacting laws for containing infectious diseases and their spread. Examples include the 1878 U.S. National Quarantine Act, the 1889 U.K. Infectious Disease Act, and the 1889 India Epidemic Diseases Act. To coordinate rules on the imposition of quarantine and other measures that restricted the flow of goods from their expanding empires into Europe and lay the groundwork for subsequent negotiations on coordinating state response to the spread of disease, the first International Sanitary Conference was held by European countries in 1851. The first International Sanitary Convention was adopted in 1892 in Venice to regulate traffic through the Suez Canal. It underwent 14 revisions until 1938 (1). From the Middle Ages through to the recent pandemic of COVID-19, legal frameworks that restrict the movement of persons and goods during suspected outbreaks of infectious diseases have been challenged by affected populations, sometimes validly but have occasionally included an inclination towards conspiracy theories. These responses highlight the role of proactive community engagement and education before and during responses, as laws created *during* a pandemic can be perceived as power grabs by authorities.

The legal framework that is in place in many countries today is more expansive and detailed, as well as convoluted and consistent with the complexities of research, confidentiality, technology, and information and data management that interrelate with the management of public health.

THE ROLE OF LAW IN OUTBREAK PREPAREDNESS

Any discourse around infectious disease outbreak preparedness and response should consider the role of law. International, regional, and national legal frameworks play a pivotal role in health emergency preparedness and response, serving as the foundation for international and national efforts to manage and mitigate the impacts of outbreaks. Legal regulation is of relevance at all stages of addressing health emergencies, from preparation through to response (2). This includes, among others, rules on surveillance, the sharing of scientific data, early detection and reporting of outbreaks, standards for the implementation of public health measures, restrictions on movement, and provisions for the equitable distribution of vaccines and therapeutics.

Infectious illnesses have no borders, and because we live in a globalised world with international movement and trade, spread quickly between countries. Due to this interconnectedness, each country is affected by the health security of other countries. Effective outbreak response is hard to achieve in isolation, with international collaboration required (3–4). The IHR is the main international agreement for governing outbreaks and international public health emergencies. Other international agreements, notably the World Trade Organisation (WTO) TRIPS Agreement, the CBD and its Nagoya Protocol, and the PIP Framework, have an influence on access to medical countermeasures.

At the national level, legal frameworks support national capacity for outbreak preparedness and response, including the ability to coordinate across different sectors. National legal frameworks both facilitate the implementation of international agreements and tailor national responses to the specific needs, customs, and circumstances of each country. National legal systems also provide governmental authorities with the powers needed for the application and enforcement of public health measures such as quarantine, travel restrictions, and vaccination mandates and incentives. This delegation of authority to government departments and institutions is not always clear-cut. There were several instances during the COVID-19 pandemic where there was conflict between government departments regarding which government body was responsible for coordinating the pandemic response (e.g., whether departments of disaster management and response or departments of health were responsible for coordinating response and relief during the outbreak). Legislative frameworks still contain such overlaps which need to be addressed to ensure clear lines of authority during the next public health challenge. Not all national frameworks are perfectly "de-conflicted", and there will be overlaps and gaps that need to be addressed to ensure a cohesive response in public health emergencies. These overlaps can lead to delays in critical decision-making processes.

Following the experiences gained over the past three decades with HIV, severe acute respiratory syndrome (SARS), H1N1, Middle East respiratory syndrome (MERS), Ebola, and COVID-19, there is a growing realisation that law plays a key role in facilitating, enabling, or undermining outbreak preparedness and response. In the absence of legal frameworks or their ambiguity, governments are forced to resolve issues on the fly during an emergency, which can hinder or delay responses. When legal frameworks are in place, a more consistent, expeditious, and effective response is possible. Thus, law underpins national, regional, and global health security.

International legal instrument	Year of adoption/ last revision	Is it legally binding?	Key obligations
IHR	1969/2024	Yes	• Reports certain diseases and public health events • Develops minimum public health capacities • Responds promptly to public health risks and emergencies
TRIPS Agreement	1994	Yes	• Protects intellectual property (IP) for pharmaceuticals and health technologies • Allows for compulsory licensing in emergencies • Implements IP rights in a manner supportive of public health
PIP Framework	2011/2019	No	• Shares influenza viruses judged to have pandemic potential • Shares vaccines and treatments during pandemics • Enhances global surveillance and response
CBD & Nagoya Protocol	1992/2010	Yes	• Conserves biological diversity • Promotes the sustainable use of components • Fairly and equitably shares the benefits from genetic resources
Universal Declaration of Human Rights (UDHR)	1948	No	• Sets out universal human rights standards • Calls for freedom, justice, and peace • Promotes equality and non-discrimination
WHO Constitution	1948	Yes	• Promotes and protects the health of all people

International legal instrument	Year of adoption/ last revision	Is it legally binding?	Key obligations
International Covenant on Economic, Social and Cultural Rights (ICESCR)	1966 (effective 1976)	Yes	• Progressively achieves the right to health • Ensures rights related to work, social security, and family life • Respects, protects, and fulfils the rights enshrined in the Covenant
International Covenant on Civil and Political Rights (ICCPR)	1966 (effective 1976)	Yes	• Ensures freedoms of speech, assembly, and religion • Protects the right to a fair trial and privacy • Prohibits torture and arbitrary detention
The Siracusa Principles	1984	No	• Specify conditions under which rights may be legally limited • Ensure that limitations are necessary and proportionate • Protect the essence of fundamental human rights

Table 4.1: Overview of key international legal instruments

INTERNATIONAL LEGAL INSTRUMENTS
The IHR

The IHR is the main international agreement governing international public health emergencies. It was revised in 2024 to address some of the shortcomings revealed during the COVID-19 pandemic.

Despite being legally binding in all WHO Member States, the IHR has faced key challenges and limitations with regard to its implementation and compliance. The implementation of core capacity requirements has been low (only about 30 per cent of Member States), revealing widespread global unpreparedness (5). This concern about country readiness in pandemic response continues to be reflected in the findings of the Global Health Security Index (GHSI) which assesses and benchmarks health security and related capabilities of State Parties to the IHR. The GHSI's 2021 indicator that looks at commitments to improve national capacity, financial plans to address gaps, and adherence to global norms (including adherence to the IHR) found an average score of 47.8 out of a possible 100 across countries, suggesting considerable room for improvement. This concern is greatest in resource-limited settings and is compounded by the challenges faced by the WHO in monitoring IHR implementation. A WHO Working Group on Amendments to the IHR was responsible for reviewing the IHR (2005) (6). Improving IHR implementation and strengthening compliance was one of the main topics on the agenda, with Member States having submitted diverse proposals to this end. The World Health Assembly (WHA) adopted a revision of the IHR in 2024 which establishes certain mechanisms for improving implementation.

Moreover, following the failure of the IHR to prevent and effectively respond to the COVID-19 pandemic, the WHO set out to negotiate a new pandemic accord, the objective of which is to address gaps and improve pandemic prevention and response. The mandate of the international negotiation body for negotiating a pandemic treaty has been extended until May 2025 (**See A new pandemic treaty?**).

IP and access to medical countermeasures: the TRIPS Agreement

While the purpose of the IHR is to regulate public health emergencies, the 1994 TRIPS Agreement is an international treaty that regulates IP rights regarding goods. It mandates the 195 WTO Member States to enforce patent and other IP protections. As such, it also has a significant impact on access to medical goods including medicines, vaccines, and other goods that are protected by patents.

In contrast to the IHR, the TRIPS Agreement contains a dispute resolution mechanism which states that violation of the Agreement may lead to legal action; this has resulted in substantial adherence to the TRIPS Agreement. Thus, while IHR has poor compliance, States hesitate to breach their TRIPS obligations.

The TRIPS Agreement has faced criticism from developing countries and public health advocates since patent protection of medicines and vaccines can result in high prices, significantly undermining the affordability of and access to medicines in developing countries. To mitigate this public health challenge, the TRIPS Agreement incorporates specific "flexibilities" regarding public health. For example, these flexibilities enable States to issue compulsory licences (7). Governments have the authority to enforce a non-voluntary licence that grants a third party the ability to utilise, manufacture, or import a patented product without the patent holder's consent, in exchange for adequate remuneration. In the wake of the AIDS pandemic, the Declaration of Doha concerning the TRIPS Agreement and Public Health reinforced countries' rights to make use of such flexibilities (8).

> **The TRIPS waiver**
>
> The COVID-19 pandemic demonstrated the limitations of TRIPS flexibilities in providing a fair and effective solution amid a worldwide public health emergency. Compulsory licensing cannot help States that lack pharmaceutical manufacturing capacity, and many vaccine innovations comprise hundreds of patents, necessitating the issuance of several compulsory licences. Thus, during the COVID-19 pandemic, South Africa and India led the efforts to reach an agreement on a TRIPS waiver—a blanket waiver that would remove its application to medical countermeasures during the pandemic, allowing developing countries to produce, import, or export SARS-CoV-2 countermeasures without the fear of being sued for IP infringement. The idea was strongly opposed by high-income countries, and a restricted waiver was eventually adopted in 2022.

That said, a legal waiver of IP protection (as advanced during COVID-19) does not solve the problem of access to medicines, given that many countries lack the necessary technology and production capacities. Although legal IP barriers would be eliminated by a waiver, many countries would remain incapable of manufacturing their own vaccines due to a lack of production facilities and expertise. As a result, there have also been discussions regarding improving local capacities, including through technology transfer. The pandemic treaty negotiations include, for example, provisions that seek to encourage the transmission of know-how, technology transfer, and voluntary licensing, as well as provisions that seek to strengthen local research and development. This would facilitate the domestic development and production of vaccines in developing nations.

Pathogen access and benefit sharing

Sharing pathogens, including pathogen genetic sequences, has profound implications for public health, particularly in the rapid identification of new pathogens and the development of medical countermeasures. For example, access to the genetic sequences of novel and emerging viruses enables researchers to understand their evolution, spread, and mechanisms of infection, which is critical for developing effective vaccines, diagnostics, and therapeutics.

On one hand, many are calling for "open science", whereby scientific data is shared freely and transparently. On the other hand, many developing countries seek to ensure that their sharing of pathogen sequences is made conditional on the receipt of medical benefits. Notably, in 2006, Indonesia refused to disclose H5N1 virus samples, claiming that it was inequitable for pharmaceutical companies to use pathogen samples in the development of new vaccines which were subsequently sold at unaffordable prices, leaving lower income countries vulnerable. It justified its refusal based on the CBD which adopts an access and benefit-sharing approach regarding biological and genetic materials. Indonesia argued that pathogen samples qualify as genetic materials safeguarded under the agreement and as such, they were entitled to just and equitable access to the benefits derived from their use (e.g., vaccines). WHO officials began discussions to resolve the matter and attempts were made to create a system for transparent, fair, and equitable benefit sharing that led to the establishment of the PIP Framework. The WHO admitted that there had been a breakdown in trust between Indonesia and the WHO's Global Influenza Surveillance Network (GISN). Indonesia only agreed to move forward after putting a Material Transfer Agreement (MTA) in place, a formality that had, up until then, been dispensed in the interests of expediency and solidarity (9).

In what follows, we lay out the main legal frameworks underpinning access and benefit concerning pathogens—the PIP Framework and the CBD's Nagoya Protocol. As we shall highlight, both frameworks have significant shortcomings, and there are now negotiations on a new pathogen access and benefit-sharing mechanism under the new pandemic treaty.

The PIP Framework

The PIP Framework (10) was established by the WHO in 2011, and an updated second version was issued in 2019. The PIP Framework was developed in response to the challenges and controversies that arose during the avian influenza H5N1 outbreak in 2005, including Indonesia's dissatisfaction with the terms of information sharing.

The PIP Framework aimed to address such disparities with the adoption of an "access and benefit" sharing multilateral mechanism. Under this system, countries share influenza viruses of pandemic potential (10) with the WHO's Global Influenza Surveillance and Response System (GISRS, formerly GISN), and in return, receive access to benefits derived from the data that are shared (e.g., vaccines, treatments, and other medical countermeasures). The transfer of the biological materials from members to the WHO GISRS, and from the

WHO GISRS to pharmaceutical companies and other recipients, is carried out under Standard Material Transfer Agreements (SMTA1 and SMTA2, respectively). Under the SMTA2, the recipient agrees to provide a percentage of their products or contribute other benefits, such as voluntary royalty-free licensing, technology transfer, and more (Article 4 of Annex 2 of the PIP Framework sets out a list of benefits the recipient can choose from). This mechanism ensures that the benefits derived from the shared viruses, such as vaccines, are made available to all countries, not just those with the ability to pay.

The PIP Framework has improved global preparedness for influenza pandemics. It has enhanced the capacity of the GISRS, improved the global surveillance network, and facilitated faster and more equitable access to pandemic influenza vaccines. That said, its actual effectiveness remains unclear. The PIP Framework has several shortcomings, including that it is not a legally binding agreement, is limited to influenza with pandemic potential (Article 3) (10), and does not cover seasonal influenza or other pathogens (11–12). Nevertheless, the multilateral model of the PIP Framework (as opposed to the bilateral model of the Nagoya Protocol), where data sharing is facilitated by the WHO, is often regarded as a best practice for rapid, fair, and equitable access and benefit sharing. Current negotiations over pathogen access and benefit-sharing mechanisms under a new pandemic treaty follow a multilateral approach as well.

The CBD and the Nagoya Protocol

The CBD was established at the Earth Summit in Rio de Janeiro in 1992 and came into effect in 1993 (13). It is a binding, international treaty focused on the conservation of biological diversity, sustainable use of its components, and the fair and equitable sharing of benefits derived from biological and genetic resources. The CBD affirms state sovereignty over biological and genetic resources found in its jurisdiction. The approach is transactional: the sovereign state is required to grant informed consent and, in exchange, must be granted access to the benefits derived, subject to mutually agreed terms.

The Nagoya Protocol on Access to Genetic Resources and the Fair and Equitable Sharing of Benefits Arising from their Utilization (14), commonly referred to as the Nagoya Protocol, is a supplementary agreement to the CBD, adopted in 2010. It aims to implement the fair and equitable sharing of benefits arising from the utilisation of biological and genetic resources, thereby contributing to the conservation and sustainable use of biodiversity.

While the Nagoya Protocol is applicable to "genetic resources", it makes no explicit mention of pathogens, though many countries understand it as applying to pathogens as well. As such, the CBD and Nagoya Protocol have become increasingly relevant in the context of public health emergencies. Indeed, Indonesia's refusal to share influenza samples rested on the CBD.

While the Nagoya Protocol promotes the sovereignty of countries over their natural resources and ensures that benefits derived from their use are shared equitably, numerous features are incompatible with the rapid and effective management of public health emergencies. The CBD and Nagoya Protocol were designed to strengthen biodiversity, not respond to public health emergencies. The bilateral transactional model of the Nagoya Protocol impedes timely access to pathogen samples during an emergency because bilateral talks may cause delays in pathogen sharing (11,15). Moreover, some contest its application to pathogens, with inconsistent national implementation. These divergences cause delays in sharing during a public health emergency. Furthermore, there are ongoing debates about applying the CBD to digital sequencing data (16). It is uncertain if the application of the CBD to digital sequences extends to pathogen sequences as well.

The pandemic treaty
Efforts to reconcile the objectives of the Nagoya Protocol with the imperatives of global health emergency response have led to negotiations at the WHO regarding creating a specialised framework (Article 4.4) (14). The pandemic treaty which is being negotiated establishes a multilateral "pathogen access and benefit-sharing system" that would allow for the swift multilateral sharing of pathogens with pandemic potential, including genetic sequence data (Article 12) (12). While there was considerable support for a new legal instrument immediately after the pandemic, access and benefit sharing has been contentious, and has been one of the main barriers in reaching an agreement on a new pandemic treaty by the 77th WHA in May 2024, as originally envisioned. The mandate of the Intergovernmental Negotiating Body (INB) to negotiate a treaty has been extended until May 2025.

HUMAN RIGHTS LAW AND OUTBREAKS
The UDHR was adopted at the United Nations (UN) General Assembly in 1948. It was drafted by diverse representatives with different legal, cultural, and geographic backgrounds. While not formally legally binding, in 30 articles translated into over 500 languages, the Declaration presents the foundation upon which current norms of international human rights were developed. Human rights apply before, during, and after outbreaks. Several main human rights issues arise during outbreaks:
- the right to health is most obviously threatened
- there will be issues involved in balancing public health measures (e.g., quarantine, isolation, travel restrictions, contract tracing, vaccination mandates) with individual human rights (e.g., freedom of movement, privacy, liberty, lack of discrimination)
- protections of marginalised populations are often threatened
- there may be derogations to human rights during a public health emergency

The right to health
The right to health is embedded in several international instruments which have been almost universally ratified. These include, among others, the 1948 WHO Constitution, the 1976 ICCPR, and the 1976 ICESCR. The WHO defines the right to health as the "enjoyment of the highest attainable standard of health" and as "one of the fundamental rights of every human being" (17). The 1948 UDHR recognises the right through language that states that "everyone has the right to a standard of living adequate for the health and well-being of himself and of his family, including food, clothing, housing and medical care, and necessary social services" (Article 25) (18). The right to health includes access to healthcare and the protection and provision of the underlying determinants of health (Para. 4) (19). If the right to health is part of public health, health system preparedness and responses should arguably reflect that in their decisions and actions.

Balancing between public health measures and human rights
Quarantine, isolation, contract tracing, mask use, vaccine regulations, safe distancing, and misinformation prevention, among others, are all public health measures that may be in

tension with human rights. Their application may result in limitations on the freedom of movement, the right of assembly and privacy, and the right to free expression. A human rights approach to outbreaks involves balancing the collective interest in limiting the spread of a harmful or contagious pathogen with individual human rights. The ICCPR, for example, recognises that public health may justify limiting the right to movement and the right to assembly (18).

In balancing collective interest with individual rights, human rights law uses proportionality and necessity tests to determine that the measure is not arbitrary, and that the limitations to human rights are acceptable in a democratic society. Such tests usually have four parts and pose the following questions (20):
- is the measure prescribed by clear and accessible law?
- does the measure have a legitimate aim?
- is the measure proportionate to the stated legitimate aim, and is the limitation necessary to achieve that aim, or could it be achieved with less stringent means?
- does the measure discriminate between certain groups or people?

Finally, during an emergency, such limitations should also be time-limited, and subject to periodic review.

This four-part test has been articulated under the framework of the Siracusa Principles on the Limitation and Derogation Provisions in the ICCPR, developed by the International Commission of Jurists (ICJ), and adopted by the UN Economic and Social Council (ECOSOC). These principles provide interpretive guidance on the limitation and derogation provisions in the ICCPR. While proportionality and necessity tests are common features of human rights law, their ultimate application depends on national courts, resulting, in practice, in divergent applications in different jurisdictions.

The IHR also includes provisions on the protection of human rights during public health emergencies of international concern. Article 3 of the IHR determines that "state parties must have full respect for dignity, human rights, and fundamental freedoms of persons, guided by the UN charter and WHO constitution ...". Article 43 determines that "state's health measures cannot be more restrictive of trade and human rights than needed to avert or reduce the risk, and if a measure causes significant interference", states must provide "the public health rationale and relevant scientific information". Further, Article 42 determines that health measures must be applied in a transparent and non-discriminatory manner (21).

Protection of marginalised groups and non-discrimination

An outbreak and its public health-associated restrictions may disproportionately affect the health or the risk profile of certain populations (**See Chapter 32, Protecting the vulnerable**). The principle of non-discrimination, however, suggests that measures need to be put in place to mitigate such disproportionate impact (20), including during a public health emergency (22).

Non-discrimination does not mean treating all populations the same. Rather, it prohibits differential treatment of specific groups solely based on personal characteristics such as gender, ethnicity, national origin, religion, age, or other personal characteristics, and which results in less preferential treatment of that group relative to the general population (23).

Derogation from human rights during public health emergencies

States can derogate from human rights (except from non-derogable rights, such as the right to life or prohibition on torture) during public health emergencies. International human rights instruments like Article 4 of the ICCPR allow derogation. To derogate, a state must meet substantive and procedural criteria. Common criteria are (22):

- the existence of an exceptional crisis or emergency
- the state must notify the treaty authority of its decision to derogate, the measures adopted, their rationale, and their application
- the proportionality and necessity of the measure, given the circumstances
- the consistency with other obligations under international law
- the measure must be uniformly applicable and non-discriminatory

When derogating, states are not given a free pass to trample on human rights; instead, they are making clear that they are to act in extraordinary and temporary circumstances, and that because of the urgency of the situation, may apply restrictions on freedoms and rights ordinarily granted to persons (24).

Be that as it may, the legality of public health measures applied during a public health emergency depends on the legal system of the respective jurisdiction, and different national and regional courts have taken divergent approaches (25–29). While states are often granted a margin of appreciation by courts in the context of emergencies, this does not give them free reign on their actions.

International human rights commitments are an important consideration in public health emergencies and outbreaks. Whether and how they are applied and interpreted depend largely on the legal systems and national courts of the respective jurisdictions that are responsible for enforcing their own constitutions and national human rights laws. Some countries are also parties to regional human rights treaties, such as the European Convention on Human Rights, the American Convention, and the African Charter on Human and People's Rights, which have their own courts. Thus, the specific recourse of individuals and the interpretation and application of human rights by national or regional courts may vary.

Indeed, despite these provisions being in place to check the arbitrary use of powers by states, some states have been charged with violating human rights in the name of outbreak control (30), including allegations of the use of arbitrary incarcerations, limits on freedom of speech, and the use of measures that disproportionately impact or target marginalised groups (e.g., migrant workers). International legal scholars, in response to some of the actions taken by states during the COVID-19 outbreak, have proposed a set of Principles and Guidelines on Human Rights and Public Health Emergencies to further articulate human rights obligations during public health emergencies (31).

THE ROLE OF NATIONAL LEGAL FRAMEWORKS

Both national and international law are key building blocks of public health emergency preparedness. National legal frameworks have two main roles. They have a role in the implementation of the international legal obligations mentioned above, such as IHR core capacity obligations, TRIPS IP protections, or pathogen sharing rules, by translating these into national legislation and embedding them within existing national structures. In practice, however, implementation often poses a problem. For example, the implementation of IHR core capacities has been generally inadequate (32). Implementation varies between countries, resulting in inconsistency. Also, mechanisms to ensure compliance and consistency with international norms and commitments within and across jurisdictions tends to be weak.

But even more critically, national law is key in regulating government authority in governing prevention, preparedness, and response to outbreaks. Such authority must be established in national law. The Global Health Security Agenda (GHSA): Legal Preparedness Action Package has sought to list the main topics that are required for national legal preparedness (33). The list includes laws for triggering public health measures (e.g., quarantine, isolation, masking, border control measures, contract tracing, vaccination) and balancing them with human rights, laws for establishing key agencies and providing them with authority and powers, laws regarding the manufacture and procurement of medical countermeasures, regulatory mechanisms for the authorisation of medicines and vaccines, and liability risk management (33).

However, the COVID-19 pandemic revealed that many countries had major gaps in national legal preparedness and lacked the necessary legal infrastructure (33–35). These gaps slowed down their response. For example, many countries lacked legal frameworks for liability risk management, resulting in delays of several months in access to vaccines and measures to offer social and economic relief to populations (**See National legal reform**). The absence of robust social security frameworks also hindered efforts to mitigate the side effects of lockdowns, leaving many individuals without adequate support during extended periods of restricted movement and economic decline.

National legal reform

Following the 2014–2016 Ebola outbreak in West Africa, several countries affected by the epidemic undertook significant legal reforms to strengthen their health systems and emergency response capabilities. Liberia, for example, revised its public health law to better align with the IHR, establishing a more robust legal foundation for disease surveillance, reporting, and response (36).

Similarly, for the COVID-19 pandemic, South Korea's effective response was supported by laws that allowed for comprehensive contact tracing, quarantine measures, and public communication strategies, rooted in lessons learned from the MERS outbreak in 2015 (37).

National legislation, informed by international law, can enhance preparedness and response to health emergencies, underscoring the importance of legal frameworks at both the national and global levels.

Liability risk management

During the COVID-19 pandemic, disparities in vaccine access between high-income and developing countries were exacerbated by various factors. A significant hurdle was the lack of pre-established liability risk management frameworks, leading to delays as countries navigated suppliers' demands for indemnification against vaccine injuries as well as specific dispute resolution provisions. This resulted in states needing to hastily develop policies and negotiate contract terms, such as indemnification scope and changes to dispute resolution mechanisms. This, in turn, caused delays in procurement.

To act swiftly, countries needed legal frameworks to deal with liability challenges, such as the U.S. Public Readiness and Emergency Preparedness (PREP) Act, and to regulate matters such as no-fault injury compensation mechanisms, indemnification for vaccine manufacturers or other providers in the vaccine supply chain, insurance mechanisms, contractual clauses that balance liability risk concerns with timely and equitable access to medical countermeasures, and so on.

This lack of liability risk management laws slowed down access to new vaccines in developing countries. The GHSA Legal Preparedness Action Package established the Liability Risk Management Sub-Working Group to develop such guidance. Examples of liability and indemnification provisions in COVID-19 vaccine procurement contracts are available in the Global Health Innovation Alliance Accelerator (GHIAA) MAPGuide (33,38–42).

A NEW PANDEMIC TREATY?

The COVID-19 pandemic exposed significant vulnerabilities in the world's ability to prevent, prepare for, and respond to pandemics (43–44). Recognising the limitations of the existing international legal frameworks addressed above, the WHO, country governments, public health experts, and international organisations advocated for a more robust and equitable instrument that is legally binding. This proposed new treaty aims to address the gaps identified, enhance international cooperation, and ensure that the world is better equipped to manage future pandemics (45–46). Key issues and objectives being considered in the pandemic treaty include:
- ensuring equitable access to vaccines, treatments, and diagnostics
- improving global surveillance and early warning systems
- enhancing transparency and information sharing among countries
- strengthening health systems worldwide

The treaty also aims to establish a more effective framework for international cooperation and solidarity, ensuring that all countries, regardless of their economic status, can respond effectively to health threats (45–46). The treaty is also aligned with the One Health approach, recognising the interconnectedness of human, animal, and environmental health, and the need for a coordinated response to zoonotic diseases (46).

Ultimately, the successful negotiation and implementation of a pandemic treaty could mark a transformative step in global health security governance, making the world safer and more resilient against future pandemics. However, for the treaty to see success that sets it apart from the existing legal frameworks, consensus among Member States will need to be achieved. Reaching an agreement is a significant challenge given the diverse political, economic, and health priorities of different countries. Countries have differing views on issues such as information sharing, IP rights, and the sharing of pathogen sequences and data. The dilemma of countries balancing national interests and political will against a greater, global public health goal must be effectively addressed. Given these difficulties, at the time of writing, the intention to conclude a pandemic treaty by the 77th WHA has not been fulfilled and the mandate of the INB to continue negotiations has been extended by one year.

THE ROLE OF REGIONAL AGREEMENTS

There are a range of regional agreements related to pandemic preparedness and capacity building. Regions are increasingly engaged in active collaboration, with the discernment that national measures against the spread of pathogens are only effective if their neighbouring countries are equally protected. In Europe, the European Union (EU) established a legal framework for joint procurement of medical countermeasures (47). This initiative was developed in response to the H1N1 pandemic and enables EU Member States to pool resources to jointly purchase vaccines and antiviral drugs for the region, thereby ensuring equitable access to essential medicines during a health crisis and enhancing the collective response to pandemics within Europe.

In the African region, the Africa Centres for Disease Control and Prevention (Africa CDC) plays a crucial role in coordinating efforts across the continent to prepare for and respond to public health emergencies (48). The Africa CDC provides technical assistance, disease surveillance, emergency response, and capacity-building programmes, demonstrating a regional approach to addressing the challenges of pandemic preparedness and response.

The Association of Southeast Asian Nations (ASEAN) adopted the Agreement on Disaster Management and Emergency Response (49). While the Agreement primarily focuses on natural disasters, its framework has been extended to cover public health emergencies, including pandemics. Following the COVID-19 pandemic (50), ASEAN leaders adopted the ASEAN Comprehensive Recovery Framework (51) and its Implementation Plan as a consolidated strategy for recovery. This framework aims to address the broad impacts of the pandemic, including health, economic, and social dimensions, and emphasises strengthening health systems and enhancing regional mechanisms for public health emergencies and future pandemics.

Key features of the success of implementing legal instruments or global guidelines are cooperation, trust, and transparency. There are many examples of efforts that strive to build these strengths regionally. For example, the Africa Pathogen Genomics Initiative (Africa PGI) (52) and Asia Pathogen Genomics Initiative (Asia PGI) (53) aim to accelerate pathogen genomic sequencing in their respective regions and foster knowledge and skills exchange by hosting workshops, training programmes, and other opportunities for researchers, scientists, and public health emergency focal points to connect and build on each other's strengths and achieve a unified response in times of emergencies.

CONCLUSION

Legal frameworks play an indispensable role in enhancing global and national responses to health emergencies, serving as the scaffolding upon which preparedness, detection, response, and recovery efforts are built.

National laws enable the implementation of international commitments, translating them into concrete actions. They are also necessary for supporting authorities to enforce public health measures, mobilise resources, protect their populations, and achieve health equity before and during infectious disease emergencies.

International frameworks provide a structure for international collaboration and impact access to medical countermeasures. The value of international agreements lies in establishing normative frameworks for international cooperation and platforms for orchestrating an international response. Reform initiatives at the WHO on a pandemic treaty and IHR revisions seek to address many of the identified gaps. At the time of writing, a few changes have been introduced to the IHR (2024) and negotiations between Member States on a pandemic treaty have been unsuccessful so far.

As the world continues to grapple with emerging health threats, strengthening these legal frameworks can assist in building a more resilient global health security system capable of protecting all people from the impact of future outbreaks.

REFERENCES:

1. Fidler DP. From international sanitary conventions to global health security: the new International Health Regulations. Chin J Int Law. 2005;4(2):325–92. https://doi.org/10.1093/chinesejil/jmi029.
2. Gostin LO, Katz R. The International Health Regulations: the governing framework for global health security. Milbank Q. 2016 Jun;94(2):264–313. https://doi.org/10.1111/1468-0009.12186 PMID:27166578.
3. WHO. "We are only as strong as the weakest", Secretary-General Stresses, at Launch of Economic Report on COVID-19 Pandemic | UN Press [Internet]. 2020. https://press.un.org/en/2020/sgsm20029.doc.htm.
4. Agyarko R, Al Slail F, Garrett DO, Gentry B, Gresham L, Kromberg Underwood ML, et al. Chapter 4 - The imperative for global cooperation to prevent and control pandemics [Internet]. McNabb SJN, Shaikh AT, Haley CJ, editors. ScienceDirect. Academic Press; 2024 [cited 2024 Mar 5]; 53–69. https://www.sciencedirect.com/science/article/abs/pii/B9780323909457000191.
5. Global Health Security Index. Advancing collective action and accountability amid global crisis [Internet]. 2021. https://ghsindex.org/wp-content/uploads/2021/12/2021_GHSindexFullReport_Final.pdf.
6. WHO. Working Group on Amendments to the International Health Regulations (2005) [Internet]. [cited 2024 Mar 14]. https://www.who.int/teams/ihr/working-group-on-amendments-to-the-international-health-regulations-(2005).
7. World Trade Organisation. WTO | Intellectual Property (TRIPS) - Agreement Text - Contents [Internet]. 2019. https://www.wto.org/english/docs_e/legal_e/27-trips_01_e.htm.
8. WTO. WTO | Ministerial conferences - Doha 4th Ministerial - TRIPS declaration [Internet]. 2016. https://www.wto.org/english/thewto_e/minist_e/min01_e/mindecl_trips_e.htm.
9. Sedyaningsih ER, Isfandari S, Soendoro T, Supari SF. Towards mutual trust, transparency and equity in virus sharing mechanism: the avian influenza case of Indonesia. Ann Acad Med Singap. 2008 Jun;37(6):482–8. https://pubmed.ncbi.nlm.nih.gov/18618060/ https://doi.org/10.47102/annals-acadmedsg.V37N6p482 PMID:18618060.
10. WHO. Pandemic influenza preparedness framework for the sharing of influenza viruses and access to vaccines and other benefits, 2nd ed [Internet]. 2022. https://www.who.int/publications/i/item/9789240024854.
11. Rourke M, Eccleston-Turner M. The Pandemic Influenza Preparedness Framework as a "Specialized International Access and Benefit-Sharing Instrument" under the Nagoya Protocol [Internet]. North Irel Leg Q. 2021;72(3):411–47. [cited 2024 Mar 5] https://heinonline.org/HOL/LandingPage?handle=hein.journals/nilq72&div=39&id=&page= https://doi.org/10.53386/nilq.v72i3.881.
12. Imamura T, Oshitani H. Global Strategy for Influenza Viral Infection: What Is the Latest Information from WHO? Respiratory Disease Series: Diagnostic Tools and Disease Managements. 2020 Nov 11;3–11.
13. Convention on Biological Diversity United Nations [Internet]. 2016. https://www.cbd.int/convention/text.
14. Convention on Biological Diversity United Nations. Nagoya Protocol on access to genetic resources and the fair and equitable sharing of benefits arising from their utilisation [Internet]. 2011. https://www.cbd.int/abs/doc/protocol/nagoya-protocol-en.pdf.
15. Hodnett DQ. Legitimising biopiracy? Fairness and efficacy of the Nagoya Protocol. York Law Review [Internet]. 2021 [cited 2024 Mar 5];2:75. https://heinonline.org/HOL/LandingPage?handle=hein.journals/yorklr2&div=8&id=&page=.
16. CBD. Compilation of views and information on digital sequence information on genetic resources submitted pursuant to Paragraphs 9 and 10 of Decision 14/20. 2020.

17. World Health Organization. Constitution of the World Health Organization [Internet]. 2006. https://www.who.int/governance/eb/who_constitution_en.pdf.
18. United Nations. Universal Declaration of Human Rights [Internet]. https://www.un.org/en/about-us/universal-declaration-of-human-rights.
19. UN Committee on Economic, Social and Cultural Rights (CESCR). UN Economic and Social Council, General Comment No. 14: The Right to the Highest Attainable Standard of Health (Art. 12 of the Covenant). 2000.
20. United Nations. Siracusa Principles on the Limitation and Derogation of Provisions in the International Covenant on Civil and Political Rights Annex, UN Doc E/CN.4/1984/4 (1984) [Internet]. https://www.uio.no/studier/emner/jus/humanrights/HUMR5503/h09/undervisningsmateriale/SiracusaPrinciples.pdf.
21. WHO. International Health Regulations (2005) Third Edition [Internet]. 2005. https://www.who.int/publications-detail-redirect/9789241580496.
22. UN Human Rights Committee. General Comment No. 29: Article 4: Derogations during a State of Emergency. UN Doc. CCPR/C/21/Rev.1/Add.11. Geneva: United Nations; 2001, para. 8.
23. UN Human Rights Committee, General Comment 18 on Non-Discrimination, 10 November 1989.
24. Office of the United Nations High Commissioner for Human Rights (OHCHR). Emergency Measures and COVID-19: Guidance. 27 April 2020. https://www.ohchr.org/sites/default/files/Documents/Events/EmergencyMeasures_COVID19.pdf.
25. Oxford Constitutional Law, The Oxford Compendium of National Legal Responses to Covid-19. https://oxcon.ouplaw.com/home/OCC19.
26. Covid-19 Litigation, Open-Access Case Law Database. https://www.covid19litigation.org/.
27. Lex-Atlas: Covid-19. A global academic project mapping legal responses to Covid-19. https://lexatlas-c19.org/.
28. COVID-19 Law Lab. Find recent legislative action to control and reduce the pandemic. https://www.covidlawlab.org/.
29. Oxford Human Rights Hub. Results for 'COVID-19'.
30. Amon J. J., Wurth M. A virtual roundtable on COVID-19 and human rights with human rights watch researchers. Health Hum Rights. 2020 Jun;22(1):399–413. PMID:32669829.
31. Principles and Guidelines on Human Rights and Public Health Emergencies. 10 May 2023. https://www.icj.org/wp-content/uploads/2024/01/Human-Rights-Public-Health-Emergencies.pdf.
32. Sodjinou VD, Ayelo PA, Douba A, Ouendo DE. Main challenges of the detection in the context of global health security: systematic review of Joint External Evaluation (JEE) reports. Pan Afr Med J. 2022 Jul;42:243. https://doi.org/10.11604/pamj.2022.42.243.26563 PMID:36303822.
33. Global Health Security Agenda. Legal Preparedness Action Package [Internet]. Retrieved March 11, 2024. https://globalhealthsecurityagenda.org/legal-preparedness/.
34. Gostin LO, Magnusson RS, Krech R, Patterson DW, Solomon SA, Walton D, et al. Advancing the right to health-the vital role of law. Am J Public Health. 2017 Nov;107(11):1755–6. https://doi.org/10.2105/AJPH.2017.304077 PMID:29019787.
35. International Development Law Organization. Preventing pandemics through the rule of law: strengthening countries' legal preparedness for public health emergencies [Internet]. 2023, September 19. https://www.idlo.int/publications/preventing-pandemics-through-rule-law-strengthening-countries-legal-preparedness-public.
36. Gupta S, Gupta N, Yadav P, Patil D. Ebola virus outbreak preparedness plan for developing nations: lessons learnt from affected countries. J Infect Public Health. 2021 Mar;14(3):293–305. https://doi.org/10.1016/j.jiph.2020.12.030 PMID:33610938.
37. Oh SY. From a 'super spreader of MERS' to a 'super stopper' of COVID-19: explaining the evolution of South Korea's effective crisis management system. Journal of Asian Public Policy, 15(2), 250–65. https://doi.org/10.1080/17516234.2020.1863540.
38. Global Health Security Agenda. (2022, October 10). Promoting legal preparedness & equity through liability risk management [Video]. YouTube. https://www.youtube.com/watch?v=fwkX3_ADtRI.
39. The Global Healthcare Innovation Alliance Accelerator (GHIAA). Master Alliance Provisions Guide. Retrieved March 11, 2024. https://ghiaa.org/mapguide-home/search-results/?qs=covid+19.
40. GHIAA. Map Guide Commentaries: Liability and Indemnification Provisions in COVID-19 Vaccine Supply Agreements. Retrieved March 11, 2024. https://ghiaa.org/mapguide-home/liability-and-indemnity-obligations-in-early-covid-19-vaccine-agreements/.

41. Halabi S, Heinrich A, Omer SB. No-fault compensation for vaccine injury - the other side of equitable access to Covid-19 vaccines. N Engl J Med. 2020 Dec;383(23):e125. https://doi.org/10.1056/NEJMp2030600 PMID:33113309.
42. U.S. Health Resources and Services Administration. National Vaccine Injury Compensation Program: Covid-19 claims. Retrieved March 11, 2024. https://www.hrsa.gov/vaccine-compensation.
43. Kavanagh MM, Wenham C, Massard da Fonseca E, Helfer LR, Nyukuri E, Maleche A, et al. Increasing compliance with international pandemic law: international relations and new global health agreements. Lancet. 2023 Sep;402(10407):1097–106. https://doi.org/10.1016/S0140-6736(23)01527-1 PMID:37678291.
44. Williamson A, Forman R, Azzopardi-Muscat N, Battista R, Colombo F, Glassman A, et al. Effective post-pandemic governance must focus on shared challenges. Lancet. 2022 May;399(10340):1999–2001. https://doi.org/10.1016/S0140-6736(22)00891-1 PMID:35588759.
45. Matsoso P, Driece R, da Silva Nunes T, Soliman A, Taguchi K, Tangcharoensathien V. Negotiating a pandemic accord: a promising start [Internet]. BMJ. 2023 Mar;380:506. https://doi.org/10.1136/bmj.p506 PMID:36863729.
46. Jamal N. One Health and the opportunity for paradigm shifts through a new WHO Pandemic Agreement. Development. 2023 Nov;66(3-4):199–206. https://doi.org/10.1057/s41301-023-00384-1.
47. WHO. Call for urgent agreement on international deal to prepare for and prevent future pandemics [Internet]. 2024 [cited 2024 Mar 25]. https://www.who.int/news/item/20-03-2024-call-for-urgent-agreement-on-international-deal-to-prepare-for-and-prevent-future-pandemics#:~:text=Nations%20set%20themselves%20the%20deadline.
48. Dzinamarira T, Dzobo M, Chitungo I. COVID-19: a perspective on Africa's capacity and response. Journal of Medical Virology [Internet]. 2020 Jun 11. https://pubmed.ncbi.nlm.nih.gov/32525568/. https://doi.org/10.1002/jmv.26159 PMID:32525568.
49. ASEAN. ASEAN Agreement on Disaster Management and Emergency Response. [Internet]. https://agreement.asean.org/media/download/20220330063139.pdf.
50. Djalante R, Nurhidayah L, Lassa J, Minh HV, Mahendradhata Y, Phuong NT, et al. The ASEAN's responses to COVID-19: a policy sciences analysis [Internet]. Rochester, NY; 2020. https://papers.ssrn.com/sol3/papers.cfm?abstract_id=3595012.
51. ASEAN. ASEAN Comprehensive Recovery Framework [Internet]. https://asean.org/book/asean-comprehensive-recovery-framework/.
52. Africa CDC. Africa Pathogen Genomics Initiative | Africa PGI 2.0 [Internet]. https://africacdc.org/africa-pathogen-genomics-initiative-africa-pgi/.
53. Asia Pathogen Genomics Initiative. Asia Pathogen Genomics Initiative | Duke-NUS Medical School [Internet]. https://www.duke-nus.edu.sg/asiapgi/.

CHAPTER 5

ETHICS TO INFORM DECISION-MAKING

by Sarah J.L. Edwards, Caitlin Gordon, Blessing Silaigwana, and Roli Mathur

Ethical considerations are an important part of decision-making processes at each stage of an infectious disease emergency. This chapter introduces the notion that ethical thinking begins with a process of clarification of the values and moral principles at work in decision-making, and evolves a set of procedures to reason morally in each decision-making context. Certain moral concepts are necessary to highlight in the ethics of infectious disease emergencies, particularly ideas of autonomy, beneficence, and justice. The chapter then works through the different phases of emergency response, introducing the key ethical issues and questions at each phase.

Ethical thinking does not provide single ideal answers, but enables decision-makers to identify and articulate the value components of decisions, so as to balance, for example, considerations of individual liberties with public health outcomes in an emergency. Elaborate processes of consideration and consultation are often in tension with the challenges of making critical decisions rapidly and under uncertainty. That is why trustworthy institutions and continued community engagement are crucial, particularly in culturally diverse settings.

The chapter concludes by emphasising the need for ongoing ethical reflection and preparedness to better manage future outbreaks, advocating for a sustained social conversation on the balance between protecting public health and respecting individual rights.

INTRODUCTION

Infectious disease emergencies present many ethical and practical challenges for stakeholders involved in outbreak preparedness and response including policymakers, public health officials, and first responders (1). For instance, as witnessed during the 2020–2023 COVID-19 public health emergency of international concern, very complex ethical decisions and trade-offs had to be made to balance the competing needs and interests of individuals, communities, and societies, especially when faced with a rapidly spreading high-mortality condition, and when speed was of the essence (2). While there could be very good reasons to move quickly to protect the health and safety of the public, in many cases, important questions of ethics seem not to have been considered fully before interventions were implemented. The impact of these interventions may not have been assessed according to how their expected benefits would be distributed or how expected costs are imposed. Those who bear the greatest costs may not be the ones who stand to benefit the most. Public health reasoning alone cannot ethically justify any such distribution of costs and benefits. Even when included, ethics is all too often considered separately from outbreak preparedness and response management rather than as an integral concern (3).

Ethics in medicine has a long history, often being traced back at least as far as ancient Greece with the Hippocratic Oath. Such early articulation of professional values in medicine, dating to before the establishment of the scientific method, stated that physicians should put the best interests of their patients first. Ethical concerns in public health involving blunt and extremely restrictive measures during acute crises outside normal medical practice are also historically familiar. The very notions of quarantine (issued to potentially infected persons) and isolation (ordered for persons known to be contagious) used to control the spread of disease go back centuries, at least to the plague outbreak in the 14th century (3). Duties of patient confidentiality also have early ethical and legal origins.

However, the rise of a more scientific understanding of disease and epidemiology occurred much later in the 19th century, as did the elaboration of professional values in respecting the autonomy of patients with consent to treatments which were physically invasive. The advance of medical diagnostics, vaccines, anti-infective treatments, and health systems infrastructure have themselves created more options for public health decision-makers, raising new ethical considerations. The professional duty to treat patients during outbreaks of known infectious diseases was well-established by the influenza pandemics of the early 20th century. While the regulation of medicines to protect public health is relatively recent and followed the widespread use of harmful products in the early 20th century, more liberal notions have brought about the considerations of further rights and interests of individual patients including privacy rights and the right to fair access to essential medicines.

This chapter seeks to outline what we mean by ethics in general as well as during outbreak emergencies. This chapter also provides an overview of ethical issues at different stages of an outbreak. We further illustrate why it is important to consider ethics as an integral part of outbreak preparedness, response, and management, and show how ethical considerations are contextual and cultural, emerging through all aspects of infectious disease emergencies. Ethics rarely provides black and white answers for decision-makers.

WHAT EXACTLY IS ETHICS, AND WHY IS IT IMPORTANT?
Identifying values
We all bring our own values to the practical decisions we make. A key task for thinking about ethics in outbreaks is to first identify those values which may otherwise be implicit (4). Public health officials make decisions all the time, either as policies or in practice, as individuals or in teams. The values at work may be revealed in codes or guidelines or may be discovered as tacit norms and customs. Sometimes, claims of fact also carry important implicit values. To say the evidence does not support a certain intervention includes evaluative judgements about the intervention itself with an implicit judgement of what balance of risks and expected benefits are acceptable under uncertainty. Ethics requires that these values be made explicit so they can be considered and balanced against other factors in the round.

Defining moral concepts and identifying moral issues
In order to identify values, we need the concepts and vocabulary to articulate them. There are many moral concepts which we might consider more or less important in public health ethics (5). These include liberty or freedoms which can be thought of as positive or negative. Liberal approaches tend to place importance on preserving negative freedoms to determine one's own conception of a good life, whereas many non-liberal approaches are not propagated by a leader or an ideology but are part of a society's value regime (e.g., "conformity is

better than individualism") (2). Related to liberty is the concept of autonomy, which stresses self-determination and is often respected through informed consent, especially to physically invasive treatment. To be able to make autonomous choices, one must have enough information on which to base a decision, be capable of understanding the information in whatever form, and weigh that information in the balance to reach a decision which is not coerced by others. Coercion can occur though obvious mechanisms such as brute force or threat of sanction, or more subtle use of deception or manipulation (e.g., inducing fear). Adults not mentally competent to make decisions may need a surrogate or representative to do so on their behalf. Children are often thought to be vulnerable and even if relatively mature and apparently capable, they deserve special protections (2). Collective decision-making requires each individual in the group to consent, while participative decision-making can be more consultative, tolerating individual veto. Solidarity is a term used to connect people to a cause or situation to show collective support and is different from shared or joint decision-making.

Traditional duties of beneficence and non-maleficence are ways of describing obligations around calculating and balancing the risks and expected benefits for affected individuals and communities. Justice often requires that we distribute risks and benefits fairly across populations and compensate those unfairly harmed. Methods for allocating resources or social goods need to be rational and may use metrics of cost-effectiveness which underline the consequentialist maxim, the greatest good for the greatest number.

When attempting to treat or prevent a new disease, different types of uncertainty are compounded. The precautionary principle advises against introducing new technologies or treatments until their safety is proven, placing the burden of proof on the developer. However, during an emergency, this principle is often challenged due to the urgent need for solutions. Risk profiles change in emergencies, especially for novel pathogens, due to the overall learning as well as treatment availability and evolving natural or vaccine-related immunity.

Those who are not themselves healthcare workers (HCWs) should recognise that professional duties of care are more stringent than the everyday duties held by the general public, and these duties can vary based on the specific roles of public health and medical professionals. These professionals have distinct responsibilities, and their decision-making processes are held to high standards to avoid negligence. Negligence occurs when a decision-maker fails to meet the expected standard, resulting in harm to individuals or populations. Ideas of wrongdoing tend to focus more on actions taken rather than omissions, though failing to act can also have severely negative consequences.

Reasoning about moral concepts to resolve issues

Armed with moral concepts such as those above, we are now able to identify some of the moral issues in decision-making in public health. A decision whether or not to isolate a patient will require considering the values associated with the patient's liberty and possible containment in hospital, their autonomy in agreeing to diagnostic tests and treatments, privacy rights in keeping their medical history confidential, and informing the public. Public health needs are primarily designed to protect others so they must be weighed against the rights and interests of the individual. These issues can usually be resolved through different methods although the answers may vary with cultural norms and contextual features such as the severity of the disease. Dilemmas are not, by definition, issues which can be definitively resolved. This chapter, therefore, seeks to give a descriptive overview of the ethical issues involved at different stages of outbreak response, and what methods are used to reach ethical decisions about those public health interventions, both singly and in combination. A review of the many arguments used to support different positions is outside the scope of this chapter.

One method used to think about ethics is moral philosophy. As a discipline, it seeks to clarify and refine moral concepts and drive systematic thinking about the questions over what one should do or the kind of person one should be in any given circumstance. However, ethics in practical decision-making can never be a straightforward application of any moral philosophy (6). There will always be imperfect information, room for interpretation, and implementation of principles in context, even if the principles themselves are considered universal. The real world is messy and multiple ethical issues may interlock and interact at any one time with no agreed universal answer to resolve them. Notwithstanding these challenges, the values guiding decisions and the moral concepts used to think about and resolve issues must be explicit. Other methods used to consider ethics are through laws, regulations, and empirical study as outlined below.

Laws and regulations

The legal rules which protect individual liberty, autonomy, and privacy may be very different in liberal compared with communitarian or patriarchal societies. Yet, under international organisations, some shared values have been agreed and background working assumptions made. Indeed, the United Nations (UN) Universal Declaration of Human Rights (UDHR), adopted in 1948, was a milestone in international relations, laying out a common legal standard for all UN Member States (7). We will consider specific human rights concerns as they relate to outbreaks in due course.

Empirical ethics

Ethics also have an empirical dimension, in the sense that we could simply ask people about their moral compass and conscience in different contexts. Such a consultative or participative approach to ethics resonates well with the moral philosophies behind the legal human rights instruments (8). Such an approach to decision-making seeks to be more inclusive of those previously disadvantaged or marginalised and helps increase awareness and engagement with public policies (9).

Developing an African-centred ethics framework

Following the West African Ebola crisis in 2014–2016, it became clear that different external researchers resolved the ethical issues associated with clinical trial designs in different incompatible ways. The U.S. favoured choosing a few drug candidates and evaluating them through placebo-controlled trials, while the U.K. was more pragmatic and favoured small screening studies of more candidate medicines to identify large effect sizes before considering large trials of the more promising candidates. The U.K. approach featured different trial designs to provide wider access to known active medicines.

> The outbreak was over before definitive results were gained for science yet provided the groundwork for clinical trials in later outbreaks in the Democratic Republic of the Congo (DRC). In order to guide future consideration of ethics within cultural context by those directly affected by the diseases, members of the European & Developing Countries Clinical Trials Partnership (EDCTP) funded the PANDORA-ID NET Consortium and worked with the newly created Africa Centres for Disease Control and Prevention (Africa CDC) to support the creation of an African-centred ethics framework for outbreaks of emerging and re-emerging infectious diseases. Considerable effort was put into convening a group of researchers, members of ethics committees and regulators from the central region, during these later outbreaks in the DRC to consider the ethics of research, especially of monoclonal antibodies. A working group comprising African bioethicists then wrote a culturally authentic and participative framework whilst acknowledging diversity across Africa. Extensive consultation was done in different African settings, including amongst public health researchers, first responders, and members of research ethics committees, to create a set of cultural values to guide research (10).

Ultimately, we might find that we should set somewhat modest aims concerning ethics in outbreaks. It may be possible to reach only an operational consensus on what values should underpin morally acceptable trade-offs or strike apparent compromises in collective negotiation. We might agree on which interventions are acceptable and yet disagree over the underlying moral reasoning. As a result, many codes of ethics will outline certain principles without wider philosophical theories and will provide general guidance over the detailed task of implementation over many different types of cases. Indeed, the major ethics codes lay out operational principles. With the help of academic and operational ethicists, the World Health Organization (WHO) has also issued ethics documents in many areas of ethics and global health with an associated training manual (1,11). While these codes may change over time, they can help describe expected norms for decision-making, have huge symbolic moral salience, and help foster public trust in decision-makers. However, ethics codes cannot cover all the ethical issues which can arise in practice, nor can they offer the fine-gained guidance needed to resolve every case.

Ethics consultations and committees

The COVID-19 pandemic also saw a rise in the provision of ethics support or consultation with ethicists as knowledge brokers or advocates of policies with some perceived moral authority and apparent expertise (12). With the values of people (including ethicists!) themselves potentially being so diverse, it is worth clarifying what expertise was sought and how it was selected in individual cases. The aim of such facilitative exercises may have been less about providing an ethical answer to given questions, and more to help decision-makers explore all relevant avenues and expose possible consequences, intended or otherwise, of different courses of action. However, the responsibilities and liabilities usually still lie with the decision-makers themselves.

In some areas of public health and medicine (e.g., research), ethics committees are well-established structures, with agreed international and domestic standards of practice, often required by law (13). Constitutions, memberships, and remits can vary but the key idea is to provide an independent opinion on research based on diverse experiences, backgrounds, and expertise to mitigate against a researcher's potentially conflicting interests, minimise risk/harm, and protect research participants from exploitation. There is usually a lay contingent included to offer a counterbalance to professional researchers. Such procedural review takes international and domestic laws into account but cannot be considered substitutes for community engagement or wider public consultation over controversial topics.

All the pillars of outbreak response (**See Chapter 1, Introduction**) will raise ethical issues and draw on the previously mentioned concepts in different ways. Some of the activities and topics have been considered by the WHO Ethics Unit, and others through academic publication or media commentary. However, there are some issues which still need careful thought. Here we provide an overview of the main ethical issues that influence decision-making in outbreak preparedness, response, and recovery.

The following three sections of the chapter review some of the main ethical issues and decisions corresponding to the different stages of infectious disease emergency response. In most cases, such a rapid survey can only identify the issues. In many cases, other chapters include the relevant ethical reasoning on key topics and are cross-referenced.

ETHICS IN PREPAREDNESS AND PREVENTION

Under International Health Regulations (IIIR), governments are obliged to invest in systems designed to pick up a seeming needle in a haystack just in case an outbreak ensues, as an outbreak always carries the potential of leading to a severe pandemic, no matter how rarely. In addition, the IHR embrace human rights, providing common ground for all Member States. However, human rights thinking fundamentally concerns the relationship between individuals and the nation state, making wider concerns of international distribution and transnational solidarity more difficult to address. Assistance from the international community to countries less able to devote resources to preparedness is still a source of ethical debate and is highly political (14). Past public health emergencies have seen existing global inequalities become entrenched due to restrictions in vaccine sharing, patent waivers, and diagnostics, as well as research and development infrastructure. As a result, there is growing recognition that there should be more capacity and expertise to prepare for and manage outbreaks *within* developing countries, to redress such global injustices (15). For example, The Nagoya Protocol restricts how biological samples can be lawfully shared internationally, protecting developing countries.

Early warning systems rely on sustainable community engagement (16). However, attempts to change risky behaviour against cultural norms or sensitivities can be counterproductive as new cases may be hidden from officials for fear of reprimand or social stigma (17). Furthermore, without support and resources for day-to-day living, tension and violence against officials could occur when they attempt to quarantine cases and isolate contacts.

Human rights thinking cannot adequately address many emerging and re-emerging infectious diseases which are zoonotic in origin. Ecological studies are providing more data on how to identify potential hotspots for zoonotic disease—especially when they are re-emerging—so that the surveillance of humans and animals can be more targeted (16). However, there has not been sufficient attention paid to our responsibilities towards animals during outbreaks of infectious diseases with zoonotic and pandemic potential. An approach in high-income countries is often to simply protect or cull groups of animals and compensate any affected animal owners (18) (**See Public health crisis associated with variant Creutzfeldt-Jakob disease**).

Realising that emerging diseases of zoonotic origin may pose global risks, there has been some international support for One Health surveillance in certain developing countries (**See Chapter 13, One Health**). At the same time, there can be reluctance to intervene early when there are strong economic and cultural interests at stake, for example, in maintaining the international meat trade or respecting religious norms in diets (17).

> **Public health crisis associated with variant Creutzfeldt-Jakob disease in the U.K.**
>
> The emergence of variant Creutzfeldt-Jakob disease (vCJD) in the U.K. was linked to cows given contaminated feed. Considering the importance of the meat industry and beef exports, it took significant time to properly investigate and take correct measures for what was known to be poor farming practices and meat processing. The public was consistently, yet falsely, reassured by politicians that consuming beef was considered safe. By safe, however, they meant "safe enough" from a policy point of view accepting a certain level of risk to some. Once there was direct and unequivocal evidence that the human disease was caused by eating beef from diseased cows, the public health approach had to change, both in terms of messaging and industry practices. Meanwhile, other countries cancelled import contracts and started to ban donations of blood from U.K. residents. Between 1996 and 2024, 178 people died from confirmed or probable vCJD, while over four million cows were eventually culled to prevent the spread of Bovine Spongiform Encephalopathy (BSE). Many more people were expected to develop the disease which has a long incubation period.

Basic research and building community trust

It is certainly possible to design response programmes ahead of public health threats, to support decision-makers as and when needed. However, there is no substitute for developing sustainable partnerships with communities and building trustworthy institutions to quickly mobilise effective and ethical responses should the need arise (19). For example, public health interventions invariably require population endorsement especially when carried out in deprived areas with populations who have recollections of past abuses and historic colonialism (16). It is never too early to improve levels of trust (**See Chapter 33, RCCE**).

ETHICS IN OUTBREAK RESPONSE
Risk assessment and strategy

Even with data from early warning systems, it can be difficult to judge when to act and what strategy to utilise. The true severity of the threat may not be recognised until there is too much community transmission to be able to implement standard contact tracing programmes. A fundamental decision in such cases is whether to let the virus spread unchecked to result—ultimately—in herd immunity from natural infection. Herd immunity is the indirect protection offered after a certain percentage of the population becomes immune. These decisions are based on the severity of the disease and speed of spread. Early models attempt to predict case fatality rates and agree on a threshold. The level of protection conferred by herd immunity must also be well understood, and this is unlikely for emerging diseases. As there is generally no consensus on how many deaths are acceptable, we often look to other endemic diseases for suitable reference points.

Cost-benefit assessments compare the consequences of intervening or not, while other approaches may better account for the idea that negative consequences may sometimes be considered more blameworthy than failures to act (or acts of omission). Negative consequences may also be distributed in ways we consider to be unfair, not reflected in a straightforward cost-benefit assessment. To compound this bias, the precautionary principle requires innovative technologies to be tested for safety before they are made widely available, whatever the prevailing need. Notions of negligence, however, judge both acts and omissions alike in preparing protocols and plans against a reasonable expected professional standard for decision-making.

Knowing where to turn for advice in a crisis is hugely important and it remains good policymaking to draw on diverse expertise and experience. Consulting a wide panel of ethicists can help open possibilities and check assumptions.

Contact tracing and privacy

In an effort to reduce transmission or control the spread of disease, the standard approach is to target contacts of cases for intervention. The principle of proportionality is key so that the severity and intrusiveness of the interventions are in proportion to the threat (20). This principle involves choosing the least restrictive method to meet the same overall objectives. Such methods may involve simply using and sharing the personal data of individual patients as part of routine surveillance programmes for possible targeted interventions later. Contact tracing, for example, monitors potential spread, warns the individuals concerned, and should offer methods of mitigation. The individuals concerned may have no choice over the use of personal data for public health purposes, yet their rights and freedoms are otherwise intact. Mandatory testing of those known to have been exposed may be required when there are no less intrusive measures available and the public health threat is severe enough (21). Necessary measures to enact such policies include a data sharing infrastructure and systems for making diagnoses notifiable to authorities often required by law when the disease is not so stigmatising that patients are dissuaded from seeking medical help.

Closing national borders

During pandemics, the decision whether and when to close national borders to international travel has major implications for economic activity and can ultimately do more harm than good. However, the COVID-19 pandemic has shown that the economy could be protected only through protecting public health. Some countries might close their borders to try to keep a pandemic disease out rather than in.

Physical distancing, quarantine

In all outbreaks, the use of quarantine is arguably one of the most drastic public health measures. It is coercive as it restricts the freedom of movement. It is universally agreed to be morally justifiable only in the most extreme circumstances when no other less restrictive measures would be effective (21). Despite its severity, it can be justified by the most liberal accounts of the state, which allow or require state interference to prevent a patient from severely harming others. This is called the harm principle (22). Over centuries and until today, this is a commonly agreed practice during the early treatment phase of patients with tuberculosis.

During the COVID-19 pandemic, most of the world became familiar with restrictions on liberty in one form or another, either for targeted communities or across mass populations, to reduce the spread of the SARS-CoV-2 virus. These restrictions—in the form of lockdowns—were designed principally to better manage surge capacities of the health services. With a virus able to spread from person to person asymptomatically, restrictions of movement, especially those enforceable by the state, are more difficult to justify using the harm principle alone. We can then appeal to thresholds of probabilities, severity of harm, and collective responsibilities or solidarity. These approaches are philosophically debatable and culturally relative if intuitively morally acceptable in some cases. Communities or states that do not endorse liberal values will generally be more favourable to such restrictions.

Other ethical concerns for the most drastic and blanket measures weigh the consequences of such measures, not all of which can be foreseen. In many countries, lockdowns had unfortunate and unintended consequences, particularly for marginalised populations with limited access to resources (23–24). Additionally, the long-term consequences of lockdowns on human rights, economic development, and social cohesion must be carefully considered. The debate on the ethics of these lockdown decisions continues to reverberate.

The doctrine of double effect (25–26) provides a framework for evaluating morally complex actions like lockdown orders, which bring both intended and unintended consequences. According to this doctrine, an action can be morally permissible if the intended effect is good while the unintended effect may be harmful, but not intrinsically evil. Many lockdowns will have been ethically justified by the application of this doctrine.

The full consequences of the COVID-19 lockdowns are only now becoming clearer, with many countries seeing additional deaths due to other diseases left untreated, delays in diagnoses, and a rise in domestic violence (27) (**See Chapter 23, Maintaining essential services**). However, the number of fatal accidents was likewise reduced. The consequences of quarantine without maintaining social security networks were clearly dire for many of the already disadvantaged (28). Some governments did not implement official lockdowns, perhaps because of the lack of government social security cover, meaning that those at high risk of severe COVID-19 (e.g., pregnant women) were still expected to go to work, often using public transport with little or no personal protection (**See Chapter 32, Protecting the vulnerable**). Entitlements to essential resources to maintain life were not met in many cases.

Conflicts, communities, and communication

Much of the previous research on health and risk communication in academic social sciences foretold ethical issues which arose later in the COVID-19 pandemic especially in relation to social or behavioural issues such as vaccine hesitancy (29) (**See Chapter 29, Vaccine implementation**). Honest communication about uncertainties and trade-offs is required. Any strategy which relays values inherent in policies as indisputable facts to sell them or manipulate people rarely pays off in the long term (30). Deception or misinformation is coercive. Without checking, informational manipulation, such as emphasising benefits and downplaying risks or uncertainties, may or may not be deceptive to motivate or change behaviour.

In addition, using risk communication to instil a culture of fear as a political device for control often leads to stigma and unintended consequences, as seen in the early HIV/AIDS campaigns (31).

Conveying science to some communities, especially those that do not have a clear perception of risk, can bring about some issues. This creates challenges in discharging duties of truth-telling (2). Generating rapport alone is not ethically sufficient to create trusting and trustworthy relationships. The methods for mobilising communities themselves can involve treading a moral tightrope. Tactics such as enlisting and employing a member of the affected community to persuade others to comply with the proposed public health measures simply because this person is trusted by them may be common practice and can be seen as a shortcut to success. For example, community engagement for clinical trials has sometimes been used merely to maximise recruitment rates without necessarily examining understanding and voluntary consent (32).

The rise of digital health

Telemedicine is increasingly being used to facilitate communication at a distance with the hope of improving access. However, there are ethical issues in rolling out telemedicine and include the development of suitable capacity, data protection, security, and sharing agreements. Over-reliance on telemedicine may disadvantage those who are not digitally literate or do not have access to equipment or the internet. If so, it only reinforces inequalities. But this concern alone is not a sufficient reason to deny everyone access to such facilities, to 'level down' rather than to work towards universal coverage.

Ethics in research and clinical practice

For outbreaks of emerging and re-emerging infectious diseases, all types of research, from basic to the behavioural sciences, are needed. While the ethics of animal experimentation and clinical research are well-trodden areas, outbreaks create unique difficulties (13). In the context of a pandemic, proper coordination is needed to avoid a situation where numerous small clinical trials compete for research participants. Standard principles of research ethics include the need for the assessments of risks and benefits to discharge the duties of non-maleficence and beneficence, respectively, independent checks by research ethics review, and consent where possible. All these requirements may be difficult in practice (13) (**See Chapter 18, Research to inform practice; See Chapter 27, Research for therapeutics**).

There are currently two competing approaches to clinical research strategies for therapeutics (**See Developing an African-centred ethics framework**). The first is to evaluate very few candidate therapeutics in placebo-controlled trials to reach definitive results as quickly as possible (33). The second is to cast the net wider to screen candidates through smaller observational work first and only begin large RCTs once candidates show clinical promise (34). The type of research and development (R&D) strategy adopted has major implications for what investigational treatments patients can try and how outcomes are monitored over time. Research ethics often rest initially on assumptions about and disagreements over how medical science can maximise social value. **See R&D strategies for clinical research and options for patients** for how the choice of scientific methods in clinical research can impact the treatments available to individual patients.

> **R&D strategies for clinical research and options for patients**
>
> Early in the COVID-19 pandemic, when the WHO convened its first meeting of experts to agree on a strategy for R&D for therapeutics, there were many more candidate medicines than could feasibly be evaluated in the SOLIDARITY study, a large pragmatic platform RCT which used adaptive ratios so patients had more chances of receiving the more promising treatment of the moment. At the time, there was little understanding of the disease. Some candidates were initially excluded but later found to be useful for severe disease once COVID-19 was better understood. In the beginning, it was not clear whether dexamethasone should be included at all, yet it turned out to be definitive, at least in certain high-income hospital settings. Additionally, tocilizumab, first developed for the treatment of overactive immune reactions and licensed for severe rheumatoid arthritis, was later found in smaller scale trials and early access schemes to be beneficial in some cases. Hydroxychloroquine was initially thought to offer some antiviral action at high doses despite possible adverse effects and so was included and mistakenly used widely outside clinical trials, despite evidence that it could not target the original virus in human cells, but only in African green monkeys. With more understanding of the virus and the disease, it was clear that antivirals are needed early in the course of the disease, yet they were pitted by randomisation against treatments for severe symptoms, possibly after the virus had begun to clear. A strategy which prioritises large RCTs while excluding observational work may be unable to offer the maximum number of individual patients the best possible combination of treatments for their particular stage and set of symptoms (35).

Protecting the healthcare workforce

Procuring adequate personal protective equipment (PPE) was an issue during the COVID-19 pandemic. However, healthcare staff also face other risks, including safety in the field (36). First responders may be received with suspicion and hostility by communities they are investigating, as was seen during Ebola outbreaks in socially unstable contexts in the DRC.

Many health professionals had not seen death on such a scale and were traumatised during the COVID-19 pandemic (37). At the height of the surge in COVID-19 patients, clinical ethics committees were helping record the context within which staff were working and documenting the impact of scarce resources. Without reassurances over professional indemnity and full recognition of the context, staff may become increasingly concerned about their liabilities and may seek advice from clinical ethics committees where they exist.

In addition, HCWs are almost universally considered a priority population for vaccination to safeguard response capacity (20). As a result, HCWs are often asked to participate in research (often clinical trials), though this participation raises questions on how trials are designed including:
- what is the expected exposure to the virus, and under what background working conditions and policies which may be more or less protective from the virus?
- what other diseases are circulating which may seem more or less severe?
- what other surveillance and intervention measures trace and reduce transmission of the virus?

There has been much debate over intended and unintended consequences of policies that make vaccination mandatory or require it as a condition of employment (38). Disciplinary measures or sanctions were sometimes applied to persistent refusers who were thereby deemed unfit to work, especially in patient-facing roles. Such sanctions may have been applied without exhausting alternative measures and exploring the reasons behind reluctance or hesitancy. In some countries particularly short of staff, HCWs may be required to work even when ill.

Human challenge studies
To speed up research into vaccines during COVID-19, many young people were willing to undergo challenge studies as they had a lower risk of severe disease from the virus yet bore the brunt of blanket restrictions on liberty. The acceptability of risk in research is often a matter of referencing other accepted activities to test consistency.

Mass and emergency vaccination programmes
The ethical issues raised by particular vaccination programmes designed by governments and health officials hinged critically on the wider response strategies, other public health measures being used, and the background conditions of the populations affected. In some countries, vaccines licensed for emergency use were widely distributed to release populations from measures which restricted freedom of movement. The ethics of vaccine passports may simply be applicable only in contexts where social restrictions on liberty are relatively accepted. Vaccine passports to enable travel and interaction with others promised a controlled and possibly incremental exit from a full lockdown. However, there could be objections to the policy on the grounds that it maintains state interference on liberty and encroaches on privacy rights irrespective of risks individuals pose to others and what level of risk people were willing to accept. Some established vaccines for endemic diseases become routine, including for people lacking mental capacity as it may be considered in their best interests as a member of a social group to reach a threshold of herd immunity.

Distributive justice and global health
There continues to be concern for justice in the distribution of risks and benefits of research in global health following vaccine nationalism and the role of commercial sectors in upholding patent protections for profits (27). In many respects, highly valuable innovations developed by the private sector always rest on prior public sector funding. We should be able to factor in how different measures affect existing inequalities to better establish fairness in these calculations.

Dealing with death
One of the most challenging aspects of an outbreak response is dealing with death. During the West African Ebola crisis, establishing a practice of safe burials was key to reducing disease transmission but sometimes required an ethical justification to override cultural norms without community agreement or against their wishes (28). Over time, though, compromises through negotiation may be reached to respect all parties. How we deal with death is inevitably symbolic. During the Black Death, many bodies were buried in mass graves but pointed in a certain direction in respect of religious beliefs (3). During COVID-19, many hospitals did

not have enough body bags to maintain usual practice and pits for mass graves and funeral pyres were reported across the world. Funerals were restricted and social distancing rules applied (39).

ETHICS IN RECOVERY
Establishing a new normal

The easing of restrictive emergency measures can occur in two incubation periods after the last case. In the case of endemic conditions, the end of the emergency is based on epidemiologic and immunologic factors which represent a threat reduction. Relaxing measures can be done incrementally to test each singly before life can return to some semblance of normality (40). Restrictive measures that are extended beyond this point become draconian.

However, the ethics of measures associated with learning to live with diseases which are becoming endemic can itself be difficult. Restoring a liberal order as soon as possible may be more pressing for some countries than others. It may simply involve accepting a certain expected death toll for the sake of regaining freedoms. Reducing the requirements to test and isolate are further indicators. Nonetheless, some diseases cannot be tolerated in human populations as they are too serious, with high case fatality rates, and are too contagious to let loose. In such cases, a policy of elimination may need to be maintained. The harm principle introduced earlier is key to assessing the ethics and legitimacy of such restrictive measures.

Extended monitoring and further research

There may need to be some continued monitoring for epidemiologic and genetic trends along with research into the long-term effects of a disease and to refine therapies, while keeping abreast of trends in case mix and management. Hospitals will still need to address the infection control policies they adapted in the emergency and to determine when, whether, and how they will revert. Booster vaccines may also be needed for staff.

Towards personal responsibilities

A new normal may be devastating for those still clinically vulnerable, unable to benefit fully from vaccination, and seemingly all but forgotten. The weight of personal responsibilities in managing risks can be heavy and stigma is hard to shake, isolating and marginalising the vulnerable. Survivors may still be left unable to work and economically dependent on their families (**See Continuing duties of care to Ebola survivors**). Such loss of livelihood could be due to complications of the disease itself, the vaccines or treatment they received, or underlying chronic diseases putting them at an increased risk.

Compensation and catch-up

Dealing with the consequences of outbreaks can be a long process. There is often little compensation for relatives of the bereaved or those injured through vaccination or working in high-risk environments especially without adequate protective equipment. There may be systems failures for which governments should be held to account (41).

Normal life will also require addressing the backlog in deferred medical treatments unrelated to the infectious disease outbreak. Staff may find themselves dealing with the fallout of frustrated populations with a rise in instances of abuse rather than welcome appreciation.

Widespread access to mental health services (**See Chapter 31, Mental health**) may be essential to smooth the way.

Children in many countries which experienced lockdowns will have missed vital schooling and social interactions which may never be fully restored to a level they would have expected if not for the outbreaks and associated public health measures (**See Chapter 32, Protecting the vulnerable**) (42). Intensive tuition during summer holidays and lengthening school days have been considered following COVID-19.

> **Continuing duties of care to Ebola survivors**
>
> Following the Ebola crisis in West Africa in 2014–2016, Ebola survivors faced numerous challenges including the loss of parents or children, the loss of livelihood, social stigma, poor health, and continued surveillance. Mental health support was critical. The offer of vaccination, with a vaccine developed by Janssen and a programme supported by the Innovative Medicines Initiative (IMI), while experimental, was still available. However, it was not clear to what extent public health officials should prioritise continuing the occasional long-term support in specific programmes for survivors when resources are generally scarce, other vital health programmes need to be reinstated, and communities may become dependent on external, possibly foreign aid, especially when they are at odds with cultural and spiritual beliefs. For example, some cultures do not accept that mental health difficulties can be treated by medicine. That stigma can only be addressed with sustained efforts to communicate current science understandings (43).

Finally, the recovery phase provides an opportunity to reflect on what has happened, reassess current and future population needs, and learn lessons to prepare for future outbreaks.

CONCLUSION

Ethics requires that decision-makers identify moral values in their cultural, religious, and political contexts, and seek to intervene in ways that are least restrictive of rights and freedoms as possible while in proportion to the threat posed. The earlier we can establish trustworthy institutions and foster equal and fair partnerships with populations in different parts of the world, the more prepared we will be for future emerging and re-emerging infectious disease emergencies.

The more liberal the rights and interests we embrace, the more ethical issues there are to consider in public health decision-making and the more complicated the balancing of individual interests against the group's public health status becomes. Fairness requires that we prioritise protecting the vulnerable, distributing the risks of research and sharing of its benefits, and treating different cultures with the respect they deserve.

REFERENCES:

1. World Health Organization. Ethics in epidemics, emergencies and disasters: research, surveillance and patient care [Internet]. Geneva; 2015 [cited 2024 Mar 20]. www.who.int/about/licensing/.
2. Mastroianni A, Kahn J, Kass N. The Oxford Handbook of Public Health Ethics [Internet]. 2019 Jan 8 [cited 2024 Mar 20]; https://academic.oup.com/edited-volume/28138.

3. Aliyu AA. Public health ethics and the COVID-19 pandemic. Ann Afr Med. 2021 Jul-Sep;20(3):157-163. https://doi.org/10.4103/aam.aam_80_20. PMID:34558443.

4. Mertz M, Prince I, Pietschmann I. Values, decision-making and empirical bioethics: a conceptual model for empirically identifying and analyzing value judgements [Internet]. Theor Med Bioeth. 2023 Dec;44(6):567–87. https://doi.org/10.1007/s11017-023-09640-4 PMID:37589807.

5. Tulchinsky TH. Ethical issues in public health. Case Studies in Public Health. 2018:277–316. https://doi.org/10.1016/B978-0-12-804571-8.00027-5.

6. Wolff J. Ethics and public policy: a philosophical inquiry. 2019 Aug 15 [cited 2024 Mar 20];1–329. https://www.taylorfrancis.com/books/mono/10.4324/9781351128667/ethics-public-policy-jonathan-wolff https://doi.org/10.4324/9781351128667.

7. Ooms G, Latif LA, Waris A, Brolan CE, Hammonds R, Friedman EA, et al. Is universal health coverage the practical expression of the right to health care? [Internet]. BMC Int Health Hum Rights. 2014 Feb;14(1):3. https://doi.org/10.1186/1472-698X-14-3 PMID:24559232.

8. Marten R, El-Jardali F, Hafeez A, Hanefeld J, Leung GM, Ghaffar A. Co-producing the covid-19 response in Germany, Hong Kong, Lebanon, and Pakistan [Internet]. BMJ. 2021 Feb;372:n243. https://doi.org/10.1136/bmj.n243 PMID:33593791.

9. Durrance-Bagale A, Marzouk M, Tung LS, Agarwal S, Aribou ZM, Ibrahim NB, et al. Community engagement in health systems interventions and research in conflict-affected countries: a scoping review of approaches [Internet]. Glob Health Action. 2022 Dec;15(1):2074131. https://doi.org/10.1080/16549716.2022.2074131 PMID:35762841.

10. Tajudeen R, Silaigwana B, Yavlinsky A, Edwards SJ. Research ethics during infectious disease outbreaks: a survey of African research stakeholders using the Ebola virus disease outbreak as a case. J Public Health Africa. 2023 Oct;14(9):1632. https://doi.org/10.4081/jphia.2023.1632 PMID:37881726.

11. World Health Organization. Global health ethics: key issues [Internet]. Geneva; 2015 [cited 2024 Mar 17]. www.who.int.

12. Wilson J, Hume J, O'Donovan C, Smallman M. Providing ethics advice in a pandemic, in theory and in practice: a taxonomy of ethics advice [Internet]. Bioethics. 2024 Mar;38(3):213–22. https://doi.org/10.1111/bioe.13208 PMID:37506261.

13. World Health Organization. Ethical standards for research during public health emergencies: distilling existing guidance to support COVID-19 R&D. 2020.

14. Mathur R. Ethics preparedness for infectious disease outbreaks research in India: a case for novel coronavirus disease 2019. Indian J Med Res. 2020 Feb & Mar;151(2 & 3):124-131. https://doi.org/10.4103/ijmr.IJMR_463_20. PMID:32362641.

15. Bennett B, Carney T. Law, ethics and pandemic preparedness: the importance of cross-jurisdictional and cross-cultural perspectives [Internet]. Aust N Z J Public Health. 2010 Apr;34(2):106–12. https://doi.org/10.1111/j.1753-6405.2010.00492.x PMID:23331351.

16. World Health Organization. WHO guidelines on ethical issues in public health surveillance. Geneva; 2017.

17. van Vliet N. "Bushmeat crisis" and "cultural imperialism" in wildlife management? Taking value orientations into account for a more sustainable and culturally acceptable wildmeat sector. Front Ecol Evol. 2018 Aug;6(AUG):393036. https://doi.org/10.3389/fevo.2018.00112.

18. van Herten J, Buikstra S, Bovenkerk B, Stassen E. Ethical decision-making in zoonotic disease control: how do one health strategies function in the Netherlands? [Internet]. J Agric Environ Ethics. 2020 Apr;33(2):239–59. https://doi.org/10.1007/s10806-020-09828-x.

19. The Independent Panel for Pandemic Preparedness and Response. Centering communities in pandemic preparedness and response. 2021.

20. Munzert S, Ramirez-Ruiz S, Çalı B, Stoetzer LF, Gohdes A, Lowe W. Prioritization preferences for COVID-19 vaccination are consistent across five countries. Humanit Soc Sci Commun. 2022;9(1):439. https://doi.org/10.1057/s41599-022-01392-1 PMID:36530547.

21. World Health Organization. Guidance for managing ethical issues in infectious disease outbreaks [Internet]. Geneva; 2016 [cited 2024 Mar 17]. http://www.who.int.

22. Stanton-Ife J, Zalta E. Stanford Encyclopedia of Philosophy. 2017 [cited 2024 Mar 20]. The Limits of Law. https://plato.stanford.edu/cgi-bin/encyclopedia/archinfo.cgi?entry=law-limits.

23. Jefferies S, French N, Gilkison C, Graham G, Hope V, Marshall J, et al. COVID-19 in New Zealand and the impact of the national response: a descriptive epidemiological study [Internet]. Lancet Public Health. 2020 Nov;5(11):e612–23. https://doi.org/10.1016/S2468-2667(20)30225-5 PMID:33065023.

24. Summers J, Cheng HY, Lin HH, Barnard LT, Kvalsvig A, Wilson N, et al. Potential lessons from the Taiwan and New Zealand health responses to the COVID-19 pandemic [Internet]. Lancet Reg Health West Pac. 2020 Nov;4:100044. https://doi.org/10.1016/j.lanwpc.2020.100044 PMID:34013216.

25. The Lancet. COVID-19 in the USA: a question of time [Internet]. Lancet. 2020 Apr;395(10232):1229. https://doi.org/10.1016/S0140-6736(20)30863-1 PMID:32305080.

26. Ruiu ML. Mismanagement of COVID-19: lessons learned from Italy [Internet]. J Risk Res. 2020 May;23(7–8):1007–20. https://doi.org/10.1080/13669877.2020.1758755.

27. Borowicz J, Zhang Z, Day G, Pinto da Costa M. Vaccine equity in COVID-19: a meta-narrative review [Internet]. BMJ Glob Health. 2022 Dec;7(12):e009876. https://doi.org/10.1136/bmjgh-2022-009876 PMID:36524409.

28. Feinmann J. The BMJ Appeal 2022-23: how safe burial helped end the 2022 Ebola epidemic [Internet]. BMJ. 2023 Jan;380:92. https://doi.org/10.1136/bmj.p92 PMID:36653034.

29. Giubilini DrA. The Ethics of Vaccination [Internet]. 1st ed. Brooks T, editor. The Ethics of Vaccination. Durham: Palgrave Pivot; 2019 [cited 2024 Mar 20]. https://www.ncbi.nlm.nih.gov/books/NBK538383/.

30. Albrecht SS, Aronowitz SV, Buttenheim AM, Coles S, Dowd JB, Hale L, et al. Lessons learned from dear pandemic, a social media–based science communication project targeting the COVID-19 infodemic [Internet]. Public Health Rep. 2022;137(3):449–56. https://doi.org/10.1177/00333549221076544 PMID:35238241.

31. Fairchild AL, Bayer R, Green SH, Colgrove J, Kilgore E, Sweeney M, et al. The two faces of fear: a history of hard-hitting public health campaigns against tobacco and AIDS [Internet]. Am J Public Health. 2018 Sep;108(9):1180–6. https://doi.org/10.2105/AJPH.2018.304516 PMID:30088996.

32. Edwards SJ, Silaigwana B, Asogun D, Mugwagwa J, Ntoumi F, Ansumana R, et al. An ethics of anthropology-informed community engagement with COVID-19 clinical trials in Africa [Internet]. Dev World Bioeth. 2023 Sep;23(3):242–51. https://doi.org/10.1111/dewb.12767 PMID:35944158.

33. Keusch GT, McAdam K, Cuff PA, Mancher M, Busta ER. Integrating clinical research into epidemic response: the Ebola experience. Integrating Clinical Research into Epidemic Response: The Ebola Experience. National Academies Press; 2017 Apr. https://doi.org/10.17226/24739.

34. Edwards S, Gordon C, Reeves M, Pitts P. How many eggs in one basket? Reconciling early or expanded access to and clinical trials of new medicines for COVID-19. Journal of Philosophy and Medicine. Under review 2024.

35. Whitty C, Smith G, Atherton F, McBride M, Vallance P, Harries J, et al. Technical report on the COVID-19 pandemic in the UK - GOV.UK [Internet]. London; 2023 Jan [cited 2024 Jun 4]. https://www.gov.uk/government/publications/technical-report-on-the-covid-19-pandemic-in-the-uk.

36. World Health Organization, International Labour Organization. Occupational health and safety in public health emergencies: a manual for protecting health workers and responders. Geneva; 2018 May.

37. De Kock JH, Latham HA, Leslie SJ, Grindle M, Munoz SA, Ellis L, et al. A rapid review of the impact of COVID-19 on the mental health of healthcare workers: implications for supporting psychological well-being [Internet]. BMC Public Health. 2021 Jan;21(1):104. https://doi.org/10.1186/s12889-020-10070-3 PMID:33422039.

38. Maneze D, Salamonson Y, Grollman M, Montayre J, Ramjan L. Mandatory COVID-19 vaccination for healthcare workers: a discussion paper. Int J Nurs Stud. 2023 Feb;138:104389. https://doi.org/10.1016/j.ijnurstu.2022.104389 PMID:36462385.

39. Suwalowska H, Amara F, Roberts N, Kingori P. Ethical and sociocultural challenges in managing dead bodies during epidemics and natural disasters [Internet]. BMJ Glob Health. 2021 Nov;6(11):6345. https://doi.org/10.1136/bmjgh-2021-006345 PMID:34740913.

40. World Health Organization. WHO/Europe publishes considerations for gradual easing of COVID-19 measures. 2020 Apr 24 [cited 2024 Mar 20]; https://www.who.int/europe/news/item/24-04-2020-who-europe-publishes-considerations-for-gradual-easing-of-covid-19-measures.

41. House of Commons Health and Social Care Committee, House of Commons Science and Technology Committee. Coronavirus: lessons learned to date [Internet]. London; 2021 Sep [cited 2024 Mar 19]. www.parliament.uk/hsccom.

42. Betthäuser BA, Bach-Mortensen AM, Engzell P. A systematic review and meta-analysis of the evidence on learning during the COVID-19 pandemic. Nat Hum Behav. 2023 Mar;7(3):375-385. https://doi.org/10.1038/s41562-022-01506-4. PMID:36717609.

43. Ambe JR, Kombe FK. Context and ethical challenges during the Ebola outbreak in West Africa. Socio-cultural dimensions of emerging infectious diseases in Africa [Internet]. 2019 Jan 1 [cited 2024 Jun 4];191. https://doi.org/10.1007/978-3-030-17474-3_14.

CHAPTER 6

TEAMWORK AND DECISION-MAKING

by Nikita Devnarain and Salim S. Abdool Karim

Action, panic, blame, and denial are common stress-driven responses in the face of any calamity, including a pandemic. When attempting concerted action as a response, doctors, nurses, scientists, politicians, and the myriad of others involved will work most effectively if they see a common purpose in coordinated action. This requires leadership to build a common vision, feasible approach, and concerted plan that can be followed by all those involved. These elements create the foundation for effective teamwork in any organisation, particularly in a pandemic response where urgency is of the essence. A key characteristic of a team is that the individual members contribute different strengths which achieve synergy when combined. Working together to realise a common objective is a requirement of effective teams, where members of a team are committed and support each other to achieve shared goals. Teamwork, whether at a family, organisation, or even country level, is a key element in preparing to navigate through a pandemic with the most effective response.

INTRODUCTION
In the face of a public health emergency such as a pandemic, there is an urgent need for national and subnational leadership, as well as both discipline-specific and multidisciplinary teams to adapt to effectively respond to imminent challenges. We need to mobilise a national health incident management system at all levels so that resources are effectively and systematically used, with the government, private sector, and non-governmental organisations acting in unison. This teamwork essential to a rapid and effective response requires that members of the team possess relevant skillsets to update their leadership and enable well-informed decisions and implementation. This chapter will describe common features of effective teams in a public health crisis. It will consider how decisions should be made and how subsequent strategies should be implemented and monitored.

QUALITIES OF EFFECTIVE TEAMS
During crises characterised by uncertainty, executives and leaders of organisations and countries need to establish teams to collect information needed to rapidly make decisions to guide the implementation of an effective response. Leaders need to empower others and form a network of teams that have a common objective to promote problem-solving and to determine and implement solutions. This approach—incident management response—has a long history in emergency response (1).

Team	Description
Incident Management Team (IMT)	Responsible for the overall management of the response to an emergency. This team is typically composed of individuals with expertise in emergency management, public health, and other relevant areas.
Clinical Response Team	Responsible for providing medical care and support to individuals affected by the emergency. The team may include physicians, nurses, and other healthcare professionals.
Public Health Team	Responsible for investigating, collecting, and analysing information, and controlling infectious disease spread, as well as implementing measures to promote public health and safety. The team may include epidemiologists, veterinarians, environmental health specialists, and health educators, among others.
Communication Team	Responsible for managing communication and information dissemination to stakeholders, the media, and the public. This team may include public relations specialists, social media experts, and crisis communication professionals.
Logistics Team	Responsible for managing the resources and supplies needed for the emergency response, including transportation, equipment, and medical supplies.
Psychosocial Support Team	Responsible for providing psychological and emotional support to individuals affected by the emergency. The team may include counsellors, social workers, and other mental health professionals.
Research and Innovation Team	Responsible for defining research priorities, mobilising research funding, and coordinating research activities.

Table 6.1: Types of teams formed in a health emergency

Other teams might be required, such as those devoted to research and innovation, ethics, or health system concerns. The goal is to create a network of effective teams comprising flexible, coordinated groups, working together, united by a common vision and displaying the qualities set out below. The most effective response teams in a pandemic are (2–3):

- often **multidisciplinary**, to better engage with experts from different fields and to address the needs of a large and highly complex outbreak response – case management, epidemiology, laboratory, risk communication, social mobilisation, and infection prevention and control specialists. This feature will be especially required of teams that take leadership or coordinate emergency responses.
- **trained** and equipped with individuals with technical expertise and experience.
- **built for purpose** – able to collect information, solve problems, and implement strategies and continuously improve them, as opposed to focusing on process issues or simply seeking the advice of experts.
- **adequately sized** – effective span of control requires that the number of subordinates managed by supervisors or managers in a team must be limited.

- **adaptable and mobile** with ready-to-deploy team members who can fill critically needed roles as circumstances change and new knowledge becomes available about the pandemic.
- **transparent and willing to collaborate** – sharing information without hesitation as appropriate.
- **coordinated** – activities must support the common objective and be coordinated with relevant stakeholders.

As much as teams in a pandemic require the support of each member to function optimally, they also require leadership to facilitate effective functioning. When a new team is formed in an outbreak response, leaders need to ensure reporting lines, time frames, mechanisms and protocols of communication, clarity of tasks and objectives, format of products, expectations, and the right mix of expertise. Teams need to be adequately resourced.

OWNERSHIP AND DECISION-MAKING IN A TEAM

Decision-making processes during a pandemic may vary over time. Early decision-making during a pandemic, where urgency is required, will tend more towards command-and-control, as opposed to a more open-ended approach. Once a pandemic or outbreak is established, decision-making will often tend to be more dispersed and negotiated between parties, rather than decided by central authorities (ideally after adequate consultation) (4).

If a process is shaped by collective decision-making, those affected by the outcomes tend to take greater ownership of final decisions. They have been given opportunities to voice their views and actively participate in determining solutions. In such cases, the group typically engages in negotiations and deliberations over potential strategies. The course of action that emerges as the most preferred or most dominant is then adopted. While this approach fosters consensus, it is time-consuming and may have limitations when urgent decision-making is required (5). It should be noted that even where decisions are made via command-and-control structures, they can still be consultative to a degree, and their execution still requires compliance with administrative rules and hierarchical protocols governing the healthcare system, even during a pandemic response (4).

The command-and-control approach has even more limitations when the healthcare system is in a poor state, for example, from structural underfinancing. In such cases, top-down decisions will have little prospect of being implemented unless they reflect the situation of those at the frontline. The situation may get worse when government authorities have questionable legitimacy. In these circumstances, healthcare workers (HCWs) and institutions can sometimes be torn between instructions from the health system leadership and the realities confronting the users of the health system (4).

Leaders empowered with authority to make decisions during crises will need to understand how to balance top-down speed with the benefits and necessities of consultative decision-making. Neither of these approaches alone is sufficient. Generally, and whenever possible, erring on the side of more consultation, ownership, and involvement in the process is the safer option, although it does slow down decisions (6).

Leaders often need to find a middle ground specific to the management of a pandemic. New and ad hoc high-level structures may be required of governments. These structures might be, inter alia, ministerial committees, intersectoral committees, and committees of differing disciplines. Without such innovative structures, leaders and policymakers may lack sufficient means of coordinating and translating intellectual exercises into policy. These structures may be grouped into four general categories (7):

i)   ad hoc arrangements
ii) existing structures adapted to the crises
iii) temporary structures provided for by crisis management plans, policies, or laws on national security
iv) a hybrid approach, combining two or three of the aforementioned mechanisms

> **Coronavirus Command Council in South Africa**
>
> In responding to the COVID-19 threat in South Africa, the government created a new temporary decision-making body that brought together the relevant ministers of government to make rapid decisions for the pandemic response. Since the Cabinet processes are slow and somewhat rigid for decision-making, a Coronavirus Command Council was created by the President with high levels of flexibility to ensure swift decision-making. Meetings occurred at short notice, chaired by the country's President, and presentations were often sought from the committee of scientists advising the government and from various government departments so that the best available evidence was made available for decision-making.

Government participation in the pandemic response team

In a pandemic situation, especially when the threat is not fully understood, response decisions are often initially focused purely on health outcomes. To achieve a sustained, high-level response that is effective during the longer run of a pandemic, a wider consideration of stakeholders is needed. Non-health players may need a pandemic response structure with their own teams and they should be represented on coordinating teams mindful of turf-protectors and petty politics (8). This can be a significant challenge when individuals in established leadership positions are not familiar with pandemic preparedness and responses and do not create space for experts in outbreaks to provide leadership. To try to deal with this, whole-of-government responses need to be implemented. This sentiment was echoed during the COVID-19 pandemic on 9 April 2020 by the Director-General of the World Health Organization (WHO), Dr Tedros Adhanom Ghebreyesus, when he stated, "this pandemic is much more than a health crisis. It requires a whole-of-government and whole-of-society response" (9).

In most countries, the central government takes the lead on policymaking and budgetary allocation, and state/provincial governments have to implement the measures on the ground. To do this effectively, states/provinces may have to set up their own coordination structures, as well as monitoring and evaluation teams, as the activities and players will likely differ between states/provinces.

Public health agencies within ministries of health often have a leading role in the whole-of-government approach (7,10). In other countries, where a stronger statement is needed, governments may create special programmes, sometimes under the direct guidance of heads of government, to emphasise the whole-of-government approach. If done well, such institutions provide for better coordination and a structured mechanism for multiple parts of government to become involved (social development, treasury, education department, border control, transportation, police, etc.). However, decisions made in each of these areas will always need to be coordinated across sectors. For example, in decisions involving school closures, input from the department of education can be sought. The department of transport should also be party to the decision-making so that school buses are made available when schools open. This approach ensures that the relevant departments are directly involved in decision-making. Whole-of-government national health response structures should ideally exist in a preparedness phase—through planning, exercises, and regular engagement.

An overarching national pandemic coordinator may need to be appointed, with the directive to steer whole-of-government coordination response, as well as preparedness (8). Furthermore, this approach allows for timely sharing of information to improve decision-making processes for coordinated action and ensures transparency across all government departments or ministries (11).

There are two important insights that power the whole-of-government approach. The first is that healthcare and public health require more actors than health departments and health service delivery organisations. The second is the acknowledgement that the social determinants of health are important, especially the multidisciplinary challenges fundamental to the social determinants of health needs. These two insights can assist in better understanding what it takes to prevail over the separateness and disjointed functioning of departments and processes, to enhance policy effectiveness and coherence (11).

MOST EFFECTIVE PANDEMIC RESPONSE TEAMS USE AN EVIDENCE-BASED DECISION-MAKING CYCLE

Evidence-based decision-making is the gold standard to be used by leaders during health emergencies (12). The national public health agency generates scientific evidence which is used by whole-of-government interministerial structures for decision-making. The various departments of government and the private sector then need to implement these decisions. As decisions are implemented, they need to be monitored so their effectiveness can be captured and fed into the next set of evidence-based decisions (**Figure 6.1**).

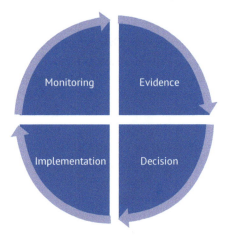

Figure 6.1: The continuous process of evidence-based decision-making

Evidence

In a public health setting, operational decision-making processes need to run efficiently for routine functionality. When operational decisions uninformed by scientific evidence are made during a crisis, the resulting policies may lead to inappropriate and ineffective actions (13–14).

Decision-making by public health agencies for policies, approaches, and interventions needs to be guided by sound scientific evidence or experience, which should be publicly available to the greatest extent possible. Sharing of evidence needs to be free of hesitancy and should include information on effectiveness and risks, as well as distribution of health benefits and burdens for different groups. Transparency and openness are important principles in a pandemic, even when there is urgency in the situation (15).

The evidence required for decision-making includes information needed for the characterisation of populations that are particularly high risk (e.g., children for measles, men who have sex with men for mpox) as well as:
- size of the at-risk population using estimations of population size
- prevalence of the infectious disease among at-risk populations
- geographic distribution of the at-risk population using mapping exercises
- risk behaviours, characteristics, and health concerns among at-risk populations using demographic, behavioural, and general health surveys
- needs of the at-risk population, significant structural factors, and challenges to be faced during response implementation, using behavioural surveys, assessments of existing legislation, policy, and practice, and discussion with members of the community and organisations headed by the community
- possible interventions – their coverage, accessibility, quality, outcome, and impact need to be assessed using administrative information, infectious disease notification registries, and integrated bio-behavioural surveys

It is noteworthy that under certain circumstances, mapping at-risk populations can inadvertently jeopardise members of these communities, that is by recognising these populations and their locations and making them vulnerable to stigma. It is imperative that evidence, and the process of gathering evidence by public health agencies, serves to protect rather than endanger the lives and privacy of at-risk populations. The process of gathering information should follow ethical guidelines. Another significant aspect of evidence collection is to assess the quality, accuracy, and potential sources of bias when analysing and interpreting data (15).

Decision

Once the relevant evidence has been collected, it is disseminated across other government departments, with an assessment of its strengths and weaknesses. Such structured information to inform policy decisions will be part of a vast flow of information (and requests for information) that comes with a public health crisis. After deliberation and negotiation with the various governmental departments and leaders, the evidence should be used by interministerial structures for decision-making on how to respond to the pandemic most effectively. Ideally, the decision-making process should take into account ethics and principles of fairness and equity, involvement of stakeholders, efficiency, and sustainability (15), but bringing all these dimensions into decision-making may be difficult in a crisis.

Implementation

Governmental departments, public sector agencies, healthcare providers, professionals, community organisations, civil society, and sometimes, the private sector, usually combine to implement the decisions as they are made or changed. Some of the decisions that need to be made by these committees when preparing to implement a national response to a pandemic involve the following:

- target the response – identify the populations that are most at risk and the guidelines, policies, and legislations that need conceptualisation or revision
- identify and prioritise interventions – where they need to be implemented, to what extent should services be dispersed and integrated for optimal service coverage, timeframe and scale-up potential, the extent of integration of services to sufficiently cover key populations, appropriate means of service delivery, and the roles of stakeholders
- resources – establish the implementation costs and the costs of procrastination; identify infrastructure and human, financial, and other resources needed, means of acquiring resources, types of healthcare required, HCWs needed, and means of recruitment and training
- risks, outcomes, and impacts – identify potential risks and susceptibilities of the response, strategies to relieve the impact of potential risks, such as domestic factors (e.g., reduction in budget, theft, HCW attrition, development of drug resistance) and external factors (e.g., natural disasters, loss of funding, political instability)
- monitor and evaluate – identify means by which an intervention can be monitored and evaluated, and how to reinforce strategic information systems to collect the information needed

Monitoring

After crisis decisions are implemented, intervention outcomes need to be monitored. This is to enable the healthcare and structural components of the response to be assessed, particularly in at-risk populations, and preferably in close to real time. The monitoring systems need to be practical and user-friendly to be able to gather information that is accurate and current. Frameworks need to be established to recommend the right national-level indicators. These factors are related to the enabling environment, determine the availability, coverage, and characteristics of specific interventions, assess the outcome and impact of the interventions, and can be used to capture progress for funders. This process requires information from several sources, such as the surveys used during the initial evidence-gathering process. This information also needs to be assessed for its quality and limitations during analysis and interpretation (15). Again, keeping the focus on policy evaluation will be difficult when circumstances are rapidly changing and new information has to be assimilated.

Monitoring the emergence of new SARS-CoV-2 variants in South Africa

When the WHO announced that the new variant EG.5 had been classified as a variant of interest and given the name Eris, three separate monitoring mechanisms were activated to assess whether it had started spreading in South Africa. First, SARS-CoV-2 polymerase chain reaction (PCR)-

positive nasopharyngeal swabs collected for diagnostic purposes in symptomatic patients as part of passive surveillance were monitored through genetic sequencing to identify the presence of Eris. Second, nasopharyngeal swabs collected through sentinel surveillance programmes were tested for SARS-CoV-2 and positive samples were submitted for genetic sequencing. Third, environmental surveillance of wastewater included genetic sequencing to determine whether Eris was present in various communities across the country. The information from these three sources of monitoring/surveillance was provided to decision-making authorities on a regular basis following the WHO announcement to enable proactive planning and prevention activities.

CONCLUSION

During a public health emergency, leadership at national and subnational levels needs to adapt to produce an effective response. New teams may be created to inform decision-making and to implement and monitor interventions at different stages of the pandemic. Responses should be able to adapt from a command-and-control approach to a more inclusive consensus-building approach as the health emergency recedes, ideally including greater civil society representation. As fatigue sets in and the costs of response measures mount, the added buy-in that comes from consultative decision-making will be more salient. Decisions need to be monitored once implemented. Effective pandemic response teams work in synergy, have shared goals and an inclusive approach to decision-making, and utilise the evidence-based cycle to guide their actions.

REFERENCES:

1. World Health Organization. Classification and minimum standards for emergency medical teams. 2021. https://www.who.int/publications/i/item/9789240029330.
2. D'Auria G, De Smet A. Leadership in a crisis: responding to the coronavirus outbreak and future challenges. Psychology (Irvine). 2020;22(2):273–87.
3. Stehling-Ariza T, Lefevre A, Calles D, Djawe K, Garfield R, Gerber M, et al. Establishment of CDC global rapid response team to ensure global health security. Emerg Infect Dis. 2017 Dec;23(13 Suppl 1):S203–9. https://doi.org/10.3201/eid2313.170711 PMID:29155672.
4. World Health Organization. The world health report 2006: working together for health. World Health Organization; 2006. https://www.who.int/publications/i/item/9241563176.
5. Hughes T, Adams L, Obijiaku C, Smith G. Democracy in a pandemic: participation in response to crisis. University of Westminster Press; 2021.
6. Greer SL, Jarman H, Rozenblum S, Wismar M. Who's in charge and why? Centralisation within and between governments. Eurohealth (Lond). 2020;26(2):99–103.
7. Co-operation OfE. Development. Building resilience to the Covid-19 pandemic: the role of centres of government. OECD Publishing; 2020.
8. Haldane V, Jung A-S, Neill R, Singh S, Wu S, Jamieson M, et al. From response to transformation: how countries can strengthen national pandemic preparedness and response systems. BMJ. 2021;375:e067507. https://doi.org/10.1136/bmj-2021-067507 PMID: 34840139.
9. World Health Organization. WHO Director-General's opening remarks at the Mission briefing on COVID-19 - 9 April 2020. https://www.who.int/director-general/speeches/detail/who-director-general-s-opening-remarks-at-the-mission-briefing-on-covid-19---9-april-2020.
10. World Health Organization. Pandemic influenza preparedness and response: a WHO guidance document. World Health Organization; 2009. https://www.who.int/publications/i/item/9789241547680.

11. Ortenzi F, Marten R, Valentine NB, Kwamie A, Rasanathan K. Whole of government and whole of society approaches: call for further research to improve population health and health equity. BMJ Glob Health. 2022 Jul;7(7):e009972. https://doi.org/10.1136/bmjgh-2022-009972 PMID: 35906017.

12. Baekkeskov E. Explaining science-led policy-making: pandemic deaths, epistemic deliberation and ideational trajectories. Policy Sci. 2016;49(4):395–419. https://doi.org/10.1007/s11077-016-9264-y.

13. Rubin O, Errett NA, Upshur R, Baekkeskov E. The challenges facing evidence-based decision making in the initial response to COVID-19. Scand J Public Health. 2021 Nov;49(7):790–6. https://doi.org/10.1177/1403494821997227 PMID:33685289.

14. Amrami K, Domnick R, Heinzen E, Helfinstine K, Jayakumar A, Johnson P, et al., editors. Deployment of an interdisciplinary predictive analytics task force to inform hospital operational decision-making during the COVID-19 pandemic. Mayo Clinic Proceedings. Elsevier; 2021.

15. World Health Organization. Developing the response: the decision-making, planning and monitoring process. Consolidated guidelines on HIV prevention, diagnosis, treatment and care for key populations. Update. 2016.

CHAPTER 7

OPERATIONAL LOGISTICS SUPPORT AND SUPPLY CHAINS

by Matthew Y.S. Lai, Pierre Boulet-Desbareau, J.C. Azé, and Robert Blanchard

Supply chain management and health logistics are a long-neglected, under-represented, and underinvested aspect of public health policy and practice. Recent disease outbreaks exposed the vulnerability of the global supply chain to the emergence of a novel health threat. There is a dearth of resources available to introduce policymakers, emergency planners, and non-logisticians to the fundamental concepts of supply chain strategy.

The following chapter explains key aspects of logistics and supply chain management and provides a set of recommendations for policymakers and stakeholders. Public health logisticians are responsible for implementing the logistics measures necessary to develop and deploy emergency preparedness and response plans. They hold a unique body of knowledge but are generally under-recognised as a profession, despite the critical nature of strategies surrounding supply chain management and the effect of disease outbreaks on international supply chain dynamics. Key investments can make supply chains more robust in the future to greatly mitigate the financial and health ramifications of epidemics. It is paramount that logisticians are integrated into decision-making authorities in crisis situations alongside other key leaders as a core pillar of outbreak response.

INTRODUCTION

The COVID-19 pandemic exposed the vulnerability of highly interdependent global health commodity supply chains to the emergence of a novel health threat. The unprecedented demand for health commodities such as personal protective equipment (PPE), biomedical supplies, and laboratory diagnostic equipment outstripped available stockpiles and the capacity to source them in sufficient quantities. Manufacturing limitations stemming from staff shortages, the inability to source raw materials, lockdowns, border closures, and protectionism led to dwindling inventories that exacerbated the disruption.

The economic burden of the COVID-19 pandemic is estimated to be US$ 16–35 trillion (1) and the World Economic Forum estimates that epidemics in the coming decades will cause an average economic loss of 0.7 per cent of global gross domestic product (GDP) (2). Investing a fraction of the economic cost of pandemics into more resilient systems to mount and sustain public health responses would save innumerable lives and significantly reduce global financial losses (3).

The need for emergency responses has only grown. In 2022, the number of people in need of humanitarian assistance worldwide was estimated at over 323 million (1 in 29 people). This represented a dramatic increase from 1 in 33 in 2020 and 1 in 45 in 2019 (4).

In the wake of the COVID-19 pandemic, there were numerous outbreaks of cholera, dengue, Ebola, measles, mpox, and yellow fever (5). Numerous factors including climate change, armed conflict, demographics, and socioeconomic issues provide new opportunities for pathogens to emerge and proliferate into disease outbreaks, underscoring the vital role of surveillance and detection activities (**See Chapter 2, What causes outbreaks?**). Infrastructure built to address long-term endemic infectious diseases can be co-opted and adapted for these emerging threats (6).

Given that the annual probability of extreme epidemics occurring could increase threefold in the coming decades (6), public health supply chains and logistics are of paramount importance to prevent, prepare, detect, and respond to health emergencies.

PROFESSIONALISATION OF PUBLIC HEALTH LOGISTICIANS

Preparedness can be defined as the "knowledge, capacities, and organisational systems developed by governments, response and recovery organisations, communities, and individuals to effectively anticipate, respond to, and recover from the impacts of likely, imminent, emerging, or current emergencies" (7).

The council of Supply Chain Management Professionals defines logistics as "that part of supply chain management that plans, implements, and controls the efficient, effective forward and reverse flow and storage of goods, services, and related information between the point of origin and the point of consumption in order to meet customers' requirements".

Tasks within the supply chain are often not considered as requiring a professional role or specialised training; this leads to inefficiencies (8). Public health logisticians play a critical yet often overlooked role in turning health emergency plans into real, actionable services. They assess a myriad of interconnected variables that will determine the successful implementation of an emergency response. For example, calculating the weight, volume, and temperature requirements of health commodities determines the type of storage facilities needed and transportation required to move commodities through the supply chain. Determining lead times from suppliers or warehouses to health facilities or final distribution points establishes realistic timeframes for emergency responses. Advanced planning by public health logisticians ensures minimal transportation disruptions and allows the development of alternatives to overcome supply constraints or long lead times in the delivery of supplies to the masses in times of public health emergencies of international concern (PHEIC). Public health logisticians are also crucial in disseminating technical skills to others, allowing the scaling up of human resources required to sustain a response to a prolonged crisis.

At present, the explicit mention of supply chain management and logistics is absent in the Association of Schools of Public Health in the European Region's list of core competencies for the public health professional (9). Professionalisation encourages commitment to ethical behaviour and allows advice to be provided in the public interest from a professional body that organisations can trust. It promotes access to information, advice, publications, and other resources that would be otherwise difficult to obtain (10).

Going forward, the importance of public health logisticians needs to be recognised and logistics prioritised as a core capability (11). A central "control tower" of logistics officers with a clear hierarchy and chain of authority would strengthen the coordination of a response in an emergency.

A core group of logistics staff with knowledge and prior experience should be strategically placed within national health supply chain systems and maintained during routine times. Operationally they would:
- understand a given geography's need for medical supplies (including vaccines) and plan for sourcing, transportation, storage, stockpiling, inventory management, and distribution (including last-mile delivery)
- draw upon the work of surveillance networks to forecast demand for medical supplies
- develop scenarios and appropriate medical surge plans
- have procurement knowledge and techniques, and monitor market competitiveness to initiate the search for supplementary or substitute suppliers
- manage relationships with suppliers and other interested stakeholders
- plan and prepare for a scale-up of logistics response from the initial stages to the resolution of a public health emergency
- conduct a risk assessment to identify potential disruptions
- develop various scenarios to anticipate the different levels of demand fluctuation and supply chain disturbance that may occur locally, nationally, or globally

Establishing training pathways through tertiary education centres can equip public health professionals with an understanding of the role of logistics in health emergencies. It is important that all staff have been adequately trained in simulations or have prior experience in emergency responses. Once trained, regular revision seminars and drills should be carried out to ensure the maintenance of skills and continuing education (e.g., having one or two days every year dedicated to emergency training) (**See Chapter 37, Stakeholder training**).

Real-time training of logistics partners during the 2014–2015 Ebola epidemic in West Africa

In 2015, during the Ebola epidemic in West Africa, the transport of samples from the collection site to the first mobile or central laboratory by road was difficult. Logistics operators from the World Health Organization (WHO) thus used several aircraft to transport staff and materials. However, pilots of the aircraft were extremely reluctant to transport poorly packaged boxes or bags with blood samples, especially if requests came on an ad hoc basis.

The WHO organised a series of briefings, in collaboration with partners such as the World Food Programme (WFP) and independent non-governmental organisations (NGOs), where public health experts explained the disease, its transmission, and the risks involved in transport, as well as ensured the use of the International Air Transport Association (IATA)-compliant triple packaging during transport, and trained logistics staff to handle such samples. This drastically reduced the number of samples refused by air crews. It is important to be mindful that the pilot has the right to refuse the transport of pathogens even if properly packaged and compliant with standard operating procedures. In epidemics, fear and a lack of understanding can prevent various parties from participating fully. The briefing and training of non-medical actors on the biological and medical aspects of disease outbreaks, in collaboration with logistics and supply chain colleagues, would allow everyone to operate at their best.

THE EMERGENCY PREPAREDNESS AND RESPONSE PLAN (EPREP)

Public health logistics planning is often minimal, last minute, and done only when demanded by national authorities. The COVID-19 pandemic hit while many procurement entities were implementing professionalisation measures after widespread international endorsement of the 2015 Sendai Framework for Disaster Risk Reduction (12–13).

Efficient emergency responses require plans tailored to the specific characteristics of the operating environment at a national, subnational, and local level, taking a One Health approach that considers the impact of human, animal, and environmental factors in disease preparedness and response (14–15) **(See Chapter 13, One Health)**. The multisectoral approach strengthens the interface between health systems, other government sectors, the private sector, NGOs, and community organisations (16). The logistics solution must be adapted to ever-changing circumstances and responsive to new technological, scientific, and administrative innovations. In an emergency, identification of the main health threats and needed commodities is crucial, as is clarifying governance of the emergency supply chain (16).

When developing these plans, the threshold at which an exceptional situation or local outbreak becomes a public health emergency must be defined; this would clarify the entry point of intervention by governments.

These considerations form part of an emergency preparedness and response plan (EPREP). The EPREP should be regularly reviewed and adjusted according to new information, changing circumstances, and budget. It is crucial to include explicit and concrete allocations of financial and human resources, and the requisite legislative and political mechanisms to provide these resources. As policy changes require both time and political capital to be implemented, planning must begin well in advance of an emergency. The following are required to optimise the establishment and operations of an EPREP:

- All EPREPs should be built and reviewed through a sequential framework that is established either in the aftermath of a major health emergency response or in anticipation of future health threats. The framework should be informed by post-crises health risk analyses and epidemiological surveillance programmes. Each scenario should be assigned its own EPREP which will include an analysis of logistics and supply chain issues, gaps, needs, and likely barriers.
- Response scenarios for the initial stage of each emergency response should be defined. This includes population size, expected minimum coverage given the population size, duration (usually 2–3 months), and emergency health facilities and teams that need to be deployed to meet the desired level of coverage.
- A resource mobilisation plan for the rapid deployment of human resources needs to be established. This includes logistics rosters and staff training, assets including strategic stockpiles, framework agreements for asset use, public supplier markets, and financial resources which encompass a preparedness budget and a three-month deployment budget. A well-defined plan maximises operational readiness and a prompt response can contain a localised outbreak.
- A scaling plan detailing the development, training, and equipping of a health emergency workforce. The plan must allow the maintenance of routine health services and the non-emergency supply chain even in the presence of an emergency **(See Chapter 23, Essential services)**.

- A risk reduction plan to augment the resilience of a nation's health system before and during an exceptional public health event. The plan should emphasise prevention measures to avoid hazards and reduce vulnerability.
- Centralised oversight and coordination of the entire healthcare supply chain to ensure coordinated allocation of healthcare supplies to the emergency response and routine health services.

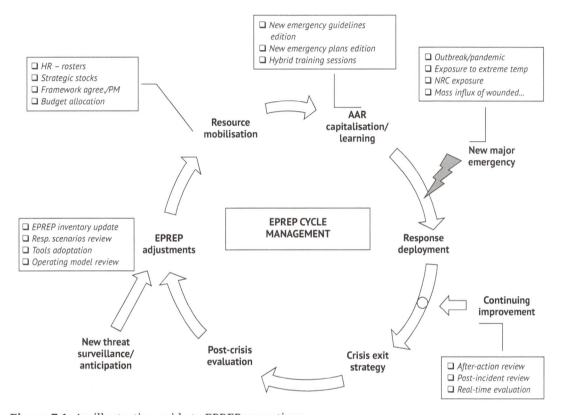

Figure 7.1: An illustrative guide to EPREP operations

EPREP: a review of a decade of planning for the unexpected

Crises over the past decade have raised the following key questions for public health logisticians to answer:
- What budget should be allocated in response to future infectious disease outbreaks?
- What hospital facilities would need to be mobilised to treat the wounded from future industrial disasters (e.g., Beirut in 2020) or multisite mass killings (e.g., Paris in 2015)?
- What should be pre-negotiated with competent authorities to ensure the respect and protection of healthcare facilities, patients, and healthcare workers who operate close to the frontlines (e.g., Ukraine in 2022), in besieged areas (e.g., Syria in 2013), or at the heart of an armed conflict (e.g., Sudan in 2023)?

The answers to these questions form an integral part of the risk analysis and deployment scenarios considered by governments and humanitarian agencies when forming their EPREPs. However, crises over the past decade have revealed persistent gaps between plans and the effectiveness of the emergency responses carried out.

During the 2014 Ebola epidemic in West Africa, treatment centres were forced to turn patients away due to the lack of available beds. The president of the International Committee of the Red Cross (ICRC) regretted that "aid is arriving on the ground too slowly, in insufficient quantities, and is not effective enough." Undersizing of strategic stocks from most countries in the European Union (EU) led to a protracted shortage of medical equipment during the COVID-19 pandemic. However, lessons were not learned and two years later, major shortages of mpox vaccines forced vulnerable groups to travel abroad to be vaccinated outside of their home countries.

Despite the exponential cost of running emergency responses to major disasters, with international humanitarian assistance funding increasing by 27 per cent to US$ 46.9 billion in 2022 (17), some governments and institutional donors remain reluctant when it comes to funding strategic stocks to cope with foreseeable threats.

An inadequate EPREP scope necessitates the costly mobilisation of last-resort logistical resources to compensate for the protracted shortages of strategic items including emergency purchases in saturated supplier markets and organising large-scale airlifts during emergency repatriations. Senior managers would benefit greatly from recognising the need for public health expertise before a public health emergency, or these resources will be exhausted trying to respond to and correct events that could have been avoided through careful planning.

EPREP budget considerations

During a public health emergency response, challenges include the assessment of financial needs and timely reallocation of resources which require transparent tracking and reporting of expenditure (18). It is good practice to structure EPREP budgets with two separate allotments of funds for emergency responses (19).

Preparedness fund	Dedicated emergency financial envelope
Covers the expenses of maintaining and updating the EPREP, storage of emergency supplies, inventory management, emergency staff payroll, and routine preparedness training.	Comprises an allotted increase to the preparedness budget anticipating several potential interventions during the year. This budget must take into account demand forecasts of essential commodities, transportation costs, cold chain capabilities, and the extra staff required to man the supply chain. The budgets should be updated frequently based on the ongoing forecasting and surveillance data.

At the national level, the Ministry of Finance should establish a public financial management system to minimise funding delays at the beginning of an emergency. The system should account for the delays required to vote for a new budget, including to respond to a major health crisis.

Most countries would have access to one or more contingency appropriations, emergency spending provisions, expenditure reprioritisation through reallocations and virements, supplementary budgets, and external grants. If national-level funding proves difficult, low-income countries can establish written contracts with international bodies, such as the World Bank or WHO contingency fund, for emergency response funds. Coordination between national and subnational levels of government would help ensure effective allocation and distribution of funding.

Ensuring the continuity of routine health services

Traditional health EPREPs in high-income countries are commonly emergency interventions that maximise the incremental capacity of hospital emergency responses. However, it is challenging to simultaneously provide the requisite numbers of staff and equipment to non-acute and primary care, testing centres, laboratories, pharmacies, and elderly care homes. Centralised coordination of emergency and routine healthcare supply chains minimises the cannibalisation of resources and disruption to service delivery.

SUPPLY CHAIN STRATEGY

The supply chain encompasses the processes and personnel involved in delivering a product or service to an end-consumer and includes demand forecasting, emergency stockpiles, cold chain systems, and last-mile planning.

The most impactful areas of supply chain investment will differ between countries and between regions within countries. While all geographies can benefit from investment in large infrastructure projects and pre-positioning of emergency supplies, economically developed countries derive comparatively greater benefit from improving personnel training and organisational capacity (19).

Demand forecasting

Predicting demand for medical goods is a function of the public health response to a pandemic (20); it is key to maintaining an adequate emergency stockpile of essential health commodities and minimising supply chain disruption. PPE and existing emergency medical goods can be rationed in accordance with fluctuating levels of hospitalisation rates and transmission rates.

It is difficult to forecast demand for emergent threats or those lacking historical data to model growth rate, behaviour, and pattern of spread. Behavioural and operational phenomena such as "phantom demand" or "panic buying" (21), and the "bullwhip" effect, where small fluctuations in consumer demand cause large disturbances in supplier stock levels and manufacturing rates (22), complicate forecasting attempts.

> **The bullwhip effect during the 2023 cholera outbreaks**
>
> The bullwhip effect describes how forecasting inaccuracies at local levels can be magnified further along the supply chain, in an analogy to the mechanics of cracking a whip. For example, a retailer overbuying stock for a particular item may send a signal that is greatly magnified when read by a distributor, who will respond by requesting even greater stock from manufacturers.

In response to the increased demand for health supplies driven by the 2023 cholera outbreaks, the WHO conducted a forecast to assess the average monthly consumption based on contemporaneous demands. The initial analysis indicated that significantly greater quantities of cholera kits were needed for pre-positioning than were required and that they had to be procured immediately. This bullwhip effect is a distortion of actual demand caused by increased signals from the point of origin of a request. Supply chain managers reviewed the initial data and identified a number of potential variables that were not considered, such as supplier ability to ramp up or increase production lines, the procurement of individual items versus entire kits, and the geographic proximity to locally available products. Once these elements were accounted for, the projected demand for the pre-positioned cholera supplies was significantly less than what was originally predicted. Decreased demand allowed suppliers to fulfil the orders directly rather than through third parties, which reduced the lead time for delivery.

Ultimately, the decision was made to procure smaller quantities to avoid disrupting the global supply chain with artificial demand and focus on filling gaps in response to the evolving demands of the outbreak. Monitoring both upstream production and downstream demands can provide key insights into the dynamics of the supply chain that can help organisations avoid the bullwhip effect and make more precise calculations with regard to the quantities of supplies needed to be held as buffer stocks.

The number of supply chain datasets grows with the increasing number of supply chain organisations with their own stockpiles. Supply chain datasets have become more complex as more data fields are added to document information, such as stock condition and date of purchase. The lack of standardised formatting for data entry has historically made it difficult for data engineers and analysts to combine datasets, thus limiting forecasting accuracy. As such, we recommend that logisticians work with relevant stakeholders to continuously identify and standardise useful datasets to enhance forecasting capabilities (23).

Predicting supply needs

While real-time and precise forecasting is difficult, there are several tools available to assist in the estimation of quantities of key commodities that will be necessary to support care delivery in the event of a public health emergency in limited contexts. The following are two interesting tools developed and used by the Operations Support and Logistics (OSL) arm of the WHO during the recent COVID-19 pandemic:

Essential Items Estimator Tool

(https://partnersplatform.who.int/essentialitemsestimator)
The primary objective of this tool is to facilitate the estimation of essential items required for the preparation and response to distinct health emergencies. This estimation is derived from user inputs, including the number of beds, average duration of hospitalisation, and the quantity of

healthcare facilities needing support. The tool employs a calculated ratio of item per patient or item per facility, grounded in empirical data accrued from past emergency responses.

WHO COVID-19 Essential Supplies Forecasting Tool (COVID-ESFT) v4.1
(https://www.who.int/publications/i/item/WHO-2019-nCoV-Tools-Essential_forecasting-2022.1)
The ESFT assists governments, partners, and other stakeholders to forecast the necessary volume of PPE, diagnostic equipment, consumable medical supplies, biomedical equipment for case management, and essential drugs for the supportive care and treatment of COVID-19. The tool provides the user with a choice among several epidemiological methods for forecasting COVID-19 cases, including an integration with the Susceptible-Exposed-Infectious-Removed (SEIR) model from Imperial College.

These tools are freely accessible and available on the WHO "partners" platform. They are merely examples of available tools; other tools probably exist through operational and governmental actors around the world. UNICEF's Emergency Supplies Calculator helps countries identify quantities required and costs during an epidemic based on several demographic factors, such as population at risk. General tools, however, will not be able to forecast the variation in demand across the regions and stages of a crisis. In addition, tools can become out of date or be rendered obsolete by improved models. Thus, it is best practice to work with experienced partners with significant modelling experience (16).

Emergency stockpiles

The national emergency stockpile has been traditionally conceived of as a capacitor. It acts as a buffer to unforeseen surges in demand for critical commodities in times of crisis. However, the maintenance of emergency stockpiles is costly and wasteful as large quantities of products expire before they can be used. For example, an audit of the Australian National Medical Stockpile found that across a decade, A$ 250 million worth of goods had expired, generating additional disposal costs of A$ 75 million (24). This creates a clear dilemma for policy- and decision-makers. However, mitigating efforts exist, and four of these are presented here (25).

Improving local production and surge capacity

One of the first proposed solutions to supply chain issues in the pandemic was to nationalise as much of the supply chain as possible, minimising dependence on the global supply chain. However, supply chains cannot be drastically altered within a short time period (26). Efforts to scale up local production were hampered by poor quality assurance. Reliance on external supply chains left some countries without adequate capacity to mass produce products such as PPE (27).

Some have suggested holding a minimum local stock of raw materials in anticipation of the need to mitigate dependence on the global supply chain (27). However, maintaining this inventory is expensive and the raw materials used in the production of medical supplies could change over time. In addition, the relative cost of manufacturing goods in certain countries is prohibitively expensive compared to outsourcing. For example, 80 per cent of antibiotics in the U.S. market are produced in China (28).

Furthermore, relying on private industry as the suppliers of an emergency stockpile and providers of surge capacity comes with a risk. Private entities may exploit loopholes and calculative techniques that allow them to meet regulatory requirements without having the genuine capacity to scale up production or meet quotas on time in health emergencies.

Outsourcing elements of stockpiling to the community and civilians
Some elements of stockpiling could be outsourced to civilians and the community under governmental guidance. However, this puts the financial and spatial burden on private citizens who will also require training to maintain such stockpiles.

A change in outlook
It is difficult to run a lean minimal system without wastage when prioritising the goal of maximising lives saved. Compromises in economic efficiency are acceptable to some degree in this situation.

Strategies to minimise wastage
One strategy integrates the emergency stockpile with routine procurement mechanisms for health supplies. The emergency stockpile would be the first-line supplier to fulfil part or all of procurement demand. This triggers a flow-on effect of "constant turnover" where products are routinely restocked and distributed while maintaining sufficient inventory buffers.

Centralising health supply procurement would promote better stock rotation at a national level. Centralised oversight encourages an all-hazards, holistic approach to emergency planning that considers a diverse range of supplies required in a health emergency and prevents duplicate purchases. Joint procurement agreements amongst large organisations allow the redistribution of surplus stockpiles, further reducing wastage.

Shelf-life extension programmes (SLEPs) are a major boon for waste reduction. Batches of medicines and PPEs nearing expiration are sent to quality standards agencies for stability and quality testing after which the batch expiry date is relabelled depending on conservative estimates for the remaining useful life of the item. In the U.S., it is estimated that every US$ 1 spent on SLEP testing saved US$ 22 in replacement costs (29).

Cold chain systems

The cold chain is a system of storing and transporting commodities at recommended temperatures from the point of manufacture to the point of use. Maintenance of the cold chain is complex throughout the distribution chain and often forms a bottleneck in delivering mass vaccination campaigns as vaccines are temperature sensitive.

Significant technological advances in cold chain solutions enable the delivery of supplies within the required temperature range. Passive cold chain systems that use phase change materials, such as water or ice to maintain temperatures, are often the least expensive but require expertise in packaging and are monitored using temperature loggers. Building a core capacity of expert staff will ensure the safe and effective distribution of cold chain products, which is vital to the success of a public health response.

Last-mile planning

Last-mile transportation describes the final part of a shipment's journey from a transportation hub to the end user. Calculation of the time and resources needed to move the product from each point in the distribution chain is required to ensure the proper delivery of supplies. Real-time distribution data enables visibility when tracking and allows for the adjustment for delays at delivery sites.

Locally available human resources and infrastructure knowledge can increase efficiency in distribution activities. Partnering with local communities strengthens the flexibility of the supply chain which increases the likelihood of success.

> **Logistics support considerations during the 2022 floods in Pakistan**
>
> Several emergency operations were established to coordinate the delivery of humanitarian aid and restore basic services in response to severe flooding in Pakistan. United Nations (UN) organisations and NGOs struggled to coordinate their initial response as the scale of the emergency escalated. As logistics professionals arrived in Pakistan, they quickly established a network of key contacts to identify what supplies were being prepared for delivery by which organisations. As the network grew, organisations could establish what items they would be best positioned to provide (e.g., the WHO focused on essential medicines).
>
> The logistics team prepared a comprehensive overview of the items and quantities on-hand, in-transit (being shipped), and in the pipeline (under production), with lead times for delivery. This information and distribution data was collated to be shared by the WHO with implementing partners, UN agencies, and NGOs. This data was vital in coordinating with warehousing and freight forwarding entities to ensure that the space and equipment were available for the smooth delivery of vital resources.
>
> The logistics support required to successfully run an emergency response is often overlooked and underestimated, leading to catastrophic supply chain failures.

INTERNATIONAL COOPERATION

There are several global frameworks for emergency preparedness, including the International Health Regulations (IHR 2005), the Sendai Framework for Disaster Risk Reduction 2015–2030, the Pandemic Influenza Preparedness (PIP) Framework, the Global Health Security Agenda (GHSA), and Universal Health Coverage (UHC) 2030 (30).

> **Fierce international competition**
>
> The IHR and the International Coordinating Group (ICG) on vaccine provision heavily regulate aspects of the vaccine supply chain but there is no such regulation for other key items in infectious disease emergencies. Furthermore, despite these regulations advocating for the equitable distribution of vaccines and emphasising the avoidance of unjustified orders and non-pertinent

> allocation, the procurement and sourcing of essential commodities in emergency contexts are complicated by "me first" ordering dynamics that have created a systemic burden on production lines. This phenomenon is not limited to the COVID-19 pandemic, as illustrated by the lack of Baxter Lactated Ringers IV solutions during the initial phase of the 2010–2011 cholera outbreak in Haiti or PPE for the 2014 Ebola outbreak in Western Africa. This competition also extends to the transport of goods as observed in the aftermath of the 2004 Indian Ocean Tsunami, where there was fierce competition and bidding wars amongst various responder groups including governments, donors, and humanitarian organisations.

Self-interested government policy at a national level influences the success of procurement and sourcing strategies for the international community. In the initial stages of the COVID-19 pandemic, government supply chain policy skewed towards nationalism and protectionism to secure stockpiles of health commodities. Governments imposed export controls on medical goods, expanded domestic production, and diversified suppliers to mitigate the risk of a perceived overdependence on major global manufacturing centres such as China (20). These measures were somewhat successful as exemplified by Scotland where pre-COVID-19, 100 per cent of National Services Scotland's PPE was sourced from overseas compared to 2021 where nearly half was manufactured in Scotland (31).

However, such responses at a national level could also negatively impact public health over the medium to long term (20). For instance:
- they ameliorate the issue of excessive demand surges
- supply security strategies do not usually translate uniformly at a national level
- diversification of suppliers can interfere with the prompt restoration of operations should disruption occur
- financial subsidies can blunt the incentives for private sector providers of medical goods to reduce costs and innovate

Abandoning established global supply chains in favour of local production could result in the disappearance of the former if they lose business, leaving behind less capable suppliers that may be less effective in future emergencies (27). Reducing, rather than eliminating, the risk of supply chain disruption is the most practical procurement and sourcing policy objective. Policy should target system-wide risk considering the contribution of supplies from abroad.

A cooperative approach to procurement would yield system-wide benefits and minimise global supply chain disruptions. Open sharing of the contents of essential stockpiles with contingent joint-purchasing and swap arrangements would allow efficient redistribution of supplies from areas of excess to areas of need.

There have been some optimistic examples of international cooperation in the EU. The Health Emergency Preparedness and Response Authority (HERA) established a centralised system for vaccine procurement during the recent pandemic that allows for more equitable vaccine distribution amongst the 36 participating countries (32).

IMPROVED INFORMATION – WORKING TOWARD A VISIBLE AND TRANSPARENT SUPPLY CHAIN

Most, if not all, countries during the COVID-19 pandemic had imperfect information regarding available supplies and demand. Governments should invest in the following to ensure real-time visibility of the supply chain:
- electronic management systems for automatic stock updates
- radio-frequency identification (RFID) technology for real-time supply chain monitoring
- standardised barcode and data-entry formats for easy identification of items
- reliable communications systems that allow the flow of information between private and public stakeholders

Improved communication technology would facilitate the timely coordination of emergency responses. In the U.S. COVID-19 response, it was difficult for the strategic national stockpile group, who manages the supply chain, to liaise with those who manage the clinical and emergency issues at the U.S. Centers for Disease Control and Prevention (U.S. CDC), Federal Emergency Management Agency (FEMA), and the U.S. Department of Health and Human Services (HHS) (26).

In the future, blockchain technologies could be exploited to support logistics in an emergency. A distributed ledger system allows for complete transparency across the supply chain, preventing tampering and corruption (33).

CONCLUSIONS AND FUTURE DIRECTIONS

Supply chain management and health logistics have been a long-neglected and under-represented aspect of public health policy. Proper investment in preparedness can mitigate the financial costs and disease burden of epidemics. While no supply chain strategy is perfect, understanding the strengths and weaknesses of each strategy allows timely adjustments in response to new information.

Greater analysis of cross-border supply chain dynamics and more robust demand forecasting and management strategies will be important in improving supply chain management for health services. Modelling and optimisation research represents the future of logistics; logisticians who understand the models and translate them into action will be vital in improving supply chain management in emergency contexts. In crisis situations, logisticians must be a part of the decision-making authorities alongside all other key stakeholders and leaders at local, national, and international levels. Collaborative, contingent, international agreements could greatly contribute to preparedness for the next pandemic and mitigate the economic and health disruption witnessed in infectious disease emergencies.

REFERENCES:

1. Charumilind S, Craven M, Lamb J, Sabow A, Singhal S, Wilson M. When will the COVID-19 pandemic end? Experts explain. World Econ Forum [Internet]. 2021;(January). https://www.weforum.org/agenda/2021/09/mckinsey-experts-offer-their-latest-analysis-on-when-covid-19-will-end/.
2. World Economic Forum. Outbreak readiness and business impact protecting lives and livelihoods across the global economy. 2019;(January):1–22. http://www3.weforum.org/docs/WEFHGHI_Outbreak_Readiness_Business_Impact.pdf%0Ahttps://www.weforum.org/whitepapers/outbreak-readiness-and-business-impact-protecting-lives-and-livelihoods-across-the-global-economy.
3. International Monetary Fund. The economics of health and well-being. Financ Dev A Q Publ Int Monet Fund. 2021;58(4).

4. Global Humanitarian Overview 2022:2021.
5. World Health Organization. Dis Outbreak News. 2022.
6. Baker RE, Mahmud AS, Miller IF, Rajeev M, Rasambainarivo F, Rice BL, et al. Infectious disease in an era of global change. Nat Rev Microbiol. 2022 Apr;20(4):193–205. https://doi.org/10.1038/s41579-021-00639-z PMID:34646006.
7. WHO. Framework for a public health emergency operations centre. WHO Libr Cat Data [Internet]. 2015;(July 27). https://www.who.int/publications/i/item/framework-for-a-public-health-emergency-operations-centre.
8. Brown AN, Prosser W, Zwinkels D. Who is preparing the next generation of immunization supply chain professionals? [Internet]. Vaccine. 2017 Apr;35(17):2229–32. https://doi.org/10.1016/j.vaccine.2016.12.076 PMID:28364936.
9. ASPHER. ASPHER's European list of core competences for the public health professional. Scand J Public Health. 2018 Nov;46(23_suppl):1–52. https://doi.org/10.1177/1403494818797072 PMID: 30421646.
10. Mokoena SK. Professionalising supply chain management as an alternative mechanism to curb corruption in the South African public institutions. 3rd Annu Int Conf Public Adm Dev Altern 04 - 06 July 2018, Stellenbosch Univ Saldahna Bay, South Africa. 2018;(July):457–68.
11. Silve B. Health logistics is a profession: improving the performance of health in developing countries". Field Actions Science Reports [Online [Internet]. 2008;1 |. http://journals.openedition.org/factsreports/109.
12. Eßig M, von Deimling CH, Glas A. Challenges in public procurement before, during, and after the COVID-19 crisis: selected theses on a competency-based approach. Eur J Public Procure Mark. 2021;1(3):65–80. https://doi.org/10.54611/PGEK9560.
13. Sendai Framework for Disaster Risk Reduction 2015-2030. UN World Conference on Disaster Risk Reduction, 2015 March 14-18, Sendai, Japan. Geneva: United Nations Office for Disaster Risk Reduction; 2015.
14. World Health Organization. Ending the neglect to attain the Sustainable Development Goals. One Health: approach for action against neglected tropical diseases 2021-2030. 2022;1–30. http://apps.who.int/bookorders.
15. The World Bank. One Health - Operational Framework. 2018. http://documents.worldbank.org/curated/en/703711517234402168/pdf/123023-REVISED-PUBLIC-World-Bank-One-Health-Framework-2018.pdf.
16. USAID. Technical Report: best practices in supply chain preparedness for public health emergencies. 2019. https://www.ghsupplychain.org/best-practices-supply-chain-preparedness-public-health-emergencies.
17. Global Humanitarian Assistance. Global Humanitarian Assistance Report 2023 [Internet]. GHA Annual Report. 2023. 1–132 p. https://devinit.org/resources/global-humanitarian-assistance-report-2023/executive-summary/.
18. Stone M. Special series on fiscal policies to respond to COVID-19 preparing public financial management systems for emergency response challenges 1. Int Monet Fund; 2020. pp. 1–6.
19. UNICEF. WFP. UNICEF/WFP Return on Investment for Emergency Preparedness Study. 2015;(January):34. http://www.unicef.org/publications/index_81164.html.
20. Evenett SJ. Trade policy and medical supplies during COVID-19. Ideas for avoiding shortages and ensuring continuity of trade. Glob Econ Financ Program [Internet]. 2021;(June). file:///Users/Andrea/Downloads/2021-04-08-trade-policy-medical-supplies-covid-19-evenettpublishedversion.pdf
21. Okeagu CN, Reed DS, Sun L, Colontonio MM, Rezayev A, Ghaffar YA, et al. Principles of supply chain management in the time of crisis [Internet]. Best Pract Res Clin Anaesthesiol. 2021 Oct;35(3):369–76. https://doi.org/10.1016/j.bpa.2020.11.007 PMID:34511225.
22. Lee HL, Padmanabhan V, Whang S. Information distortion in a supply chain: the bullwhip effect. Manage Sci. 1997;43(4):546–58. https://doi.org/10.1287/mnsc.43.4.546.
23. Seyedan M, Mafakheri F. Predictive big data analytics for supply chain demand forecasting: methods, applications, and research opportunities [Internet]. J Big Data. 2020;7(1):53. https://doi.org/10.1186/s40537-020-00329-2.
24. Laing S, Westervelt E. Canada's National Emergency Stockpile System: time for a new long-term strategy. CMAJ. 2020 Jul;192(28):E810–1. https://doi.org/10.1503/cmaj.200946 PMID:32586836.
25. Folkers A. Freezing time, preparing for the future: the stockpile as a temporal matter of security. Secur Dialogue. 2019;50(6):493–511. https://doi.org/10.1177/0967010619868385.
26. Handfield R, Finkenstadt DJ, Schneller ES, Godfrey AB, Guinto P. A commons for a supply chain in the Post-COVID-19 era: the case for a reformed strategic national stockpile. Milbank Q. 2020 Dec;98(4):1058–90. https://doi.org/10.1111/1468-0009.12485 PMID:33135814.

27. Feinmann J. PPE: what now for the global supply chain? [Internet]. BMJ. 2020 May;369(May):m1910. https://doi.org/10.1136/bmj.m1910 PMID:32414747.

28. Piatek OI, Ning JC, Touchette DR. National drug shortages worsen during COVID-19 crisis: proposal for a comprehensive model to monitor and address critical drug shortages. Am J Health Syst Pharm. 2020 Oct;77(21):1778–85. https://doi.org/10.1093/ajhp/zxaa228 PMID:32716030.

29. Rizvi A, Gera M, Thind A. Eyes on the Supplies: Improving Canada's National Emergency Stockpile System (NESS). Western Public Health Casebook 2021. London: Public Health Casebook Publishing; 2022.

30. World Health Organization. Operational framework for deployment of the World Health Organization smallpox vaccine emergency stockpile in response to a smallpox event [Internet]. 2017. https://apps.who.int/iris/bitstream/handle/10665/259574/9789241513418-eng.pdf.

31. Feinmann J. What happened to our national emergency stockpiles? BMJ. 2020 May;2021(375):2020–2. https://doi.org/10.1136/bmj.n2849 PMID:34848399.

32. European Commission. Health Union: commission signs Joint Procurement contract with HIPRA for COVID-19 vaccines [Press Release]. 2022.

33. Chang SE, Chen Y. When blockchain meets supply chain: a systematic literature review on current development and potential applications. IEEE Access. 2020;8:62478–94. https://doi.org/10.1109/ACCESS.2020.2983601.

CHAPTER 8

BORDER CONTROLS AND PUBLIC HEALTH EMERGENCIES OF INTERNATIONAL CONCERN

by Vivianne Ihekweazu, Sarin K.C., and David L. Heymann

The international spread of infectious diseases and the measures taken to control and prevent their transmission across borders has driven disease control efforts, starting from the implementation of quarantine during the 14th century plague by the city-state of Venice. The subsequent international agreements that evolved, from the International Sanitary Regulations (ISR) in 1951 to the current International Health Regulations (IHR) of 2005, were in a bid to control the spread of infectious diseases. The revision of the IHR in 2005 introduced a new approach and focused on detecting and stopping disease outbreaks at their source and maintaining open borders, along with developing core public health capacities to effectively respond to public health events. Communication plays a very important role during public health emergencies, empowering populations and disseminating information, and the declaration of public health emergencies of international concern (PHEICs) and the unique communication challenges associated with each instance provides important lessons. Various measures are often put in place to control the spread of infectious diseases. The COVID-19 pandemic witnessed the closure of borders and varying requirements by countries that led to confusion about international travel, highlighting the need for coordinated international efforts and consistent communication to minimise confusion and ensure the safety of international travel and trade.

INTRODUCTION

Historically, national borders have been the focus for protection against the spread of infectious disease. Though certain measures at borders, such as vector control, have remained key to protection, there has been a gradual understanding that controls at borders alone are not sufficient to protect against the international spread of infectious diseases. In fact, though they offer a quick solution for political leaders, border control measures are often misused or misadvised, and result in false assurance that protection measures are in place. Understanding of the most effective means of preventing the international spread of infectious diseases has evolved slowly since the 14th century as outlined below.

International spread of infectious diseases

Concern about the risk of the spread of infectious disease from one country to another has been described since the beginning of written history. This concern was clearly demonstrated in the 14th century when the city-state of Venice required trading ships to anchor in port for a period of 40 days before crews could come ashore, in an attempt to keep plague from entering the city, an action that became known as quarantine. By the 19th century, when industrialisation, colonisation, and empire-building were in full swing and trade and commerce led to large-scale social changes and population movements, concern about the increased risk of spread of infectious diseases from one country to another increased in political importance. This led the governments of major European countries and the U.S. to seek agreement on standardised measures to attempt to control the spread of infectious diseases across international borders. A series of negotiations through formal International Sanitary Conferences followed suit.

Despite shared interests in controlling the international spread of disease, negotiations proved prolonged and difficult. For example, France proposed the first international meeting to negotiate a way forward in 1834 amid the world's second known cholera pandemic, but governments did not meet until the middle of the third pandemic in 1851. It would take another 40 years before these governments would reach an agreement and adopt the first International Sanitary Convention in 1892, in part due to evolving scientific understanding about infectious disease causation. The main delays in negotiation, however, came from concerns to minimise disruption to international travel and trade. As Maglen describes, "economic and political agendas impeded negotiations that should have been focused on reaching international consensus on disease control (1)."

INTERNATIONAL SANITARY REGULATIONS

A series of conventions followed in which countries where disease was occurring agreed to notify other countries of their occurrence. By 1951, the World Health Assembly, the plenary body of the newly established World Health Organization (WHO), had consolidated the patchwork of conventions into the International Sanitary Regulations (ISR). The ISR focused on six then notifiable diseases—cholera, plague, relapsing fever, smallpox, typhoid, and yellow fever. Under the ISR, countries were required to report by telegram to the WHO when one of these diseases was identified. The WHO, in turn, provided this information to all its Member States so that if persons arrived at international borders, they could be placed under surveillance and quarantined if they developed signs and symptoms (2). At the same time, countries were required to take measures to minimise the risk of vector proliferation at airports, land borders, and seaports.

INTERNATIONAL HEALTH REGULATIONS 1969

The ISR were revised in 1969 with a decreased focus to four infectious diseases, and were given their current name, the International Health Regulations (IHR). The aim of the IHR 1969 was to provide maximum security against the international spread of disease with minimum interference in travel and trade. In addition to a requirement to maintain measures at airports, land crossings, and seaports to prevent the proliferation of vectors such as insects and rodents, countries were required to report to the WHO when one of four diseases—cholera, smallpox, plague, and yellow fever—occurred within their territories, with the WHO keeping Member

States informed through the WHO Weekly Epidemiologic Report (WER). If other countries noted the report, they were able, under the IHR, to take maximum pre-described measures at their borders in an effort to keep the infection out. When, for example, yellow fever was reported by a member country to the WHO, other countries could apply pre-described measures which included a requirement of a yellow fever vaccination for passengers arriving from the reporting country.

By 1996, it had been clearly demonstrated that there was widespread non-compliance with the IHR, and countries were not immediately reporting when outbreaks occurred, or failing to report at all, because of potential economic consequences. Cholera outbreaks in Peru and Chile (3) and plague in India (4) are notable examples when reporting countries suffered severe economic loss because of protective trade embargoes and decreased tourism.

India reports an infectious disease outbreak – Damned if you do, damned if you don't

In 1994, the western Indian city of Surat was struck with a plague (5). It was declared an international public health emergency by Indian government officials. This was in compliance with the IHR which listed cholera as a notifiable disease of concern, as it posed a health threat and had to be stopped before it became an epidemic. The outbreak led to panic, with residents fearing the city would be quarantined, and it led to residents fleeing to neighbouring cities. Health facilities were on high alert, other major cities were impacted, schools and public entertainment areas were closed as a precaution, and people stayed indoors.

The United Arab Emirates (UAE) stopped cargo shipments of agricultural products coming from India. The share value of agricultural products fell in the local stock exchange and thousands of trips to India were cancelled, with many countries placing trade restrictions on India. Travellers from India to the U.S. and Rome faced plague-related travel restrictions and they had to complete separate forms and undergo additional checks on arrival. The country suffered a significant economic toll; however, the disease was quickly suppressed and prevented from spreading.

In addition, the high media profile of a major Ebola outbreak in 1995, and the silent international spread of HIV during the preceding decade, demonstrated to political leaders that other diseases were also a concern in an increasingly globalised world (6). As a result, a resolution was passed by the World Health Assembly in May 1996 requesting that the WHO Secretariat begin negotiations on a revision of the IHR 1969 (7).

INTERNATIONAL HEALTH REGULATIONS 2005

Negotiations to revise the IHR 1969 languished until after the severe acute respiratory syndrome (SARS) outbreak in 2003. The spread of SARS to over 28 countries worldwide helped political leaders understand the need to step up negotiations for revision of the IHR 1969. Negotiations were intensified during late 2003 and 2004, and the revision focused on broader disease coverage and the importance of detecting and stopping disease outbreaks when and where they occurred, thus preventing or minimising their national and international spread.

This was in contrast to attempting to stop their spread at international borders, as was the basis of the IHR 1969.

The IHR 2005 bears limited resemblance to the IHR 1969 and earlier conventions. The requirement of countries to report to the WHO continues in the IHR 2005 but was broadened to the reporting of any disease with the potential to spread internationally, as discerned by using a standardised decision tree analysis that permits countries to identify and report to the WHO a disease that is a potential PHEIC. The Director-General of the WHO then decides whether this disease is a true PHEIC by consulting with expert groups, including an emergency committee (EC) set up under the IHR 2005 framework. If the EC recommends that the disease occurrence is a PHEIC, it also provides temporary recommendations, based on its risk assessment, that would meet the aim of the IHR 2005 to prevent the international spread with minimum interruption in travel and trade. The Director-General then decides, based on the recommendations of the EC and other advisory bodies which have been consulted, whether to declare a PHEIC.

A new element in the IHR 2005, and perhaps the most important, is the requirement of countries to develop and maintain core public health capacities for surveillance, response, and communication (**Figure 8.1**) (8). This is an attempt to ensure that all countries have the infrastructure, human resources, and procedures in place to ensure the identification, risk assessment, and response to public health events that will prevent them from national and international spread that leads them to becoming a PHEIC. As such, the PHEIC becomes a safety net that provides recommendations to limit international spread by temporary recommendations on international travel and trade, and a call for international collaboration.

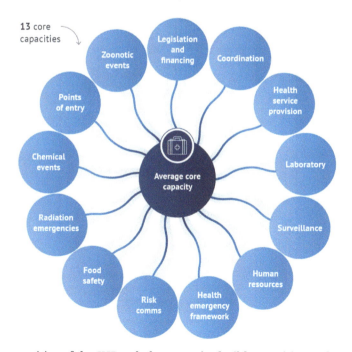

Figure 8.1: Core capacities of the IHR to help countries build capacities to detect, assess, and report public health events
(adapted from "The Triple Billion targets: a visual summary of methods to deliver impact", WHO)

COMMUNICATION DURING A PANDEMIC

In the event of a PHEIC, health communication plays an important role in ensuring that information is shared at local, national, regional, and global levels to influence the appropriate public health actions (9). Creating and sustaining a reliable means to communicate to large populations using communication methods that reach various audiences is an important part of preparedness for health emergencies and is a part of the public health core capacity requirement under the IHR 2005. Information is shared with a view to empower populations to make informed choices and take preventative measures, and often serves as a warning of potential danger of infectious disease outbreaks. It is also critical in soliciting compliance to control measures.

PHEICs are only declared by the Director-General of the WHO when an event is considered "an extraordinary event, determined to constitute a public health risk to other states through the international spread of diseases and to potentially require a coordinated international response (10)." Given the relatively high threshold, PHEICs have been declared only seven times since the IHR 2005 came into place (11). As described above, a PHEIC can only be declared after extensive consultation with the EC that is made up of a group of carefully selected international experts who provide advice to the Director-General of the WHO before a decision is taken (**Figure 8.2**). The importance of the news of the outcome of the deliberations and decisions of a PHEIC has grown in relevance over the past few years, especially with the COVID-19 pandemic and the mpox epidemic. The WHO is increasingly leveraging different platforms to disseminate the news of the decisions taken to international governments and national public health institutes, but some of the means through which information flows are not within its control.

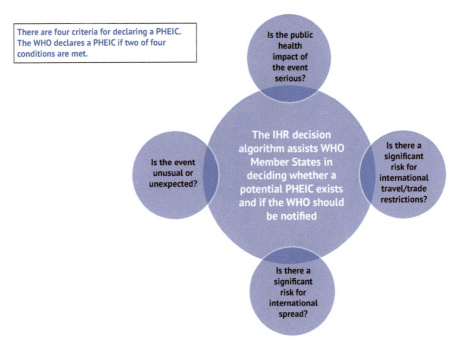

Figure 8.2: Criteria for declaring a PHEIC
(adapted from Wilder-Smith A, Osman S. Public health emergencies of international concern: a historic overview. Journal of Travel Medicine. 2020 Dec;27(8):taaa227)

Being able to accurately and effectively communicate with large populations enables the relevant public health officials to take action themselves, as well as inform populations of actions that they need to take to limit the spread of any pathogen with serious public health consequences. The urgency and gravity of declaring a PHEIC requires that consistent and accurate communication by the relevant health authorities keeps the public informed. Declaring a PHEIC also requires that preventative measures are put in place to mitigate any effects of an outbreak.

However, there are unique communication challenges that arise when a PHEIC is declared and there are important lessons that can be learnt from all seven PHEICs that have been declared to date. The first thing to remember is that the purpose of a PHEIC is not as an early warning mechanism as many people often assume. The purpose of a PHEIC declaration is to serve as a safety net to enable international coordination, streamline funding, accelerate the advancement of the development of countermeasures, catalyse timely evidence-based action, and limit the public health and societal impacts of emerging and re-emerging disease risks, while preventing unwarranted travel and trade restrictions (11).

The outbreak of the H1N1 influenza virus was the first incident declared a PHEIC in June 2009 following early reports of its spread in North America (11). The virus spread across the world at an unprecedented pace as international travel enabled the rapid transmission to different countries. By November 2009, over 6,250 deaths had been reported (12). The initial communication around the influenza pandemic caused fear as there were projections from academic epidemiological models that there would be a high number of deaths, given what was known of the impact of previous pandemics of novel influenza viruses. However, as the outbreak evolved, it became clear that while there would be widespread infection, the associated mortality was likely to be lower than anticipated. People stopped adhering to some of the public health and safety measures that had been put in place (13). Some people even accused the WHO of "shouting wolf" too early as stockpiles of vaccines and other medical countermeasures were left unused (14).

The second PHEIC was declared in 2014 following an outbreak of wild poliovirus (15). This proved to be challenging because wild poliovirus was not a new problem, given its continued existence in at least three countries. However, it was an important disease that had been earmarked for eradication. A large outbreak in West Africa threatened these efforts. The significant challenge on this occasion was how to communicate a PHEIC for an event that was not a new or acute disease. The communication challenge was related to how to heighten the sense of urgency for a disease that was well established, and to communicate that the urgency to act was only in specific places, and in a very specific way. However, for a vast majority of people around the world, there was nothing extra that they needed to do.

The third PHEIC was declared later in the same year, in 2014, for an Ebola outbreak in West Africa. This was in a part of the continent where the disease had not been widely seen before, and where there was no experience in mounting a response. The PHEIC was perceived by many to have been declared too late in the outbreak and so subsequent communication around the preventative measures came late. Against a backdrop of low community trust, resistance from communities due to established cultural practices, and poor health literacy, it was clear that alternative communication strategies were needed to enable active community engagement **(See Chapter 33, RCCE)**. Also, it appeared as if the rest of the world only took interest when sporadic cases appeared outside of Africa. This incident presented the challenge of communicating global risk when the outbreak itself was local.

The fourth PHEIC declaration was for Zika virus in February 2016. This presented unique challenges (16). It was difficult to put across the fact that the concerning public health outcome was not acute infection, but ensuing microcephaly in children. This was difficult to explain clearly, partly because the pathway of causation was not yet fully understood. The viral link to the particular outcome in pregnancy was difficult to establish given the non-specific nature of the infection and the long duration to the outcome. The way to communicate this to an already sceptical public complicated pathogenesis, against a backdrop of ongoing uncertainty. This was compounded by the lack of initial understanding of appropriate countermeasures.

The fifth PHEIC declared was for Ebola again, but this time in the Democratic Republic of the Congo (DRC). This outbreak was complicated by significant security challenges that limited access to traditional means of communication, and public health authorities, including the WHO, had to find ways of working with local communities, including those involved in the insecurity situation. Poor community cohesion and low public trust made public health messaging and dissemination very challenging. Communication in a hostile environment with security issues presents several challenges during a PHEIC, as channels of communication are limited and free access to key populations is impeded.

The sixth PHEIC declared was for the COVID-19 pandemic in 2020. Given the overwhelming nature of the pandemic and its impact globally, there has been much written about communication challenges at all levels and the response through the different phases of the outbreak in the different geographies affected. Possibly the biggest lesson to be learnt is that science communication is by definition evolving and that the evolution of public health response from precautionary to more evidence-based recommendations because of new scientific evidence is not "flip flopping" (17), but exactly how science works. The other lesson that has persisted throughout the pandemic is that populations are unwilling and sometimes unable to accept restrictions on their lives over prolonged periods of time.

The seventh and most recent PHEIC was for mpox in 2022. One unique communication challenge for this PHEIC was the primary focus on a specific population group that already feels stigmatised. Lessons learnt from HIV showed that stigmatisation has severe consequences on public health outcomes, so there was a need to develop a communication strategy that would involve information dissemination through trusted groups that most affected communities' trust.

Year	Event	Communication challenge	Border measures
2009	H1N1 influenza	Rapid spread of the virus and high predicted number of deaths. Given what is known about the novel influenza virus, mortality was lower than anticipated.	Border entry screening measures were put in place, but no border closures.
2014	Wild poliovirus	Challenge of communicating the threat of a virus that was not new or acute. There was a need to communicate a sense of urgency for the disease.	No border closures.

Year	Event	Communication challenge	Border measures
2014	Ebola virus disease	Communicating the virus against low community trust, resistance from communities due to established cultural practices, and poor health literacy.	Border controls and migration management around the world to control traffic to affected countries.
2016	Zika virus	Communication was challenged as microcephaly occurred through a pathway that was not fully understood.	No border closures.
2019	Ebola virus disease	Communication was in the midst of low public trust, poor community cohesion, and security challenges.	Rwanda closed its border with the DRC.
2020	COVID-19 pandemic	Communication was challenged by the rapid evolution of the virus and the provision of evidence-based recommendations, while dealing with the prolonged nature of the virus and maintaining public trust.	Border closures took place globally in countries that experienced COVID-19 virus transmission.
2022	Mpox	Communicating the threat of the virus that was primarily focused on a specific population.	No border closures.

Table 8.1: The declaration and communication of PHEICs and border measures

In summary, it is evident that each PHEIC presents unique communication challenges, and that there are important lessons to be learnt from each of them. Public health communication was previously an insignificant and neglected responsibility and was not often incorporated in any public health response. The most significant underlying factor through all the PHEICs declared, which is necessary for the success of public health responses, is the role that trust (18) plays in communication. Therefore, it is also essential to note how important communication is in building trust.

IHR 2005 AND THE FUTURE OF HEALTH SECURITY AND INTERNATIONAL TRAVEL AND TRADE

On 30 January 2020, after having previously convened seven days earlier and requesting more information for its risk assessment, the EC of the IHR had what it considered sufficient additional information to recommend to the Director-General of the WHO that the outbreak of COVID-19 should be classified as a PHEIC. Temporary recommendations that were made by the experts on the EC to the Director-General, after having reviewed all available information at this time, included a statement that the Committee did not recommend any travel or trade restrictions based on the information they had available, and emphasised infection prevention and control in healthcare settings and the protection of health workers.

At a following meeting of the EC on 30 April 2020, the EC recommended to the Director-General that because many countries had closed their international borders, essential travel needed for pandemic response, humanitarian relief, repatriation, and cargo operations should be enabled. They also recommended that the WHO update its recommendations on appropriate travel measures and analyse their effects on the international transmission of COVID-19, with a consideration of the balance between benefits and unintended consequences, including entry and exit screening, education of travellers on responsible travel behaviour, case finding, contact tracing, isolation, and quarantine.

By the time of the meeting of the EC on 31 July 2020, it had become clear that countries were not following the guidance of the Director-General regarding travel, and that there was great confusion about the safety of international travel. The EC recommended that the WHO work with partners to revise the WHO travel guidance in order to reinforce evidence-informed measures that would avoid unnecessary interference with international travel. The EC also recommended that WHO Member States proactively and regularly share information with the WHO on appropriate and proportionate travel measures and advise, based on risk assessments, to implement necessary measures, including at points of entry, in order to mitigate the potential risks of international transmission of COVID-19, and to facilitate international contact tracing.

Despite the temporary recommendations associated with the announcement of the PHEIC, over 1,000 international border closures occurred in nearly all countries in 2020 and 2021 in an attempt to decrease the importation of SARS-CoV-2 (19). Though research continues at the time of writing this chapter, most peer-reviewed reports to date suggest that closing international borders during late January and February 2020, the first two months when international spread is thought to have begun, slowed the international spread to Asian countries that had closed their borders (**Figure 8.4**). Conversely, in other parts of the world including Europe and North America, inaction allowed the infections to take hold and spread during those months, and later border closures did not appear to slow the spread of SARS-CoV-2 (20).

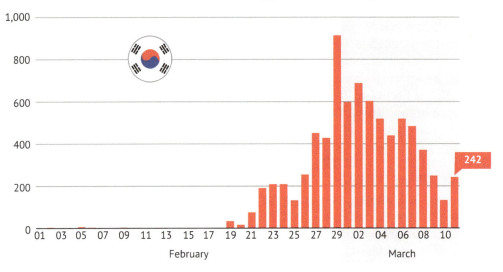

Figure 8.3: Reported COVID-19 cases in South Korea in February–March 2020
(adapted from the Korea Centers For Disease Control and Prevention)

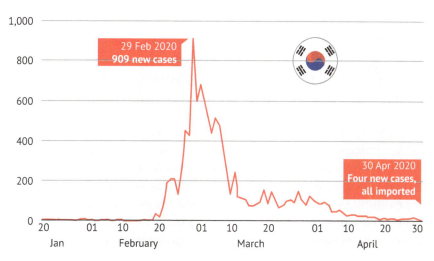

Figure 8.4: Reported COVID-19 cases in South Korea in January–April 2020
(adapted from the Korea Centers For Disease Control and Prevention)

As a result of uncoordinated and independent decisions of countries and subnational regions on border closures, and inconsistent requirements of international carriers and of countries for passengers who crossed their international borders, there was an interruption and great confusion regarding the safety of international travel and trade.

Border closures and COVID-19

The COVID-19 pandemic saw the implementation of lockdowns, border closures, and travel restrictions globally in a bid to slow down the transmission of the virus (21). In January 2020, the government of China imposed a lockdown in Wuhan, the city where the first case of COVID-19 was reported, in a bid to control the spread of the virus to other cities (22). Entry bans were then quickly imposed on Chinese visitors to other countries that were reporting cases of COVID-19. Border closures and travel bans then quickly expanded to include further countries that were experiencing a rapid spread of COVID-19. Lockdown and border closures were seen as extreme, though at the time, a necessary policy response to the spread of the virus (21). The border closures had varying impacts on countries. In high-income countries, governments provided economic support for families through rental assistance and unemployment compensation, and financial support for businesses through furlough schemes (23–24). However, in low-income countries where a large informal sector existed and many families survive on a daily wage, border closures disrupted trade and placed a significant financial burden on families (25).

It is hard to distinguish the longer term impact of border closures on the spread of COVID-19, as countries imposed different degrees of border shutdowns and these were in conjunction with other interventions, such as non-pharmaceutical interventions.

CONCLUSION

During the COVID-19 pandemic, many public health and political leaders sought simple and highly visible solutions to stop the international spread of infection in order to reassure populations that everything possible was being done for their protection. One of these measures was to close national borders, sometimes with the misunderstanding that by doing so they could prevent international spread. While such measures may have been reassuring to populations, they provide a false sense of security. This insight has been learned over centuries since efforts to stop disease at borders were first recorded in the 14th century.

The IHR 2005 encapsulate the current understanding that international borders cannot stop the international spread of disease, and so require countries to develop core capacities in public health that will detect and respond to disease outbreaks where and when they occur, thus saving lives and preventing national and international spread. The IHR 2005 also provide a safety net when countries have not stopped the spread of a disease outbreak. This includes the recommendations of a PHEIC and about international travel and trade. During the COVID-19 pandemic, several weaknesses in the IHR 2005 were recognised, and negotiations are currently underway to revise the Regulations. At the same time, a pandemic treaty is being negotiated by WHO member countries, the outcome of which will become clear in the coming years.

No matter to what actions the negotiations of these two political instruments lead, the IHR 2005 requirement for all countries to develop their public health core capacities to rapidly detect, respond to, and communicate about public health emergencies remains cardinal. Disease outbreaks must be detected and responded to rapidly to save lives, prevent or slow national and international spread, and decrease the negative impact of public health emergencies on people and economies, while minimising their impact on international travel and trade.

REFERENCES:

1. Maglen K. MSJAMA. Politics of quarantine in the 19th century. JAMA. 2003 Dec;290(21):2873–3. https://doi.org/10.1001/jama.290.21.2873 PMID:14657074.
2. Howard-Jones N. The scientific background of the International Sanitary Conferences, 1851-1938. 5. The ninth conference: Paris, 1894 [Internet]. WHO Chron. 1974 Oct;28(10):455–70. [cited 2023 Jul 4]. https://pubmed.ncbi.nlm.nih.gov/4607249/ PMID:4607249.
3. Ganesan D, Gupta SS, Legros D. Cholera surveillance and estimation of burden of cholera. Vaccine. 2019;(Jul):38. PMID:31326254.
4. Cash RA, Narasimhan V. Impediments to global surveillance of infectious diseases: consequences of open reporting in a global economy [Internet]. Bull World Health Organ. 2000;78(11):1358–67. https://www.ncbi.nlm.nih.gov/pmc/articles/PMC2560626 PMID:11143197.
5. The Surat plague and its aftermath - insects, disease, and history | Montana State University [Internet]. www.montana.edu. https://www.montana.edu/historybug/yersiniaessays/godshen.html.
6. Jones KE, Patel NG, Levy MA, Storeygard A, Balk D, Gittleman JL, et al. Global trends in emerging infectious diseases. Nature. 2008 Feb;451(7181):990–3. https://doi.org/10.1038/nature06536 PMID:18288193.
7. World Health Organization. Fifty-First World Health Assembly, Geneva, 11-16 May 1998: resolutions and decisions, annexes [Internet]. 1998. https://apps.who.int/iris/handle/10665/258896.
8. World Health Organization. International Health Regulations (2005) assessment tool for core capacity requirements at designated airports, ports and ground crossings [Internet]. 2009. https://apps.who.int/iris/bitstream/handle/10665/70839/WHO_HSE_IHR_LYO_2009.9_eng.pdf.
9. Regidor E, de la Fuente L, Gutiérrez-Fisac JL, de Mateo S, Pascual C, Sánchez-Payá J, et al. The role of the public health official in communicating public health information. Am J Public Health. 2007 Apr;97(Suppl 1 Suppl 1):S93–7. https://doi.org/10.2105/AJPH.2006.094623 PMID:17413063.

10. World Health Organization. Emergencies: international health regulations and emergency committees [Internet]. 2019. https://www.who.int/news-room/questions-and-answers/item/emergencies-international-health-regulations-and-emergency-committees.
11. Wilder-Smith A, Osman S. Public health emergencies of international concern: a historic overview. J Travel Med. 2020 Dec;27(8):taaa227. https://doi.org/10.1093/jtm/taaa227 PMID:33284964.
12. World Health Organization. Evolution of a pandemic 2nd edition [Internet]. 2009. https://apps.who.int/iris/bitstream/handle/10665/78414/9789241503051_eng.pdf.
13. Lin L, Savoia E, Agboola F, Viswanath K. What have we learned about communication inequalities during the H1N1 pandemic: a systematic review of the literature. BMC Public Health. 2014 May;14(1):484. https://www.ncbi.nlm.nih.gov/pmc/articles/PMC4048599/?report=classic https://doi.org/10.1186/1471-2458-14-484 PMID:24884634.
14. Watson R. WHO is accused of "crying wolf" over swine flu pandemic. BMJ. 2010 Apr;340 apr06 2:c1904. https://doi.org/10.1136/bmj.c1904 PMID:20371580.
15. World Health Organization. WHO statement on the second meeting of the International Health Regulations Emergency Committee concerning the international spread of wild poliovirus [Internet]. 2014. https://www.who.int/news/item/03-08-2014-who-statement-on-the-second-meeting-of-the-international-health-regulations-emergency-committee-concerning-the-international-spread-of-wild-poliovirus.
16. Heymann DL, Hodgson A, Sall AA, Freedman DO, Staples JE, Althabe F, et al. Zika virus and microcephaly: why is this situation a PHEIC?. Lancet. 2016 Feb;387(10020):719–21. https://www.ncbi.nlm.nih.gov/pmc/articles/PMC7134564/ https://doi.org/10.1016/S0140-6736(16)00320-2 PMID:26876373.
17. CBS News. Causing coronavirus confusion again, CDC flip-flops on guidance regarding COVID-19 spread [Internet]. 2020. https://www.cbsnews.com/sacramento/news/causing-coronavirus-confusion-again-cdc-flip-flops-on-guidance-regarding-covid-19-spread/.
18. Holroyd TA, Oloko OK, Salmon DA, Omer SB, Limaye RJ. Communicating recommendations in public health emergencies: the role of public health authorities. Health Secur. 2020;18(1):21–8. https://doi.org/10.1089/hs.2019.0073 PMID:32078416.
19. Shiraef MA, Friesen P, Feddern L, Weiss MA; COBAP Team. Did border closures slow SARS-CoV-2? Sci Rep. 2022 Feb 1;12(1):1709. https://doi.org/10.1038/s41598-022-05482-7. PMID: 35105912.
20. Hale T, Angrist N, Goldszmidt R, Kira B, Petherick A, Phillips T, et al. A global panel database of pandemic policies (Oxford COVID-19 Government Response Tracker). Nature Human Behaviour [Internet]. 2021 Mar 8;5:529–38. https://www.nature.com/articles/s41562-021-01079-8.
21. Kang N, Kim B. The effects of border shutdowns on the spread of COVID-19. J Prev Med Public Health. 2020 Sep;53(5):293–301. https://doi.org/10.3961/jpmph.20.332 PMID:33070499.
22. Guo X, Zhong S, Wu Y, Zhang Y, Wang Z. The impact of lockdown in Wuhan on residents confidence in controlling COVID-19 outbreak at the destination cities. Front Public Health. 2022 Aug;10:902455. https://doi.org/10.3389/fpubh.2022.902455 PMID:36045730.
23. Working Families. Coronavirus (COVID-19) – What financial support is there for working families? [Internet]. Working Families. https://workingfamilies.org.uk/articles/coronavirus-support/.
24. U.S. Department of the Treasury. Assistance for American families and workers [Internet]. 2021. https://home.treasury.gov/policy-issues/coronavirus/assistance-for-American-families-and-workers.
25. Emeto TI, Alele FO, Ilesanmi OS. Evaluation of the effect of border closure on COVID-19 incidence rates across nine African countries: an interrupted time series study. Trans R Soc Trop Med Hyg. 2021 Oct;115(10):1174–83. https://doi.org/10.1093/trstmh/trab033 PMID:33690835.

CHAPTER 9

SURVEILLANCE, OUTBREAK DETECTION, AND EARLY WARNING

by Rachel Peh, Geoffrey Namara, Oyeronke Oyebanji, and Chikwe Ihekweazu

Public health surveillance is important for outbreak detection and overall health security. An agile surveillance system can prevent the escalation of an outbreak locally and potentially prevent a pandemic. Over the years, humankind has encountered outbreaks of various scales with varying impacts, and improvements have been made to disease surveillance systems to detect outbreaks early and enable a timely response. An effective and functional disease surveillance system requires actors at many different levels—community, subnational, national, regional, and international—to perform their roles and responsibilities. However, this is not without challenges, and resources are needed to sustain and streamline surveillance efforts. Trust within and between countries is critical for the sharing of surveillance information for global health security. To further enhance and strengthen disease surveillance against the changing dynamics of infectious diseases, more coordination and multisectoral partnerships are required.

INTRODUCTION

Surveillance is the backbone of infectious disease control and prevention. Surveillance systems monitor population health status and reveal unusual health events. An effective and agile disease surveillance system can prevent disease outbreaks from developing into costly infectious disease emergencies.

Public health surveillance can be defined as the ongoing systematic collection, analysis, and interpretation of health-related data essential to the planning, implementation, and evaluation of public health practice, combined with the timely dissemination of these results to those who need to know (1).

In this chapter, we provide the history of disease surveillance, how it has evolved, and what an ideal surveillance system for timely outbreak detection and response could be. The barriers to sustain effective disease surveillance for global health security are also discussed. We provide insights on developing an agile surveillance system for detection, monitoring, and response, and the way forward.

This chapter builds on existing literature on infectious disease surveillance, both from peer-reviewed materials as well as from intergovernmental and non-governmental organisations (NGOs), governmental agencies such as the World Health Organization (WHO), regional public health agencies like the African and European Centres for Disease Prevention and Control, and national public health agencies like the U.S. Centers for Disease Control and Prevention (U.S. CDC) and Nigeria Centre for Disease Control and Prevention (NCDC).

EVOLUTION OF DISEASE SURVEILLANCE

The concept of public health surveillance has been shaped over centuries by many major events. Systematic collection of surveillance data goes back at least as far as 1532, with the town council of London collecting mortality data to keep track of the number of persons dying from the plague (2). By the 19th century, British physician William Farr collected and reported mortality data of different populations in England and Wales, again to investigate the cause of plague outbreaks. His contributions to disease surveillance methodology earned him recognition as the founder of the modern concept of disease surveillance (3).

The WHO, established in 1948, plays a major role in coordinating global response efforts to outbreaks alongside its normative role. The concept of surveillance was recognised formally as an essential function of public health practice in the 1960s (4). The International Health Regulations (IHR) 1969, preceded by the Sanitary Health Regulations and revised from time to time, required Member States to monitor and inform the WHO of outbreaks of a specific list of "notifiable" diseases. In 2003, the severe acute respiratory syndrome (SARS) pandemic, also the first global public health emergency in the 21st century, led to another IHR revision in 2005 (5). In light of the increasing number of new and re-emerging diseases circulating, the scope and surveillance obligations of Member States expanded in IHR 2005. Countries were required to build national surveillance capacity and report any potential health emergencies.

> **International Health Regulations (IHR) 2005**
>
> Under the IHR, disease surveillance is not limited to specific diseases, but any illness or medical condition that can pose significant harm to humans. Furthermore, Member States have the responsibility to develop and strengthen public health core capacities. The WHO also established National IHR Focal Points (NFPs), a network of 24/7 two-way communication nodes in each country. Through NFPs, members are obligated to report promptly any local event potentially of public health emergency of international concern (PHEIC) (5).

At the regional level, with changing disease dynamics, disease-specific surveillance systems have also been established. They promote collaboration among countries from the same geographical region to monitor potential cross-border health threats, further reinforcing national compliance with the IHR and strengthening global health security (6). These are regional public health agencies with the political mandate to bolster disease surveillance and response and include the European and African Centres for Disease Prevention and Control.

In many countries, disease surveillance at a national level is implemented by a ministry of health. Over the years, several countries have established a national public health agency that leads local disease monitoring amongst other functions. The U.S. CDC is the model upon which many other public health agencies are based, including the Korea Disease Control and Prevention Agency (KDCA) and the NCDC. The U.S. CDC's concepts and approaches to public health service and surveillance have also been adapted in several countries, supported through the U.S. CDC's global health programmes (10).

> **Regional surveillance activities in Europe and Africa**
>
> The European Centre for Disease Prevention and Control (ECDC) was created in 2005, a public health agency among the countries of the European Union (EU) and European Economic Area (EEA). The agency works with national health institutions and other partners within the region to strengthen Europe's public health capacity (7). Similarly, the African Centres for Disease Control and Prevention (Africa CDC) was officially launched in 2017 to support African Union Member States. Its long-term vision is to strengthen the network of national public health agencies, recruit trained staff, and build regional public health capabilities towards a "New Public Health Order" for Africa (8–9).

Types of disease surveillance

Traditionally, most forms of surveillance begin with indicator-based surveillance (IBS). Clinicians or public health workers are typically key in such outbreak detection (11). When a patient is suspected of an infectious disease that is endemic or prone to re-emergence, a biological sample is sent for diagnostic confirmation before reporting to the central agency (**Figure 9.1**) (12). In areas with limited resources, and for highly pathogenic infections, suspected cases should be reported immediately. While outbreak information detected through IBS is mostly accurate, information collection may be slow. IBS is dependent on the presence of public health structures and health-seeking behaviours. Those who seek alternative treatments may be missed. Events in low-resource or rural settings are usually identified late (12–13).

Complementing IBS in outbreak detection is the use of event-based surveillance (EBS). Unstructured information and rumours from witnesses, NGOs, and government agencies and news outlets may identify an emerging outbreak (**Figure 9.2**). Both IBS and EBS enhance the sensitivity and timeliness of disease surveillance for outbreak detection and response.

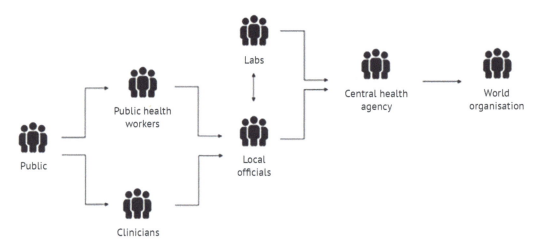

Figure 9.1: Sources and flow of information for outbreak detection in an indicator-based surveillance system

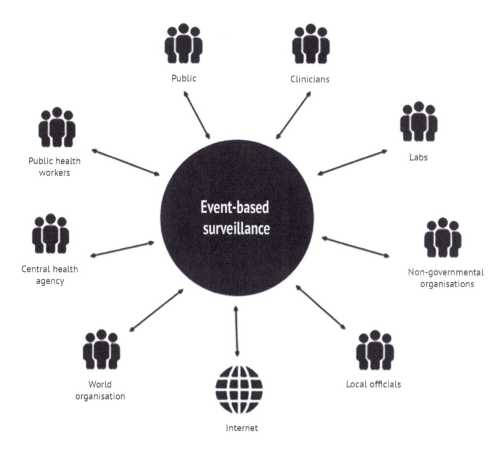

Figure 9.2: Sources and flow of information for outbreak detection in an event-based surveillance system
(adapted from O'Shea J. Digital disease detection: a systematic review of event-based internet biosurveillance systems. Int J Med Inform. 2017 May;101:15–22. https://doi.org/10.1016/j.ijmedinf.2017.01.019 PMID:28347443)

Emergence of digital technology for disease surveillance

Social media and web-based platforms have expanded the number and kind of information sources that can be used to detect unusual events. New technology also helps support public health experts in navigating huge amounts of information more efficiently.

In 2017, the Global Health Security Initiative (GHSI), the Joint Research Centre (JRC) of the European Commission, and the WHO spearheaded the development of the Epidemic Intelligence from Open Sources (EIOS) initiative. It works with various public health stakeholders and uses a One Health all-hazards approach to detect, verify, assess, and disseminate public health threats early, using publicly available information. The EIOS initiative leverages ongoing research advances in natural language processing and machine learning to sieve and identify important events early, working towards zero impact from health threats. EIOS has since proven to be successful in identifying outbreaks in a timely fashion (14).

Surveillance systems continue to become increasingly sophisticated with innovation and more collaboration. Technology has greatly changed how disease surveillance is conducted.

> **Early outbreak detection in the COVID-19 pandemic episode**
>
> The EIOS system actively extracts a wide range of publicly available online sources and collates information from other public health intelligence tools. It collects several thousand articles per hour and categorises them according to public health threats and topics. On 31 December 2019, it picked up the first signal, a media source, which reported the pneumonia cluster in Wuhan, China. The signal was complemented shortly after by other sources connected to the EIOS system, such as ProMED and HealthMap. This kicked off the EIOS community to collaborate for immediate verification and risk assessment processes (14).

However, the advances achieved thus far are still insufficient. At different levels of society, surveillance systems must adapt continuously to respond to infectious disease threats. A local outbreak of a newly emerging or re-emerging disease may escalate locally or evolve into a global pandemic depending on the transmissibility and impact on human health (3). This calls for increasing regional and international coordination in detection, prevention, and response efforts. An ideal system is agile and can provide early identification and notification.

AN IDEAL DISEASE SURVEILLANCE SYSTEM FOR OUTBREAK DETECTION, MONITORING, AND RESPONSE

Roles and responsibilities of key actors

Clinicians, community health workers, representatives, and volunteers play a key role at the community level in data collection and reporting (15). Community key informants need health training to be able to identify diseases and unusual events of public health importance. They need to be well acquainted with the reporting systems and communication channels, and follow the guidance set by local health authorities to deliver information or data to the next level. In addition, community volunteers should have a strong sense of responsibility for community health to perform their role with dedication (13).

Subnational health officers (holding positions as epidemiologists, surveillance officers, etc.) are responsible for compiling data collected from IBS and EBS systems, performing epidemiological analysis, and interpreting the data before passing an alert to the next level (17). Recognising an outbreak or a disease pattern and investigating the cause are to be done at this level. Subnational health officers also create active reporting linkages and motivate the work of health facilities and community through routine feedback (17). They provide support to facilities and community health workers to ensure that they are engaging in data collection (18). Furthermore, governments and partners at the subnational level are often responsible for cascading capacity building initiatives and action plans from national to subnational levels as part of outbreak preparedness efforts.

An active community-based surveillance-response system for Buruli ulcer in Ghana

The mode of transmission of *Mycobacterium ulcerans*, which causes Buruli ulcer, is unknown, and hence, the control of the disease relies largely on case detection and treatment. In Ghana, the implementation of a community-based surveillance-response system for early case detection, diagnosis, and treatment was feasible due to the training given to community-based volunteers, disease control officers, and clinicians. Upon suspecting a case, community volunteers refer the potential case to the nearest health facility for diagnosis and treatment. Volunteers were motivated with a token gift and provided with bicycles that aided their monthly rounds for case detection, encouraging their efforts in surveillance rounds (16).

Country-level government health leaders develop and adapt global and regional surveillance guidelines to their country's particular context (17). This is usually the responsibility of the national public health agency—where it exists—or a ministry of health. The government institution oversees and monitors the overall functioning of a surveillance system through evaluations and assessments (19). In most cases, the government institution analyses overall disease trends, and allocates manpower, logistical, and financial resources necessary for capacity building and sustainability. National governments collaborate and exchange information with other countries and international agencies, as per their IHR 2005 obligations (17).

Regional agencies and networks facilitate cooperation between neighbouring countries, sharing both data and expertise on surveillance and investigation of unusual events. They are an avenue for countries lacking in surveillance capacity to gain assistance from neighbouring countries in their implementation (20). Furthermore, they are usually viewed as neutral platforms committed to the objectives of their set up (i.e., combating health threats, even in difficult political environments) (6).

Middle East Consortium on Infectious Disease Surveillance (MECIDS)

MECIDS is a regional surveillance network between Jordan, the Palestinian Authority, and Israel. The intergovernmental partnership among the ministries of health has been effective in harmonising diagnostic and reporting methodologies, training, data sharing, and analysis. It has improved the detection of infectious diseases and facilitated cross-border communication. When avian influenza among poultry hit the region in 2006, the reporting system, open lines of communication, and cooperative control measures were critical in alleviating the impact of the outbreak (6,21).

The WHO provides leadership with regards to global health matters. It sets protocols for surveillance systems and provides technical expertise that strengthens countries' capacity to detect and respond to outbreaks. This leadership is exercised mainly through the IHR which defines the standards countries must meet to be able to prevent, detect, and respond to public health threats. The WHO also communicates closely with its members for information exchange through national focal points (NFPs) (5). In addition, the WHO leads policy dialogue and convenes stakeholders for surveillance initiatives such as the Global Influenza Surveillance and Response System (GISRS) (22).

In an ideal surveillance system, there is smooth communication of surveillance data and feedback between government levels (**Figure 9.3**).

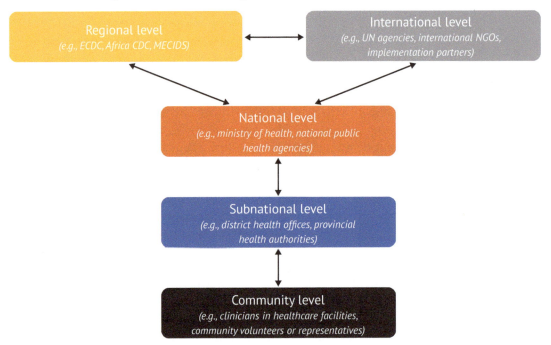

Figure 9.3: General overview of surveillance information flow or exchange across the different levels of a global surveillance system

Verification of signals detected and risk assessment for outbreak response

In order to rapidly respond to an event, timely verification must follow detection. A risk assessment of the potential significance is then required to determine appropriate action (23).

When an unusual event is detected, field investigators are expected to verify whether it is an outbreak. In the case of routine data, comparisons will be made with past surveillance records in a comparable time and area. When local data are unavailable, state-level or national data may be used. Interviews with health workers might be conducted to determine if the number of cases observed is typical. Eliminating other potential causes of an increased number of cases (such as changes in case definition or increased awareness and improvements in diagnostic procedures) is required before confirming the existence of an outbreak (**See Chapter 10, Field epidemiology**).

Following that, a risk assessment will help prioritise and assign resources (24). Any event potentially of public health importance as listed in the IHR is reported to the WHO rapidly through the NFPs (5). The WHO looks at four criteria to evaluate the threat of an event:
- the health impact or illness and death rate
- the potential for cross-border spread
- the potential for disrupting international travel or trade
- national capacity to contain the outbreak

Public health resources are precious, so confirming the signals and evaluating the risk of disease spread are necessary to inform outbreak response. Timely verification contributes to an agile system for outbreak detection and response (25).

RESOURCES NEEDED TO DEVELOP AGILE DISEASE SURVEILLANCE SYSTEMS

Resources are needed for disease surveillance and outbreak detection. An agile disease surveillance system can be characterised by several attributes such as timeliness, stability, simplicity, and data quality (26–27). In this section, we will discuss the resources needed for an agile disease surveillance system and the challenges that inhibit attaining that system. These challenges are grouped into those that are cross-cutting at every level and those that are level-specific.

Cross-cutting challenges

Human resources. A trained technical team is required to collect, report, and synthesise surveillance data. In addition to clinicians at healthcare facilities, community health workers or volunteers trained in case detection, management, and investigation are required (13). Epidemiologists are needed for outbreak investigation and data analysis. Public health officers supervise, organise capacity building activities at various levels, partake in developing technical products and communication activities, and evaluate surveillance system functionality (18). Other professionals such as statisticians, mathematical modellers, natural language processing specialists, anthropologists, and data analytics programmers are also needed (28). Coordination of partners across different levels enables monitoring and support to sentinel sites, which are designated health facilities or reporting sites, in the recording, reporting, and management of case data.

The list is not exhaustive but it highlights the importance of multidisciplinary and multi-skilled teams to ensure the proper functioning of a surveillance system at different levels. Frequent turnover of staff and limited knowledge and skills, along with limited opportunities for continuous capacity building, can hamper the effectiveness of the surveillance systems for timely detection (29).

Ebola outbreak in Nigeria and in Guinea, Sierra Leone, and Liberia

By April 2016, the Ebola epidemic had taken over 11,000 lives and crippled the economies in affected countries—Guinea, Sierra Leone, and Liberia. The economic impact was estimated as a US$ 2.2 billion drop in gross domestic product (GDP). However, the Ebola outbreak in Nigeria in July 2014 had only 20 cases, including 11 deaths. Different factors combine to explain this variation in impact. In Guinea, Sierra Leone, and Liberia, surveillance systems were limited and there was an insufficient number of skilled public health professionals. Data were often delayed and missing. Undetected initial spread between December 2013 and March 2014 slowed the early outbreak response. Nigeria leveraged resources from its polio response and had trained and capable health professionals and infrastructure, coordinated through Emergency Operations Centres, all of which enabled disease monitoring and outbreak response (30).

Financial resources. Sustainable, stable, and sufficient funding is required to maintain an effective surveillance system, including the recruitment of health professionals and provision of tools and equipment. Establishing the infrastructure for surveillance operations is costly. Suboptimal funding for surveillance affects activities such as training programmes, supervisory visits, and information systems infrastructure, all of which are critical (31–32).

Level-specific challenges

Digital technology has improved the speed of disease detection, communications, and response in general. Electronic forms can be completed by data collectors to expedite information flow. The use of electronic health records, which decreases paperwork and human errors during data transfer and management, can improve the quality and efficiency of surveillance (33). However, in places where technology penetration and digital literacy are low, it remains a challenge to leverage the benefits of digital technology for timely reporting. The rollout of digital technology at the community level is often hampered by capacity and the provision and maintenance of the digital hardware required at this level.

There are ethical concerns to surveillance data collected which may contain identifiable and private information that exposes individuals to harm such as intrusion on privacy, discrimination, and stigmatisation. Data might be collected without consent. Further public mistrust and a lack of transparency on how data is collected, stored, and used can be a hindrance to case reporting and timely detection (34).

A surveillance system is most effective when collection methods and software are standardised. Often, national disease surveillance data are collected by several bodies with different areas of interest. Government authorities, academic institutes, private sector partners, and NGOs may operate multiple surveillance systems in parallel or independently. This usually results in a poorly coordinated, inefficient, and disjointed national surveillance function. Surveillance officers reporting to multiple systems tend to get overwhelmed, resulting in a decline in the quality of data collected and the ability to analyse (35).

The different levels of autonomy that the reporting entities (districts/provinces/regions) have in different government systems have been shown to impact the effectiveness of a national surveillance system. The autonomy of subnational units can hinder the development of centralised approaches to national challenges. Federal governments might not be able to collect data when subnational governments fail to cooperate, hindering the downstream process of harmonised outbreak response and control (36). Furthermore, when data collection is not standardised, with inconsistencies in data formats or case definition, pooling data for nationwide analysis or making comparisons becomes challenging (37).

A lack of trust and transparency between countries remains a major challenge to the sharing of information vital for timely outbreak detection and response (38). This distrust can lead to the introduction of legal frameworks to protect the nation's interest and prevent sharing of data at the regional or international level (39). When countries fear the negative political and economic consequences of sharing important data, such as risks linked to travel and trade restrictions, they become reluctant to comply with the IHR. The IHR are currently without an enforcement mechanism (38).

> **Indonesia's response to the inequitable use of H5N1 virus samples**
>
> Distrust can arise from the inequitable sharing of benefits associated with data sharing, with wealthier states gaining more advantage. Between 2005 and 2007, Indonesia reported the highest number of Influenza A(H5N1) human cases in the world. After the H5N1 outbreak, Indonesia shared virus samples with WHO-affiliated laboratories under the GISRS Network. However, when Indonesia realised that these samples were shared outside of the WHO, and pharmaceutical companies were patenting modified strains of viruses from Indonesia, it stopped sharing samples to protect state sovereignty and Indonesian citizens' rights and interests in vaccine development (38).

STRENGTHENING SURVEILLANCE SYSTEMS

Human travel, changes in human and ecosystem behaviour, and adaptive survival strategies of microbial pathogens increase our vulnerability to infectious diseases globally (**See Chapter 2, What causes outbreaks?**). Harmonising disease surveillance efforts as much as possible is extremely important as outbreaks often spread across geographical boundaries within or beyond a country. To prevent, detect, and respond effectively to outbreaks and avert the next pandemic, countries must enhance their national surveillance capacity and collaborate multi-laterally with other nations and sectors.

Harmonising efforts and collaborating between all levels

Within countries, national capacities need to be strengthened at subnational and community levels. Compared to high-income countries, low- and middle-income countries often face greater challenges building this capacity, especially when they have to devote a portion of their surveillance resources to ongoing disease-specific challenges like HIV, tuberculosis, and other endemic diseases with significant donor funding. Political commitment and budgetary allocation and disbursement to public health surveillance are needed. Donors should not be the only source of such funding, and where donor funding is available, it should be used for system-wide development (40). Government or donor-funded resources could be used to train a capable workforce and create a stable infrastructure for surveillance activities set out through a careful evaluation process. Furthermore, close partnerships at all levels need to be established for smooth communication and timely information flow. A national health agency or its equivalent needs to work towards integrating multiple vertical surveillance systems into a single surveillance unit, detecting outbreaks and monitoring endemic diseases. This integrated approach coordinates data collection, analysis, interpretation, and dissemination, streamlining efforts and harmonising surveillance systems across all levels.

Strengthened coordination between countries will enhance health security individually and collectively. Globally, we are only as strong as our weakest link in the surveillance chain (30). Collaboration between countries for systems for outbreak detection, monitoring, and response includes optimal and ethical data sharing and building together in surveillance capacity (41).

International and regional networks help facilitate the exchange of expertise and best practices for surveillance activities. Those with strong capacities should support those who are developing. The WHO offers support to developing countries and countries with economies in transition when they request for assistance in building, strengthening, and maintaining public health capacities (5).

Multisectoral partnerships

Most infectious diseases that emerge in humans originate from animals (42). Hence, collaboration and consistent information sharing between human, animal, and environment sectors and disciplines, known as the One Health approach, are critical to better detect emerging epidemics (**See Chapter 13, One Health**). Identifying unusual events in animals and the environment can forecast infectious disease outbreaks in humans (43). NGOs involved in animal health can augment surveillance systems to facilitate early detection and response.

> **Multisectoral collaboration for global health security**
>
> The Global Health Security Agenda (GHSA) is an international collaborative effort, working multilaterally among governments and across sectors to improve country capacity to prevent, detect, and respond to infectious disease threats. It focuses on laboratory systems, surveillance systems, workforce development, and emergency management and response (30).

CONCLUSION

Advancements in surveillance systems have led to better disease detection and an increase in the identification of events that might have gone undetected. Quiet periods are not for idling or rest, but should be used to better prepare for the next outbreak. Global health systems must continue to evolve to respond swiftly and prevent the next infectious disease emergency. Much work is still required. Sustained monitoring must continue, even as national detection capacity is increased, as should collaboration across borders and between sectors.

REFERENCES:

1. Gregg MB. Field Epidemiology. 3rd ed. Oxford: Oxford University Press; 2008.
2. Choi BC. The past, present, and future of public health surveillance. Scientifica (Cairo). 2012;2012:875253. https://doi.org/10.6064/2012/875253 PMID:24278752.
3. Langmuir AD. William Farr: founder of modern concepts of surveillance. Int J Epidemiol. 1976 Mar;5(1):13–8. https://doi.org/10.1093/ije/5.1.13 PMID:770352.
4. Declich S, Carter AO. Public health surveillance: historical origins, methods and evaluation. Bull World Health Organ. 1994;72(2):285–304. PMID:8205649.
5. World Health Organization. International Health Regulations. 2005. https://www.who.int/publications/i/item/9789241580496.
6. Kimball AM, Moore M, French HM, Arima Y, Ungchusak K, Wibulpolprasert S, et al. Regional infectious disease surveillance networks and their potential to facilitate the implementation of the international health regulations [xii.]. Med Clin North Am. 2008 Nov;92(6):1459–71. https://doi.org/10.1016/j.mcna.2008.06.001 PMID:19061762.
7. European Centre for Disease Prevention and Control. What we do [cited 26 September 2022]. https://www.ecdc.europa.eu/en/about-us/what-we-do.
8. Watts G. John Nkengasong: long-term vision for Africa CDC. Lancet. 2019 Jun;393(10191):2581. https://doi.org/10.1016/S0140-6736(19)31420-5 PMID:31258119.
9. Africa CDC. About Us [cited 2023 29 July 2023]. https://africacdc.org/about-us/.

10. Thacker SB, Stroup DF. Origins and progress in surveillance systems. Infectious Disease Surveillance; 2013. pp. 21–31. https://doi.org/10.1002/9781118543504.ch2.
11. Isere EE, Fatiregun AA, Ajayi IO. An overview of disease surveillance and notification system in Nigeria and the roles of clinicians in disease outbreak prevention and control. Niger Med J. 2015;56(3):161–8. https://doi.org/10.4103/0300-1652.160347 PMID:26229222.
12. O'Shea J. Digital disease detection: a systematic review of event-based internet biosurveillance systems. Int J Med Inform. 2017 May;101:15–22. https://doi.org/10.1016/j.ijmedinf.2017.01.019 PMID:28347443.
13. McGowan CR, Takahashi E, Romig L, Bertram K, Kadir A, Cummings R, et al. Community-based surveillance of infectious diseases: a systematic review of drivers of success. BMJ Glob Health. 2022 Aug;7(8):e009934. https://doi.org/10.1136/bmjgh-2022-009934 PMID:35985697.
14. World Health Organization. Epidemic Intelligence from Open Sources (EIOS) World Health Organization [cited 2023 30 January 2023]. https://www.who.int/initiatives/eios.
15. Byrne A, Nichol B. A community-centred approach to global health security: implementation experience of community-based surveillance (CBS) for epidemic preparedness. Glob Secur Health Sci Policy. 2020;5(1):71–84. https://doi.org/10.1080/23779497.2020.1819854.
16. Ahorlu CS, Okyere D, Ampadu E. Implementing active community-based surveillance-response system for Buruli ulcer early case detection and management in Ghana. PLoS Negl Trop Dis. 2018 Sep;12(9):e0006776. https://doi.org/10.1371/journal.pntd.0006776 PMID:30208037.
17. World Health Organization Regional Office for Africa. Integrated Disease Surveillance in the African Region: A Regional Strategy for Communicable Disease 1999-2003. 1999. Report No.: AFR/RC/48/8.
18. World Health Organization. Integrated Disease Surveillance and Response Technical Guidelines. WHO Regional Office for Africa; 2019. https://www.who.int/publications/i/item/WHO-AF-WHE-CPI-05-2019.
19. World Health Organization. Protocol for the Assessment of National Communicable Disease Surveillance and Response System: Guidelines for Assessment Teams. World Health Organization; 2001. https://iris.who.int/handle/10665/66787?&locale-attribute=ar.
20. Bond KC, Macfarlane SB, Burke C, Ungchusak K, Wibulpolprasert S. The evolution and expansion of regional disease surveillance networks and their role in mitigating the threat of infectious disease outbreaks. Emerg Health Threats J. 2013;6(1):6. https://doi.org/10.3402/ehtj.v6i0.19913 PMID:23362414.
21. MECIDS. About us 2023 [cited 2023 29 July 2023]. http://mecidsnetwork.org/about.
22. Hay AJ, McCauley JW. The WHO global influenza surveillance and response system (GISRS)-a future perspective. Influenza Other Respir Viruses. 2018 Sep;12(5):551–7. https://doi.org/10.1111/irv.12565 PMID:29722140.
23. Heymann DL, Rodier GR; WHO Operational Support Team to the Global Outbreak Alert and Response Network. Hot spots in a wired world: WHO surveillance of emerging and re-emerging infectious diseases. Lancet Infect Dis. 2001 Dec;1(5):345–53. https://doi.org/10.1016/S1473-3099(01)00148-7 PMID:11871807.
24. Tam C, Haas W; Outbreak investigations. In: Abubakar I, Stagg HR, Cohen T, Rodrigues LC, editors. Infectious Disease Epidemiology: Oxford University Press; 2016.
25. Grein TW, Kamara KB, Rodier G, Plant AJ, Bovier P, Ryan MJ, et al. Rumors of disease in the global village: outbreak verification. Emerg Infect Dis. 2000;6(2):97–102. https://doi.org/10.3201/eid0602.000201 PMID:10756142.
26. Centers for Disease Control (CDC). Guidelines for evaluating surveillance systems. MMWR Suppl. 1988 May;37(5):1–18. PMID:3131659.
27. German RR, Lee LM, Horan JM, Milstein RL, Pertowski CA, Waller MN; Guidelines Working Group Centers for Disease Control and Prevention (CDC). Updated guidelines for evaluating public health surveillance systems: recommendations from the Guidelines Working Group. MMWR Recomm Rep. 2001 Jul;50 RR-13:1–35. PMID:18634202.
28. Drehobl PA, Roush SW, Stover BH, Koo D; Centers for Disease Control and Prevention. Public health surveillance workforce of the future. MMWR Suppl. 2012 Jul;61(3):25–9. PMID:22832994.
29. Phalkey RK, Yamamoto S, Awate P, Marx M. Challenges with the implementation of an Integrated Disease Surveillance and Response (IDSR) system: systematic review of the lessons learned. Health Policy Plan. 2015 Feb;30(1):131–43. https://doi.org/10.1093/heapol/czt097 PMID:24362642.
30. Wolicki SB, Nuzzo JB, Blazes DL, Pitts DL, Iskander JK, Tappero JW. Public health surveillance: at the core of the Global Health Security Agenda. Health Secur. 2016;14(3):185–8. https://doi.org/10.1089/hs.2016.0002 PMID:27314658.

31. Joseph Wu TS, Kagoli M, Kaasbøll JJ, Bjune GA. Integrated Disease Surveillance and Response (IDSR) in Malawi: implementation gaps and challenges for timely alert. PLoS One. 2018 Nov;13(11):e0200858. https://doi.org/10.1371/journal.pone.0200858 PMID:30496177.
32. Mandyata CB, Olowski LK, Mutale W. Challenges of implementing the integrated disease surveillance and response strategy in Zambia: a health worker perspective. BMC Public Health. 2017 Sep;17(1):746. https://doi.org/10.1186/s12889-017-4791-9 PMID:28950834.
33. Ibrahim LM, Okudo I, Stephen M, Ogundiran O, Pantuvo JS, Oyaole DR, et al. Electronic reporting of integrated disease surveillance and response: lessons learned from northeast, Nigeria, 2019. BMC Public Health. 2021 May;21(1):916. https://doi.org/10.1186/s12889-021-10957-9 PMID:33985451.
34. World Health Organization. WHO guidelines on ethical issues in public health surveillance. World Health Organization; 2017. https://www.who.int/publications/i/item/9789241512657.
35. World Health Organization. An integrated approach to communicable disease surveillance. Weekly Epidemiological Record. 2000;75(01):1–7. https://www3.paho.org/english/dd/ais/EB_v21n1.pdf.
36. Wilson K, McDougall C, Upshur R; Joint Centre for Bioethics SARS Global Health Ethics Research Group. The new International Health Regulations and the federalism dilemma. PLoS Med. 2006 Jan;3(1):e1. https://doi.org/10.1371/journal.pmed.0030001 PMID:16354103.
37. Gordon SH, Huberfeld N, Jones DK. What federalism means for the US response to coronavirus disease 2019. JAMA Health Forum. 2020 May;1(5):e200510. https://doi.org/10.1001/jamahealthforum.2020.0510 PMID:36218490.
38. Lencucha R, Bandara S. Trust, risk, and the challenge of information sharing during a health emergency. Global Health. 2021 Feb;17(1):21. https://doi.org/10.1186/s12992-021-00673-9 PMID:33602281.
39. Aarestrup FM, Koopmans MG. Sharing data for global infectious disease surveillance and outbreak detection. Trends Microbiol. 2016 Apr;24(4):241–5. https://doi.org/10.1016/j.tim.2016.01.009 PMID:26875619.
40. Calain P. From the field side of the binoculars: a different view on global public health surveillance. Health Policy Plan. 2007 Jan;22(1):13–20. https://doi.org/10.1093/heapol/czl035 PMID:17237490.
41. Edelstein M, Lee LM, Herten-Crabb A, Heymann DL, Harper DR. Strengthening global public health surveillance through data and benefit sharing. Emerg Infect Dis. 2018;24(7):1324–30. https://doi.org/10.3201/eid2407.151830.
42. Taylor LH, Latham SM, Woolhouse ME. Risk factors for human disease emergence. Philos Trans R Soc Lond B Biol Sci. 2001 Jul;356(1411):983–9. https://doi.org/10.1098/rstb.2001.0888 PMID:11516376.
43. Ajuwon BI, Roper K, Richardson A, Lidbury BA. One Health approach: a data-driven priority for mitigating outbreaks of emerging and re-emerging zoonotic infectious diseases. Trop Med Infect Dis. 2021 Dec;7(1):4. https://doi.org/10.3390/tropicalmed7010004 PMID:35051120.

CHAPTER 10

FIELD EPIDEMIOLOGY AND OUTBREAK INVESTIGATION

by Alexander Spina, Erika Valeska Rossetto, and Neale Batra

This chapter introduces the principles and practice of epidemiology for disease control as applied to outbreak response through the lens of "field epidemiology". Applied or "field" epidemiology is primarily concerned with producing timely contextual information to intervene when public health problems arise, often using messy primary data. To advance beyond the military and colonial legacies of the discipline, the term "field epidemiology" will likely, and should, be phased out in favour of terms such as "applied" or "intervention" epidemiology. We will nevertheless, for the purpose of this chapter, use the term "field epidemiology".

The role of a field epidemiologist in investigating and responding to outbreaks of any aetiology can be summarised in ten common steps: preparing for field work, confirming the diagnosis, determining the existence of an outbreak, identifying and registering cases, descriptive analysis, statistical analysis, drawing conclusions, communicating findings, implementing interventions, and evaluating the response as well as continued surveillance. We demonstrate these steps using a hypothetical outbreak scenario, with questions for the reader, and highlight that in practice, these steps do not necessarily happen in succession, multiple steps can happen simultaneously or not at all, and outbreak response is an iterative process.

INTRODUCTION

Definitions of epidemiological practice are separated into two broad categories, academic and applied epidemiology (1). Academic epidemiology is primarily practised in research settings and often uses complex methodologies on high-quality data from controlled circumstances (often secondary data) to further the understanding of disease aetiology or make predictions. Applied epidemiology is primarily practised for government public health institutions, or non-governmental or international organisations, and is primarily concerned with delivering timely, contextualised information to implement interventions against public health problems, often using messy primary data (1–4). In this chapter, we will introduce the principles and practice of epidemiology for disease control as applied to outbreak response, the so-called "field epidemiology".

The canonical origin story of field epidemiology describes John Snow as the archetypical figure who in 1854, used a dot map to identify and remove the Broad Street pump as the source of a cholera outbreak in London, England (5). In reality, as described in Jim Downs' *Maladies of Empire*, field epidemiology more likely took root in less acceptable circumstances, in closed population studies among non-consenting participants primarily for the economic benefit of Western colonising nations including plantations, slave trading ships, and war camps (6). To advance beyond the military and colonial legacies of the discipline, the term "field epidemiology" will likely, and should, be phased out in favour of terms such as "applied" or "intervention epidemiology". We will nevertheless, for the purpose of this chapter, use the term "field epidemiology".

In 1951, the U.S. Centers for Disease Control and Prevention (U.S. CDC) and Alexander Langmuir established the U.S. Epidemic Intelligence Service (EIS) as the first field epidemiology training programme (FETP). This model of intensive, field-based learning to create a workforce capable of responding to local and international public health threats (7) has underpinned 91 FETPs and arguably had a substantial impact on disease amelioration globally (8–9). However, most public health and medical personnel confronting epidemics operate outside the FETP sphere and lack formal training in field epidemiology.

OVERVIEW OF THE 10 STEPS OF OUTBREAK INVESTIGATION

Field epidemiologists are most often involved in the "response" pillar of the outbreak cycle (**See Chapter 1, Introduction**). The role of a field epidemiologist in investigating and responding to outbreaks of any aetiology can be summarised in a few common steps. There are various interpretations in the number, order, and naming of these steps including from the U.S. CDC (10) and the European Centre for Disease Prevention and Control (ECDC) (11), as well as others in textbooks (1). For the purpose of this chapter, we synthesised from these various sources to create ten steps which most closely fit the reality of outbreak response, as outlined in **Table 10.1**.

It is important to note that in practice, these steps do not necessarily happen in succession, multiple steps can happen simultaneously or not at all, and outbreak response is an iterative process (meaning that steps need to be revised and repeated). The role of a field epidemiologist will differ depending on the context and their role within the healthcare system. Generally, a field epidemiologist working closer to the "frontline" of the outbreak, in a local or regional position, is more likely to undertake the steps in a hands-on fashion, whereas one at the national or international level may perform different tasks and will likely require an invitation to operate at the local level. The remainder of this chapter will introduce an outbreak scenario to demonstrate these ten steps, with questions for the reader.

Step	Description
1. Prepare for field work	• Initial request and invitation to local response • Assemble a team and clarify roles • Confirm logistical aspects (travel, accommodation, *per diem*) and personal arrangements (family, pets, pills, bills) • Gather appropriate guidelines and templates
2. Confirm the diagnosis	• Collect appropriate samples and information • Clinical and laboratory diagnosis
3. Determine the existence of an outbreak	• Compare disease counts to established local baseline • Consider alternate explanations such as surveillance system changes or population movements

Step	Description

4. Identify and register cases	• Construct a case definition by time, place, and person
	  o Use pre-approved definitions where possible (such as from the World Health Organization [WHO])
	  o Consider multiple levels (e.g., suspected, probable, confirmed, discarded)
	• Design a questionnaire to collect data
	• Search for cases through passive or active surveillance
	• Capture data in a line list

5. Descriptive analysis: generate hypotheses	• Analyse data by time, place, and person • Synthesise what cases have in common and suggest possible exposures to test
6. Statistical analysis: test hypotheses	• Design an analytical study (case-control or retrospective cohort) • Investigate if hypotheses withstand statistical testing, controlling for relevant confounders and effect modifiers and following the principle of parsimony
7. Draw conclusions: compare results with established facts, consider additional studies	• Consider the biological plausibility of the analytic results • Compare analytic results to what is already known for the disease • Combine results with findings from other sources (i.e., clinical, laboratory, environmental, local community knowledge) and establish a source or factors associated with disease • If necessary, make adjustments and conduct further studies or analysis
8. Communicate findings	• Share your findings with local authorities, stakeholders, and the local community • Discuss the relevance and ensure consensus on the appropriate interventions
9. Implement control and prevention measures	• Using the conclusions and community consensus, action culturally appropriate and evidence-based disease specific interventions to mitigate the outbreak
10. Evaluate response, initiate or maintain surveillance	• Planning for how to ensure interventions are working should start with step 4 (identify and register cases) • Use existing outbreak or surveillance data, or conduct surveys to see if interventions are working as planned • Continue monitoring case trends for early detection of further outbreaks

Table 10.1: Ten steps of an outbreak investigation (2,10–11)

OUTBREAK SCENARIO

This scenario demonstrates the application of the ten steps. Maximal learning will come from reflecting upon the scenario developments, answering and critiquing the questions, and comparing them with outbreaks that will likely be confronted.

Setting the scene

You are the government epidemiologist serving a district comprising a population of 100,000, and are responsible for the maintenance of disease surveillance systems, investigation of potential outbreaks, and support for health promotion activities such as vaccination campaigns. Indicator-based surveillance (IBS) data (12) (routinely reported case counts) arrive weekly from 12 public clinics, the public hospital, and a private hospital, with suspect cases of epidemic-prone diseases reported within 24 hours. Careful cultivation of relationships with the local community and religious and business leaders has resulted in a robust event-based surveillance (EBS) system (12), such that alerts of unusual health events are reported quickly by SMS. Routine activities are coordinated with medical laboratory and vector control teams, although simulated exercises of outbreak response are infrequent due to budget constraints.

The alert

In the first week of January 2018, after a strong rainstorm, you receive an email from the nurse at the district hospital who perceives an increase in patients presenting with acute watery diarrhoea. You recall seeing complaints on social media about the closure of a popular local business, reportedly due to staff being ill. In the evening, you receive a text message from a religious leader serving rural town "C" (population of 2,000) who is alarmed after performing funerals for a child and an unrelated elderly adult, both of whom had suffered from severe diarrhoea.

1. Prepare for field work

The district health officer informs you that several years ago, town C experienced an outbreak of cholera. She suggests that you first conduct phone calls with the district hospital, business owners, and leaders of town C to validate the alerts and gather more information. A call with the medical laboratory and the water, sanitation, and hygiene (WASH) unit results in plans for an in-person joint investigation the following day.

Which personnel, supplies, and equipment should be included in the joint outbreak investigation?

The team needs personnel with experience in community engagement, clinical medicine, environmental sanitation, laboratory specimen collection, field epidemiology, data management, logistics, and language translation. Local points of contact are also extremely important. Bring rapid appropriate personal protective equipment, hand sanitiser, diagnostic tests, specimen collection and storage material, questionnaires, and data collection instruments (with backups for offline use), capability to collect GPS coordinates, first aid supplies, and emergency communication devices. Also consider finances, human resource management, personal supplies (including food and water), and security (**See Chapter 6, Teamwork**).

2. Confirm the diagnosis

> Your investigation substantiates the alerts and raises further concern. In the last week, 40 town C residents, half of the business' employees, and 75 patients presenting to the district hospital have experienced debilitating fatigue and diarrhoea. At town C, the investigation team observed damaged sanitation infrastructure, interviewed relatives of deceased and hospitalised individuals, collected samples of stool with "rice-water" appearance for laboratory culture and polymerase chain reaction (PCR) testing, and advised community leaders and caregivers of precautionary isolation measures to reduce disease transmission.

Which diseases are you concerned about based on clinical presentation? What further information would be useful and how would you collect it?

Diarrhoea has many possible infectious (and non-infectious) aetiologies including the concerning possibility of *Vibrio cholerae*. Information about patient demographics, residence, the consistency, frequency, and presence of blood in the stool, travel history, and sources of environmental exposure can help indicate the seriousness of the situation even before specimens are analysed.

What are useful measures of a diagnostic test and how are these calculated?

	Reference result	
Test result	Disease present	Disease absent
Positive	**TP**	**FP**
Negative	**FN**	**TN**

Table 10.2: Two-by-two table comparing counts of a test with a reference result

T = True; F = False; P = Positive; N = Negative

Sensitivity, specificity, and positive and negative predictive values are calculated for a test by comparing it to a reference result (or "gold standard") where the presence or absence of disease can be confirmed (**Tables 10.2 and 10.3**). Sensitivity and specificity are usually used for epidemiological purposes, whereas positive and negative predictive values are more often used in clinical practice. In general, a screening test should have high sensitivity and a diagnostic test should have high specificity (**See Chapter 9, Surveillance; See Chapter 20, Diagnostics**).

Measure	Explanation	Formula
Sensitivity	Proportion of true cases detected (i.e., if the disease is present, what is the chance of detection)	$\dfrac{TP}{TP + FN}$
Specificity	Proportion of true negative results (i.e., if the disease is not present, what is the chance of ruling it out appropriately)	$\dfrac{TN}{FP + TN}$
Positive predictive value	Likelihood of having the disease with a positive test result	$\dfrac{TP}{TP + FP}$

Measure	Explanation	Formula
Negative predictive value	Likelihood of not having the disease with a negative test result	$\dfrac{TN}{TN + FN}$

Table 10.3: Definitions and equations for calculating sensitivity, specificity, and positive and negative predictive values

The investigation team performs cholera rapid diagnostic tests (RDTs), some of which return positive results for the O1 serogroup. What are the possible uses of RDTs in outbreak investigation? In this scenario, how are the RDTs being used?

The use of RDTs can serve surveillance purposes, and in select scenarios, can inform patient care. The Global Task Force on Cholera Control advises that cholera RDTs be used only for early outbreak detection (to be confirmed by culture or PCR) and not for individual diagnosis (13).

3. Determine the existence of an outbreak

Your initial data analysis suggests that the volume of patients presenting with acute watery diarrhoea at health facilities throughout the district clearly exceeds the expected range based on five years of historical data.

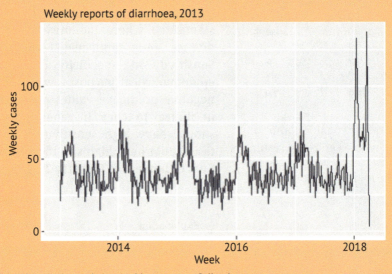

Figure 10.1: Historical trends in weekly reports of diarrhoea

The first PCR results arrive—*V. cholerae* was detected in eight of ten stool specimens. Your data uses unique patient identifiers, so you can link this laboratory data to your line listing and GPS data. For cholera specifically, confirmation of an ongoing outbreak expands the surveillance case definition to include any person presenting with or dying from acute watery diarrhoea (13).

Review the 2001 Morbidity and Mortality Weekly Report (MMWR) article on updated guidelines for evaluating public health surveillance systems (14) on the attributes of a robust surveillance system, and Chapter 9, Surveillance. How do each of the system attributes impact outbreak detection and response?

Attribute	Summary	Impact on outbreak detection and response
Acceptability	The willingness of persons and organisations to participate in the system	These attributes contribute to the ability of the system to accurately track underlying disease trends
Data quality	The completeness and validity of the data	
Representativeness	The coverage by geography, demographics, and variation in clinical manifestation	
Sensitivity	The sensitivity as applied to case definition, case detection, and outbreak detection	
Stability	The reliability and availability	These attributes have consequences for the ability of the system to survive shocks such as loss of personnel, changing epidemiologies, or natural hazards that undermine internet connectivity
Flexibility	The ability for the system to adapt	
Simplicity	The structure and ease of use	
Timeliness	The speed or delay between steps	This can determine whether the system generates actionable information at the speed necessary for effective response
Positive predictive value (PPV)	The probability that outbreaks detected are of public health significance and require response	These attributes impact the long-term sustainability of the system
Cost-effectiveness	Including direct, indirect, and societal costs	

Table 10.4: Attributes of disease surveillance systems (14) and their impact on outbreak detection and response

Which actors in a health ecosystem are frequently missed by standard disease surveillance systems?
Private medical and pharmacy facilities, traditional or non-certified providers, veterinary or animal disease surveillance, and home-based diagnostic tests.

How might you determine whether an increase in case reports constitutes a departure from normal?
You will need to assess how this event compares to historical trends in temporal, spatial, and demographic distribution of the disease, in light of seasonality and recent population exposures or movement.

What are other possible causes for an observed increase in the number of cases of a given disease reported from one area, aside from an epidemic?
Increases in the number of reported cases can also occur due to increases in the serviced population, planned changes to case definition or reporting requirements, unexpected changes in reporting patterns such as a new clinician or a malfunction of diagnostic equipment, or simple data entry errors.

4. Identify and register cases

With an outbreak now confirmed, the response team determines that all health centres are to be queried daily by phone and receive frequent site visits with a manual review of patient records for missed cases. The network of local community health workers (CHWs) is re-oriented to conduct active case finding (15) via household interviews. A public call line is established, and rapid response teams are trained to investigate alerts. This intensified operational cadence and expansion of activities demands significant human resources, and your district struggles to find sufficient qualified personnel.

You have compiled a line listing of known cases (**Figure 10.2**) and an accompanying "data dictionary" which details the eligible values for each variable.

case_id	town	sex	age_years	date_onset	prior_vax	dehy	preg	blood_stool	rdt	outcome
A46	C		10	2018-01-07	No	Severe		No	Pos	Death
A296	C	F	36	2018-01-08	No	Moderate	No	No	Pos	Death
A1	C		62	2018-01-21	No	Severe		No	Neg	Death
A16	C	F	17	2018-01-25	No	Severe	No	No	Pos	Death
A129	C		7	2018-01-27		Severe		No		Death
A78	C	M	21	2018-01-31	No	Severe		No	Pos	Death

Figure 10.2: Select rows and columns of a line list of suspect cases

Review the definitions for cholera cases and outbreak declarations (13). Create definitions for confirmed, probable, suspected, and discarded cases, incorporating concepts for time, place, and person, as well as clinical and laboratory criteria.
Consider the challenges of recognising "loose or watery (non-bloody) stools". In a declared cholera outbreak, will most counted cases be suspect or confirmed?

How will you record information gathered about the cases?
A line listing containing information on each patient should be recorded electronically, using either the existing health information platform, a temporary data collection platform (e.g., ODK), or directly into a spreadsheet using value validation checks (16). Another tool is the WHO Go.Data platform.

Why is it important to designate a unique identification number (UID) for each patient?
UIDs can facilitate the alignment of surveillance, laboratory, contact tracing, and medical outcome data without relying on the manual matching of names and dates of birth. Similarly, consider facility IDs to avoid variation in the spelling of clinic names.

What complications in epidemiological interpretation may arise from implementing door-to-door active case finding?
Approaches for case finding are outlined in different technical guidelines from the WHO (15). However, if pressures, incentives, or other enhanced case detection activities are unevenly applied across the affected area, observed differential increases in case reporting may not reflect true shifts in disease burden but may instead reflect variation in the implementation of active surveillance techniques. It is also important to establish a population denominator, particularly in situations with mobile populations (**See Chapter 35, Volunteers**).

How might responders arriving from outside your jurisdiction (or country) complicate or even negatively impact your response operations?
Persons willing to assist in outbreak response should await a request from the affected jurisdiction, offer needed skills and experience, and be trained in the incident management system (IMS) used in the response.

5. Descriptive analysis: generate hypotheses
Field epidemiologists often wrestle with uncertainty, relying on relatively simple descriptive analysis of outbreak data by person, time, and place to provide insight and generate hypotheses (2,17). William Foege coined the term "consequential epidemiology" (1) and Mike Ryan succinctly described this during the COVID-19 response: "If you need to be right before you move, you will lose. Speed trumps perfection. Perfection is the enemy of good when it comes to emergency management" (18).

Analysis by person
Descriptive analysis of the persons affected typically begins with tables and a demographic (age–sex) pyramid, best compared to a baseline population. Tables are often expanded to include clinical outcomes and response indicators such as a delay to case detection.

Further analysis by person may include calculations of overall and group case fatality ratios (CFRs), i.e., the proportion of cases that died. Confidence intervals (CIs) for these estimates are cumbersome by hand but simple to do with common statistical software (2,19).

Calculating the attack rate (AR) per 10,000 population allows more accurate comparisons between relevant groups (e.g., age, hospitals, or regions). Consideration of population denominators can sometimes reveal that groups with fewer reported cases may still be experiencing significant disease burden relative to their size (2,19).

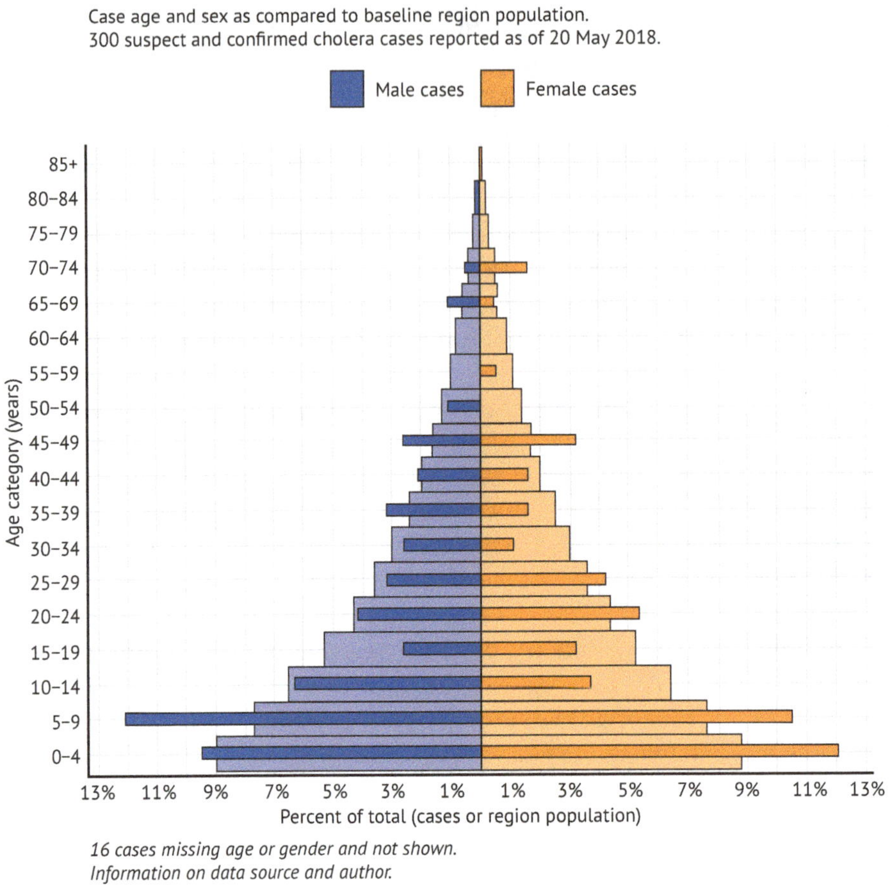

Case age and sex as compared to baseline region population.
300 suspect and confirmed cholera cases reported as of 20 May 2018.

■ Male cases ■ Female cases

16 cases missing age or gender and not shown.
Information on data source and author.

Figure 10.3: Demographic (age–sex) pyramid of cases as compared to a baseline population

Group	Deaths (n)	Cases (N)	CFR (%)
Male	a	b	$\frac{a \times 100}{b}$
Female	c	d	$\frac{c \times 100}{d}$

Table 10.5: Calculation of case fatality ratios (CFRs)

Group	Cases (n)	Population	AR (per 10,000)
Region A	a	b	$\frac{a \times 10,000}{b}$
Region B	c	d	$\frac{c \times 10,000}{d}$

Table 10.6: Calculation of attack rates (ARs)

Analysis by time

The time dimension of an outbreak is typically presented as an epidemic curve ("epicurve"), with the distribution of dates of symptom onset displayed as a histogram, using an appropriate time interval, often differentiated by case status. Close analysis of epidemic curves, with attention to data quality limitations, can highlight the source, propagation characteristics, and serial interval of the disease.

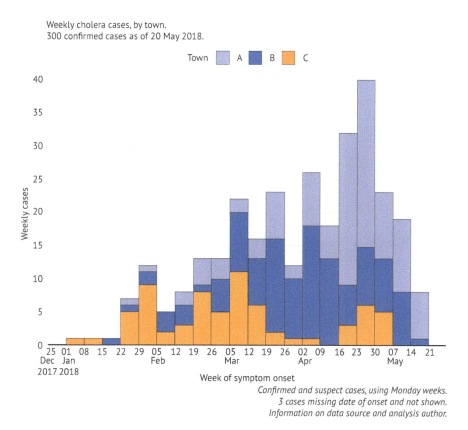

Figure 10.4: An example of an epidemic curve, shown by geographic subdivision

Analysis by place
Geographical analysis can be used to illuminate patterns in many facets of outbreak response including disease burden, access to healthcare services, environmental sampling, and operational activities. Despite the attraction of maps, such analyses can often also be communicated via tables (20).

Which data management techniques will be critical as you handle the increasing number of data types and sources and attempt to consolidate them into actionable information?
To facilitate efficient updates to the analytics, epidemiologists should consider a free tool such as R which enables reproducible and collaborative workflows, deduplication and joining of multiple datasets, geographic information system (GIS) mapping, and production of dashboards and automatically generated reports via scripted commands. If this is not possible, analytics can be achieved with less versatility via Microsoft Excel or software such as DHIS2, Go.Data, and Kobo.

What hypotheses might you be interested in testing?
Field epidemiologists are interested in information for action. This involves finding associations between groups of people or particular exposures to the disease in order to implement targeted control measures. In our example, we might want to test whether a particular age group or gender is more likely to have cholera, or whether one town has a disproportionate

case burden. While not available in our data, we might be interested in certain professions or water sources. What other potential exposures can you think of?

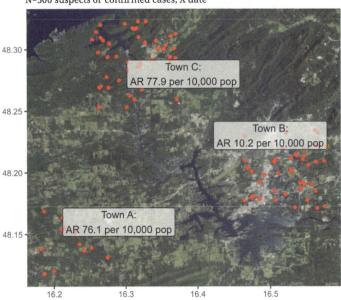

Figure 10.5: An example of a fictional point map showing case locations and calculated ARs per population, by town (20)
(Basemap source: USGS The National Map: Orthoimagery)

6. Statistical analysis: test hypotheses

Well-conducted analytical studies provide actionable context-specific information with relatively low logistical and financial burden (21–22). These are most often observational studies investigating disease risks (or mortality) among people with exposures of interest. Randomised controlled studies have been used in outbreak scenarios for impact evaluation of interventions such as vaccines (23) or treatments (24), but often fall under the auspice of operational research (**See Chapter 17, Integrated outbreak analytics; See Chapter 18, Research to inform practice; See Chapter 27, Research for therapeutics**). Novel approaches have a place in outbreak response but should not replace analytical studies (**See Chapter 16, Modelling to inform strategy; See Chapter 21, Genomics**) (17).

What possible study designs would you consider to test the hypothesis from the previous section?

Field epidemiologists mostly conduct observational studies (**Figure 10.5**) using outbreak line list data. We can subset our line list to those who attended hospital and had an RDT in order to conduct a case-control study. A cohort study would be appropriate if all residents were tested; however, this is rare and usually occurs in closed settings such as gatherings, hospitals, schools, or camps. If we had widespread testing and could perform a cohort analysis, we could be more confident interpreting the statistical results, as we would not need to worry about sampling bias. When investigating a rare or unknown disease, publication of case reports or a case series should be considered.

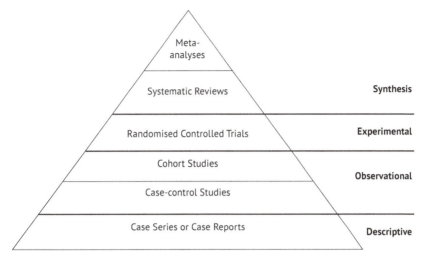

Figure 10.6: Types of studies

What is the most appropriate control group in your setting?
Among our discarded cases are those with a negative RDT. This would be an ideal control group, making this a case test-negative study.

What simple statistical tests could you use to compare groups?
Simple statistical tests can be useful in highlighting differences, particularly potential sampling bias when only analysing a subset of your population. In our scenario, we might be interested in comparing the demographics of those tested to the overall population of the region to see if there were differences in testing uptake which might bias our results. The most commonly used tests are listed below along with the types of variables for which they are appropriate. We have not included the formulas as calculating these by hand can be quite tedious; however, any statistical software will have implementations of these. Another useful test not listed below is the Shapiro–Wilk test for normality. This is important as several other tests assume that data are normally distributed in order to be valid.

Outcome	Exposure	Test	Notes
Categorical	Categorical	Chi-squared	Differences in observed and expected frequencies are often used to compare proportions. With small samples, consider Fisher's exact test instead.
Categorical	Continuous	T-test	Difference in means of a continuous variable between two groups. Requires variables to be normally distributed (parametric test).

Outcome	Exposure	Test	Notes
Categorical	Continuous	Kruskal–Wallis	Difference in distribution of a continuous variable between two groups. Does not require variables to be normally distributed (non-parametric test). When only two samples are used, the results will be identical to a Wilcoxon rank-sum test.

Table 10.7: The most commonly used statistical tests

What are the different measures of association you can calculate for various study designs? Which one is the most appropriate for the chosen study design?

Odds ratios (ORs) and risk ratios (RRs) are the most commonly used estimates of effect size (or association). ORs are the appropriate estimate for a case-control study as there is no denominator to calculate the risk (this requires a cohort). ORs are often inferior estimates to RRs as they exaggerate the size of the effect (both above and below 1). At lower risk (or odds), the OR may more closely approximate the risk ratio (2,19,25).

Study design	Estimate	Notes	Regression
Case-control	Odds ratio (OR)	Odds of exposure among cases divided by controls	Logistic
Cohort	Risk ratio (RR)	Risk of outcome (usually disease) among the exposed divided by unexposed	Poisson or negative binomial
	Incidence rate ratio (IRR)	Rate (frequency divided by person-time) of outcome (usually disease or mortality) among the exposed divided by the unexposed * Note that this requires knowing how many days each individual was observed to be able to calculate person-time for the group. This can approximate the hazard ratio for binomial non-time-varying exposures (26).	

Table 10.8: Measures to estimate effect sizes

How would you interpret the results of the univariate analysis?

The odds of the exposure among cases is a certain number of times higher than among the controls. In **Table 10.9**, the odds of having severe dehydration was 7.51 (95 percent CI, 3.48–18.7) times higher in cases compared to controls. While it makes sense that confirmed cholera cases are more likely to be dehydrated, unfortunately, none of these associations provide us with actionable insight, which can often happen when dealing with messy real-world data. We should therefore focus on using the information from descriptive time, place, and person analyses. Note that there has been a move away from describing results as "significant or not" based on p-values and CIs. Instead, these should be considered as measures of uncertainty

(27). Many of our results show wide CIs which cross one, so we cannot be confident about these observed associations.

Characteristic	Control, N = 239[1]	Case, N = 61[1]	OR[2]	95% CI[2]	p-value
Sex					
Female	82 (49%)	24 (65%)	–	–	
Male	85 (51%)	13 (35%)	0.52	0.24, 1.08	0.086
Unknown	72	24			
Age group					
0–4	36 (15%)	9 (15%)	–	–	
5–9	41 (17%)	16 (26%)	1.56	0.62, 4.09	0.3
10–19	49 (21%)	13 (21%)	1.06	0.41, 2.83	>0.9
20–29	63 (26%)	10 (16%)	0.63	0.23, 1.74	0.4
30–39	23 (9.6%)	4 (6.6%)	0.70	0.17, 2.41	0.6
40–49	20 (8.4%)	5 (8.2%)	1.00	0.28, 3.32	>0.9
50+	7 (2.9%)	4 (6.6%)	2.29	0.51, 9.45	0.3
Dehydration					
Moderate	113 (50%)	7 (12%)	–	–	
Severe	114 (50%)	53 (88%)	7.51	3.48, 18.7	<0.001
Unknown	12	1			
Oedema					
1	112 (47%)	32 (52%)	–	–	
0	127 (53%)	29 (48%)	0.80	0.45, 1.40	0.4

[1] n (%)

[2] OR = Odds ratio; CI = Confidence interval

Table 10.9: An example of analysis interpretation

What further analysis could you consider?
You could investigate confounding and effect modification by calculating stratified and Mantel–Haenszel (a pooled estimate from both strata) estimates, compared to crude estimates

(19). In our case, as is often the case in outbreaks, there may be insufficient data available for this; however, it may uncover associations that were previously masked. Multivariable models using regression (**Table 10.8** shows regression types) can also be used to control for the above and covariates. Note that it is no longer recommended to select variables based on statistically significant univariate associations followed by stepwise selection (28–29). When constructing a multivariable model, consider again biological plausibility and Occam's razor (or the principle of parsimony) which states that the simplest model will be the best one.

7. Draw conclusions: compare results with established facts, consider additional studies

> As the outbreak response becomes more complex, you interface with a variety of partners to interpret your epidemiological findings. You regularly monitor events such as the opening and closing of cholera treatment centres, shortages of critical personnel at health facilities, environmental and sanitation interventions, logistics updates, public education campaigns, rumour tracking, and population movements.

Alongside the quantitative data from the clinical, vaccination, and logistics arms of the response, which qualitative data may aid the outbreak response?
Qualitative information produced by interviews and surveys of healthcare workers, patients, and other stakeholders can contextualise and inform action (**See Chapter 17, Integrated outbreak analytics**). How would these pieces of information add to the conclusions you can draw from the data presented in descriptive and analytical studies?

8. Communicate findings

> As the lead local epidemiologist, you are tasked with validating, analysing, and synthesising many data streams into actionable information. You prepare daily situation reports ("sitreps") for the response coordination team; these sitreps must be succinct, informative, timely, and place recent developments in context. You further work with outreach professionals to disseminate evidence-based community health messaging and speak to policymakers to enlist their support for interventions.

What information should you include in an outbreak sitrep?
A sitrep will vary by the type and stage of the emergency, but summary statements accompanied by succinct analyses of person, time, and place trends are the minimum expectations.

How might you handle pressures from policymakers to provide clear answers on the outbreak source, trends, and risk factors?
A sitrep might not strictly adhere to scientific writing standards as communicating uncertainty in outbreak contexts can be nuanced when data quality is poor, yet decision-makers seek straightforward answers. You must find a balance that maintains scientific rigour but also provides useful interpretation.

9. Implement control and prevention measures

After the outbreak declaration, a cholera vaccination campaign begins, potable water and chlorination mechanisms are provided to affected communities, damage to infrastructure is repaired, and locally adapted communication about safety and hygiene best practices is delivered by trusted local voices. Daily new reported cases begin to decrease.

What strategies can be deployed to prepare for outbreak mass vaccination campaigns?

The WHO has published guidance on response and preparedness for cholera outbreaks (30). Routine vaccination campaigns can be opportunities to exercise systems such as cold chain and waste management.

What are the relative benefits of structural interventions as compared to person-level interventions?

Interventions which address contextual socioeconomic constraints to shift default behaviours, such as ensuring access to sanitation and healthcare services, may require more upfront investment but can have a more broad impact than individual-level interventions such as counselling (31).

10. Evaluate response, initiate or maintain surveillance

As the outbreak concludes, questions arise regarding evaluation, documentation, and adaptation of the surveillance systems.

What considerations have an impact when the outbreak is declared "over"?

Consider the incubation period of the disease, delays to reporting, and the robustness and extensiveness of the detection capabilities of your surveillance system. You might wait two or more incubation periods with no reported cases before declaring the outbreak ended.

How can you assess response performance and prepare for future outbreaks?

After-action review (AAR) conferences and reports can identify areas for improvement. Regular exercises with clear objectives can test specific response components (a drill), decision-making (a tabletop exercise), multi-agency coordination (a functional exercise), or physical mobilisation (a full-scale exercise). One common mistake is the exclusion of elected political leaders from planning and exercises.

Have you experienced or observed "burnout"? What harm can come from such overwork?

Public health is a discipline often associated with self-motivated workers, yet safety of the personnel must include considerations of overwork and mental health (32).

CONCLUSION

Field epidemiology is a demanding, thrilling, and rewarding profession. More than any complex modelling endeavour, successful epidemic and pandemic response rests upon the capability, agility, and creativity of local-level field epidemiologists. This discipline stands upon the cusp of dramatic change as scripted analytics, GIS mapping, One Health, electronic data entry, and other innovations are increasingly adopted at the ground level (33). To solidify these advancements, sustained investment in training (FETPs) and national and subnational health agencies is paramount (34). Moreover, the discourse directing such investment must centre the voices and expressed needs of frontline public health responders.

REFERENCES:

1. Koo D, Thacker SB. In Snow's footsteps: commentary on shoe-leather and applied epidemiology. Am J Epidemiol. 2010 Sep;172(6):737–9. https://doi.org/10.1093/aje/kwq252 PMID:20720100.
2. Gregg MB. Field Epidemiology. Oxford University Press; 2008. https://doi.org/10.1093/acprof:oso/9780195313802.001.0001.
3. Griffith MM, Parry AE, Housen T, Stewart T, Kirk MD. COVID-19 and investment in applied epidemiology. Bull World Health Organ. 2022 Jul;100(7):415–415A. https://doi.org/10.2471/BLT.22.288687 PMID:35813518.
4. Perrocheau A, Jephcott F, Asgari-Jirhanden N, Greig J, Peyraud N, Tempowski J. Investigating outbreaks of initially unknown aetiology in complex settings: findings and recommendations from 10 case studies. Int Health. 2023 Sep;15(5):537–46. https://doi.org/10.1093/inthealth/ihac088 PMID:36630891.
5. Snow J. On the Mode of Communication of Cholera. 2nd ed. London: John Churchill; 1855.
6. Downs J. Maladies of Empire: How Colonialism, Slavery, and War Transformed Medicine. Cambridge (Massachusetts): Harvard University Press; 2021. https://doi.org/10.2307/j.ctv3405vth.
7. Thacker SB, Dannenberg AL, Hamilton DH. Epidemic intelligence service of the Centers for Disease Control and Prevention: 50 years of training and service in applied epidemiology. Am J Epidemiol. 2001 Dec;154(11):985–92. https://doi.org/10.1093/aje/154.11.985 PMID:11724713.
8. Martin R, Fall IS. Field Epidemiology Training Programs to accelerate public health workforce development and global health security. Int J Infect Dis. 2021 Oct;110 Suppl 1:S3–5. https://doi.org/10.1016/j.ijid.2021.08.021 PMID:34518062.
9. About FETPs | TEPHINET. [cited 9 Oct 2022]. https://www.tephinet.org/about/about-fetps.
10. Rasmussen SA, Goodman RA, editors. The CDC Field Epidemiology Manual. Oxford, New York: Oxford University Press; 2019. https://doi.org/10.1093/oso/9780190933692.001.0001.
11. Outbreak investigations 10 steps, 10 pitfalls. [cited 10 Sep 2022]. https://wiki.ecdc.europa.eu/fem/Pages/Outbreak%20investigations%2010%20steps,%2010%20pitfalls.aspx.
12. World Health Organization; 2014. Early detection, assessment and response to acute public health events: implementation of early warning and response with a focus on event-based surveillance. https://apps.who.int/iris/bitstream/handle/10665/112667/WHO_HSE_GCR?sequence=1.
13. Interim Guidance Document on Cholera Surveillance; Global Task Force on Cholera Control (GTFCC) Surveillance Working Group. 2017. https://www.gtfcc.org/wp-content/uploads/2019/10/gtfcc-interim-guidance-document-on-cholera-surveillance.pdf.
14. German RR, Lee LM, Horan JM, Milstein RL, Pertowski CA, Waller MN; Guidelines Working Group Centers for Disease Control and Prevention (CDC). Updated guidelines for evaluating public health surveillance systems: recommendations from the Guidelines Working Group. MMWR Recomm Rep. 2001 Jul;50 RR-13:1–35. PMID:18634202.
15. Technical Guidelines for Integrated Disease Surveillance and Response in the WHO African Region, Booklet Two: Sections 1, 2, and 3. Brazzaville: WHO Regional Office for Africa; 2019.
16. Keating P, Murray J, Schenkel K, Merson L, Seale A. Electronic data collection, management and analysis tools used for outbreak response in low- and middle-income countries: a systematic review and stakeholder survey. BMC Public Health. 2021 Sep;21(1):1741. https://doi.org/10.1186/s12889-021-11790-w PMID:34560871.
17. Polonsky JA, Baidjoe A, Kamvar ZN, Cori A, Durski K, Edmunds WJ, et al. Outbreak analytics: a developing data science for informing the response to emerging pathogens. Philos Trans R Soc Lond B Biol Sci. 2019 Jul;374(1776):20180276. https://doi.org/10.1098/rstb.2018.0276 PMID:31104603.
18. Ryan M. World Health Organization Emergency Coronavirus Press Conference Transcript. 2020. https://www.who.int/docs/default-source/coronaviruse/transcripts/who-transcript-emergencies-coronavirus-press-conference-full-13mar2020848c48d2065143bd8d07a1647c863d6b.pdf.
19. Lash LT, VanderWeele JT. Haneuse, Sebastien, et al. Modern Epidemiology. 4th ed. Philadelphia: Lippincott Williams and Wilkins; 2021.
20. USGS The National Map: Orthoimagery. Data refreshed December, 2021. USGS.

21. Grandesso F, Allan M, Jean-Simon PS, Boncy J, Blake A, Pierre R, et al. Risk factors for cholera transmission in Haiti during inter-peak periods: insights to improve current control strategies from two case-control studies. Epidemiol Infect. 2014 Aug;142(8):1625–35. https://doi.org/10.1017/S0950268813002562 PMID:24112364.
22. Spina A, Lenglet A, Beversluis D, de Jong M, Vernier L, Spencer C, et al. A large outbreak of Hepatitis E virus genotype 1 infection in an urban setting in Chad likely linked to household level transmission factors, 2016-2017. PLoS One. 2017 Nov;12(11):e0188240. https://doi.org/10.1371/journal.pone.0188240 PMID:29176816.
23. Ebola ça Suffit Ring Vaccination Trial Consortium. The ring vaccination trial: a novel cluster randomised controlled trial design to evaluate vaccine efficacy and effectiveness during outbreaks, with special reference to Ebola. BMJ. 2015 Jul;351:h3740. https://doi.org/10.1136/bmj.h3740 PMID:26215666.
24. Horby P, Lim WS, Emberson JR, Mafham M, Bell JL, Linsell L, et al.; RECOVERY Collaborative Group. Dexamethasone in hospitalized patients with Covid-19. N Engl J Med. 2021 Feb;384(8):693–704. https://doi.org/10.1056/NEJMoa2021436 PMID:32678530.
25. Davies HT, Crombie IK, Tavakoli M. When can odds ratios mislead? BMJ. 1998 Mar;316(7136):989–91. https://doi.org/10.1136/bmj.316.7136.989 PMID:9550961.
26. Hernán MA. The hazards of hazard ratios. Epidemiology. 2010 Jan;21(1):13–5. https://doi.org/10.1097/EDE.0b013e3181c1ea43 PMID:20010207.
27. Greenland S, Senn SJ, Rothman KJ, Carlin JB, Poole C, Goodman SN, et al. Statistical tests, P values, confidence intervals, and power: a guide to misinterpretations. Eur J Epidemiol. 2016 Apr;31(4):337–50. https://doi.org/10.1007/s10654-016-0149-3 PMID:27209009.
28. Greenland S. Modeling and variable selection in epidemiologic analysis. Am J Public Health. 1989 Mar;79(3):340–9. https://doi.org/10.2105/AJPH.79.3.340 PMID:2916724.
29. Harrell FE, Harrell FE. Regression Modeling Strategies: With Applications to Linear Models, Logistic Regression, and Survival Analysis. 2nd ed. New York: Springer; 2006.
30. Cholera Outbreak Response. Field Manual. Global Task Force on Cholera Control (GTFCC) Surveillance Working Group; 2019. https://www.gtfcc.org/wp-content/uploads/2020/05/gtfcc-cholera-outbreak-response-field-manual.pdf.
31. Frieden TR. A framework for public health action: the health impact pyramid. Am J Public Health. 2010 Apr;100(4):590–5. https://doi.org/10.2105/AJPH.2009.185652 PMID:20167880.
32. Burnout: a silent crisis in global health. In: Forbes [Internet]. [cited 7 Dec 2022]. https://www.forbes.com/sites/madhukarpai/2020/07/20/burnout-a-silent-crisis-in-global-health/.
33. Bedford J, Farrar J, Ihekweazu C, Kang G, Koopmans M, Nkengasong J. A new twenty-first century science for effective epidemic response. Nature. 2019 Nov;575(7781):130–6. https://doi.org/10.1038/s41586-019-1717-y PMID:31695207.
34. Parry AE, Kirk MD, Durrheim DN, Olowokure B, Colquhoun SM, Housen T. Shaping applied epidemiology workforce training to strengthen emergency response: a global survey of applied epidemiologists, 2019-2020. Hum Resour Health. 2021 Apr;19(1):58. https://doi.org/10.1186/s12960-021-00603-1 PMID:33926469.

CHAPTER 11

THE EVOLUTION OF CONTACT TRACING

by Zheng Jie Marc Ho, Vernon Lee, and Yang Luo

Contact tracing has been a pillar of managing infectious disease outbreaks for many years. This chapter describes the instances when contact tracing is useful and the challenges faced in overwhelming contexts, such as during the COVID-19 pandemic. Many countries have developed innovative tools for minimising human resource requirements, but these can bring about new challenges. With vast amounts of data generated by contact tracing technologies, public health officials need to ensure data security and privacy in order to gain and maintain public trust in their use.

INTRODUCTION

Contact tracing has come a long way, having served as a vital component in responses to infectious disease outbreaks since the 1930s, starting with the syphilis outbreak in the U.S. (1). It is a key strategy in controlling disease transmission through early identification, risk stratification, and quarantine of exposed individuals before they become infective and spread the disease to others. During the recent COVID-19 pandemic, innovative tools emerged to facilitate contact tracing in the context of wide and rapid virus spread in an urbanised and interconnected society. However, these are not without challenges and setbacks. This chapter discusses recent experiences and provides an overview of the strengths and weaknesses of emerging contact tracing strategies.

THE EVOLUTION OF CONTACT TRACING
Conventional approaches

Traditionally, contact tracing starts with case identification and investigation by the local health authority. This involves interviewing the case to map places visited and activities undertaken within the infectious period and identifying close contacts encountered by establishing the type and duration of contact. The transmission characteristics of the pathogen in question will guide the definition of a contact. A good public health understanding of the disease would be helpful for interviewers who may need to counsel close contacts or patients. Contact tracers will be put in the position of answering questions that their subjects may have (e.g., their own prognosis, anxieties around spread to loved ones). Interviews can also be challenging; for example, contact details of the identified individuals may not always be available, especially if the contact was transient or the identities of people encountered were not clear. Some cases may be too ill to give a comprehensive description of their recent activities and interviews may need to be undertaken over multiple sessions. Contacts also may not always be reachable (e.g., those who have left the jurisdiction). Some cases or contacts may withhold information or not convey the truth in view of stigmatising behaviours or fear of implicating themselves or others (1–2), especially if illegal or inappropriate behaviour was involved.

Thereafter, the contacts traced are notified and their exposure broadly confirmed (e.g., that they were at the place of exposure at that date and time). They are provided with information regarding the disease, transmissibility and incubation periods, and next steps of action. This could be in the form of testing, quarantine, requests to reduce social interactions, monitoring for symptoms, and/or post-exposure prophylaxis. At times, for highly transmissible diseases, details of a contact's contacts are also collected ("spring-loading") to speed up disease control efforts should the person become a case. The privacy of the patient is commonly protected, and identities are not usually revealed to the contacts unless necessary. Activity maps and network linkages (**Figure 11.1**) may be employed to track movements and identify clusters. Such work, including visual diagrams showing linkages between cases (**Figure 11.2**), has been recently facilitated by using information technology platforms, which could either be bespoke or commercial off-the-shelf options.

*Date from (dd/mm/yy)	*Time from (hhmm)	*Date to (dd/mm/yy)	*Time to (hhmm)	Description of activity	*Name of places visited	Address
20/03/21	0000	21/03/21	1100	Case stayed at home, no visitors reported during this period.	Home	2 Rose Road, Singapore 111202
21/03/21	1100	21/03/21	1130	Case walked alone to Rose Road Market to buy takeaway lunch before walking home thereafter. Case wore a mask throughout and reported he did not interact with anyone during this period.	Rose Road Market	11 Rose Road, Singapore 111202
–	–	–	–	–	–	–
22/03/21	1010	22/03/21	1430	Case was at work. He worked as a waiter at XYZ Restaurant in ABC Hotel, in a team of five waiters (including case). At the start of his shift, he attended a 15-min briefing held by his supervisor (all restaurant staff on duty attended). He also reported multiple instances of casual contact (~3-5 minutes per episode) with the restaurant kitchen staff. Case wore a mask throughout his shift.	XYZ Restaurant @ ABC Hotel	2 Riverfront Road, #02-220, Singapore 123001
22/03/21	1430	22/03/21	1530	Case had his break in the Level 2 staff pantry (shared with other hotel staff). During this time, he consumed his lunch (provided by XYZ Restaurant) and rested at the pantry. One hotel security guard was reported to have been in the staff pantry from 1430hrs to 1500hrs. Case wore his mask, except while eating his lunch.	ABC Hotel	2 Riverfront Road, Level 2, Singapore 123001
22/03/21	1530	22/03/21	2000	Case resumed work (wore a mask while at work). At approximately 2000hrs, case felt feverish and reported his symptoms (37.7°C) to his supervisor, and was advised to leave work early and see a doctor (5 mins contact with supervisor).	XYZ Restaurant @ ABC Hotel	2 Riverfront Road, #02-220, Singapore 123001
–	–	–	–	–	–	–
24/03/21	1200	24/03/21	1300	Case was conveyed via MOH-arranged ambulance to Northern General Hospital. Case was warded at isolation Ward 6B, Bed 27. All ambulance and hospital staff in full PPE (goggles, N95 respirator, gown, gloves).	XYZ Restaurant @ ABC Hotel	25 Northern General Hospital Avenue, Singapore 939303

Figure 11.1: Example of an activity map for contact tracing

Although case interviews were the mainstay for contact tracing in previous outbreaks such as severe acute respiratory syndrome (SARS) and Ebola, it can be a very manual and laborious process for diseases that are highly contagious and have a high basic reproduction number (R_0) or for outbreaks that have reached immense caseloads (**See Lockdown and an overwhelmed system**). This is especially so if the disease has very short incubation periods, or if infectiousness begins early in the course of illness, including during an asymptomatic or pre-symptomatic phase. Indeed, during the COVID-19 pandemic, the absolute number of cases grew to tens of thousands per day in many countries due to these characteristics, especially for later subvariants. Manually tracking down individual contacts and conducting case interviews often involves specialised skills. Under such conditions, it was simply not practicable to conduct case interviews en masse and within the necessary very rapid turnaround time. Furthermore, it takes time to train competent personnel, and keeping a large resource pool of dedicated contact tracers on standby is not feasible. A list of key traits for contact tracers is shown in **Table 11.1**.

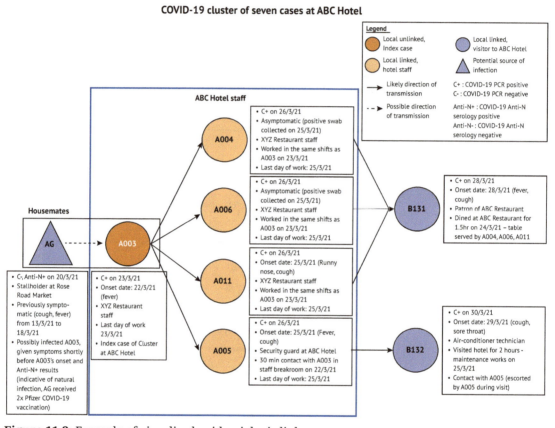

Figure 11.2: Example of visualised epidemiologic linkages

Analytical and problem-solving skills	• Adaptable to changes in processes and able to handle a range of different cases • Able to think on their feet to identify gaps and follow up accordingly • Able to think outside the box and explore different/innovative solutions (e.g., obtain a comprehensive activity map, work with difficult-to-contact stakeholders/people resistant to sharing information, overcome language barriers) • Able to analyse information obtained through contact tracing and make appropriate assessments on the recommended public health actions
Organisational skills	• Able to organise and manage large amounts of data for complete and accurate documentation of contact tracing information • Able to multi-task, including handling and following up on multiple cases concurrently

Communication and interpersonal skills	• Strong interpersonal skills (e.g., communicate in a tactful manner, exercise empathy) • Able to practise active listening and identify possible underlying issues/concerns that may affect downstream actions • Able to handle people who may be anxious, distressed, unwell, or otherwise challenging to engage with, in an assertive, polite, and professional manner • Able to engage and work closely with external agencies to coordinate actions and achieve public health objectives
Work ethics	• Able to work under time pressure for expeditious public health action implementation • Able to work independently and a good team player • Able to maintain confidentiality of information obtained during contact tracing (no unnecessary disclosure beyond what is needed for public health actions) • Dedicated (e.g., working extended hours and on weekends, when required)

Table 11.1: What makes a good contact tracer?

Lockdown and an overwhelmed system

As the number of cases surged globally in early 2020, contact tracing was unable to keep up to contain the spread of COVID-19. Many countries implemented lockdowns to bring the number of cases to manageable levels. In the U.S., lockdown measures were implemented from March–May 2020 and managed to significantly reduce transmission rates and case volume. Specific guidelines were put in place by the White House before a state could evaluate standing down such measures. These guidelines included the state's ability to provide hospital care for infected persons, conduct testing of cases, and manage overall caseloads (3). However, it was reported that many states reopened prior to meeting these guidelines, leading to concerns over resurgence. Public health and social measures must work hand-in-hand with contact tracing efforts when outbreak containment of a highly transmissible disease remains the overarching intent.

Strategies to overcome the challenges of mass contact tracing

Given the limitations of individual case and contact interviews, emerging technologies and artificial intelligence supplemented the role of contact tracing, especially during the COVID-19 pandemic. This included broader digital tools to aid in the management of case and contact data during outbreak investigations, such as Go.Data, a platform developed by WHO and GOARN partners. For example, Singapore widely utilised the Bluetooth-aided exchange of anonymised data via the government-developed *TraceTogether* mobile phone app or portable token device to record potential interactions and exposure to places with high transmission (**See Singapore's digital contact tracing strategy**). One advantage of Bluetooth is that it allows for pings with multiple devices, and the short-range service can be tailored to limit this to those within a proximity where transmission is more likely, say within a two-metre radius. It is a popular technology widely adopted for tracking purposes in many countries, and was used in systems such as *COVIDSafe* in Australia, *Stopp Corona* in Austria, and *Aarogya Setu* in India (4–5).

Aside from Bluetooth, satellite-based Global Positioning System (GPS) services have also been deployed to help with contact tracing, particularly to identify the location of users (to an accuracy of within metres in most circumstances). In Norway, GPS technology was used as an adjunct to Bluetooth via the algorithm-based app *Smittestopp*, coupling both technologies to accurately identify contacts (6). Likewise, *Rakning C-19* was an app provided by the Iceland government where GPS was used to track users' activities and movements over the preceding 14 days (6). The data was stored in the users' phones and the government could retrieve it for contact tracing purposes upon the users' agreement.

Quick response (QR) codes were another commonly used technology (4), employed at gantry points when entering and leaving a particular location. During the peak of the COVID-19 pandemic, many governments introduced a check-in (with or without a check-out) system which was conducted via scanning QR codes specific to the premises. This helped to account for visitors over a specific period and was particularly helpful for contact tracing of persons at higher risk locations (e.g., crowded, poorly ventilated places) or at "superspreading" events. Location-based contact tracing was sometimes also paired with policies to deny entry to those who posed a risk to themselves or others (e.g., unvaccinated individuals, individuals under quarantine orders, suspected or infected COVID-19 cases). In Singapore, QR codes and Bluetooth-based location check-ins were integrated with the aforementioned *TraceTogether* platform (7–8). Similarly, China employed a Health Code system developed by Alipay and WeChat (9). Residents would be required to fill up a questionnaire with their contact information and declaration of COVID-19 symptoms daily. This then generated a check-in QR code with three colours indicating varying risk of exposure, with the green code allowing entry to public spaces.

Singapore's digital contact tracing strategy during the COVID-19 pandemic

Singapore rolled out the *TraceTogether* platform (both the mobile app and tokens) during the COVID-19 pandemic (7). Tokens were issued free of charge to all residents upon request and were particularly useful for those who were not familiar with smartphones or those who did not have mobile connection services.

TraceTogether used Bluetooth technology which exchanged anonymous data with neighbouring devices and tokens, and the date and time of the exchange. This was through exchanging temporary IDs generated by encrypting a randomly assigned user ID with a private key held by the Ministry of Health (MoH). These data were stored in the user's device for a set period. Data stored on government databases were the registered user's contact number, identification details, and the user ID. Once a person contracted COVID-19, the stored data within the app or token would be shared with the MoH with the consent of the case. The individuals whom the Bluetooth contact had taken place would then be alerted to self-isolate.

TraceTogether also pulled information, such as proof of vaccination status, from central sources, which was in turn used for check in to public spaces or events either through Bluetooth or by scanning a QR code. This was primarily to reduce undue risk to unvaccinated individuals, but also supported a high adoption rate of the *TraceTogether* platform among the local population.

Mapping of contacts through genetics

Apart from technological advances, genomic studies of the SARS-CoV-2 virus provided valuable insights into the spread of COVID-19, especially when combined with epidemiologic information from contact tracing. This provided evidence of actual spread between persons and improved assessments of transmission risk in different settings. In one instance, genetic evidence in the viruses sampled from initially unlinked cases —people who had visited a poorly ventilated bar at different times—showed that there had been transmission despite a lack of direct interaction or overlapping exposure times. Similarly, an outbreak at a nursing home was initially thought to be due to resident-to-resident transmission, but disparate genomic strains suggested multiple introductions from staff or visitors. In other instances, there may be changes in single nucleotide polymorphisms (SNPs) over time and transmission directionality can be derived **(See Chapter 21, Genomics)**. This data helps sharpen the knowledge of risk factors which can allow for tailoring of public health and social measures accordingly, including prioritising resources for future contact tracing and disease control (10–11).

CHALLENGES MOVING FORWARD
Disease factors

Even with technological advancements, many governments around the world still face challenges in the prevention and control of outbreaks. During the recent COVID-19 pandemic, one challenging factor was asymptomatic and pre-symptomatic transmission of the disease, which in some studies, accounted for more than 50 per cent of all transmissions **(See Face masks mandatory)** (12). Some other diseases, such as tuberculosis and HIV, have long latencies with symptoms that may appear more insidiously.

When countries shifted to only picking up symptomatic cases, including through contact tracing, many secondary transmissions could have been missed, resulting in emerging clusters and seemingly unlinked cases. Therefore, robust approaches to detecting these other cases (e.g., testing of contacts at appropriate intervals, even if asymptomatic) are essential for a full picture. For instance, in COVID-19, to identify the asymptomatic cases, some countries introduced the polymerase chain reaction (PCR) test at the start and towards the end of contacts' quarantine. PCR tests were invasive, resource intensive, and costly, and the availability of antigen rapid tests (ARTs) **(See Antigen rapid testing)** provided a convenient alternative to testing and case detection, especially among contacts (13). For tuberculosis, contact investigations to pick up asymptomatic and latent cases often require a combination of chest radiographs, sputum smear and cultures, Mantoux skin tests, and interferon gamma release assay tests.

Face masks mandatory

In view of the increasing evidence of asymptomatic and pre-symptomatic transmissions in early 2020, the U.S. Centers for Disease Control and Prevention recommended the universal wearing of face masks. Many states and other countries followed up with face mask mandates in public spaces, especially once masking was endorsed by the World Health Organization as a means to reduce spread. This achieved a significant reduction in transmission rates of COVID-19 (14).

> Face mask studies, including epidemiological investigations showing mode of spread between cases and contacts, highlight how such studies on contact transmissions can influence strategy.

> **Antigen rapid testing and how it shaped contact tracing and management**
>
> Antigen rapid testing works by detecting traces of viral proteins. The user collects a nasal specimen and mixes it with the buffer solution before placing drops of the mixture on a lateral flow test strip. The result usually takes up to 15 minutes, allowing it to be done at point of care. ART kits could be purchased over the counter or were issued by authorities.
>
> Antigen rapid testing was widely adopted and changed the way contact management was carried out during COVID-19. For instance, some authorities encouraged daily ARTs for contacts before leaving home. Towards the end of quarantine, having a negative ART and the absence of symptoms could better ensure safety. This helped reduce the socioeconomic burden by reducing absenteeism.
>
> Although relatively good sensitivity and specificity was demonstrated, particularly if samples were taken within the first seven days of symptom onset (15), one of the downsides was false negative results that could give false assurances and allow further spread by unidentified cases. Given such leakiness, antigen rapid testing for contact management tends to be more useful in mitigation rather than in containment phases.

Population factors

In some populations, the penetration rate of smartphones, useful for contact tracing efforts, was low. For digital contact tracing platforms to be effective, sufficiently high adoption rates are needed. Users needed to own phones that could support the app, install it, keep it on in the background, allow notifications and alerts, carry the phone with them, and agree to the sharing of information with contact tracing authorities should they test positive.

In some developed countries, smartphone ownership rates are over 80 per cent. However, in countries with high population density but relatively lower smartphone penetration, contact tracing through digital tools would be less effective.

Moreover, many countries adopted a voluntary approach, which in some cases did not succeed in creating a critical mass of adoption, whether due to the inconvenience of installation, increased usage of phone data and storage, battery consumption, or concerns regarding privacy (1).

Technology factors

The overly sensitive nature of these contact tracing tools may produce false-positive detections, where brief encounters of minimal transmission risk are flagged up as potential contacts. Bluetooth signals may also ping across solid barriers that inherently prevent disease spread (e.g., through full-height walls) (16). This may lead to unnecessary anxiety and isolation of persons who are not at risk.

Apps based on GPS location services have also faced concerns with privacy (16). Some were seen as being intrusive, and that on the principle of data minimisation (elaborated below), exact locations of users were not required to establish contact. Furthermore, the accuracy of GPS signals may not be high in certain locations and situations, such as in underground tunnels or during stormy weather. GPS services tend to exhaust smartphone batteries faster, which is a potential disincentive for users.

Data storage and appropriate use issues

The generation of large amounts of data with the adoption of such contact tracing tools poses challenges related to the storage and utilisation of data and the related risks around privacy breaches.

Broadly, governments adapted centralised or decentralised approaches to the storage of contact tracing data (4,6). In centralised storage, a specific authority, usually the health ministry or the government, is granted direct access to the information. On the other hand, a decentralised model maintains storage of data with the end users themselves, usually encrypted and/or anonymous. Under conditions of potential contact, the users would be asked to release the data to the authority, whether under a mandate or as an option. This decentralised approach may offer greater privacy, a sense of control for users over their own data, and may reduce the perception of excessive state oversight. Other technologies that have helped to augment storage include big data services (e.g., health information systems that could retrieve user's updated vaccination or infection status) and the use of blockchain technology for the encryption and storage of data (5).

Data minimisation is another way to reduce privacy breach risks. This principle involves using the least amount of data needed to achieve a specific purpose, in this instance, for contact tracing. During data generation, governments or app developers may place careful considerations on the necessity of certain data fields and whether they are truly relevant to contact tracing, the period of storage of these data, and proper disclosure on the utilisation of these data to users. One concern that surfaced during the COVID-19 pandemic was whether governments would use contact tracing data for other purposes, such as the investigation of criminal activities reported in countries such as Singapore and Germany (17). Public trust in the contact tracing apps may be at risk and could be hard to regain if data were found to be used for purposes beyond the originally announced intent.

Data protection laws and policies can and should be used to enforce the need for data minimisation and delineate the usage of data collected. With these in place, users may have greater trust in the authorities on ensuring data security. This will increase the adoption of digital technology solutions for contact tracing.

CONCLUSION

The COVID-19 pandemic has led to an increased reliance on technology for contact tracing, bypassing human resource limitations posed by traditional methods of contact tracing when faced with enormous demands. In low-income countries, such technology-mediated contact tracing systems were not feasible. A challenge now is to consider how these capacities can be built globally and shared across countries in preparation for future pandemics or even outbreak responses at the national and subnational levels. We should not wait for the next emergency response before establishing how contact tracing technology can be adapted in all countries.

Where technology is implemented, health authorities will need to find ways to address the challenges outlined in this chapter, including garnering public acceptance for digital solutions, by ensuring privacy and the appropriate utilisation of data. If this can be achieved, we can be more confident that contact tracing can be scaled by orders of magnitude to enable this pillar of outbreak response to most effectively contribute its important role.

REFERENCES:

1. Brandt AM. The history of contact tracing and the future of public health. Am J Public Health. 2022 Aug;112(8):1097–9. https://doi.org/10.2105/AJPH.2022.306949 PMID:35830671.
2. Sevimli S, Sevimli BS. Challenges and ethical issues related to COVID-19 contact tracing teams in Turkey. J Multidiscip Healthc. 2021 Nov;14:3151–9. https://doi.org/10.2147/JMDH.S327302 PMID:34803383.
3. Ngonghala CN, Iboi EA, Gumel AB. Could masks curtail the post-lockdown resurgence of COVID-19 in the US? Math Biosci. 2020 Nov;329:108452. https://doi.org/10.1016/j.mbs.2020.108452 PMID:32818515.
4. Shahroz M, Ahmad F, Younis MS, Ahmad N, Kamel Boulos MN, Vinuesa R, et al. COVID-19 digital contact tracing applications and techniques: A review post initial deployments. Transp Eng. 2021 Sep;5:100072. https://doi.org/10.1016/j.treng.2021.100072.
5. Mbunge E. Integrating emerging technologies into COVID-19 contact tracing: Opportunities, challenges and pitfalls. Diabetes Metab Syndr. 2020;14(6):1631–6. https://doi.org/10.1016/j.dsx.2020.08.029 PMID:32892060.
6. Alshawi A, Al-Razgan M, AlKallas FH, Bin Suhaim RA, Al-Tamimi R, Alharbi N, et al. Data privacy during pandemics: a systematic literature review of COVID-19 smartphone applications. PeerJ Comput Sci. 2022 Jan;8:e826. https://doi.org/10.7717/peerj-cs.826 PMID:35111915.
7. TraceTogether – Community-driven contact tracing [Internet]. https://www.developer.tech.gov.sg/products/categories/digital-solutions-to-address-covid-19/tracetogether/overview.html.
8. World Health Organization. About Go.Data [Internet]. https://www.who.int/tools/godata/about.
9. Liang F. COVID-19 and health code: how digital platforms tackle the pandemic in China. Soc Media Soc. 2020 Aug;6(3):2056305120947657. https://doi.org/10.1177/2056305120947657 PMID:34192023.
10. Zella D, Giovanetti M, Cella E, Borsetti A, Ciotti M, Ceccarelli G, et al. The importance of genomic analysis in cracking the coronavirus pandemic. Expert Rev Mol Diagn. :1–16. https://doi.org/10.1080/14737159.2021.1917998.
11. Wang JT, Lin YY, Chang SY, Yeh SH, Hu BH, Chen PJ, et al. The role of phylogenetic analysis in clarifying the infection source of a COVID-19 patient. J Infect. 2020 Jul;81(1):147–78. https://doi.org/10.1016/j.jinf.2020.03.031 PMID:32277969.
12. Johansson MA, Quandelacy TM, Kada S, Prasad PV, Steele M, Brooks JT, et al. SARS-CoV-2 transmission from people without COVID-19 symptoms. JAMA Netw Open. 2021 Jan;4(1):e2035057. https://doi.org/10.1001/jamanetworkopen.2020.35057 PMID:33410879.
13. Candel FJ, Barreiro P, San Román J, Abanades JC, Barba R, Barberán J, et al. Recommendations for use of antigenic tests in the diagnosis of acute SARS-CoV-2 infection in the second pandemic wave: attitude in different clinical settings. Rev Esp Quimioter. 2020 Dec;33(6):466–84. https://doi.org/10.37201/req/120.2020 PMID:33070578.
14. Guy GP. Association of state-issued mask mandates and allowing on-premises restaurant dining with county-level COVID-19 case and death growth rates — United States, March 1–December 31, 2020. MMWR Morb Mortal Wkly Rep [Internet]. 2021 [cited 2023 Jan 17];70. https://www.cdc.gov/mmwr/volumes/70/wr/mm7010e3.htm.
15. Wang YH, Wu CC, Bai CH, Lu SC, Yang YP, Lin YY, et al. Evaluation of the diagnostic accuracy of COVID-19 antigen tests: A systematic review and meta-analysis. J Chin Med Assoc. 2021 Nov;84(11):1028–37. https://doi.org/10.1097/JCMA.0000000000000626 PMID:34596082.
16. Min-Allah N, Alahmed BA, Albreek EM, Alghamdi LS, Alawad DA, Alharbi AS, et al. A survey of COVID-19 contact-tracing apps. Comput Biol Med. 2021 Oct;137:104787. https://doi.org/10.1016/j.compbiomed.2021.104787 PMID:34482197.
17. Maras MH, Miranda MD, Scott Wandt A. The use of COVID-19 contact tracing app data as evidence of a crime. Sci Justice. 2023 Mar;63(2):158–63. https://doi.org/10.1016/j.scijus.2022.12.008 PMID:36870696.

CHAPTER 12

NON-PHARMACEUTICAL INTERVENTIONS

by Caitriona Murphy and Benjamin J. Cowling

At the start of an epidemic or pandemic, before vaccines or targeted antivirals are available, non-pharmaceutical interventions (NPIs) help to slow transmission, reducing the burden on healthcare systems. Drawing on experiences during the COVID-19 pandemic, this chapter reviews the evidence of different interventions and their possible implications. We consider four categories of interventions— personal protective measures, environmental measures, targeted response measures, and community-wide response measures.

INTRODUCTION

Non-pharmaceutical interventions (NPIs) are also known as public health and social measures (PHSMs) and play a key role in the control of emerging and re-emerging infections. NPIs such as quarantine and isolation have a long history of use in public health (1). Large-scale use of NPIs in the 1918/1919 influenza pandemic likely saved many lives in some U.S. cities, while the late application of NPIs in other cities had the opposite impact (2–3). There was a renewed interest in NPIs following the emergence of highly pathogenic avian influenza A(H5N1) in 1997, with the goal of improving the evidence base for influenza pandemic planning. However, the 2009 H1N1 influenza A pandemic had a lower health impact than the three influenza pandemics of the 20th century, and NPIs such as isolation and school closures were only used in the early months of the pandemic (4). More recently, the response to the COVID-19 pandemic in 2020 involved prolonged application of stringent NPIs intended to slow or even stop transmission. In this chapter, we review a range of NPIs and discuss their potential impact as well as some of their drawbacks. Beyond directly transmitted respiratory pathogens, NPIs also play a role in the control of many other infectious diseases, and we briefly review these at the end of the chapter. NPIs can be categorised into five groups:
- personal protective measures
- environmental measures
- targeted response measures
- community-wide response measures
- international travel measures (**See Chapter 8, Border controls**)

NPIs include measures such as community face mask use, school closures, and gathering restrictions (**Table 12.1**).

Infectious Disease Emergencies: Preparedness & Response

Category	NPIs discussed
Personal protective measures (undertaken by individuals)	• Hand hygiene • Respiratory etiquette • Face masks
Environmental measures	• Surface and object cleaning • Improving ventilation
Targeted response measures	• Isolation of sick individuals • Contact tracing • Quarantine of exposed individuals • Rapid testing
Community-wide response measures	• Physical distancing • Domestic travel restrictions • Restrictions on gatherings • School and workplace measures and closures • Stay-at-home orders
International travel-related measures	**See Chapter 8, Border controls**

Table 12.1: Categories of NPIs

NPIs are the most attainable interventions to implement at the start of an epidemic or pandemic when faced with an emerging or re-emerging disease when there is no vaccine or targeted treatment (e.g., antivirals) available. NPIs can be implemented in a community with several objectives in mind, as illustrated in **Figure 12.1**. The most common stated objective of NPIs is to "flatten the curve", i.e., to reduce the height of the peak in number of cases, likely also delaying the peak and spreading cases over a longer period of time (5).

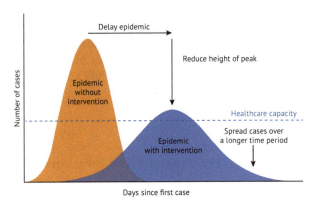

Figure 12.1: The effect of NPIs on the epidemic curve
The idea of NPIs is to "flatten the curve", reducing pressure on the healthcare system at peak. Note that delaying the epidemic could also buy more time for expansion of healthcare capacity (blue dashed line) which is not necessarily constant over time, as shown here. The "flattened" epidemic curve may not necessarily have a smaller area (total number of infections) than the unmitigated curve but spreading the infections over a longer period of time will improve patient outcomes and reduce public health impact.

In late 2019, the SARS-CoV-2 coronavirus emerged and subsequently caused a pandemic that had an enormous impact on global economies and public health. When outbreaks began worldwide, many nations responded by implementing a variety of NPIs. Wuhan was the first city to issue a stay-at-home order as well as a cordon sanitaire around the city, immobilising its 11 million residents. Food was delivered to homes and sick individuals were isolated in centralised facilities (6–7). This was implemented for 76 days and was shown to decrease the growth rate of cases (8), ultimately bringing the incidence of cases down to zero. As the pandemic progressed, bans on mass gatherings such as festivals and capacity limits for weddings were seen worldwide, aiming to reduce the number of people's social contacts. Many businesses introduced or expanded teleworking options, while critical services that remained open enhanced cleaning frequency and carried out temperature or symptom checks upon entry. To reduce social mixing further, caps were placed on the number of people who could dine together or the number of households that could interact at one time. Movement was restricted to local areas or a certain distance from the home (9). These measures were implemented alongside school closures. This sparked debate, with some arguing there was a lack of evidence on the importance of children in SARS-CoV-2 transmission. Additionally, COVID-19 severity was lowest in children aged 1–18 years (10–11).

The timing and stringency of interventions can depend on whether the goal is to eliminate or mitigate the outbreak. In the early stages of the COVID-19 pandemic, countries such as South Korea, China, Australia, New Zealand, and Singapore opted for an elimination strategy which aimed to stop transmission, reducing cases in the community to zero or close to it (12). To effectively stop or minimise transmission, timely identification and contact tracing were carried out, followed by strict isolation and quarantine. Efforts were made to increase capacity, train new personnel, and even build new testing laboratories and isolation facilities (13). These measures can be resource heavy and may not be easily enforced in nations with fewer resources. In the absence of sufficient capacity, testing resources could be concentrated towards high-risk groups such as healthcare workers and the elderly.

Mitigation strategies, on the other hand, include NPIs that aim to slow down transmission, flattening the curve as illustrated above, until population immunity is reached (14). It is not necessary to reduce the total number of cases, but the goal is rather to spread cases over a longer period to reduce pressure on the healthcare system and protect the vulnerable. In practice, measures to achieve mitigation and elimination overlap. Mitigation also relies on measures such as isolation, quarantine, ventilation, and physical distancing, but implementation may be less stringent. Ultimately, transmission could not be contained, and mitigation was the only possible approach in many settings, where surveillance was limited, a majority were living hand to mouth, or in overcrowded settings with severe resource constraints.

The success of interventions depends on human behaviour as well as the dynamics and natural history of a pathogen. Some key features to understand are the incubation period and routes of transmission of a pathogen. The length of time individuals are quarantined is determined by the incubation period of a pathogen. In some cases, due to the natural history of the disease, varying transmissibility, and healthcare settings, symptom monitoring may suffice (15). For the initial strains of SARS-CoV-2, the incubation period ranged from 5–14 days (16). Consequently, to capture all possible cases and out of an abundance of caution, some countries implemented up to 21 days of quarantine.

Compliance with NPIs drives their effectiveness, and authorities may choose between recommending or mandating measures to change human behaviours. The chosen approach depends on the severity of the epidemic, control strategy, cultural practices, and levels of social trust in the community. During the COVID-19 pandemic, compliance changed over time, and by the second wave of infections, both recommendations and mandates were more frequently disregarded, due to 'fatigue' or an erosion in public trust (17). In general, mandates will have a bigger impact on public trust. Critically, this loss of trust may not be visible immediately or in the short term but could erode trust towards public health authorities for future outbreaks.

The route of transmission informs us on whether an intervention is appropriate to reduce the spread of disease. Some interventions are capable of reducing transmissibility via specific transmission routes and not others. Multiple interventions may be implemented concurrently to target different transmission routes (18). Transmission risks may also differ across settings and consequently, so will the appropriate NPIs. During the severe acute respiratory syndrome (SARS) outbreak in 2003, disease progression was acute, viral load peaked in the second week of illness, and many cases occurred in nosocomial settings. Interventions strengthening hospital infection control were likely the most important measures in that epidemic, alongside early isolation (19). During the COVID-19 pandemic, institutions such as long-term care homes were at particular risk and NPIs, such as the use of personal protective equipment and isolation rooms and wards, formed a major part of infection control protocols in hospitals. Such measures are likely to be strengthened during pandemics. In this chapter, we specifically focus on the application and impact of NPIs in the community for infectious disease emergencies, which excluded community-based long-term care facilities.

PERSONAL PROTECTIVE MEASURES

Measures that individuals can take to protect themselves from contracting an infection include maintaining hand hygiene, good respiratory etiquette, and wearing face masks. Hand hygiene is an inexpensive and relatively straightforward measure to implement. It is well established that hand hygiene is effective in reducing diarrhoea and the spread of gastrointestinal diseases (20). What is less clear is its effect on reducing the spread of respiratory viruses. Evidence from six of eight randomised controlled trials (RCTs) assessing the efficacy of hand hygiene interventions on laboratory-confirmed influenza showed no significant effect for hand hygiene alone (21–26). Transmission routes may differ across settings and the two RCTs that did show significant effects were in primary and elementary schools, while those without effects were in households or university residential halls (27–28). Despite the variable evidence, hand hygiene is highly recommended throughout an epidemic or pandemic, due to its biological plausibility and experimental studies showing it can reduce the amount of viable virus on hands (29).

Face masks cover the nose and mouth. When worn by infectious individuals, face masks can reduce transmission through controlling the source. Masks can also provide protection for uninfected individuals by filtering the air being breathed in and reducing the frequency that individuals touch their face (30). The effectiveness of face masks to prevent the transmission of SARS-CoV-2 in the community was highly disputed leading to conflicting advice in the early stages of the pandemic (31). Some nations opted to recommend masks for indoor public spaces, while others mandated mask wearing indoors and outdoors. A number of RCTs for face masks have assessed the protective effect against influenza virus infection, and all except one trial found no statistically significant effects (32). A review carried out earlier in the COVID-19 pandemic, which included observational studies and two trials, found evidence for a 6–15 per cent reduction in the risk of infection with the use of face masks in the community setting (33). Another review of 39 studies estimated that face masks compared to no face masks would reduce the risk of infection by 14.3 per cent (95 per cent confidence interval [CI], 10.7–15.9) (34). More recently, another review assessing the comparative effectiveness of face masks in both community and healthcare settings for Middle East respiratory syndrome (MERS), SARS, and COVID-19 reported that N95 masks were the most effective, providing protection across viruses and settings (35). Even if the effects are relatively small, face masks are less disruptive for a population, and their affordability compared to other measures provides sufficient rationale for implementation (36). The acceptability of wearing masks has differed culturally in the past and achieving high uptake may be challenging in some locations (37).

ENVIRONMENTAL MEASURES

Surface and object cleaning is a widely used environmental measure, aiming to kill pathogens on objects to avoid fomite transmission. Studies have shown that cleaning can reduce the detection of respiratory viruses on surfaces and objects, but there is limited evidence that transmission is subsequently reduced (32). As cleaning reduces the microbial presence in the environment and is a simple measure to implement, it is still recommended throughout an epidemic or pandemic (29). However, indiscriminate environmental spraying or the spraying of humans using disinfection tunnels was used in some locations during the COVID-19 pandemic, without supporting evidence of its effectiveness. This was not recommended by the World Health Organization (WHO) (38) due to the possible adverse effects of exposure to the chemicals used for disinfection. Ultraviolet light is another environmental measure that has so far mainly been used in laboratory settings to kill pathogens on surfaces. It has been more difficult to implement in the community due to feasibility, cost, and possible safety concerns, although there is certainly scope for further research on this approach (29).

The importance of having an inflow of fresh air has long been recognised as a positive measure, and it is built into building regulations in many countries. These may specify a minimum ventilation rate (rate at which the volume of air in an enclosed space is replaced with outdoor air) (39). Ventilation was much discussed during the COVID-19 pandemic, especially for higher-risk settings. Indoor environments are riskier, as the concentration of SARS-CoV-2 particles will be higher indoors than outdoors (40). There is general agreement that close-range transmission plays an important role in the spread of SARS-CoV-2; however, there is a lack of consensus on the contribution of longer range (>2 m) airborne transmission in indoor environments (41). A review of 18 outbreak investigation studies for indoor community settings, such as churches, buses, and gyms, concluded that long-range transmission was likely in 16 of them and inadequate airflow may have been a contributing factor (42). However, evidence for the cost-effectiveness of directing limited resources to tackle longer range transmission is limited. Ventilation can also be undertaken for personal protection in households by opening windows and circulating fresh air where possible. In such cases, it is simple to implement and should be used.

TARGETED RESPONSE MEASURES

Some NPIs aim to reduce transmission through identifying cases and their contacts, breaking transmission chains in a targeted manner. Isolation of cases is a fundamental strategy for many infections; however, the approach to isolation varies substantially. Some locations opt for voluntary or even mandatory isolation of cases outside the home, to minimise the possibility of onward transmission in the household. However, this strategy requires the availability of isolation facilities, which have their own benefits and drawbacks (**See Community isolation facilities**). During the COVID-19 pandemic, university student residences (43), hotels, or purpose-built facilities were all used as isolation facilities (44). Many other locations recommended or mandated home isolation for durations that changed as time progressed during the pandemic. The WHO recommended a minimum isolation period of 13 days (45), though over time, many countries reduced this to 10 days or even 5 days. This was based on the growing understanding that peak infectiousness was earlier in the course of infection (46). These reductions were also about finding a balance between the risk of onward transmission and limiting societal disruption and maintaining sufficient staff in essential public services (47). As vaccination roll-out began a year into the pandemic, authorities sometimes mandated different isolation and quarantine periods for vaccinated and unvaccinated individuals (44).

One feature recognised quickly during the COVID-19 pandemic was the occurrence of pre-symptomatic transmission, as well as delays in identifying cases. As a consequence, isolation of cases sometimes had a limited impact on transmission because onward transmission had already occurred by the time the case was isolated. To "get ahead" of the virus, contact tracing can identify exposed individuals who are then recommended or mandated to quarantine themselves, reducing the chance that they spread infection further if they have been infected. Contact tracing may also aim to identify where or how a case was infected, as a way to identify clusters (**See Chapter 11, Contact tracing**). Focusing efforts on reducing the cluster can help reduce transmission and the risk of superspreading events (48). However, these tracing efforts substantially increase the number of people to be quarantined. Isolation facilities may quickly fill up if there are no concurrent measures in the community to limit transmission and therefore, infections.

While there is evidence indicating that contact tracing and quarantine are effective at reducing epidemic spread (3,49–51), these measures can be challenging to implement at scale and also have legal and ethical dimensions to consider. The principle behind isolation is very clear—hindering transmission by separating infected individuals from the susceptible population—and as such, is more easily accepted. Quarantine, on the other hand, restricts the movements of non-infectious individuals and has provoked resentment throughout history, as seen in the 1600s for a smallpox epidemic in New York (1663) or the plague in Moscow (1664) (1). Without clear scientific evidence, the perception of utility decreases and a trust deficit could be exacerbated by mandates on behaviours and movements, damaging the reserve of trust in public health actions for future epidemics. Additionally, other measures may need to be implemented to support quarantined individuals. For instance, compensating employees who are unable to work remotely is both ethical and can enhance compliance.

Community isolation facilities during the COVID-19 pandemic: learning from the Hong Kong case

The creation of community isolation facilities for the isolation of infected persons outside their home can be particularly useful for high-risk or vulnerable and marginalised populations that may be unable to isolate from home, have no home, or live in crowded homes, as is the case in Hong Kong. For the first two years of the COVID-19 pandemic, all cases were hospitalised for up to 14 days. When public hospital resources became strained in February 2022, additional facilities such as hotels or holiday camps were repurposed, and quarantine facilities that had been purpose-built for the quarantine of exposed individuals were converted to isolation facilities (52), providing isolation beds for individuals at no cost. The use of these facilities may have reduced within-household transmission, which could be particularly concerning in multi-generation households in which some individuals, if infected, were particularly vulnerable to more severe COVID-19.

While isolation facilities can be beneficial to limit community transmission, ethical concerns arose. In Hong Kong, many children under the age of ten were separated from their families during isolation and treatment, raising public concerns and possibly leading to underreporting of infections (53–54). Breaches of isolation orders led to US$ 650 fines for some. Designing, building, and operating community isolation facilities required a multidisciplinary effort and quick mobilisation of a very large number of resources (55).

As the incidence of infections in the community increased, the use of community isolation facilities in Hong Kong was restricted to families living in accommodation with just one shared bathroom for the family, while those living in multi-bathroom homes were permitted to isolate at home (56). In a future respiratory virus pandemic, the creation of community isolation facilities could be valuable to provide a minimal level of care to mild cases while reducing transmission in the community, particularly when individuals live in crowded settings or where social inequities lead vulnerable and marginalised population groups unable to protect themselves. In other parts of the world, community isolation facilities were made available for use on a voluntary basis (57–58).

Another targeted response measure is the use of rapid antigen testing (RAT), also called lateral flow tests in some locations. These point-of-care kits allow members of the community to test themselves if they are not seeking medical attention. Given the social and economic burden of stringent NPIs, mass testing using RATs can help identify mild cases occurring in the community and allow infected people to isolate themselves more quickly, helping to reduce the impact of the epidemic. This was especially advantageous during the COVID-19 pandemic as many had mild or asymptomatic cases and would not seek further healthcare or testing. Between October and November 2020, 45 counties in Slovakia implemented two rounds of mass testing using nasopharyngeal swab RATs administered by medical personnel (followed up with isolation if infected) and found a 58 per cent decrease in observed prevalence within a week (59). Despite RATs being less sensitive than polymerase chain reaction (PCR) tests, they are cheaper and take 10–15 minutes to generate a result, becoming beneficial in identifying and isolating cases in a timely manner, informing sick individuals when to stop isolating, or allowing exposed individuals exemptions from self-quarantine.

> **RATs to reduce isolation and quarantine periods**
>
> Isolation and quarantine can have considerable social costs, increasing loneliness and negatively impacting physical activity and mental health (60–62), especially over prolonged periods. RATs indicate actively contagious individuals, and so help to inform sick individuals when to stop isolating. In late December 2021, the U.K. recommended self-isolation be reduced from 10 days to 7 days if individuals tested negative via RAT on the 6th and 7th day consecutively (63). This decision was based on modelling that assessed the impact of different isolation strategies and the reduced infectious period as the pandemic progressed (63). An RCT carried out in England also estimated that daily contact testing was non-inferior to self-quarantine, indicating that the use of RATs to support self-quarantine could reduce secondary infections while also reducing the adverse effects of self-quarantine (64).

COMMUNITY-WIDE RESPONSE MEASURES

Many NPIs apply to members of the community regardless of their infection or exposure status. These include physical distancing, gathering restrictions, domestic travel restrictions, school or workplace measures, and closures. Physical distancing aims to reduce transmission by increasing the average distances between individuals, which was recommended to be at least one metre during the COVID-19 pandemic. As such, food and beverage businesses in some locations were required to implement physical distancing between tables, maintain a capacity limit, or close entirely by a designated hour. Public transport imposed physical distancing where possible, or completely banned travelling outside certain areas or regions within a country. Mass gatherings were also associated with a high risk of transmission as physical distancing is difficult to maintain in crowds and people may travel from different regions to attend (65). Activities such as music and sporting events were subsequently restricted to a decreased number of attendees or banned altogether in many locations. These restrictions tended to change with caseloads, tightening when cases were high and relaxing when they were lower. As countries began reopening, events such as concerts in some locations required negative RATs within 24 hours to reduce transmission within the event (66). A sporting event of note was the Beijing Winter Olympics that successfully avoided large community outbreaks by creating a 'bubble' or 'closed loop system' in the Olympic village. This allowed athletes to be exempt from on-arrival quarantine at the cost of daily testing requirements and restrictions to certain venues, preventing any contact with the community.

Segments of the community may have more stringent measures applied to them, due to their higher susceptibility or increased transmission risk. In particular, transmission of many respiratory viruses, such as influenza, is more frequent in school settings, and school closures have been used in past influenza pandemics to slow the spread of infections (67–68). The timing and duration of implementation is important to get right. In past epidemics, closing schools after the peak had little impact on the overall attack rates, while reopening schools contributed to transmission surges, therefore both delaying the end of the epidemic and not working to reduce the height of the epidemic peak (69–70). During the early phase of the COVID-19 pandemic, multiple studies suggested that reopening schools when transmission in the community was low and alongside other preventative measures would have a minor impact on community transmission (71). Throughout the pandemic, school closures were generally mandated regionally or nationwide in a proactive manner. However, school closures can disproportionately affect communities that are unable to learn online or which rely on schools to feed children (**See Impact of school closures**). As such, closures are likely to be accompanied by additional fiscal measures. Prolonged periods of closure might also have more negative long-term effects such as reduced exposure to other viruses which then resurge when schools reopen.

The most stringent community-wide measure is a "blanket" stay-at-home order sometimes also called a lockdown. When such measures are used, adjustments to their stringency should be updated based on continuous situational reports that may include indicators such as the healthcare capacity and local epidemiology of the epidemic or pandemic. Being the most extreme intervention, implementation should be justified by taking public health, economy, and legal aspects into consideration. Restricting a population's mobility can result in job loss, slow down the economy, and negatively impact mental health and children's education. Alternatively, a lockdown could be conceptualised as "a circuit breaker" which is implemented on a scale of weeks rather than months, long enough to break transmission chains and delay the epidemic peak, but not so long as to damage the economy. Importantly, this could be done to buy time to increase capacity for testing, contact tracing, or isolation facilities as cases will begin to increase again once a lockdown is relaxed (72–73). Strategies for lifting lockdowns differed across nations as balancing the healthcare system, access to vaccines, and social and economic factors proved challenging in various ways across different locations (74).

Impact of school closures in Italy during the COVID-19 pandemic

In early 2020, Italy was one of the first countries outside of China that experienced a major cluster of COVID-19 infections. In response, authorities closed schools nationwide, beginning March 2020, for 13 weeks followed by the summer break (75). This became one of the longest school closure periods in Europe. While the lockdown during the first wave was generally accepted, the second wave of infections ignited protests, including some by students outside their schools, demanding that the schools remain open (76). A study estimated that reopening schools in September 2020 was associated with an increase in COVID-19 cases in the community (77). This indicated that school closures had an impact on transmission, not solely due to transmission among children within schools, but also the subsequent social circumstances that come about from having schools open, including more crowded commutes and parents no longer working from home (77). Despite helping to reduce transmission in the community, school closures came at a high cost to children's education and exacerbated social inequities (78–79). In Italy, a learning loss in mathematics was estimated among primary school children post-COVID-19. This learning loss was larger among students whose parents had lower education levels (78).

Higher COVID-19 death rates were reported among minority or low-income groups in numerous countries during the pandemic, including among Non-Hispanic Black and Hispanic populations in America (80), as well as indigenous populations in New Zealand (81) and lower income areas in Chile (82). Meta-analyses have since estimated that the risk of infection was also highest among minority groups (83–84). However, they suggest that the risk of hospitalisation and death following infection was not significantly different to their majority counterparts (83–84), indicating the increased risk of infection as the main driver of disproportionate outcomes. Differential risks of infection are driven by pre-existing differences in the social determinants of health which can be exacerbated by the implementation of NPIs. For instance, individuals who were unable to work from home and worked in adverse conditions with configurations that made physical distancing impossible had a higher risk of exposure. Additionally, low wages made it challenging for them to take the recommended precautionary measures to protect themselves. This was evident in India, where a 21-day lockdown was imposed with four hours notice, causing migrant workers to lose their income and walk, in some cases, hundreds of kilometres to their home villages (85). In response, the government took several measures, such as setting up relief camps and later arranging transportation (85).

NPIS FOR OTHER INFECTIOUS DISEASES

The above-mentioned NPIs may require adaptation for pathogens with different routes of transmission. Blood-borne diseases, for example, may be contracted by intravenous drug use or high-risk sexual behaviours. Authorities could target high-risk groups and provide clean equipment for injecting drug users or promote safe sex by providing free condoms. Engagement with the community through health promotion and educational campaigns can be particularly important to drive behaviour changes in a community.

Ebola virus disease, on the other hand, spreads through direct or indirect contact with bodily fluids. Community engagement during the 2014 epidemic went beyond educational programmes, requiring a greater component of cultural competency in communications.

For vector-borne diseases, a principal intervention is to control the vector population. The use of insecticides to reduce the mosquito population has successfully prevented malaria infections (86). However, without eradication of the vector, infections will continue to persist and other concurrent interventions, such as the wide availability of mosquito nets, are also necessary (87). Both HIV and malaria have drugs to prevent disease, but there are currently no licensed vaccines for these diseases and NPIs remain the key tools available to reduce their public health burden.

NPIs utilised during the Ebola virus outbreak in West Africa

During the large Ebola virus disease epidemic in West Africa (2014–2016), targeted response measures were an important bundle of interventions to help control transmission. Case isolation and contact tracing were carried out by isolating patients in healthcare facilities, although not all regions had isolation wards and sufficient treatment capacity (88). This, as well as slow identification of cases, aided in the spread of disease. Due to the severity of the outbreak, schools closed for 6–8 months (89). This caused socioeconomic issues and led to an increase in violence and child labour (90). Interventions required working within cultural practices. In 2014, the Ministry of Health of Guinea estimated that 60 per cent of Ebola cases were linked to traditional burial practices and WHO staff in Sierra Leone approximated that 80 per cent of cases were linked to these practices (88). This insight led to the promotion of safe burial measures, including disinfecting the exterior of body bags and coffins. Community engagement was an integral part of the response strategy to aid in maintaining trust towards the public health authorities and the subsequent actions that were taken.

CONCLUSION

The COVID-19 pandemic highlighted the importance of implementing NPIs to reduce transmission, especially in its early stages, before vaccines were available. NPIs were able to alleviate pressure on healthcare systems and saved many lives. There is growing evidence that countries which implemented an elimination strategy—where feasible—were estimated to have better health and economic outcomes then those that opted for a mitigation strategy (13,91). However, an elimination strategy is difficult to sustain for long periods and is not possible for low resourced or highly interconnected countries (91). The COVID-19 pandemic was also particularly severe, and an elimination strategy may not be appropriate for respiratory viruses that have higher transmission rates or shorter infectious periods. One priority for research is to identify the best combination of measures, taking into account their cost and sustainability as well as their effectiveness for mitigation or elimination over different timescales. Optimum measures might have a lower cost and be sustainable for longer, while having a higher impact on transmission. NPIs will continue to form an integral part of pandemic preparedness plans and as their success hinges on widespread compliance, building public trust and understanding better reasons people may not comply with such measures are both important for future implementation.

REFERENCES:

1. Conti AA. Quarantine through history. International Encyclopedia of Public Health [Internet]Elsevier; 2008. pp. 454–62. https://doi.org/10.1016/B978-012373960-5.00380-4.
2. Bootsma MC, Ferguson NM. The effect of public health measures on the 1918 influenza pandemic in U.S. cities [Internet]. Proc Natl Acad Sci USA. 2007 May;104(18):7588–93. https://doi.org/10.1073/pnas.0611071104 PMID:17416677.
3. Markel H, Lipman HB, Navarro JA, Sloan A, Michalsen JR, Stern AM, et al. Nonpharmaceutical interventions implemented by US cities during the 1918-1919 influenza pandemic [Internet]. JAMA. 2007 Aug;298(6):644–54. https://doi.org/10.1001/jama.298.6.644 PMID:17684187.
4. European Centre for Disease Prevention and Control. The 2009 A(H1N1) pandemic in Europe. A review of the experience.; 2010. https://www.ecdc.europa.eu/en/publications-data/2009-ah1n1-pandemic-europe-review-experience.
5. Qualls N, Levitt A, Kanade N, Wright-Jegede N, Dopson S, Biggerstaff M, et al.; CDC Community Mitigation Guidelines Work Group. Community mitigation guidelines to prevent pandemic influenza - United States, 2017 [Internet]. MMWR Recomm Rep. 2017 Apr;66(1):1–34. https://doi.org/10.15585/mmwr.rr6601a1 PMID:28426646.
6. Chen W, Wang Q, Li YQ, Yu HL, Xia YY, Zhang ML, et al. Early containment strategies and core measures for prevention and control of novel coronavirus pneumonia in China. Zhonghua Yu Fang Yi Xue Za Zhi. 2020 Mar;54(3):239–44. https://doi.org/10.3760/cma.j.issn.0253-9624.2020.03.003 PMID:32064856.
7. Lai S, Ruktanonchai NW, Zhou L, Prosper O, Luo W, Floyd JR, et al. Effect of non-pharmaceutical interventions to contain COVID-19 in China [Internet]. Nature. 2020 Sep;585(7825):410–3. https://doi.org/10.1038/s41586-020-2293-x PMID:32365354.

8. Lau H, Khosrawipour V, Kocbach P, Mikolajczyk A, Schubert J, Bania J, et al. The positive impact of lockdown in Wuhan on containing the COVID-19 outbreak in China [Internet]. J Travel Med. 2020 May;27(3):taaa037. https://doi.org/10.1093/jtm/taaa037 PMID:32181488.
9. Guidelines for non-pharmaceutical interventions to reduce the impact of COVID-19 in the EU/EEA and the UK. 24 September 2020. ECDC: Stockholm; 2020.
10. Ladhani SN; sKIDs Investigation Team. Children and COVID-19 in schools [Internet]. Science. 2021 Nov;374(6568):680–2. https://doi.org/10.1126/science.abj2042 PMID:34735251.
11. European Centre for Disease Prevention and Control. COVID-19 in children and the role of school settings in transmission - second update. Stockholm; 2021. https://www.ecdc.europa.eu/en/publications-data/children-and-school-settings-covid-19-transmission.
12. De Foo C, Grépin KA, Cook AR, Hsu LY, Bartos M, Singh S, et al. Navigating from SARS-CoV-2 elimination to endemicity in Australia, Hong Kong, New Zealand, and Singapore [Internet]. Lancet. 2021 Oct;398(10311):1547–51. https://doi.org/10.1016/S0140-6736(21)02186-3 PMID:34619099.
13. Wu S, Neill R, De Foo C, Chua AQ, Jung AS, Haldane V, et al. Aggressive containment, suppression, and mitigation of covid-19: lessons learnt from eight countries [Internet]. BMJ. 2021 Nov;375:e067508. https://doi.org/10.1136/bmj-2021-067508 PMID:34840136.
14. OECD. Flattening the covid-19 peak: Containment and mitigation policies. 2020
15. Peak CM, Childs LM, Grad YH, Buckee CO. Comparing nonpharmaceutical interventions for containing emerging epidemics [Internet]. Proc Natl Acad Sci USA. 2017 Apr;114(15):4023–8. https://doi.org/10.1073/pnas.1616438114 PMID:28351976.
16. Xin H, Wong JY, Murphy C, Yeung A, Taslim Ali S, Wu P, et al. The incubation period distribution of coronavirus disease 2019: a systematic review and meta-analysis [Internet]. Clin Infect Dis. 2021 Dec;73(12):2344–52. https://doi.org/10.1093/cid/ciab501 PMID:34117868.
17. Franzen A, Wöhner F. Fatigue during the COVID-19 pandemic: Evidence of social distancing adherence from a panel study of young adults in Switzerland. Zia A, editor. PLoS ONE [Internet]. 2021 Dec 10;16(12):e0261276. https://doi.org/10.1371/journal.pone.0261276.
18. Leung NH. Transmissibility and transmission of respiratory viruses [Internet]. Nat Rev Microbiol. 2021 Aug;19(8):528–45. https://doi.org/10.1038/s41579-021-00535-6 PMID:33753932.
19. Liu JW, Lu SN, Chen SS, Yang KD, Lin MC, Wu CC, et al. Epidemiologic study and containment of a nosocomial outbreak of severe acute respiratory syndrome in a medical center in Kaohsiung, Taiwan [Internet]. Infect Control Hosp Epidemiol. 2006 May;27(5):466–72. https://doi.org/10.1086/504501 PMID:16671027.
20. Ehiri J, Ejere H. Hand washing for preventing diarrhoea [Internet]. Ehiri J, editor. Cochrane Database of Systematic Reviews. John Wiley & Sons, Ltd; 2003. https://doi.org/10.1002/14651858.CD004265.
21. Cowling BJ, Chan KH, Fang VJ, Cheng CK, Fung RO, Wai W, et al. Facemasks and hand hygiene to prevent influenza transmission in households: a cluster randomized trial [Internet]. Ann Intern Med. 2009 Oct;151(7):437–46. https://doi.org/10.7326/0003-4819-151-7-200910060-00142 PMID:19652172.
22. Cowling BJ, Fung RO, Cheng CK, Fang VJ, Chan KH, Seto WH, et al. Preliminary findings of a randomized trial of non-pharmaceutical interventions to prevent influenza transmission in households. Yang Y, editor. PLoS ONE [Internet]. 2008 May 7;3(5):e2101. https://doi.org/10.1371/journal.pone.0002101.
23. Larson EL, Ferng YH, Wong-McLoughlin J, Wang S, Haber M, Morse SS. Impact of non-pharmaceutical interventions on URIs and influenza in crowded, urban households [Internet]. Public Health Rep. 2010;125(2):178–91. https://doi.org/10.1177/003335491012500206 PMID:20297744.
24. Simmerman JM, Suntarattiwong P, Levy J, Jarman RG, Kaewchana S, Gibbons RV, et al. Findings from a household randomized controlled trial of hand washing and face masks to reduce influenza transmission in Bangkok, Thailand [Internet]. Influenza Other Respir Viruses. 2011 Jul;5(4):256–67. https://doi.org/10.1111/j.1750-2659.2011.00205.x PMID:21651736.
25. Stebbins S, Cummings DA, Stark JH, Vukotich C, Mitruka K, Thompson W, et al. Reduction in the incidence of influenza A but not influenza B associated with use of hand sanitizer and cough hygiene in schools: a randomized controlled trial [Internet]. Pediatr Infect Dis J. 2011 Nov;30(11):921–6. https://doi.org/10.1097/INF.0b013e3182218656 PMID:21691245.
26. Ram PK, DiVita MA, Khatun-e-Jannat K, Islam M, Krytus K, Cercone E, et al. Impact of intensive handwashing promotion on secondary household influenza-like illness in rural Bangladesh: findings from a randomized controlled trial. Doherty TM, editor. PLoS ONE [Internet]. 2015 Jun 11;10(6):e0125200. https://doi.org/10.1371/journal.pone.0125200.

27. Talaat M, Afifi S, Dueger E, El-Ashry N, Marfin A, Kandeel A, et al. Effects of hand hygiene campaigns on incidence of laboratory-confirmed influenza and absenteeism in schoolchildren, Cairo, Egypt [Internet]. Emerg Infect Dis. 2011 Apr;17(4):619–25. https://doi.org/10.3201/eid1704.101353 PMID:21470450.

28. Biswas D, Ahmed M, Roguski K, Ghosh PK, Parveen S, Nizame FA, et al. Effectiveness of a behavior change intervention with hand sanitizer use and respiratory hygiene in reducing laboratory-confirmed influenza among schoolchildren in Bangladesh: a cluster randomized controlled trial [Internet]. Am J Trop Med Hyg. 2019 Dec;101(6):1446–55. https://doi.org/10.4269/ajtmh.19-0376 PMID:31701861.

29. The World Health Organization. Non-pharmaceutical public health measures for mitigating the risk and impact of epidemic and pandemic influenza. Geneva; 2019. https://www.who.int/publications/i/item/non-pharmaceutical-public-health-measuresfor-mitigating-the-risk-and-impact-of-epidemic-and-pandemic-influenza.

30. Leung NH, Chu DK, Shiu EY, Chan KH, McDevitt JJ, Hau BJ, et al. Respiratory virus shedding in exhaled breath and efficacy of face masks [Internet]. Nat Med. 2020 May;26(5):676–80. https://doi.org/10.1038/s41591-020-0843-2 PMID:32371934.

31. The World Health Organization. Advice on the use of masks in the context of COVID-19: interim guidance, 5 June 2020. 2020. https://apps.who.int/iris/handle/10665/332293.

32. Xiao J, Shiu EY, Gao H, Wong JY, Fong MW, Ryu S, et al. Nonpharmaceutical measures for pandemic influenza in nonhealthcare settings-personal protective and environmental measures [Internet]. Emerg Infect Dis. 2020 May;26(5):967–75. https://doi.org/10.3201/eid2605.190994 PMID:32027586.

33. Brainard J, Jones NR, Lake IR, Hooper L, Hunter PR. Community use of face masks and similar barriers to prevent respiratory illness such as COVID-19: a rapid scoping review [Internet]. Euro Surveill. 2020 Dec;25(49):2000725. https://doi.org/10.2807/1560-7917.ES.2020.25.49.2000725 PMID:33303066.

34. Chu DK, Akl EA, Duda S, Solo K, Yaacoub S, Schünemann HJ, et al.; COVID-19 Systematic Urgent Review Group Effort (SURGE) study authors. Physical distancing, face masks, and eye protection to prevent person-to-person transmission of SARS-CoV-2 and COVID-19: a systematic review and meta-analysis [Internet]. Lancet. 2020 Jun;395(10242):1973–87. https://doi.org/10.1016/S0140-6736(20)31142-9 PMID:32497510.

35. Kim MS, Seong D, Li H, Chung SK, Park Y, Lee M, et al. Comparative effectiveness of N95, surgical or medical, and non-medical facemasks in protection against respiratory virus infection: a systematic review and network meta-analysis [Internet]. Rev Med Virol. 2022 Sep;32(5):e2336. https://doi.org/10.1002/rmv.2336 PMID:35218279.

36. Cowling BJ, Leung GM. Face masks and COVID-19: don't let perfect be the enemy of good [Internet]. Euro Surveill. 2020 Dec;25(49):2001998. https://doi.org/10.2807/1560-7917.ES.2020.25.49.2001998 PMID:33303063.

37. Lu JG, Jin P, English AS. Collectivism predicts mask use during COVID-19 [Internet]. Proc Natl Acad Sci USA. 2021 Jun;118(23):e2021793118. https://doi.org/10.1073/pnas.2021793118 PMID:34016707.

38. The World Health Organization. Cleaning and disinfection of environmental surfaces in the context of COVID-19. 2020. https://www.who.int/publications-detail/cleaning-and-disinfection-of-environmental-surfaces-inthe-context-of-covid-19.

39. Nejc Brelih and Olli Seppänen. Ventilation rates and IAQ in European standards and national regulations Brussels, Belgium. 2011. https://www.aivc.org/sites/default/files/1a5.pdf.

40. Centers for Disease Control and Prevention. Ventilation in buildings. 2021. https://www.cdc.gov/coronavirus/2019-ncov/community/ventilation.html.

41. Dancer SJ. Airborne SARS-CoV-2 [Internet]. BMJ. 2022 Jun;377:o1408. https://doi.org/10.1136/bmj.o1408 PMID:35768134.

42. Duval D, Palmer JC, Tudge I, Pearce-Smith N, O'Connell E, Bennett A, et al. Long distance airborne transmission of SARS-CoV-2: rapid systematic review [Internet]. BMJ. 2022 Jun;377:e068743. https://doi.org/10.1136/bmj-2021-068743 PMID:35768139.

43. Quezon City Government Philippines. QC to transform buildings to isolation facilities. 2021. https://quezoncity.gov.ph/qc-to-transform-buildings-to-isolation-facilities/.

44. De Foo C, Haldane V, Jung AS, Grépin KA, Wu S, Singh S, et al. Isolation facilities for covid-19: towards a person centred approach [Internet]. BMJ. 2022 Jul;378:e069558. https://doi.org/10.1136/bmj-2021-069558 PMID:35882391.

45. The World Health Organization. Criteria for releasing COVID-19 patients from isolation. 2020. https://www.who.int/news-room/commentaries/detail/criteria-for-releasing-covid-19-patients-from-isolation.

46. Centres for Disease Control and Prevention. CDC updates and shortens recommended isolation and quarantine period for general population. 2021. https://www.cdc.gov/media/releases/2021/s1227-isolation-quarantine-guidance.html.
47. Mahase E. Covid-19: is it safe to reduce the self-isolation period? [Internet]. BMJ. 2021 Dec;375(3164):n3164. https://doi.org/10.1136/bmj.n3164 PMID:34969702.
48. Adam DC, Wu P, Wong JY, Lau EH, Tsang TK, Cauchemez S, et al. Clustering and superspreading potential of SARS-CoV-2 infections in Hong Kong [Internet]. Nat Med. 2020 Nov;26(11):1714–9. https://doi.org/10.1038/s41591-020-1092-0 PMID:32943787.
49. Dighe A, Cattarino L, Cuomo-Dannenburg G, Skarp J, Imai N, Bhatia S, et al. Response to COVID-19 in South Korea and implications for lifting stringent interventions [Internet]. BMC Med. 2020 Oct;18(1):321. https://doi.org/10.1186/s12916-020-01791-8 PMID:33032601.
50. Bushman M, Worby C, Chang HH, Kraemer MU, Hanage WP. Transmission of SARS-CoV-2 before and after symptom onset: impact of nonpharmaceutical interventions in China [Internet]. Eur J Epidemiol. 2021 Apr;36(4):429–39. https://doi.org/10.1007/s10654-021-00746-4 PMID:33881667.
51. Ali ST, Wang L, Lau EH, Xu XK, Du Z, Wu Y, et al. Serial interval of SARS-CoV-2 was shortened over time by nonpharmaceutical interventions [Internet]. Science. 2020 Aug;369(6507):1106–9. https://doi.org/10.1126/science.abc9004 PMID:32694200.
52. The Government of the Hong Kong Special Administrative Region. Government signed co-operation agreement for eight projects to construct community isolation and treatment facilities. 2022. https://www.info.gov.hk/gia/general/202202/24/P2022022400742.htm.
53. The Government of the Hong Kong Special Administrative Region. SB's response to media enquiries on community isolation facilities (with photos). 2022. https://www.info.gov.hk/gia/general/202203/07/P2022030700027.htm.
54. Sun F. 'Up to 2,000 children under age 10 separated from parents in Hong Kong hospitals over past 6 weeks after catching Covid-19'. South China Morning Post. 2022. https://www.scmp.com/news/hong-kong/health-environment/article/3172180/2000-children-under-age-10-separated-parents-hong.
55. South China Morning Post. The billions spent on isolation facilities in Hong Kong must not go to waste. 2023. https://www.scmp.com/comment/opinion/article/3209176/billions-spent-isolation-facilities-hong-kong-must-not-go-waste.
56. Tsang J. Coronavirus Hong Kong: who is eligible for home quarantine and how does it work? All you need to know about the new isolation rules for close contacts. South China Morning Post. 2022. https://www.scmp.com/news/hong-kong/health-environment/article/3166238/coronavirus-hong-kong-who-eligible-home.
57. Zweig SA, Zapf AJ, Beyrer C, Guha-Sapir D, Haar RJ. Zweig SA, Zapf AJ, Beyrer C, Guha-Sapir D, Haar RJ. Ensuring rights while protecting health: the importance of using a human rights approach in implementing public health responses to COVID-19. Health Hum Rights. 2021 Dec;23(2):173–86. PMID:34966234.
58. Public Health Agency of Canada. Government of Canada announces funding for new COVID-19 safe voluntary isolation centre in Ottawa, Ontario. 2020. https://www.canada.ca/en/public-health/news/2020/12/government-of-canada-announces-funding-for-new-covid-19-safe-voluntary-isolation-centre-in-ottawa-ontario.html.
59. Pavelka M, Van-Zandvoort K, Abbott S, Sherratt K, Majdan M, Jarčuška P, et al.; CMMID COVID-19 working group; Inštitút Zdravotných Analýz. The impact of population-wide rapid antigen testing on SARS-CoV-2 prevalence in Slovakia [Internet]. Science. 2021 May;372(6542):635–41. https://doi.org/10.1126/science.abf9648 PMID:33758017.
60. Butterworth P, Schurer S, Trinh TA, Vera-Toscano E, Wooden M. Effect of lockdown on mental health in Australia: evidence from a natural experiment analysing a longitudinal probability sample survey [Internet]. Lancet Public Health. 2022 May;7(5):e427–36. https://doi.org/10.1016/S2468-2667(22)00082-2 PMID:35461593.
61. Yamamoto T, Uchiumi C, Suzuki N, Sugaya N, Murillo-Rodriguez E, Machado S, et al. Mental health and social isolation under repeated mild lockdowns in Japan [Internet]. Sci Rep. 2022 May;12(1):8452. https://doi.org/10.1038/s41598-022-12420-0 PMID:35589930.
62. Stockwell S, Trott M, Tully M, Shin J, Barnett Y, Butler L, et al. Changes in physical activity and sedentary behaviours from before to during the COVID-19 pandemic lockdown: a systematic review [Internet]. BMJ Open Sport Exerc Med. 2021 Feb;7(1):e000960. https://doi.org/10.1136/bmjsem-2020-000960 PMID:34192010.
63. UK Health Security Agency. Using lateral flow tests to reduce the self-isolation period. 2022. https://ukhsa.blog.gov.uk/2022/01/01/using-lateral-flow-tests-to-reduce-the-self-isolation-period/.

64. Love NK, Ready DR, Turner C, Verlander NQ, French CE, Martin AF, et al. Daily use of lateral flow devices by contacts of confirmed COVID-19 cases to enable exemption from isolation compared with standard self-isolation to reduce onward transmission of SARS-CoV-2 in England: a randomised, controlled, non-inferiority trial [Internet]. Lancet Respir Med. 2022 Nov;10(11):1074–85. https://doi.org/10.1016/S2213-2600(22)00267-3 PMID:36228640.
65. Centres for Disease Control and Prevention. Interim guidance: get your mass gatherings or large community events ready for Coronavirus Disease 2019 (COVID-19). 2020. https://ncs4.usm.edu/pdf/covid-resources/cdc-interim-guidance.pdf.
66. Revollo B, Blanco I, Soler P, Toro J, Izquierdo-Useros N, Puig J, et al. Same-day SARS-CoV-2 antigen test screening in an indoor mass-gathering live music event: a randomised controlled trial [Internet]. Lancet Infect Dis. 2021 Oct;21(10):1365–72. https://doi.org/10.1016/S1473-3099(21)00268-1 PMID:34051886.
67. Chu Y, Wu Z, Ji J, Sun J, Sun X, Qin G, et al. Effects of school breaks on influenza-like illness incidence in a temperate Chinese region: an ecological study from 2008 to 2015 [Internet]. BMJ Open. 2017 Mar;7(3):e013159. https://doi.org/10.1136/bmjopen-2016-013159 PMID:28264827.
68. Chowell G, Towers S, Viboud C, Fuentes R, Sotomayor V. Rates of influenza-like illness and winter school breaks, Chile, 2004-2010 [Internet]. Emerg Infect Dis. 2014 Jul;20(7):1203–7. https://doi.org/10.3201/eid2007.130967 PMID:24963800.
69. Fong MW, Gao H, Wong JY, Xiao J, Shiu EY, Ryu S, et al. Nonpharmaceutical measures for pandemic influenza in nonhealthcare settings-social distancing measures [Internet]. Emerg Infect Dis. 2020 May;26(5):976–84. https://doi.org/10.3201/eid2605.190995 PMID:32027585.
70. Jackson C, Vynnycky E, Hawker J, Olowokure B, Mangtani P. School closures and influenza: systematic review of epidemiological studies [Internet]. BMJ Open. 2013 Feb;3(2):e002149. https://doi.org/10.1136/bmjopen-2012-002149 PMID:23447463.
71. Walsh S, Chowdhury A, Braithwaite V, Russell S, Birch JM, Ward JL, et al. Do school closures and school reopenings affect community transmission of COVID-19? A systematic review of observational studies [Internet]. BMJ Open. 2021 Aug;11(8):e053371. https://doi.org/10.1136/bmjopen-2021-053371 PMID:34404718.
72. Rawson T, Huntingford C, Bonsall MB. Temporary "circuit breaker" lockdowns could effectively delay a COVID-19 second wave infection peak to early spring [Internet]. Front Public Health. 2020 Dec;8:614945. https://doi.org/10.3389/fpubh.2020.614945 PMID:33365299.
73. Wilder-Smith A, Bar-Yam Y, Fisher D. Lockdown to contain COVID-19 is a window of opportunity to prevent the second wave [Internet]. J Travel Med. 2020 Aug;27(5):taaa091. https://doi.org/10.1093/jtm/taaa091 PMID:32478396.
74. Han E, Tan MM, Turk E, Sridhar D, Leung GM, Shibuya K, et al. Lessons learnt from easing COVID-19 restrictions: an analysis of countries and regions in Asia Pacific and Europe [Internet]. Lancet. 2020 Nov;396(10261):1525–34. https://doi.org/10.1016/S0140-6736(20)32007-9 PMID:32979936.
75. United Nations Educational Scientific and Cultural Organization. COVID-19 Education Response. 2022. https://covid19.uis.unesco.org/global-monitoring-school-closures-covid19/country-dashboard/.
76. Giuffrida A. Italian children take lessons outside school in protest at Covid closures. The Guardian. 2020. https://www.theguardian.com/world/2020/nov/21/italian-protests-covid-school-closures-anita-iacovelli-turin.
77. Alfano V, Ercolano S. Back to school or … back to lockdown? The effects of opening schools on the diffusion of COVID-19 in Italian regions [Internet]. Socioecon Plann Sci. 2022 Aug;82:101260. https://doi.org/10.1016/j.seps.2022.101260 PMID:35197654.
78. Contini D, Di Tommaso ML, Muratori C, Piazzalunga D, Schiavon L. The COVID-19 pandemic and school closure: learning loss in mathematics in primary education. SSRN Journal [Internet]. 2022. http://dx.doi.org/10.2139/ssrn.4114323.
79. Scarpellini F, Segre G, Cartabia M, Zanetti M, Campi R, Clavenna A, et al. Distance learning in Italian primary and middle school children during the COVID-19 pandemic: a national survey [Internet]. BMC Public Health. 2021 Jun;21(1):1035. https://doi.org/10.1186/s12889-021-11026-x PMID:34078328.
80. Centers for Disease Control and Prevention (CDC). Health disparities: provisional death counts for COVID-19, Race and Hispanic origin. https://www.cdc.gov/nchs/nvss/vsrr/covid19/health_disparities.htm.
81. Manatū Hauora Ministry of Health. COVID-19 mortality in Aotearoa New Zealand: inequities in risk. 2022. https://www.health.govt.nz/publication/covid-19-mortality-aotearoa-new-zealand-inequities-risk.

82. Gozzi N, Tizzoni M, Chinazzi M, Ferres L, Vespignani A, Perra N. Estimating the effect of social inequalities on the mitigation of COVID-19 across communities in Santiago de Chile [Internet]. Nat Commun. 2021 Apr;12(1):2429. https://doi.org/10.1038/s41467-021-22601-6 PMID:33893279.

83. Pan D, Sze S, Irizar P, George N, Chaka A, Lal Z, et al. Are clinical outcomes from COVID-19 improving in ethnic minority groups? [Internet]. EClinicalMedicine. 2023 Jul;61:102091. https://doi.org/10.1016/j.eclinm.2023.102091 PMID:37483547.

84. Agyemang C, Richters A, Jolani S, Hendriks S, Zalpuri S, Yu E, et al. Ethnic minority status as social determinant for COVID-19 infection, hospitalisation, severity, ICU admission and deaths in the early phase of the pandemic: a meta-analysis [Internet]. BMJ Glob Health. 2021 Nov;6(11):e007433. https://doi.org/10.1136/bmjgh-2021-007433 PMID:34740916.

85. Agoramoorthy G, Hsu MJ. How the coronavirus lockdown impacts the impoverished in India [Internet]. J Racial Ethn Health Disparities. 2021 Feb;8(1):1–6. https://doi.org/10.1007/s40615-020-00905-5 PMID:33104967.

86. The World Health Organization. Global Malaria Programme, vector control. 2023. https://www.who.int/teams/global-malaria-programme/prevention/vector-control#:~:text=From%202000%20through%202020%2C%20the,2010%20to%202.6%25%20in%202020.

87. Killeen GF, Tatarsky A, Diabate A, Chaccour CJ, Marshall JM, Okumu FO, et al. Developing an expanded vector control toolbox for malaria elimination [Internet]. BMJ Glob Health. 2017 Apr;2(2):e000211. https://doi.org/10.1136/bmjgh-2016-000211 PMID:28589022.

88. The World Health Organization. Factors that contributed to undetected spread of the Ebola virus and impeded rapid containment. 2015. https://www.who.int/news-room/spotlight/one-year-into-the-ebola-epidemic/factors-that-contributed-to-undetected-spread-of-the-ebola-virus-and-impeded-rapid-containment.

89. The World Bank. Back to school after the Ebola outbreak. 2015. https://www.worldbank.org/en/news/feature/2015/05/01/back-to-school-after-ebola-outbreak.

90. Chavez Villegas C, Peirolo S, Rocca M, Ipince A, Bakrania S. Impacts of health-related school closures on child protection outcomes: A review of evidence from past pandemics and epidemics and lessons learned for COVID-19 [Internet]. Int J Educ Dev. 2021 Jul;84:102431. https://doi.org/10.1016/j.ijedudev.2021.102431 PMID:34025016.

91. Oliu-Barton M, Pradelski BS, Algan Y, Baker MG, Binagwaho A, Dore GJ, et al. Elimination versus mitigation of SARS-CoV-2 in the presence of effective vaccines [Internet]. Lancet Glob Health. 2022 Jan;10(1):e142–7. https://doi.org/10.1016/S2214-109X(21)00494-0 PMID:34739862.

CHAPTER 13

ONE HEALTH: THE ANIMAL-HUMAN INTERFACE

by Sai Arathi Parepalli, Archith Kamath, John S. Mackenzie, and Mahmudur Rahman

---

Infectious diseases can move to human populations from an animal reservoir. Recognising and acting upon the factors that drive such spillover events can prevent the sorts of human infections of individuals we see with avian influenza H5N1 or pandemics such as the plague, H1N1 influenza, Middle East respiratory syndrome (MERS), severe acute respiratory syndrome (SARS), and COVID-19. Understanding the natural and man-made influences that promote zoonotic infections in humans and defining interventions are known as the One Health approach.

INTRODUCTION

A 2008 report estimated that around 60 per cent of emerging human infections are zoonotic in origin, reinforcing the role of the animal-human interface and the impact of their shared environment in infectious disease outbreaks (1).

> **Definition:**
> **One Health** is an integrated, unifying approach that aims to sustainably balance and optimise the health of people, animals, and ecosystems. It recognises that the health of humans, domestic and wild animals, plants, and the wider environment (including ecosystems) are closely linked and interdependent.
>
> The approach mobilises multiple sectors, disciplines, and communities at varying levels of society to work together to foster well-being and tackle threats to health and ecosystems, while addressing the collective need for healthy food, water, energy, and air, taking action on climate change, and contributing to sustainable development.
>
> **Key underlying principles include:**
> - **equity** between sectors and disciplines
> - sociopolitical and multicultural **parity** (the doctrine that all people are equal and deserve equal rights and opportunities) and inclusion and engagement of communities and marginalised voices
> - socioecological **equilibrium** that seeks a harmonious balance between human–animal–environment interaction and acknowledging the importance of biodiversity, access to sufficient natural space and resources, and the intrinsic value of all living things within the ecosystem
> - **stewardship** and the responsibility of humans to change behaviour and adopt sustainable solutions that recognise the importance of animal welfare and the integrity of the whole ecosystem, thus securing the well-being of current and future generations

- **transdisciplinarity** and multisectoral collaboration, which includes all relevant disciplines, both modern and traditional forms of knowledge, and a broad representative array of perspectives

Figure 13.1: One Health definition and key underlying principles
The new revised One Health definition, as per the One Health High-Level Expert Panel in June 2022. (adapted from Adisasmito WB, Almuhairi S, Behravesh CB, Bilivogui P, Bukachi SA, et al. One Health: a new definition for a sustainable and healthy future. PLoS Pathog. 2022;18(6):e1010537)

'Zoonotic spillover' is the term used to describe the transmission of pathogens between different species, typically from vertebrate animals to humans, whereas the reverse (pathogen moving from human to animal) is referred to as 'spillback' or 'reverse zoonosis'. The transfer of pathogen from reservoir to recipient host can occur directly (such as via an animal lick or bite, through manipulation of viscera, raw meat, or blood, or through an intermediate host, such as a flea) or indirectly (mediated through the environment) (2). The process of zoonotic spillover can be thought of as a consequence of two functional phases, pre-emergence and emergence, including spillover and subsequent widespread transmission. Scrutinisation of each phase through a One Health lens allows us to better appreciate the interaction of factors, their effect on spillover events, and how investigating each stage can impact outbreak source identification and control.

With an increasing appreciation of the animal-human interface, projects such as the U.S. Agency for International Development's (USAID) Pandemic Preparedness for Global Health Security (PREDICT) have been established in the last two decades to integrate disciplines and investigative efforts to detect zoonotic threats with a potential global threat. A One Health approach is utilised by bringing together experts in specialties including wildlife ecology, epidemiology, genetics, virology, informatics, and veterinary medicine. The project uses predictive modelling to identify regions and wildlife hosts that are most likely to propagate the next emerging zoonosis. Within these regions, polymerase chain reaction (PCR) testing with high throughput screening is used to detect known and novel pathogens. This system has identified over 900 novel viruses. This information is then used to build the infrastructure to combat emerging zoonoses at a local level in collaboration with country governments and USAID's Emerging Pandemic Threats programme partners (1). The integration of disciplines has enabled seamless control of zoonoses across the phases of spillover.

PRE-EMERGENCE

In this first phase, the focus is on the degree of human disease risk posed by a zoonotic pathogen whilst within its natural reservoir, and the kind of interactions between reservoir and recipient host that could result in zoonotic spillover. Many factors determine the degree of risk, including how easy it is for a pathogen to infect humans, the dynamics of its movement within and release from reservoir hosts, and the potential for exposure to humans at any given point in space and time. Patterns of animal host distribution within the environment, interactions with other species, and pathogen shedding determine the geographical spread of the pathogen, and so the possible risk posed by proximity to humans. The amount of time a pathogen can survive in the environment, an intermediate host, or a vector further impacts the likelihood of spillover to humans. These factors are all influenced by human and ecosystem-related factors which may increase the risk of interaction. The One Health approach encourages an integrated understanding of all these factors and is crucial in attempting to prevent spillovers from happening, rather than managing outbreaks after this stage (3).

Zoonotic pathogen reservoirs

The core strategy in target surveillance strategies is identifying organisms capable of zoonotic disease. A recent study found that species richness of animal groups was proportional to the observed number of zoonoses. Bats and rodents were found to exhibit the greatest species richness, helping to explain their importance as zoonotic reservoirs (4). Furthermore, animal hosts phylogenetically similar to humans are more likely to support transmissible pathogens. Upon analysis of 420 virus-mammal associations, including 67 zoonotic viruses and 278 mammalian hosts, a higher risk of spillover was associated with greater phylogenetic proximity. This is likely due to similarities in physiology and cellular and receptor similarity. Notably however, the authors found that phylogenetically similar animal reservoirs hosted zoonotic pathogens with less associated human morbidity and mortality (5).

Rich biodiverse ecosystems help to avoid spillover. A balance of animal species, those that can host a pathogen and those that do not, dilutes the chance of spillover events (6) (**See The dilution effect**). Areas with decreasing biodiversity flag a potential increase in subsequent zoonotic risk. This is known as the dilution effect.

The dilution effect

The West Nile virus (WNV) in the U.S. primarily replicates within birds and spreads between hosts through mosquito vectors. As the number of infected birds increases within a population, the chance of mosquito vectors incidentally infecting humans also increases.

In 1999, WNV was observed in the U.S., with the first WNV human epidemic occurring in 2002. Counties with greater avian diversity were associated with a lower incidence of human infection. Many mechanisms have been associated with higher host diversity, including a reduced transmission of disease to vectors, and from infected vectors to hosts, as well as a reduction in the number of susceptible hosts (7).

Biogeographic analysis, combined with knowledge of areas lacking in public health infrastructure and other socioeconomic, environmental, and ecological factors, has allowed identification of specific regions that would benefit from being the focus of surveillance strategies (1). These include parts of Asia and Equatorial Africa.

Conditions promoting spillover

Conditions that facilitate increased contact between species also carry greater zoonotic disease potential. New modes of mixing of species can expose pathogens to novel host types, allowing host switching events and, with progressive exposure to the new host, may lead to pathogens acquiring traits that sustain transmission within the new species (8). Such conditions also enable viral reassortment, a phenomenon describing genetic recombination through co-infection of a vessel with multiple viral strains, as seen in influenza outbreaks (9). Contexts with such animal-dense conditions include live-animal markets (or wet markets) and intensive livestock farming. Identification of geographical hotspots will help ensure surveillance is resource effective. Epidemiological studies following spillover can characterise outbreaks and provide an insight into the behavioural and environmental factors aligning as pathogens switch to human hosts (**Table 13.1**).

Factors defining spillover		Established examples
Land use change		Deforestation/reforestation, intensive agriculture, encroachment of human settlements on to wildlife habitats
Environmental change		Flood, drought, weather extremes, global warming
Human behaviour	Cultural	Wild/domestic animal capture, trade, production/handling, and consumption
	Social	Breakdown of or inadequate public health measures, war or civil conflict, humanitarian emergencies, international travel
	Industry	Overuse of pesticides and antibiotics, poor stewardship of antibiotics, globalisation of trade, pollution
Demographic		Poor sanitation, housing, increased population growth and overcrowding, poverty
Human host susceptibility		Immunocompromised states (e.g., concurrent infection, poor health)
Microbial adaptation		Evolution of pathogens naturally or accelerated as a result of factors above; greater species richness resulting in greater zoonoses

Table 13.1: Drivers of spillover
Both ecological and anthropogenic factors can place humans at an increased risk of contracting zoonotic pathogens. These factors can impact ecosystem health, encourage novel human and animal interactions, and create favourable host environments.

Anthropogenic change has a significant effect on ecosystem health and can give rise to zoonoses. As humans and animals are pushed closer together and the pre-existing balance of ecosystems is challenged, spillover events can increase.

Land use changes create opportunity for more competent pathogens to exist and transmit to new species (10). Anthropogenic change, and its effects on biodiversity, can impact spillover; these factors can therefore serve as indications of potential infectious disease emergence hotspots. Deforestation and agricultural expansion saw the destruction of bat habitats in Australia. The movement of bat colonies closer to livestock and humans in urban and periurban areas is thought to have led to an emergence of bat-associated viruses, such as the Hendra, Lyssa, and Menangle viruses (11).

Behaviours that alter patterns of contact between animals and humans can also affect zoonoses. Different methods of handling meat, the presence of wet markets for trade in animals, and hunting or poaching all increase our exposure to a variety of different species and, with that, different pathogens. Intensive agriculture is increasing worldwide and is driven by the demands of urbanisation and population growth. The closer proximity of bats and pigs is a key example of the consequences of these pressures (**See One Health approaches**). In addition to creating favourable environments for pathogen host switching and variants of risk to humans, there is an increased risk of transmission to humans interacting with this animal population (12).

Temperature, rainfall, and humidity can affect the migration patterns and behaviour of animals, including reservoir hosts, recipients, and intermediate hosts. Once a pathogen enters the environment, the risk of recipient infection is further modified by factors such as wind speed and humidity. For example, Hendra virus excretion in horse paddocks was found to be related to temperature and potential evaporation. Minor changes, such as the length of grass, changed the microclimate in which these viruses operated and influenced transmission risk (13).

Climate change has brought new pressures, challenging normal patterns and modifying the natural risk of spillover events (**Figure 13.2**). A systematic review assessing the impact of climate anomalies in Latin America and the Caribbean found that extreme events, including long periods of drought or extreme rainfall, can alter rodent populations. As rodents host the hantavirus, human hantavirus infection rates are affected by climate. Investigation of spillover events in regions affected by environmental disturbance, secondary to climate change, can be of value in targeting surveillance and management strategies (14).

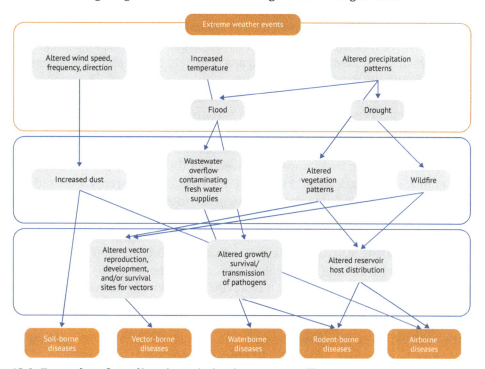

Figure 13.2: Examples of geoclimatic variation impact on spillover
A few of the geoclimatic disturbances resulting from climate change are explored. As seen, interactions are complex and downstream consequences can interact with each other.
(adapted from Rupasinghe R, Chomel BB, Martínez-López B. Climate change and zoonoses: a review of the current status, knowledge gaps, and future trends. Acta Trop. 2022 Feb;226:106225)

SPILLOVER AND TRANSMISSION

As discussed above, the recognition of zoonotic risk in particular settings, and watchfulness for localised cases, is the first level of outbreak investigation. When infections emerge, the risk of subsequent amplification increases the stakes. Once zoonotic spillover has occurred and is confirmed, two mechanisms can enable disease amplification: spread among the human population through human-to-human transmission (as with COVID-19) or establishment of a highly competent vector. Without these mechanisms, 'dead-end spillover' occurs, and the pathogen is unable to spread further than its recipient host. For example, mosquito vectors do not carry the yellow fever virus after biting humans infected by the virus.

Confirming a spillover event

Effective interventions after spillover initially rely on early detection of high-risk outbreaks. Early warning systems, such as the Human Animal Infections and Risk Surveillance (HAIRS) group in the U.K. (15), allow for detection of emerging risks prior to their amplification. This system combines reporting from a wide range of organisations, such as the Food Standards Agency and Department of Agriculture. Surveillance can be disease-specific, in which high-risk pathogens are monitored for outbreak potential, syndromic, in which non-specific health data (e.g., school absenteeism, nurse calls) are surveyed for indicators of outbreak, or event-based, in which specific alerts are investigated further (16) (**See Chapter 9, Surveillance**). This local and national level data can be formally shared between global stakeholders through established networks. The Global Public Health Intelligence Network (GPHIN) (17), a World Health Organization (WHO) electronic public health early warning system, monitors internet media in nine languages to help detect potential disease or other health threats around the world.

Identification of the causative pathogen relies on laboratory capacity and diagnostic techniques, access to which remains challenging in resource-limited areas (18) (**See Chapter 19, Laboratory capacity**). Microbiological diagnostic techniques within both human and animal populations have helped characterise filoviral outbreaks. Quick testing of primary cases of Marburg infection in young male miners allowed identification of the infection site at the Goroumbwa mine, Democratic Republic of the Congo (DRC). Vertebrate tissue and arthropod suspensions from the mine's fauna were analysed for filoviral proteins using reverse transcription-PCR (RT-PCR) which helped identify the natural reservoirs of the virus, insectivorous and fruit bats (19). Similarly, a study testing small vertebrate samples collected during the 2003 Ebola virus disease (EBOD) outbreak in Gabon and the DRC showed asymptomatic infection in three species of fruit bat (20). Serological surveys supported this finding and showed that a species of bat, implicated in being a reservoir, lives close to human settlements and is a source of wild meat in some communities (21). Primates have also been implicated in index human cases, but likely as intermediate rather than reservoir hosts (22). Primary cases of EBOD in the 2003 Congo outbreak were associated with close contact with wild meat, in this case dead or killed non-human primates and other mammals (23).

A One Health approach to the management of this outbreak would have recognised that intermediate host infection could have served as an important early marker of subsequent human infection. A study assessing non-human primate morbidity and mortality associated with EBOD showed that animal outbreaks precede human outbreaks of the disease (24). Animal surveillance can help detect disturbances in ecosystem balance and may indicate heightened human surveillance and intervention. Joint animal-human surveillance during localised emergence may provide greater insight into the movement of disease within a geographical area, as with EBOD in human and non-human primates.

Transmission dynamics

Genomic surveillance data can be used to elucidate the origin and transmission dynamics of a pathogen. By conducting genome sequencing on patients with confirmed EBOD, it was found that the 2014 West African outbreak was likely sustained within the human population after a single spillover event. Rapid intra- and interhost genetic variation was observed, allowing for characterisation of viral transmission patterns within the first few weeks of the outbreak (25) (**See Chapter 21, Genomics**).

The management of vector transmission differs from that of human-to-human transmission. With some vector-borne diseases, such as Japanese encephalitis or West Nile fever, humans are referred to as 'dead-end hosts'. WNV is sustained through a mosquito-bird-mosquito cycle, whilst infection in a human does not cause a high enough viral load for subsequent onward vector transmission. In this scenario, interventions are focused on the interaction between vectors and humans, and vector surveillance is crucial. Individual and community-based avoidance strategies such as wearing light-coloured, long clothing and reducing outdoor activities at peak times were amongst the most effective interventions, as was the use of larvicides (26). At a regional level, interventions were centred around controlling outbreaks; regular monitoring of vectors and WNV levels is used to assess when control measures are required. The data are used to inform choice of intervention, including source reduction through habitat modification, larval control, or pesticide use for adult mosquito control, though the impact of increasing insecticide resistance must also be considered (27).

Conditions promoting amplification

The mode of pathogen spread between humans is well established. Transmission can occur via direct contact, fomites, droplets, aerosol (airborne), oral (ingestion), or be vector borne (28). Transmissibility within the recipient host population is thought to be influenced by both external factors allowing for greater interconnectedness between hosts, and pathogen characteristics that enable successful transmission.

Various mathematical models can accurately predict the movement of a pathogen through the human population, via analysis of pathogen dynamics, transmission routes, and human factors (e.g., population density, local public health measures) (29) (**See Chapter 16, Modelling to inform strategy**). Dense populations have greater risk of amplification than sparser ones. Increasing global interconnectedness for trade and travel has provided multiple avenues for the transmission of pathogens across borders (30). Infections introduced through air travel have been found to become endemic in their new territories, such as Chikungunya virus in Latin America (31). Vector colonisation is also an important consideration; the introduction of new infection-free vectors can result in the vector becoming endemic to a new area and enable future pathogen transmission, as seen in several arbovirus infections.

Transmissibility of viruses amongst recipient hosts has a significant effect on the morbidity and mortality caused by the disease. As such, the characterisation of biological features that contribute to successful transmission can help identify emerging disease threats. A study looking at over 200 RNA/DNA human viruses identified various characteristics that had strong associations with sustained human-to-human transmission, such as low host mortality (32). Such studies can enable the assessment of emerging pathogens.

THE ONE HEALTH APPROACH TO PREVENTING SPILLOVER EVENTS AND INVESTIGATING EMERGING/RE-EMERGING PATHOGENS

The One Health approach builds upon the principle that human, animal, and ecosystem health are interdependent; disruption of one has consequences for the rest **(Figure 13.1)**. While in the past these were often studied in isolation in the investigation of emerging diseases, there is a greater understanding now that it is beneficial to investigate these factors together. This facilitates a coordinated approach to preventing and controlling disease outbreaks (33).

The factors affecting zoonotic spillover and local emergence have been discussed in isolation earlier. However, the practical implementation of this knowledge in a formally integrated effort using the One Health framework can help aid dynamic disease response. Knowledge of intermediate species, such as vectors or intermediate animal hosts, and local emergence transmission dynamics, with the added effects of anthropogenic change, can shape the understanding of the course a pathogen takes. As an example, Nipah virus (NiV) outbreaks in Asia are determined by both the method of spillover and subsequent onward transmission.

One Health approaches have been successfully implemented for NiV control

The reservoir for NiV is the fruit bat (flying fox), and spillover occurs via consumption of date palm sap contaminated by bats, direct contact with bats' secretions, or domestic animals infected via bats' saliva (34). Intermediate species (e.g., pigs) may act as 'amplifiers', increasing disease concentration (35). The first spillover in 1998 resulted in 265 cases in Malaysia, including 105 human deaths; 1 million pigs were slaughtered to control this (36).

Spillover from bats to pigs then humans may have occurred due to livestock intensification in an area with high population density (37). Farmers planted fruit trees for additional income, but these also housed NiV-infected bats which contaminated pig feed (33). Limiting bats' access to trees reduced humans' risk of NiV exposure (38). Spillover may have been worsened by deforestation and droughts, pushing bats' habitats and piggeries closer (39).

The 2008 Bangladesh outbreak was managed by studying the behaviour of human cases, and the team identified date sap consumption as the source of infection, combining laboratory data with ecological studies on bat movement patterns (40). Infrared cameras provided evidence that bats could contaminate the sap collection while feeding, so collection containers were redesigned to prevent future contamination.

The response to the 2018 re-emergence of NiV in India included multidisciplinary teams utilised at every level from district to state, and coordinated in daily meetings with health ministers, enabling local contact tracing and isolation while ensuring all teams worked towards a common goal (41). This successful collaboration was reintroduced to control a 2019 outbreak at the index case; no subsequent spread was reported, which was evidence of the efficacy of a One Health approach.

Drivers of disease emergence and spread vary significantly depending on geography and climate. As such, we must consider their consequential impact on host and vector health, such as breeding patterns and population size, and finally how human behaviour may play into the dynamic between these factors. Surveillance will be more effective when all such factors are combined and considered. Traditional post hoc analysis relies on historic data that may not be comprehensive, therefore masking any relationships that would otherwise have been revealed during investigative efforts during pathogen activity.

Management of an outbreak is reliant on the successful adoption of planned interventions by stakeholders. One Health epidemiology assessments incorporate the social, economic, and cultural ramifications of interventions on stakeholders at every level, in a community or nationwide. Strategies that exert pressure upon communities can sometimes lead to aversion behaviours that are high risk and can worsen the situation, highlighting the importance of stakeholder-supportive strategies.

Applying One Health surveillance strategies to Rift Valley fever virus (RVFV) outbreaks

RVFV primarily affects livestock and is seen sporadically in humans that handle animals (e.g., farmers and veterinarians). It is transmitted to humans directly, or indirectly via vectors, and there is no record of human-to-human transmission (42).

RVFV surveillance requires a One Health framework due to the interactions between the environment, livestock, and humans affecting its activity, and this varies geographically. For instance, in Eastern and Southern Africa, outbreaks occur in intervals of up to 15 years, associated with flooding of dambos (mosquito breeding areas), while in Northern and Western Africa, outbreaks seem unrelated to rainfall, and are linked to mosquito breeding in rivers and dams (43). Human behaviours also influence the risk of spillover events (e.g., raw milk consumption has been suggested as a driver of RVFV in Kenya) (44). Livestock movement and human-livestock proximity have also been demonstrated as influencing factors in disease outbreaks (45).

Climate data revealed that warm sea-surface temperatures in the Pacific Ocean and Indian Ocean resulted in above-normal rainfall in the Horn of Africa. The associated upsurge in mosquito numbers may have facilitated RVFV transmission. Risk-mapping models developed here provided a two to six week warning period for the Horn of Africa, allowing upscaling of outbreak prevention/response measures (46). Epidemiological risk assessment benefits from One Health-based surveillance, as all stakeholders are identified prior to interventions. Joint sampling of livestock and humans revealed this spatiotemporal association that would have been hidden in post hoc analyses (47).

Anthrax in western Uganda: managing perverse incentives

The natural reservoir of anthrax is grass-eating animals and it can be transmitted through contact with infected animals or meat; human-to-human transmission is rare. Anthrax outbreak responses have traditionally been based on sentinel case reporting to local public health authorities. However, the barriers to infection reporting can transcend the threats posed by the disease and include social, economic, and cultural ramifications. The 2011 Ugandan outbreak, for example, temporarily closed meat, dairy, and livestock markets, understandably having negative economic effects.

A One Health-based epidemiology assessment of anthrax management in Western Uganda investigated the impact of the disease on human livelihoods. The socioeconomic drain the disease exerts upon a community was found to result in high-risk behaviours, which further hinder early outbreak intervention. Though education was flagged as an issue, the study highlighted that this alone would not change behaviour. Individuals adopted short-term solutions to offset losses; the real barrier to change was the socioeconomic impact an outbreak had on communities (48).

A One Health approach allows identification of sentinel barriers to outbreak prevention, alert, and response, allowing us to plan investment and change. Stakeholder-supportive strategies, such as pairing disease control with poverty management, or implementation of practical solutions, such as the use of plastic bags for carcasses rather than expecting communities to employ high agency/cost methods of disposal (49), may be beneficial in such cases.

CONCLUSION

One Health is a relatively young component in the portfolio of approaches to preventing and responding to spillover events. Our understanding of the ramifications of the animal-human interface has progressed significantly in recent years, and while there are good examples of exercising these approaches, more communities must be empowered to adopt this knowledge. The forces that drive urbanisation, alteration of animal habitats, and close, often high-risk, interactions between humans and animals will not go away, but neither should our efforts to counter these and other interacting factors.

Where spillover events cannot be prevented, heightened human-animal surveillance in targeted locations is the best defence against an event turning into a larger outbreak. Surveillance featuring inter-sectoral collaboration can better enable early detection which can instigate interventions that prevent outbreaks. Effective communication and engagement of all stakeholders in these areas are key to obtaining invaluable information and facilitating interventions.

With a more detailed appreciation of the spillover events behind previous outbreaks, with better tactics to mitigate risk, and with One Health collaborations providing effective outbreak detection, response, and control, we now have a stronger framework for avoiding the health, social, and economic impacts of future outbreaks and pandemics.

REFERENCES:

1. Pathogen detection & viral discovery [Internet]. PREDICT Project. https://p2.predict.global/discovery.
2. Ellwanger JH, Chies JA. Zoonotic spillover: understanding basic aspects for better prevention [Internet]. Genet Mol Biol. 2021 Jun;44(1 Suppl 1):e20200355. https://doi.org/10.1590/1678-4685-gmb-2020-0355 PMID:34096963.
3. Members of the One Health High-Level Expert Panel (OHHLEP); Markotter W, Mettenleiter TC, Adisasmito WB, Almuhairi S, Barton Behravesh C, Bilivogui P, Bukachi SA, Casas N, Cediel Becerra N, Charron DF, Chaudhary A, Ciacci Zanella JR, Cunningham AA, Dar O, Debnath N, Dungu B, Farag E, Gao GF, Hayman DTS, Khaitsa M, Koopmans MPG, Machalaba C, Mackenzie JS, Morand S, Smolenskiy V, Zhou

L. Prevention of zoonotic spillover: from relying on response to reducing the risk at source. PLoS Pathog. 2023 Oct 5;19(10):e1011504. https://doi.org/10.1371/journal.ppat.1011504 PMID: 37796834.

4. Mollentze N, Streicker DG. Viral zoonotic risk is homogenous among taxonomic orders of mammalian and avian reservoir hosts [Internet]. Proc Natl Acad Sci USA. 2020 Apr;117(17):9423–30. https://doi.org/10.1073/pnas.1919176117 PMID:32284401.

5. Guth S, Visher E, Boots M, Brook CE. Host phylogenetic distance drives trends in virus virulence and transmissibility across the animal-human interface. Philos Trans R Soc Lond B Biol Sci [Internet]. 2019 Sep 30;374(1782):20190296. http://doi.org/10.1098/rstb.2019.0296.

6. Khalil H, Ecke F, Evander M, Magnusson M, Hörnfeldt B. Declining ecosystem health and the dilution effect [Internet]. Sci Rep. 2016 Aug;6(1):31314. https://doi.org/10.1038/srep31314 PMID:27499001.

7. Swaddle JP, Calos SE. Increased avian diversity is associated with lower incidence of human West Nile infection: observation of the dilution effect [Internet]. PLoS One. 2008 Jun;3(6):e2488. https://doi.org/10.1371/journal.pone.0002488 PMID:18575599.

8. Engering A, Hogerwerf L, Slingenbergh J. Pathogen-host-environment interplay and disease emergence [Internet]. Emerg Microbes Infect. 2013 Feb;2(2):e5. https://doi: 10.1038/emi.2013.5 PMID:26038452.

9. Neumann G, Noda T, Kawaoka Y. Emergence and pandemic potential of swine-origin H1N1 influenza virus [Internet]. Nature. 2009 Jun;459(7249):931–9. https://doi.org/10.1038/nature08157 PMID:19525932.

10. Mendoza H, Rubio AV, García-Peña GE, Suzán G, Simonetti JA. Does land-use change increase the abundance of zoonotic reservoirs? Rodents say yes [Internet]. Eur J Wildl Res. 2020 Feb;66(1):6. https://doi.org/10.1007/s10344-019-1344-9.

11. Halpin K, Young PL, Field H, Mackenzie JS. Newly discovered viruses of flying foxes [Internet]. Vet Microbiol. 1999 Aug;68(1-2):83–7. https://doi.org/10.1016/S0378-1135(99)00063-2 PMID:10501164.

12. Baker RE, Mahmud AS, Miller IF, Rajeev M, Rasambainarivo F, Rice BL, et al. Infectious disease in an era of global change [Internet]. Nat Rev Microbiol. 2022 Apr;20(4):193–205. https://doi.org/10.1038/s41579-021-00639-z PMID:34646006.

13. Martin G, Webb RJ, Chen C, Plowright RK, Skerratt LF. Microclimates might limit indirect spillover of the bat borne zoonotic Hendra virus [Internet]. Microb Ecol. 2017 Jul;74(1):106–15. https://doi.org/10.1007/s00248-017-0934-x PMID:28091706.

14. Douglas KO, Payne K, Sabino-Santos G, Agard J. Influence of climatic factors on human hantavirus infections in Latin America and the Caribbean: a systematic review. Pathog (Basel, Switzerland) [Internet]. 2021 Dec 23;11(1). https://doi.org/10.3390/pathogens11010015.

15. Health England P. Human Animal Infections and Risk Surveillance (HAIRS) group processes of risk assessment [Internet]. 2018. www.facebook.com/PublicHealthEngland.

16. Abat C, Chaudet H, Rolain JM, Colson P, Raoult D. Traditional and syndromic surveillance of infectious diseases and pathogens [Internet]. Int J Infect Dis. 2016 Jul;48:22–8. https://doi.org/10.1016/j.ijid.2016.04.021 PMID:27143522.

17. Dion M, AbdelMalik P, Mawudeku A. Big Data and the Global Public Health Intelligence Network (GPHIN) [Internet]. Can Commun Dis Rep. 2015 Sep;41(9):209–14. https://doi.org/10.14745/ccdr.v41i09a02 PMID:29769954.

18. Wilson ML, Fleming KA, Kuti MA, Looi LM, Lago N, Ru K. Access to pathology and laboratory medicine services: a crucial gap [Internet]. Lancet. 2018 May;391(10133):1927–38. https://doi.org/10.1016/S0140-6736(18)30458-6 PMID:29550029.

19. Swanepoel R, Smit SB, Rollin PE, Formenty P, Leman PA, Kemp A, et al.; International Scientific and Technical Committee for Marburg Hemorrhagic Fever Control in the Democratic Republic of Congo. Studies of reservoir hosts for Marburg virus [Internet]. Emerg Infect Dis. 2007 Dec;13(12):1847–51. https://doi.org/10.3201/eid1312.071115 PMID:18258034.

20. Leroy EM, Kumulungui B, Pourrut X, Rouquet P, Hassanin A, Yaba P, et al. Fruit bats as reservoirs of Ebola virus [Internet]. Nature. 2005 Dec;438(7068):575–6. https://doi.org/10.1038/438575a PMID:16319873.

21. Hayman DT, Emmerich P, Yu M, Wang LF, Suu-Ire R, Fooks AR, et al. Long-term survival of an urban fruit bat seropositive for Ebola and Lagos bat viruses [Internet]. PLoS One. 2010 Aug;5(8):e11978. https://doi.org/10.1371/journal.pone.0011978 PMID:20694141.

22. Hayman DT. African primates: likely victims, not reservoirs of Ebolaviruses [Internet]. J Infect Dis. 2019 Oct;220(10):1547–50. https://doi.org/10.1093/infdis/jiz007 PMID:30657949.

23. Formenty P, Libama F, Epelboin A, Allarangar Y, Leroy E, Moudzeo H, et al. Outbreak of Ebola hemorrhagic fever in the Republic of the Congo, 2003: a new strategy?. Méd Trop (Mars). 2003;63(3):291–5. PMID:14579469.

24. Rouquet P, Froment JM, Bermejo M, Kilbourn A, Karesh W, Reed P, et al. Wild animal mortality monitoring and human Ebola outbreaks, Gabon and Republic of Congo, 2001-2003 [Internet]. Emerg Infect Dis. 2005 Feb;11(2):283–90. https://doi.org/10.3201/eid1102.040533 PMID:15752448.

25. Gire SK, Goba A, Andersen KG, Sealfon RS, Park DJ, Kanneh L, et al. Genomic surveillance elucidates Ebola virus origin and transmission during the 2014 outbreak [Internet]. Science. 2014 Sep;345(6202):1369–72. https://doi.org/10.1126/science.1259657 PMID:25214632.

26. Hongoh V, Campagna C, Panic M, Samuel O, Gosselin P, Waaub JP, et al. Assessing Interventions to manage West Nile virus using multi-criteria decision analysis with risk scenarios [Internet]. PLoS One. 2016 Aug;11(8):e0160651. https://doi.org/10.1371/journal.pone.0160651 PMID:27494136.

27. Division of Vector-Borne Diseases West Nile Virus in the United States. Guidelines for Surveillance, Prevention, and Control [Internet]. https://www.cdc.gov/westnile/resources/pdfs/wnvGuidelines.pdf.

28. Stull JW, Bjorvik E, Bub J, Dvorak G, Petersen C, Troyer HL. 2018 AAHA Infection Control, Prevention, and Biosecurity Guidelines*. Journal of the American Animal Hospital Association [Internet]. 2018 Nov 1;54(6):297–326. http://dx.doi.org/10.5326/JAAHA-MS-6903.

29. Hosseini P, Sokolow SH, Vandegrift KJ, Kilpatrick AM, Daszak P. Predictive power of air travel and socio-economic data for early pandemic spread [Internet]. PLoS One. 2010 Sep;5(9):e12763. https://doi.org/10.1371/journal.pone.0012763 PMID:20856678.

30. World Health Organization. Transmission of SARS-CoV-2: implications for infection prevention precautions. 2020. https://www.who.int/news-room/commentaries/detail/transmission-of-sars-cov-2-implications-for-infection-prevention-precautions.

31. Findlater A, Bogoch II. Human mobility and the global spread of infectious diseases: a focus on air travel [Internet]. Trends Parasitol. 2018 Sep;34(9):772–83. https://doi.org/10.1016/j.pt.2018.07.004 PMID:30049602.

32. Geoghegan JL, Senior AM, Di Giallonardo F, Holmes EC. Virological factors that increase the transmissibility of emerging human viruses [Internet]. Proc Natl Acad Sci USA. 2016 Apr;113(15):4170–5. https://doi.org/10.1073/pnas.1521582113 PMID:27001840.

33. Ogden NH, Wilson JR, Richardson DM, Hui C, Davies SJ, Kumschick S, et al. Emerging infectious diseases and biological invasions: a call for a One Health collaboration in science and management [Internet]. R Soc Open Sci. 2019 Mar;6(3):181577. https://doi.org/10.1098/rsos.181577 PMID:31032015.

34. Skowron K, Bauza-Kaszewska J, Grudlewska-Buda K, Wiktorczyk-Kapischke N, Zacharski M, Bernaciak Z, et al. Nipah virus-another threat from the world of zoonotic viruses [Internet]. Front Microbiol. 2022 Jan;12:811157. https://doi.org/10.3389/fmicb.2021.811157 PMID:35145498.

35. McLean RK, Graham SP. The pig as an amplifying host for new and emerging zoonotic viruses. One Heal [Internet]. 2022 Jun 1 [cited 2022 Dec 20];14:100384. https://doi.org/10.1016/j.onehlt.2022.100384.

36. Enserink M. New virus fingered in Malaysian epidemic. Science (80-) [Internet]. 1999 Apr 16 [cited 2022 Dec 20];284(5413):407–10. https://doi.org/10.1126/science.284.5413.407.

37. Jones BA, Grace D, Kock R, Alonso S, Rushton J, Said MY, et al. Jones BA, Grace D, Kock R, Alonso S, Rushton J, Said MY, et al. Zoonosis emergence linked to agricultural intensification and environmental change [Internet]. Proc Natl Acad Sci USA. 2013 May;110(21):8399–404. https://doi.org/10.1073/pnas.1208059110 PMID:23671097.

38. Khan MS, Hossain J, Gurley ES, Nahar N, Sultana R, Luby SP. Use of infrared camera to understand bats' access to date palm sap: implications for preventing Nipah virus transmission [Internet]. EcoHealth. 2010 Dec;7(4):517–25. https://doi.org/10.1007/s10393-010-0366-2 PMID:21207105.

39. Bing Chua K. Hui Chua B, Wen Wang C. Anthropogenic deforestation, El Niño and the emergence of Nipah virus in Malaysia [Internet]. [cited 2022 Dec 20]. http://www.gov.sg/.

40. Rahman MA, Hossain MJ, Sultana S, Homaira N, Khan SU, Rahman M, et al. Date palm sap linked to Nipah virus outbreak in Bangladesh, 2008 [Internet]. Vector Borne Zoonotic Dis. 2012 Jan;12(1):65–72. https://doi.org/10.1089/vbz.2011.0656 PMID:21923274.

41. Singhai M, Jain R, Jain S, Bala M, Singh S, Goyal R. Nipah virus disease: recent perspective and One Health approach. Ann Glob Heal [Internet]. 2021 Oct 12 [cited 2022 Dec 20];87(1). https://annalsofglobalhealth.org/articles/10.5334/aogh.3431/.

42. World Health Organization. Rift Valley fever. 2018. https://www.who.int/news-room/fact-sheets/detail/rift-valley-fever.

43. Paweska JT. Rift Valley fever [Internet]. Emerg Infect Dis. 2014 Jan;73–93. https://www.sciencedirect.com/science/article/pii/B9780124169753000066 PMID:34808090.

44. Grossi-Soyster EN, Lee J, King CH, LaBeaud AD. The influence of raw milk exposures on Rift Valley fever virus transmission [Internet]. PLoS Negl Trop Dis. 2019 Mar;13(3):e0007258. https://doi.org/10.1371/journal.pntd.0007258 PMID:30893298.

45. Kim Y, Métras R, Dommergues L, Youssouffi C, Combo S, Le Godais G, et al. The role of livestock movements in the spread of Rift Valley fever virus in animals and humans in Mayotte, 2018-19 [Internet]. PLoS Negl Trop Dis. 2021 Mar;15(3):e0009202. https://doi.org/10.1371/journal.pntd.0009202 PMID:33684126.

46. Anyamba A, Chretien JP, Small J, Tucker CJ, Formenty PB, Richardson JH, et al. Prediction of a Rift Valley fever outbreak [Internet]. Proc Natl Acad Sci USA. 2009 Jan;106(3):955–9. https://doi.org/10.1073/pnas.0806490106 PMID:19144928.

47. Rostal MK, Ross N, Machalaba C, Cordel C, Paweska JT, Karesh WB. Benefits of a One Health approach: an example using Rift Valley fever. One Heal [Internet]. 2018 Jan 1 [cited 2022 Dec 21];5:34–6. https://doi:10.1016/j.onehlt.2018.01.001. PMID: 29911162.

48. Coffin JL, Monje F, Asiimwe-Karimu G, Amuguni HJ, Odoch T. A One Health, participatory epidemiology assessment of anthrax (Bacillus anthracis) management in Western Uganda [Internet]. Soc Sci Med. 2015 Mar;129:44–50. https://doi.org/10.1016/j.socscimed.2014.07.037 PMID:25066946.

49. Kock R, Haider N, Mboera LE, Zumla A. A One-Health lens for anthrax. Lancet Planet Heal [Internet]. 2019 Jul 1 [cited 2022 Dec 21];3(7):e285–6. https://doi.org/10.1016/S2542-5196(19)30111-1.

CHAPTER 14

HEALTHY POPULATIONS AND STRONG HEALTH SYSTEMS FOR OUTBREAK RESILIENCE

by Thomas Bentley, Anders Nordström, and Helena Legido-Quigley

Infectious disease outbreaks are unpredictable events that put health systems under strain. Resilient health systems are capable of responding to novel challenges whilst maintaining core functions. The COVID-19 pandemic has clearly demonstrated that health systems, even those with substantial funding, were not adequately prepared for a global outbreak. The concept of resilience has recently been used in the context of disaster risk reduction. While this concept has only recently been applied to health systems, it is now increasingly understood that investing in resilience is key to prepare health systems to adapt to crises. In this chapter, we describe three components of health system resilience, highlighting specific examples from previous pandemics, and discuss how nations can integrate these components. The three building blocks of resilience are government capacity, a strong and well-supported healthcare workforce, and the system's effective reach into the nation's most vulnerable communities.

INTRODUCTION

The COVID-19 pandemic has had a devastating effect on health, economies, and societies across the world. The pandemic stretched the resources of even the most well-funded health systems and has highlighted the strengths and weaknesses of the global approach to health security.

The coming decades may prove that COVID-19 is far from a black swan event. Increasing agricultural intensification means that the risk of zoonoses is greatly increased, whilst advances in synthetic biology may lead to the ability of rogue actors or states to easily weaponise man-made pathogens. As international travel and trade continue to grow, our vulnerability to pandemic disease will increase if no course correction is made. Climate change and environmental degradation will exacerbate vector-borne disease outbreaks such as dengue, malaria, and yellow fever, whilst the ongoing HIV/AIDS crisis still claims almost one million lives each year (1).

WHAT DEFINES A RESILIENT HEALTH SYSTEM?

A resilient health system has the capacity to prepare for and respond to crises, to maintain core functions during times of extraordinary demand, and to learn, recover, and improve from past crises (2). Research examining a range of national responses to the COVID-19 pandemic demonstrated that resilient health systems share a number of key characteristics (3).

First, successful countries adopted a whole-of-government approach. This included working across departments to address multisectoral economic, social, and cultural challenges, engaging with scientific experts, and building and maintaining trust throughout the pandemic. Second, successful countries expanded and supported their health workforce. They made use of existing community networks and expertise and provided psychological, financial, and material support. Finally, successful countries identified vulnerable groups and expanded health coverage, with the aim of ensuring that low income did not act as a barrier to COVID-19 detection and management. Global health security principles were well integrated into public health functions and private sector services were contracted to meet additional service need.

Investment in preparedness can be the difference between a successful public health response to a pandemic and a catastrophic one. It is essential that national governments and international organisations invest in more resilient health systems now, and not when the next emergency happens.

HOW TO ACHIEVE RESILIENCE?
Governance, trust, and scientific advice

COVID-19 has laid bare the relationship between health, economics, and governance. It has also demonstrated that governments must walk a careful tightrope to preserve the trust of their populations. Countries must draw on the expertise of multiple government departments with the aim of balancing public health measures, such as lockdowns, with economic, social, and cultural considerations.

National responses are dependent on multiple interacting factors. During the COVID-19 pandemic, more successful responses typically included a multisectoral, whole-of-government approach (4). In contrast, less successful responses were typically delayed, or less coordinated, with calls to act on COVID-19 often undermined by the actions of political leadership (5). It is important that national government departments engage in two-way communication and cooperation with regional governance and health directorates to maximise political capacity. Furthermore, input from government ministries not focused on health is essential to mitigate non-disease-related welfare risks during the pandemic, including economic damage and increases in domestic violence.

Nations that relied upon scientific consensus and evidence collated by expert committees typically performed better than those that did not (5). However, these committees were typically dominated by professionals with a biomedical background. Responses with input from too narrowly constituted composition might miss key social and political factors. Some of the recommendations enacted by different governments were subsequently found to have violated human rights (6) (**See Human rights and public health measures**). Others may not have taken entrenched health inequalities into account, and so led to less positive outcomes. Decisions need to consider social context, especially inequality, and must seek to holistically maintain national well-being. Successful advisory groups are multidisciplinary and engage the general public as well as government. For example, during the COVID-19 pandemic, Uruguay and Mozambique rapidly established collaborative scientific committees which provided information both to the executive leadership and directly to the public. This allowed for rapid health policy changes to be justified in a public forum (7).

> **Human rights and public health measures during an outbreak**
>
> Although quarantine measures are often essential to control the spread of an outbreak, they frequently necessitate a trade-off between individual rights and population rights.
>
> During the COVID-19 pandemic, public health concerns were used to justify the curtailment of human rights across many areas of society. Many governments have been accused of detaining critical pro-opposition journalists and activists under the guise of pandemic response (8–9). Turkmenistan was reported to have outlawed the use of the word 'coronavirus' on social media platforms (10). The Department of Justice in the U.S. sought the ability to detain people indefinitely without trial during public health emergencies (11). Police violence against civilians has been reported in at least 59 countries, and detentions and arrests linked to public health measures in at least 66 countries (12). Some governments used extreme surveillance methods to ensure that citizens did not break quarantine, including installing CCTV cameras outside homes (13), mandating the use of trackable wrist bands (14), and stamping coronavirus contacts with indelible ink (15).
>
> It is essential that quarantine measures are effective and necessary, infringe on individual liberties as little as possible, are proportional to the public health threat faced, have humane supportive services for individuals affected, and are justified in a public forum with transparent decision-making (16).

Once evidence-based policy has been formulated, political will is needed to garner support for its implementation. Although high-income countries often have internal capacity to generate high-quality advice, there must be a commitment to implement this advice and to communicate it effectively to the public (5). Some governments, especially those facing upcoming elections, placed their political agendas over an evidence-based pandemic response (17). This led to higher infection and fatality rates, the politicisation of public health, and fractured trust in the health system.

The majority of policies implemented by countries in response to COVID-19 were enacted at a national level, while most metrics tracking coronavirus impact operated at both a national and subnational resolution. However, infectious diseases do not respect borders, and international collaboration will be essential to combat future pandemics. For discrete outbreaks, it is crucial that countries communicate information not only with their neighbours, but also with nations at high risk of transmission. This includes countries that have significant trade, travel, and community connections. However, for multi-country pandemic events, relying solely on national and subnational reporting becomes unwieldy and resource intensive. A harmonised international approach, steered by institutions such as the World Health Organization (WHO) and supported by frameworks such as the International Health Regulations, is crucial. Technical networks such as the Global Outbreak Alert and Response Network (GOARN) offer a platform for nations to combine resources and share expertise, allowing for coordination before and during crises.

During an outbreak, trust in three types of actors is required (18):
- governments who are responsible for proposing policies
- citizens whose cooperation is needed for implementing measures
- scientists who provide the evidence on which policies are based

Trust between marginalised communities and governments must be built prior to pandemic events. Communities that have previously experienced racial prejudice are more hesitant to follow public health advice (19). Surveys performed in Liberia during the 2014–2015 Ebola virus disease (EBOD) outbreak demonstrated that a lack of trust in the government is correlated with the reluctance to adhere to EBOD control policies (20).

Community cohesion played a significant role in determining how well nations adapted to measures to prevent the spread of COVID-19. Countries such as Singapore, where the government had previously demonstrated an ability to effectively control severe acute respiratory syndrome (SARS), had populations who were broadly compliant with public health measures (5). Non-pharmaceutical measures to reduce transmission of COVID-19, including social distancing and face masks, rely on a sense of shared identity and social cohesion (21). Furthermore, existing cultural norms, such as mask wearing for health and fashion reasons in countries such as South Korea and Japan, removed friction when imposing stringent public health rules (22).

COVID-19 is the first epidemic since the emergence of social media to have more than one million deaths. This new media ecology has transformed how we interact and share information with each other. Engagement with social media sites allowed for governments and health authorities to convey reliable and real-time information about risks and preventative actions. Social media has been used to try and promote collective responsibility, such as the #TakeResponsibility campaign in Nigeria by the Nigeria Centre for Disease Control (NCDC) and the #NationalMask campaign in China (23).

While social media allowed for the widespread dissemination of health information, it has also been a major contributor to coronavirus-related misinformation. Misinformation has been demonstrated to spread more rapidly and widely than accurate information (24) (**See Chapter 34, Infodemics**). It has proved impossible to regulate the sources of this information given the very low barrier of entry to posting information online. In addition, as scientific knowledge regarding COVID-19 rapidly evolved, new evidence that contradicted previously held beliefs fuelled scepticism amongst the general public about the validity of public health measures and even about the pandemic itself. Governments should work proactively with social media services to mitigate the harm that misinformation and disinformation can cause, whilst simultaneously recognising the benefits that the effective use of social media can bring.

Invest in health professionals and communities

The health workforce is essential for carrying out most frontline pandemic response and it may be necessary during an outbreak to plan for and rapidly expand workforce capacity. Multiple strategies exist, including the reallocation of healthcare professionals, temporarily increasing the scope of practice, and introducing strategies for training. During the COVID-19 pandemic, it quickly became necessary to reallocate professionals from specialist areas to emergency care wards, intensive care units, and diagnosis and surveillance activities. Other strategies to expand the workforce included the establishment of recruitment agencies to directly target healthcare workers and recruit laypeople for different types of support activity, and asking retired doctors and nurses to re-enter the workforce. In Germany, the U.K., Spain, and Vietnam, final year nursing and medical students were allowed to work in different capacities as part of the nation's response (3).

Online training courses for contact tracing, laboratory protocols for analysing samples, assessment of critical patients, and management of patients on ventilators proved to be effective across many countries during the COVID-19 pandemic (3). These will also be useful in the future, ensuring that professionals gain the skills required whilst minimising potential infection exposure.

Recruiting members of the community to assist in the delivery of services can increase trust and a sense of ownership with regard to health services. Community workers in Liberia, Thailand, and Vietnam undertook training in disease identification, contact tracing, and supporting isolating community members (5). These workers often already had jobs within, or adjacent to, the health sector, which emphasises that community engagement is a continuous process to foster resilience and not a knee-jerk response to a crisis. Forming partnerships with social workers or local community and religious leaders has led to an increase in community trust in many different contexts. These partnerships are important to ensure that health messaging is adapted to local culture and health literacy (25).

Alongside recruitment, it is important to protect the existing workforce. Health workers were disproportionately affected by the pandemic (26) and were at risk of both physical and psychological harm. Support measures should include continued protection protocols, organisation of shifts in order to avoid extended hours without rest, periods of leave from duty for mental and physical recovery, accommodation near the workplace in order to protect the families of health workers, and free childcare. Psychological support for frontline staff and their families, such as counselling and trauma support, was provided by some countries, including Singapore, South Korea, Sweden, China, the U.S., Liberia, Japan, Fiji, Pakistan, Nigeria, and India (3). The provision of economic support, as well as the classification of infections as an occupational injury, provided an incentive for healthcare staff to continue to work, whilst safeguarding them from economic stress.

Support for healthcare staff also means adequate provisioning of necessary equipment. Stockpiling of ample medical products has positive short- and medium-term effects. Prior to the COVID-19 outbreak, Singapore maintained a national stockpile of medical products that could last for six months (27). In contrast, the U.K. decommissioned their stockpiles prior to the pandemic, which led to health workers working without adequate personal protective equipment (PPE) in the early stages of the pandemic. This resulted in higher rates of infection and burnout in health workers (28). Legal frameworks must be introduced to prevent individual stockpiling and price gouging and should be responsive to strategies used to evade regulation. Rational-use guidelines in health facilities help conserve supplies of essential products.

Where stockpiles are insufficient, it is important to rapidly accelerate the availability of medical products at the beginning of an outbreak. During the COVID-19 pandemic, some nations converted existing industries to produce important equipment. For example, India used automobile industry infrastructure to produce ventilators and PPE (29). Round-the-clock production in Japan resulted in a threefold increase in medical product manufacturing (30). Financial incentives, such as pre-purchase agreements between governments and manufacturing firms, can make overproduction profitable for firms in a more cautious economic climate. Governments must also provide technical and capacity support to industries that are rapidly adjusting to new manufacturing processes.

Invest in systems

Although infection control and emergency health services are often the focus during outbreaks, maintenance of primary, geriatric, and long-term care is essential for safeguarding the health of populations, both during and after an outbreak. A strong primary care system enables surveillance and early detection with important triage facilitating case management and control of transmission. Geriatric care is often a focal point for both infection and mortality. Although traditionally considered outside of the remit of healthcare, resilient systems need to consider greater integration of social care to ensure health equity across the population.

Similarly, long-term care cannot be neglected. Aside from their significant health burden, chronic conditions may also impair immunity. Metabolic conditions such as diabetes (31) and obesity (32) lead to dysfunctional innate and adaptive immune responses. Malnutrition due to caloric or micronutrient deficit is also known to impair immunity (33). Although current evidence is limited, diabetes, obesity, and malnutrition appear to be risk factors for COVID-19 infection and mortality. Resilient health systems focus on multimorbidity and disease interactions. Communities with a high prevalence of (undermanaged) chronic disease have a heightened vulnerability to an outbreak. Neglect of chronic and non-communicable diseases in an outbreak will establish a "health debt" that will need addressing post-pandemic. For example, it is estimated that 50,000 cancer diagnoses were missed during the COVID-19 pandemic in the U.K. (34) and that the National Health Service (NHS) will take 10 years to address this backlog maintaining activity levels five per cent above pre-pandemic levels (35).

A foundation of health system resilience is the provision of universal health coverage (UHC), which is the comprehensive delivery of quality health services that can be accessed without financial burden. Removing financial barriers to healthcare establishes a culture of health-seeking behaviour (2). This is especially important in the context of infectious disease outbreaks, where aversion to engaging with medical professionals and services can hamper detection and containment activities and strategies. Furthermore, regular positive interactions with health services promote trust in medical professionals. Providing healthcare with no or little cost can also bolster trust in the health system, even in the absence of citizens' trust in their government.

Marginalised and vulnerable communities have been found to experience worse health outcomes during pandemics (36) and their neglect can lead to the undetected and uncontrolled spread of disease. It is essential that policymakers identify and include these communities to prevent the widening of health inequities.

UHC can significantly reduce the burden of disease in the most vulnerable communities. After South Korea eliminated all costs associated with COVID-19 detection and treatment, no difference in mortality was found between those who could and could not afford to pay health insurance premiums (37). Although UHC is a pillar of comprehensive and equitable health services, global health security (GHS) dimensions such as surveillance, risk communication, and coordination have often been neglected (38) and may be highly salient during an outbreak emergency.

Countries with UHC had a case fatality rate twice that of countries without UHC during the COVID-19 pandemic (37), demonstrating that our current conception of UHC is woefully inadequate to deal with infectious disease outbreaks. During the COVID-19 pandemic, countries with strong investment in global health security but no UHC, such as the U.S. and Nigeria, performed less well than countries with integrated UHC and GHS systems, such as Taiwan, South Korea, and Thailand (39). An overemphasis on GHS at the expense of UHC can be catastrophic. During the 2014–2016 EBOD outbreak in West Africa, more people died from untreated malaria than from EBOD (38). Although countries lacking GHS principles are more vulnerable to epidemics, effective GHS is impossible without UHC. Policymakers should focus on incorporating ideas of pandemic control into existing UHC concepts.

The involvement of the private sector can increase national capacity for service provision. For example, governments can contract pandemic-related services such as testing, contact tracing activities, and hospital-level treatment. Countries can leverage their national-scale purchasing powers to negotiate with domestic manufacturers for rapid scale-up of the supply of essential products. Setting up a dedicated oversight body to ensure accountable usage of pandemic-related contracts can ensure that money is being spent efficiently and effectively and that public trust is preserved.

The COVID-19 pandemic has identified various areas that would benefit from further research and development The design of face masks and other PPE has barely changed for many decades. Current protective suits are mobility restricted (40), prone to overheating (41), very expensive, and have limited reusability. The development of PPE that is highly effective, easy to use, and cheap to distribute would greatly improve pandemic resilience. The development of sequencing programmes screening for potential pathogens in key areas such as airports, water supplies, and large urban centres will help prevent the international spread of disease and will provide early warning to clinicians and scientists of evolving biological threats. Platforms that allow the rapid development of vaccines are essential for reducing community transmission (**See Technical and regulatory innovations**). Built environment modifications, such as far-UVC irradiation (42) and improvements in ventilation, can be used to reduce transmission in high-risk or high-importance areas, such as hospitals or vaccine development laboratories.

Technical and regulatory innovations during COVID-19

The rapid development and deployment of vaccines, diagnostics, and therapeutics during a pandemic is essential to maintain health system functions. Prior to the COVID-19 pandemic, the average time it took for an experimental drug to progress from bench to market was 12 years (43). The necessity of a vaccine against COVID-19 drove both technical and regulatory innovations in drug development. Operation Warp Speed, which incorporated multiple vaccine candidates, parallel processing, and free technical support to industry in the U.S. (44), facilitated the production of a coronavirus vaccine 11 months after COVID-19 was first declared a public health emergency. Alvea, a U.S.-based startup biotechnology company, created a coronavirus omicron-variant vaccine from scratch, with the entire process taking 196 days (45). Accelerated vaccine development that does not compromise safety, efficacy, or product quality is associated with substantial financial risks when compared to conventional sequential developmental approaches, but was shown to be indispensable in curbing the international spread of COVID-19. Future investment in platform technologies will significantly increase health system resilience against respiratory viruses.

CONCLUSION

This chapter has identified the necessary components of resilience in the context of an infectious disease outbreak and identified specific successes and failings of national responses during the COVID-19 pandemic and the West African EBOD outbreak.

Multisectoral, whole-of-government responses that are informed by multidisciplinary scientific advice are crucial to mounting an effective response to outbreaks. Advisory groups should have balanced gender and ethnic representation and input from community groups. Governments must work to build and maintain public trust and use social media effectively to inform their populations. Making information publicly available can assist in both evidence-based decision-making and gaining the trust of populations.

Healthcare professionals are disproportionately affected by infectious disease outbreaks. New strategies need to be considered and implemented to address staff recruitment and geographical maldistribution. Psychological and financial support should be provided to ensure the well-being of the workforce, and they should be equipped properly. An integrated health systems approach, both horizontally and vertically, is required to prevent and manage chronic conditions and ensure continuing control of communicable disease, with primary healthcare placed at the forefront. Primary healthcare must be integrated with social care alongside strengthened public health systems at the local level that can be rapidly scaled up when needed. The integration of UHC and GHS principles should ensure that financial barriers do not hinder public health efforts.

Governments should partner with industry to ensure adequate access to essential products and services. Where new technologies are created, it is important that international policies promote equitable access for low- and middle-income countries. Sustainable financing mechanisms must be designed to prepare for new pandemics and foster health system resilience prior to pandemic events.

COVID-19 has highlighted the need for integration between sub-systems and across systems to prevent outbreaks. The different components described in this chapter are interrelated and dependent on legal and political frameworks to ensure their sustainability. For example, public health measures are neutered without ensuring trust and financial security in the communities that are targeted for engagement. Maintaining the public health workforce relies on reciprocal support from the government and the provision of modern infrastructure and medical technologies. Health systems need to be integrated with social care and other public institutions and must be supported by sustainable financing strategies. Systems must be adaptive to meet peaks and troughs in demand, as well as able to respond to regional variability.

Although outbreaks necessitate a population-focused public health response, hyperopic policymaking can lead to the neglect of marginalised and vulnerable groups. Investment in individuals and local communities is essential to ensure health equity during a pandemic and results in improvements in accurately mapping disease burden. A resilient health system is not defined by an ability to increase service provision—instead, it is measured by how effectively it can maintain health during a crisis. Investments in individuals include addressing socioeconomic conditions that contribute to disease and prioritising UHC. Ongoing and meaningful dialogue with communities should ensure that services are appropriate and that ownership of health rests with individuals. Attempts must be made to address structural determinants of health to reduce inequities in risk of infection and burden of mental health disorders, as well as safeguard individuals from domestic violence and neglect.

To create truly resilient health systems, new types of relationships must be developed between patients, health professionals, and researchers, supported by political commitment and sustainable funding. To ensure that people stay healthy, it is essential to address wider social and economic conditions affecting health, whilst providing holistic, people-centred health services.

The varying national outcomes of COVID-19 did not occur by chance. Countries which performed poorly during the pandemic despite having access to significant resources must learn from countries which had far fewer deaths per capita despite having more poorly resourced health systems. Global collaboration and the exchange of knowledge, technology, and resources are fundamental to our ability to guard against future pandemics.

Although national and local contexts vary across the world, there are key commonalities that can be applied by policymakers. It is essential that governments and healthcare providers invest in developing more resilient systems and communities as a bedrock of pandemic preparedness.

REFERENCES:

1. Roser M, Ritchie H. HIV/AIDS 2018. https://ourworldindata.org/hiv-aids.
2. Kruk ME, Myers M, Varpilah ST, Dahn BT. What is a resilient health system? Lessons from Ebola. Lancet. 2015 May;385(9980):1910–2. https://doi.org/10.1016/S0140-6736(15)60755-3 PMID:25987159.
3. Haldane V, De Foo C, Abdalla SM, Jung AS, Tan M, Wu S, et al. Health systems resilience in managing the COVID-19 pandemic: lessons from 28 countries. Nat Med. 2021;27(6):964–80. https://doi.org/10.1038/s41591-021-01381-y PMID:34002090.
4. Heymann DL, Legido-Quigley H. Two years of COVID-19: many lessons, but will we learn? Euro Surveill. 2022 Mar;27(10):2200222. https://doi.org/10.2807/1560-7917.ES.2022.27.10.2200222 PMID:35272747.
5. Tan MM, Neill R, Haldane V, Jung AS, De Foo C, Tan SM, et al. Assessing the role of qualitative factors in pandemic responses. BMJ. 2021;375:e067512. https://doi.org/10.1136/bmj-2021-067512 PMID:34840137.
6. Action SSiH. Key considerations: quarantine in the context of COVID-19. 2020.
7. Haldane V, Jung AS, Neill R, Singh S, Wu S, Jamieson M, et al. From response to transformation: how countries can strengthen national pandemic preparedness and response systems. BMJ. 2021;375:e067507. https://doi.org/10.1136/bmj-2021-067507 PMID:34840139.
8. Azerbaijan: crackdown on critics amid pandemic. Human Rights Watch; 2020. https://www.hrw.org/news/2020/04/16/azerbaijan-crackdown-critics-amid-pandemic.
9. Bangladesh: mass arrests over cartoons, posts. Human Rights Watch; 2020. https://www.hrw.org/news/2020/05/07/bangladesh-mass-arrests-over-cartoons-posts.
10. Brown L. Turkmenistan government outlaws any mention of the word 'coronavirus'. New York Post; 2020. https://nypost.com/2020/03/31/turkmenistan-government-outlaws-use-of-word-coronavirus/.
11. Woodruff Swan B. DOJ seeks new emergency powers amid coronavirus pandemic. Politico (Pavia); 2020. https://www.politico.com/news/2020/03/21/doj-coronavirus-emergency-powers-140023.
12. Repucci S, Slipowitz A. Democracy under lockdown. Freedom House; 2020. https://freedomhouse.org/report/special-report/2020/democracy-under-lockdown.
13. Kharpal A. Use of surveillance to fight coronavirus raises concerns about government power after pandemic ends. CNBC; 2020. https://www.cnbc.com/2020/03/27/coronavirus-surveillance-used-by-governments-to-fight-pandemic-privacy-concerns.html.
14. Saiidi U. Hong Kong is putting electronic wristbands on arriving passengers to enforce coronavirus quarantine. CNBC; 2020. https://www.cnbc.com/2020/03/18/hong-kong-uses-electronic-wristbands-to-enforce-coronavirus-quarantine.html.
15. Srivastava R, Nagaraj A. Privacy fears as India hand stamps suspected coronavirus cases. Reuters; 2020. https://www.reuters.com/article/us-health-coronavirus-privacy/privacy-fears-as-india-hand-stamps-suspected-coronavirus-cases-idUSKBN21716U.
16. Rothstein MA. From SARS to Ebola: legal and ethical considerations for modern quaratine. Indiana Health Law Rev. 2015;12(1):227–80. https://doi.org/10.18060/18963.

17. Pulejo M, Querubín P. Electoral concerns reduce restrictive measures during the COVID-19 pandemic. J Public Econ. 2021;198:104387. https://doi.org/10.1016/j.jpubeco.2021.104387 PMID:33776156.
18. Abdalla SM, Koya SF, Jamieson M, Verma M, Haldane V, Jung AS, et al. Investing in trust and community resilience: lessons from the early months of the first digital pandemic. BMJ. 2021;375:e067487. https://doi.org/10.1136/bmj-2021-067487 PMID:34840130.
19. Quinn S, Jamison A, Musa D, Hilyard K, Freimuth V. Exploring the continuum of vaccine hesitancy between African American and White adults: results of a qualitative study. PLoS Curr. 2016:8. https://doi.org/10.1371/currents.outbreaks.3e4a5ea39d8620494e2a2c874a3c4201 PMID:28239512.
20. Blair RA, Morse BS, Tsai LL. Public health and public trust: survey evidence from the Ebola Virus Disease epidemic in Liberia. Soc Sci Med. 2017;172:89–97. https://doi.org/10.1016/j.socscimed.2016.11.016 PMID:27914936.
21. Bonell C, Michie S, Reicher S, West R, Bear L, Yardley L, et al. Harnessing behavioural science in public health campaigns to maintain 'social distancing' in response to the COVID-19 pandemic: key principles. J Epidemiol Community Health. 2020;74(8):617–9. https://doi.org/10.1136/jech-2020-214290 PMID:32385125.
22. Han E, Tan MM, Turk E, Sridhar D, Leung GM, Shibuya K, et al. Lessons learnt from easing COVID-19 restrictions: an analysis of countries and regions in Asia Pacific and Europe. Lancet. 2020;396(10261):1525–34. https://doi.org/10.1016/S0140-6736(20)32007-9 PMID:32979936.
23. Jiang Q, Liu S, Hu Y, Xu J. Social media for health campaign and solidarity among Chinese fandom publics during the COVID-19 pandemic. Front Psychol. 2021;12:824377. https://doi.org/10.3389/fpsyg.2021.824377 PMID:35126267.
24. Burel G, Farrell T, Alani H. Demographics and topics impact on the co-spread of COVID-19 misinformation and fact-checks on Twitter. Inf Process Manage. 2021;58(6):102732. https://doi.org/10.1016/j.ipm.2021.102732 PMID:34511703.
25. Gilmore B, Ndejjo R, Tchetchia A, de Claro V, Mago E, Diallo AA, et al. Community engagement for COVID-19 prevention and control: a rapid evidence synthesis. BMJ Glob Health. 2020;5(10):e003188. https://doi.org/10.1136/bmjgh-2020-003188 PMID:33051285.
26. Bandyopadhyay S, Baticulon RE, Kadhum M, Alser M, Ojuka DK, Badereddin Y, et al. Infection and mortality of healthcare workers worldwide from COVID-19: a systematic review. BMJ Glob Health. 2020;5(12):e003097. https://doi.org/10.1136/bmjgh-2020-003097 PMID:33277297.
27. Chua AQ, Tan MM, Verma M, Han EK, Hsu LY, Cook AR, et al. Health system resilience in managing the COVID-19 pandemic: lessons from Singapore. BMJ Glob Health. 2020;5(9):e003317. https://doi.org/10.1136/bmjgh-2020-003317 PMID:32938609.
28. Feinmann J. What happened to our national emergency stockpiles? BMJ. 2021;375(2849):n2849. https://doi.org/10.1136/bmj.n2849 PMID:34848399.
29. Mukherjee S. Maruti Suzuki to help produce ventilators, masks and protective equipment to fight against COVID-19. The Economic Times; 2020. https://economictimes.indiatimes.com/news/company/corporate-trends/maruti-suzuki-to-help-produce-ventilators-masks-and-protective-equipment-to-fight-against-covid-19/articleshow/74859601.cms?from=mdr.
30. Ministry of Economy TaI. Current status of production and supply of facemasks, antiseptics and toilet paper. https://www.meti.go.jp/english/covid-19/mask.html.
31. Daryabor G, Atashzar MR, Kabelitz D, Meri S, Kalantar K. The effects of type 2 diabetes mellitus on organ metabolism and the immune system. Front Immunol. 2020;11:1582. https://doi.org/10.3389/fimmu.2020.01582 PMID:32793223.
32. Zhou Y, Chi J, Lv W, Wang Y. Obesity and diabetes as high-risk factors for severe coronavirus disease 2019 (Covid-19). Diabetes Metab Res Rev. 2021;37(2):e3377. https://doi.org/10.1002/dmrr.3377 PMID:32588943.
33. Fedele D, De Francesco A, Riso S, Collo A. Obesity, malnutrition, and trace element deficiency in the coronavirus disease (COVID-19) pandemic: an overview. Nutrition. 2021;81:111016. https://doi.org/10.1016/j.nut.2020.111016 PMID:33059127.
34. The impact of COVID-19 on cancer care 2022. https://www.macmillan.org.uk/get-involved/campaigns/we-make-change-happen/we-shape-policy/covid-19-impact-cancer-report.html#:~:text=The%20cancer%20backlog&text=Macmillan%20estimates%20that%20across%20the,have%20been%20diagnosed%20with%20cancer.
35. Iacobucci G. Cancer backlog could take till 2033 to clear without more consultants, says report. BMJ. 2021;374(2352):n2352. https://doi.org/10.1136/bmj.n2352 PMID:34561214.

36. Shadmi E, Chen Y, Dourado I, Faran-Perach I, Furler J, Hangoma P, et al. Health equity and COVID-19: global perspectives. Int J Equity Health. 2020 Jun 26;19(1):104. https://doi.org/10.1186/s12939-020-01218-z PMID:32586388.

37. Dongarwar D, Salihu HM. Implementation of universal health coverage by South Korea during the COVID-19 pandemic. Lancet Reg Health West Pac. 2021;7:100093. https://doi.org/10.1016/j.lanwpc.2021.100093 PMID:33532746.

38. Erondu NA, Martin J, Marten R, Ooms G, Yates R, Heymann DL. Building the case for embedding global health security into universal health coverage: a proposal for a unified health system that includes public health. Lancet. 2018;392(10156):1482–6. https://doi.org/10.1016/S0140-6736(18)32332-8 PMID:30343862.

39. Lal A, Erondu NA, Heymann DL, Gitahi G, Yates R. Fragmented health systems in COVID-19: rectifying the misalignment between global health security and universal health coverage. Lancet. 2021;397(10268):61–7. https://doi.org/10.1016/S0140-6736(20)32228-5 PMID:33275906.

40. Kasloff SB, Marszal P, Weingartl HM. Evaluation of nine positive pressure suits for use in the biosafety level-4 laboratory. Applied Biosafety [Internet]. 2018 Aug 21;23(4):223–32 https://doi.org/10.1177/1535676018793151.

41. Potter AW, Gonzalez JA, Xu X. Ebola response: modeling the risk of heat stress from personal protective clothing. PLoS One. 2015;10(11):e0143461. https://doi.org/10.1371/journal.pone.0143461 PMID:26575389.

42. Buonanno M, Welch D, Shuryak I, Brenner DJ. Far-UVC light (222 nm) efficiently and safely inactivates airborne human coronaviruses. Sci Rep. 2020;10(1):10285. https://doi.org/10.1038/s41598-020-67211-2 PMID:32581288.

43. Kraljevic S, Stambrook PJ, Pavelic K. Accelerating drug discovery. EMBO Rep. 2004;5(9):837–42. https://doi.org/10.1038/sj.embor.7400236 PMID:15470377.

44. Slaoui M, Hepburn M. Developing safe and effective covid vaccines - Operation Warp Speed's strategy and approach. N Engl J Med. 2020;383(18):1701–3. https://doi.org/10.1056/NEJMp2027405 PMID:32846056.

45. Alvea. Alvea set the record for fastest startup to take a new drug into a phase 1 clinical trial, from founding to first-in-human 2023. https://www.alvea.bio/alvea-set-the-record-for-the-fastest-startup-to-take-a-new-drug-into-a-phase-1-clinical-trial-from-founding-to-first-in-human-date/.

CHAPTER 15

COMPLICATING HUMANITARIAN EMERGENCIES

by Kate McNeil, Joycelyn Soo, and Myriam Henkens

Humanitarian emergencies may create conditions for infectious disease outbreaks, and outbreaks in turn can make humanitarian emergencies more difficult and complicated. This chapter reviews the humanitarian system including humanitarian principles, the humanitarian space, and significant actors in relation to how outbreaks can occur and be managed during humanitarian emergencies. Topics covered here include early warning and alert systems, water, sanitation, and hygiene (WASH) initiatives, nutrition, and vaccination. Comprehensive response to a health crisis in a humanitarian emergency or disaster setting often requires a strategic compromise between clinical and public health protocols and pragmatic considerations. Responses will usually involve strategies to cope with laboratory incapacity (e.g., rapid diagnostic tests), appropriate case management strategies, ample logistics planning, and community engagement for effective infection prevention and control.

INTRODUCTION

A humanitarian emergency is "an event or series of events that represents a critical threat to the health, safety, security, or wellbeing of a community or other large group of people, usually over a wide area" (1). Response to humanitarian emergencies is often understood as external support and assistance from actors in the national or international community in order to meet basic life-sustaining population needs (2).

The notion of a humanitarian emergency is closely intertwined with notions of crisis and disaster. While there are several typologies of disaster—and multiple competing ways of understanding the role of temporal and spatial components in disaster management (3)—these events should ultimately be understood as a "social product" (4). Disasters are not natural events—they are the product of a combination of risk factors encompassing hazards, vulnerability, and exposure (5). A flood in a country with poor infrastructure may have more drastic consequences than in one with resilient infrastructure. Environmental factors, such as exposure to animals, poor living conditions and crowding, economic insecurity, and conflict can also play a significant role, with risk factors compounding each other to increase the risk of outbreaks and disease transmission (6).

An infectious disease outbreak can cause or contribute to the development of a humanitarian emergency. For example, the Ebola outbreak in West Africa was also influenced by a history of civil war, specific cultural practices, mobile populations, and weak health infrastructure (7). More commonly, a humanitarian emergency can be complicated by the emergence of disease outbreaks. For example, the aftermath of flooding in Mozambique in 2008 saw cholera outbreaks and an increase in the incidence of malaria notifications, alongside population displacement (8). Specific additional challenges are linked with the management of outbreaks in humanitarian settings. These include the difficulties of working with moving populations, the lack of population or census data (or even knowledge of population size, which often precludes the calculation of basic epidemiological indicators), logistical and access challenges due to the destruction of infrastructure or ongoing conflict, and safety concerns for staff and populations (which may prevent basic investigations or response actions from being implemented). Those contributing to public health responses in humanitarian settings must consequently be in a position to identify and respond quickly in the context of an already complex situation (9).

THE HUMANITARIAN SYSTEM

Humanitarian action, whether in the aftermath of disasters or in areas experiencing political violence or conflict, operates within the context of a set of common guiding humanitarian principles which have been worked out over the years by the international community. These require humanitarian actors to ensure that the work is underpinned by "humanity, impartiality, neutrality, and independence" (10). In the context of political violence and conflict, these principles are accompanied by additional core protection principles which have been identified and codified in international law (11). These protection principles address topics including the separation of civilians from armed actors involved in the conflict, vulnerable populations, women, and children, and post-conflict issues including disarmament, de-mining, justice, reconciliation, and reintegration (12).

Alongside the humanitarian principles, medical actors contributing to responses within humanitarian contexts also bring pre-existing values and principles grounded within the medical ethics and bioethical standards of their professions. Efforts have been made to develop an ethical framework for health workers providing humanitarian assistance, which is guided by three overarching axioms: "recognising shared humanity (in the context of global disparity) ... acknowledging limits and risks ... [and] providing competent, practical assistance" (13).

In applying the humanitarian principles of independence and neutrality to their work, humanitarian organisations often rely upon the idea of humanitarian space. The basic notion is the creation of a distinct, independent operating arena in which humanitarian actors can carry out their work to meet the needs of a vulnerable population without interference. Creating and maintaining humanitarian space has both "tangible" and "normative" components as it involves creating both physical spaces in which humanitarian organisations can safely interact with affected populations, as well as ideological spaces for the implementation of international legal principles (14). For those providing healthcare to those impacted by humanitarian crises, the enaction of humanitarian space includes the creation of safe, accessible spaces for the delivery of healthcare services.

In practice, maintaining humanitarian space for healthcare provision can prove difficult. Efforts by military actors to contribute to healthcare delivery have been described as an "increasing blurring of roles between actors delivering health care in insecure environments" (15). Furthermore, it is often not enough to create space for healthcare workers to carry out their work through the creation of temporary hospitals in refugee camps or safe routes for ambulances. This space must extend to the safe and secure provision of logistical aspects of humanitarian response including transport and maintaining supply chains for food and medical products (16). Population access to health services should also be guaranteed.

Needs assessments inform decisions associated with humanitarian responses and must consider the context and realities of affected populations. This involves assessing risks, capabilities, and resources, including those specific to health (17). Health-specific needs assessments focus on immediate risks and public health priorities, including those related to malnutrition and outbreaks. More broadly, these assessments focus on understanding the extent of need and priorities for intervention, with the goal of understanding how to most appropriately plan, design, and implement a response. It should be noted that population needs will change over time and that effective needs assessments must be timely, useful, and result in actionable outcomes (18). One way of conducting these assessments is to use the Humanitarian Emergency Settings Perceived Needs Scale (HESPER) which is a methodological tool for understanding population needs (19).

The nature of the involvement of the various actors responding to humanitarian emergencies depends upon the context and nature of the specific emergency at hand. Relevant actors may include local governments and policymakers, stakeholders from within affected populations, actors from within the international system such as the United Nations High Commissioner for Refugees (UNHCR), the World Health Organization (WHO), the World Food Programme, the United Nations Children's Fund (UNICEF), the United Nations Office for the Coordination of Humanitarian Affairs (UN OCHA), the Red Cross, and the Red Crescent, and non-governmental organisations (NGOs) such as Oxfam, Médecins Sans Frontières (MSF), and CARE International (20).

RISK FACTORS AND ASSESSMENT
Why outbreaks happen

Infectious disease outbreaks can occur in the aftermath of disaster events and in humanitarian crises. This is because of the emergence of heightened vulnerability and increased risks associated with such events, be they conflict-related or the result of natural disasters such as floods, earthquakes, cyclones, or tsunamis. During and after these events, increased risks to human health can be posed by disruptions to or destruction of infrastructure, including water and sanitation systems, facilities, and their equipment, as well as by population displacement, damage to housing, and disruptions in patterns of human exposure to pathogens in animals and/or the environment (21).

Floods causing disease outbreaks

Documented links between the aftermath of flooding and epidemics such as Rift Valley fever, malaria, and West Nile fever have demonstrated that flooding can create new grounds for mosquito breeding, leading to an increased risk of vector-borne illnesses (22). The U.S. Centers for Disease Control and Prevention reported that the 1997/1998 El Niño-associated flood correlated

> with the largest ever Rift Valley fever outbreak in Kenya, as stagnant waters became breeding grounds for floodwater *Aedes* mosquitoes, resulting in approximately 89,000 infections and 478 deaths. There was also a peak of malaria parasites along the Kenya coast between 1974 and 2014 during periods of increased rainfall and flooding. Additionally, it was suggested that high rainfall influenced plant and rodent community compositions and the risk of rodent-borne pathogens.
>
> Early warning systems for infectious diseases based on flooding trends can be useful in reducing outbreaks. For example, effective predictions and timely precautionary measures helped mitigate a malaria outbreak in Botswana in 2018. Importantly, early warning systems should be coupled with public awareness to support the adoption of measures to curb disease outbreaks.

Population displacement is a significant factor in increased health risk in the aftermath of disasters, especially in conflict-affected populations. International outbreaks of measles in displaced populations in Asia and Africa, compounded by low vaccination coverage in the area of arrival, further increase the risk of outbreaks (23). Population displacement in humanitarian emergencies may exacerbate the risk of vaccine-preventable diseases, including measles, polio, yellow fever, cholera, and meningitis (24).

Inadequate (temporary) shelter and overcrowding have been linked to the spread of acute respiratory infections and outbreaks of malaria (25). The issue of shelter can interact with other risk factors—for example, elderly refugees who are less capable of carrying water for long distances will be at greater risk of obtaining waterborne communicable diseases (26).

Some heightened infectious disease risks are predictable, such as outbreaks of hepatitis E in areas where it is endemic, in the aftermath of flooding or a tsunami (27). However, other outbreaks may involve the importation of a disease to an area where it was not historically endemic, as occurred when cholera was likely imported into Haiti by international workers (28–29). Such events are rarer but should not be excluded from risk assessment in humanitarian settings and vaccination recommendations in humanitarian guidance documents, for example, those created by the Sphere (30).

Ultimately, it should be recognised that the risks posed in humanitarian settings are synergistic and compounding. This was highlighted by the experience of displaced Afghan refugees whose poor health outcomes were attributed to the compounding of exposure to multiple risk factors including "poor sanitation and nutrition, overcrowding, and inaccessibility of healthcare facilities" (31). Risks and efforts at prevention need to be managed through a holistic, systems-driven approach to humanitarian aid provision where possible.

Risk assessment

Cholera has resulted in seven great pandemics and is responsible for 1.3–4 million cases and 21,000–143,000 deaths globally each year. The first cholera pandemic originated in the Ganges delta, India, in the 19th century, while the current pandemic started in South Asia in 1961, reaching Africa in 1971, and the Americas in 1991. According to WHO recommendations, when a suspect case definition is met, a cholera alert is made and a risk assessment undertaken. The same is so for several other outbreak-associated pathogens in humanitarian settings (32).

Within healthcare facilities, risk and readiness assessment involves estimating treatment resource needs considering the number of patients expected, peak bed capacity, and treatment supplies based on existing stocks and quantities required (details and proposed calculations can be found in MSF guidance) (33). Based on rapid analysis of data collected, the potential benefit of vaccination can be assessed, and recommendations made as per evaluation.

Outside of healthcare facilities, risk assessment is based on local demographic data and various factors contributing to an epidemic such as high population density, gathering places with congregation, potential contamination of water sources, poor water quality, poor sanitation, and local meteorological conditions.

The WHO also proposes separate definitions for the end of an epidemic in endemic areas with annual or year-round transmission and non-endemic countries and endemic areas with sporadic epidemics.

Cholera risk assessment by MSF

NGOs such as MSF regularly undertake risk assessments for outbreaks of cholera in humanitarian settings (33). Data is collected and analysed to estimate the likely scale, impact, and response needs. Risk factors implicating a more severe outbreak include:

- history of outbreaks, high mortality rates, or large geographical involvement
- no outbreak two to three years prior (loss of innate immunity from a previous outbreak)
- divergence from the pattern typical of previous outbreaks (i.e., onset before usual season, outbreak in areas without prior history of disease, early involvement of a large number of individuals affected, early geographic extension, or outbreaks in several locations)
- disease emergence in communities with high population density (e.g., slums, refugee camps) or in mobile populations, either displaced from an area without history of cholera (no natural immunity) or from a cholera-endemic area (asymptomatic carriers import *Vibrio cholerae*)
- abnormal meteorological conditions (either very rainy or very dry)
- poor water and sanitation systems or healthcare access, or inadequate human resources to manage the outbreak due to humanitarian emergencies of various types

---

RISK MANAGEMENT
Early warning and alert

Early Warning, Alert and Response Networks (EWARN) and Early Warning, Alert and Response Systems (EWARS) play critical roles in identifying and supporting timely responses to infectious disease outbreaks in the context of humanitarian emergencies, particularly in fragile contexts (**See Chapter 9, Surveillance**). These systems can capture and monitor information about a range of potential health threats, such as malaria, influenza, and Ebola (34). EWARS, which is a WHO Emergencies system, collects data from primary health and community sources, manages this data via standardised systems drawing upon both qualitative and quantitative indicators, and analyses this data to produce findings which are then communicated in a routine and regular fashion (34).

> **Alert and warning systems in Haiti supported the response to cholera in 2010**
>
> Following the 2010 earthquake, the first documented cholera outbreak in Haiti further devastated the nation and spread throughout all ten departments and into neighbouring Dominican Republic (35). An alert and response (A&R) system was developed as a collaborative effort by the WHO and the Haiti Ministry of Health to complement the existing local surveillance network. This involved three components:
> - an early warning/alert function with rapid detection of cholera events
> - protocols for the verification and assessment of information collected
> - a response function coordinated by a national hub
>
> This system also informed the exit strategy. The early warning system utilised an epidemic intelligence process comprising indicator-based (data from routine surveillance systems and healthcare facilities) and event-based (unstructured information from official and unofficial sources) components. The sensitivity of the A&R system was demonstrated by the accurate prediction of areas vulnerable to cholera spread, which was later confirmed by an increased number of cases and immediate implementation of control measures. Subsequently, the A&R system strengthened the national surveillance system and built local capacities to monitor and respond to outbreaks. More than a decade later, the system is still operating.

Human knowledge networks, including through community contacts and social media, are also used as a way of obtaining local and temporally specific information. Social media monitoring informed part of the emergency response to Hurricane Maria in Puerto Rico. However, misleading rumours and misinformation may also occur with these communication channels (36).

Increasingly, as highlighted by evidence from the responses to monitoring the risk of cholera during the recent humanitarian crisis in Yemen, electronic and internet-based approaches to surveillance have played a vital role in identifying infectious disease outbreaks during the early stages of humanitarian emergencies, creating the opportunity to minimise disease spread during outbreaks (37–38). These types of electronic disease early warning systems (eDEWS) are affordable, efficient tools which can be rapidly deployed during the acute stages of an emergency and integrated into routine health surveillance systems in the aftermath of emergencies (39). Implementing electronic systems involves robust data collection from health facilities using mobile apps to facilitate easy routine reporting of health information (40).

Wastewater testing has been used to identify and monitor outbreaks of poliovirus (41) and SARS-CoV-2 (42). One Health surveillance (**See Chapter 13, One Health**) faces challenges with regards to implementation in humanitarian settings and among displaced populations. However, wastewater techniques have the potential to play a role in identifying potential zoonotic disease outbreaks (42–43).

While surveillance systems to identify potential infectious disease outbreaks are a valuable tool during a humanitarian emergency, experience from the field suggests that there are ongoing challenges to implementation, including capacities in the affected countries. Cross-country analysis of EWARN systems in the Eastern Mediterranean Region has emphasised these systems work best when simplicity is maintained by focusing on highest risk conditions (44).

The role of WASH in humanitarian emergencies
WASH initiatives are used in the prevention, control, and mitigation of potential infectious disease outbreaks in humanitarian arenas (45–46). While there remain some evidence gaps surrounding the usage of WASH during humanitarian emergencies (47), these programmes can be quick and are straightforward ways of consistently reducing both the risk of disease and transmission in outbreak contexts (45). Implementing WASH initiatives encompasses behavioural and community interventions on hygiene best practices. These include the provision of access to hygiene items—including culturally appropriate menstrual products, soap, and water containers—and the facilitation of appropriate infrastructure and supply chains related to the provision of clean water and the disposal of wastewater (46).

According to the WHO, 20 litres of water per person per day is the recommended safe minimum for meeting all basic needs. Sphere guidelines provide more detailed information on the basic acceptable standards for water provision at different time points in a humanitarian intervention, as well as the maximum acceptable distance between water points and shelters, a distance which should never exceed one kilometre (48). Different approaches may be used to provide necessary water to meet WASH standards, with emergency water trucking sometimes used as a short-term, life-saving intervention.

Nutrition
Poor nutrition can be an underlying risk factor contributing to the emergence of an infectious disease outbreak or poor outcomes during an outbreak, or it can be a consequence of an outbreak. Poor underlying nutrition is one of several factors linked to the emergence of outbreaks of measles, hepatitis A, and Leishmaniasis amongst Syrian refugees in Lebanon (49). Furthermore, measles outbreaks can have severe consequences on the nutritional status of children, particularly vitamin A deficiency (50). A high rate of existing malnutrition in a population affected by a humanitarian emergency is a well-recognised marker for poor outcomes from infection (51).

Risk management efforts related to nutrition in humanitarian settings entail assessments of the prevalence of food insecurity and extent of malnutrition, assessment of infant and young child feeding practices, and management of both micronutrient deficiencies and overall malnutrition through provision of food and nutrition assistance which meets Sphere standards (52).

Vaccination
The WHO has developed guidance for decision-makers seeking support on how to determine vaccination strategies in the context of a humanitarian emergency. It encompasses a range of factors, including an assessment of the epidemiological risk and considerations in vaccine delivery and implementation (53). This framework can guide urgent action which prevents outbreaks and has been used, for example, in guiding the delivery of meningococcal meningitis and cholera vaccines by MSF in South Sudan (54).

While there are barriers to vaccine distribution in complex humanitarian crisis settings (e.g., cost, access, logistics, and vaccine acceptability), recent research has emphasised the potential general value of increased vaccination against pneumonia, influenza, and rotavirus in reducing both morbidity and mortality (55). Other vaccines beyond those routinely scheduled may also be appropriate depending upon context-specific risks and realities within the humanitarian setting. A recent review of vaccine provision during humanitarian emergencies suggested that existing vaccination programming, while reflecting context-specific risks and disease, was insufficient (56). Furthermore, complex humanitarian crises can result in the breakdown of pre-existing immunisation services increasing the risk of these vaccine-preventable illnesses (57).

OUTBREAK RESPONSE

Identifying the outbreak and its cause will enable strategies for mitigating its impact, implementing prevention and control measures (**See Chapter 26, IPC**), and developing risk communications and community engagement strategies (**See Chapter 33, RCCE**). Humanitarian workers need to exercise clinical judgement when laboratory testing is not locally available, resources are limited, and diagnostic tools have not been developed.

Laboratory testing

Whilst laboratory confirmation is most ideal for accurate diagnosis, capacities can be limited or non-existent during health emergencies. Such circumstances may benefit from rapid diagnostic tests (RDTs) to support the quick diagnosis of disease in suspected cases and subsequent timely prevention and control measures. When used within appropriate frameworks and algorithms, public health decisions can still be guided by imperfect sensitivity and specificity of diagnostic tools. Groups such as the WHO Prequalification of In Vitro Diagnostics programme utilise rigorous prequalification processes considering the performance of these tests as well as their manufacturing conditions to ensure consistency of performance over time. However, there are no clear criteria outlined to select between competing RDTs. Several imperfect rapid diagnostic tools, via testing of faecal specimens, are also available for cholera—with such imperfect tools being considered most useful for early identification of an outbreak, rather than for diagnosis in individual patient cases, due to less-than-optimal test specificity and sensitivity (58). To be appropriately deployed in humanitarian settings, RDTs ideally need to fulfil certain criteria.

Criteria for selecting field-friendly RDTs in public health emergency settings
- RDTs quality assured according to international standards (performance independently assessed and remaining reliable over time)
- Acceptable cost
- Ease of use
- Need for limited training, equipment, or supplies
- Reliable procurement from the manufacturer
- Long shelf life (≥1 year)
- Storage without refrigeration
- Acceptable waste

Clinical management

Local constraints may shape case management strategies in humanitarian settings (**See Chapter 22, Clinical care**). For example, case management during the 2016–2018 cholera outbreak in Yemen involved setting up diarrhoea treatment centres and oral rehydration corners in or near existing health facilities due to a shortage of staff and volunteers (**See Chapter 25, Infrastructure**) (59). Moreover, for some infectious diseases including cholera, there are standard targets defined in the relevant guidance document which can be used in quality control monitoring during case management. For other diseases, including acute respiratory infections, there are no standard indicators available (60).

The examples above illustrate that to cope with an outbreak in most humanitarian circumstances, standard treatment protocols must be established as soon as possible, with single-dose treatment preferred (or at least one dose daily). Simplified protocols should allow for ambulatory treatment and decentralisation of care with task shifting.

Additionally, humanitarian aid providers are sometimes forced to grapple with the ethics of providing time-sensitive access to experimental medications, as during the 2014 Ebola outbreak (61). Intellectual property and patent constraints in accessing medications may also become fraught issues.

Strategic compromise in Cox's Bazar during the 2018 diphtheria outbreak

In 2017, an estimated 720,000 Rohingya refugees were displaced from Rakhine to the district of Cox's Bazar, Bangladesh (62). Together with pre-existing refugees, this added up to a total of 930,000 people living in refugee camps by the end of that year. Within this population, several outbreaks of diphtheria were detected, with 8,179 cases reported by August 2018, including 44 deaths. Humanitarian actors used a protocol which provides care to those with a "probable clinical diagnosis". Most patients in this setting never received a confirmatory diagnosis as laboratory capacity was limited. Oral azithromycin was chosen as the primary antibiotic because it is a once-daily dose, viewed to be more feasible in a resource-limited setting, as opposed to oral penicillin and erythromycin which are typically recommended for first-time treatment but require administration up to four times a day (62). Diphtheria antitoxin treatments, contrary to standard treatment protocol, were only used in severe cases instead of in all probable cases of respiratory diphtheria due to a limited supply of the antitoxin globally with concurrent outbreaks in Yemen, Indonesia, Venezuela, and Haiti. This type of response has been described by humanitarian practitioners as a strategic compromise, that is, a modification to a response to allow feasibility and scalability of an outbreak response in a humanitarian emergency.

Infection prevention and control (IPC)

While the IPC principles all apply, in humanitarian contexts, there is sometimes a need to prioritise to implement large-scale interventions. The ideal will in any case be compromised so there is a need to distinguish the 'must have' from the 'nice to have'. As an example, the use of a footbath in cholera treatment centres has never proven to be efficacious. Home disinfection programmes proved to be a costly intervention diverting resources from other more important measures such as the provision of sufficient quantities of clear water to the population.

Logistics
An already complex logistics challenge is made even more challenging when an infectious disease outbreak occurs within a humanitarian emergency context (**See Chapter 7, Logistics**). Disruptions to transportation and communication networks need to be overcome to understand needs and manage the supply chain. The provision of WASH interventions should also be accompanied by health kits in cases of waterborne disease outbreaks, such as cholera and typhoid fever.

Some components of logistical management may also be emergency-specific, with pragmatic operational approaches being deployed where there are shortages of needed goods or resources. For example, in October 2022, a global shortage of cholera vaccines resulted in the transition from a two-dose to a single-dose approach to administering cholera vaccines, despite the single-dose approach shortening the duration of immunity (63).

Community engagement
Community engagement has the goal of increasing understanding and building trust (**See Chapter 33, RCCE**). A community engagement working group was created in the Philippines during Typhoon Bopha in 2012 and persisted as a core humanitarian activity through the next few humanitarian emergencies in the Philippines in 2013 namely the Zamboanga Siege, Bohol Earthquake, and Typhoon Haiyan.

Risk communications and community engagement (RCCE) strategies will have to take into account population displacement and that emergency living conditions may shift individual priorities away from specific disease control measures (e.g., food and drinking water being prioritised over washing hands).

CONCLUSION
Humanitarian emergencies have a devastating impact on the local population and wider community, often involving population displacement. Densely populated temporary lodging, poor sanitation and nutrition, and breakdowns in healthcare systems and public health services predispose disaster settings to infectious disease outbreaks. Even if outbreaks in such settings can be predicted, they pose specific challenges in the surveillance required for detection and monitoring, as well as in mounting the needed response. Through the 2020s, an increasing number of countries are experiencing cholera outbreaks due to climate change. Other countries can attribute outbreaks of cholera to political instability and conflict. These cholera outbreaks often do not occur in isolation, with mpox, dengue, chikungunya, measles, and COVID-19 outbreaks confounding responses.

Health services and their functionality are often severely compromised during disasters and lack adequate resources (e.g., staff, supplies, and finance). Humanitarian disaster response teams and the leadership of countries affected will increasingly need to be more proficient in risk assessment and preventative efforts for infectious disease outbreaks. This includes surveillance and preparedness efforts recognising that such outbreaks can be predictable and potentially preventable.

REFERENCES:

1. The Humanitarian Coalition. What is a Humanitarian Emergency. https://www.humanitariancoalition.ca/what-is-a-humanitarian-emergency.
2. Anderson M, Gerber M. Introduction to Humanitarian Emergencies. In: Townes D, editor. Health in Humanitarian Emergencies: Principles and Practice for Public Health and Healthcare Practitioners [Internet] Cambridge: Cambridge University Press; 2018. pp. 1–8. https://www.cambridge.org/core/books/health-in-humanitarian-emergencies/introduction-to-humanitarian-emergencies/D2A8592F97497D7C786B4EF4B19E081F.
3. Hsu EL. Must disasters be rapidly occurring? The case for an expanded temporal typology of disasters. Time Soc. 2019 Aug;28(3):904–21. https://doi.org/10.1177/0961463X17701956.
4. Britton NR. Developing an understanding of disaster. Aust N Z J Sociol. 1986 Aug;22(2):254–71. https://doi.org/10.1177/144078338602200206.
5. Vulnerability. UNDDR PreventionWeb. https://www.preventionweb.net/understanding-disaster-risk/component-risk/vulnerability.
6. Hammer CC, Brainard J, Hunter PR. Risk factors and risk factor cascades for communicable disease outbreaks in complex humanitarian emergencies: a qualitative systematic review. BMJ Glob Health. 2018 Jul;3(4):e000647. https://doi.org/10.1136/bmjgh-2017-000647 PMID:30002920.
7. Piot P, Muyembe JJ, Edmunds WJ. Ebola in west Africa: from disease outbreak to humanitarian crisis. Lancet Infect Dis. 2014 Nov;14(11):1034–5. https://doi.org/10.1016/S1473-3099(14)70956-9 PMID:25282665.
8. Sidley P. Floods in southern Africa result in cholera outbreak and displacement. BMJ. 2008 Mar;336(7642):471. https://doi.org/10.1136/bmj.39503.700903.DB PMID:18309996.
9. Ager A, Burnham G, Checchi F, Gayer M, Grais RF, Henkens M, et al. Strengthening the evidence base for health programming in humanitarian crises. Science. 2014 Sep;345(6202):1290–2. https://doi.org/10.1126/science.1254164 PMID:25214616.
10. Humanitarian principles. UNHCR Emergency Handbook. https://emergency.unhcr.org/entry/44765/humanitarian-principles.
11. Françoise Bouchet-Saulnier. The Practical Guide to Humanitarian Law; Rowman and Littlefield, 2007.
12. Wisner B. Violent conflict, natural hazards, and disaster. The Routledge Handbook of Hazards and Disaster Risk Reduction. Routledge; 2012.
13. Hunt MR, Schwartz L, Sinding C, Elit L. The ethics of engaged presence: a framework for health professionals in humanitarian assistance and development work. Dev World Bioeth. 2014 Apr;14(1):47–55. https://doi.org/10.1111/dewb.12013 PMID:23279367.
14. ICRC. Humanitarian space – or spaces – must be protected, without exception. International Committee of the Red Cross. 2021. https://www.icrc.org/en/document/humanitarian-space-must-be-protected-without-exception.
15. Birch M. Delivering health care in insecure environments: UK foreign policy, military actors and the erosion of humanitarian space. Med Confl Surviv. 2010;26(1):80–5. https://doi.org/10.1080/13623690903553277 PMID:20411857.
16. Larson PD. Security, sustainability and supply chain collaboration in the humanitarian space. Journal of Humanitarian Logistics and Supply Chain Management. 2021;11(4):609–22. https://doi.org/10.1108/JHLSCM-06-2021-0059.
17. Garfield R, von Schreeb J, Eriksson A, Chataigner P. Needs Assessments. In: Townes D, editor. Health in Humanitarian Emergencies: Principles and Practice for Public Health and Healthcare Practitioners Cambridge: Cambridge University Press; 2018. pp. 79–90. https://www.cambridge.org/core/books/health-in-humanitarian-emergencies/needs-assessments/226DEA0E626A7E82762291B18705C6F8 https://doi.org/10.1017/9781107477261.008.
18. Deitchman S. What have we learned? Needs assessment. Prehosp Disaster Med. 2005;20(6):468–70. https://doi.org/10.1017/S1049023X00003149 PMID:16496639.
19. Hugelius K. Measurement of perceived needs in humanitarian contexts using the HESPER scale: a scoping study with reflections on the collaboration between researchers and humanitarian actors. Confl Health. 2022 Aug;16(1):44. https://doi.org/10.1186/s13031-022-00478-6 PMID:36028872.
20. UN and intergovernmental actors. https://phap.org/PHAP/PHAP/Themes/UN and intergov.aspx.
21. Charnley GE, Kelman I, Gaythorpe KA, Murray KA. Traits and risk factors of post-disaster infectious disease outbreaks: a systematic review. Sci Rep. 2021 Mar;11(1):5616. https://doi.org/10.1038/s41598-021-85146-0 PMID:33692451.

22. Okaka FO, Odhiambo BD. Relationship between flooding and out break of infectious diseases in Kenya: a review of the literature. J Environ Public Health. 2018 Oct;2018:5452938. https://doi.org/10.1155/2018/5452938 PMID:30416526.
23. Kouadio IK, Kamigaki T, Oshitani H. Measles outbreaks in displaced populations: a review of transmission, morbidity and mortality associated factors. BMC Int Health Hum Rights. 2010 Mar;10(1):5. https://doi.org/10.1186/1472-698X-10-5 PMID:20298611.
24. Connolly MA, Gayer M, Ryan MJ, Salama P, Spiegel P, Heymann DL. Communicable diseases in complex emergencies: impact and challenges. Lancet. 2004 Nov;364(9449):1974–83. https://doi.org/10.1016/S0140-6736(04)17481-3 PMID:15567014.
25. Topluoglu S, Taylan-Ozkan A, Alp E. Impact of wars and natural disasters on emerging and re-emerging infectious diseases. Front Public Health. 2023;11:1215929. https://doi.org/10.3389/fpubh.2023.1215929 PMID:37727613.
26. Burton A, Breen C. Older refugees in humanitarian emergencies. Lancet. 2002 Dec;360 Suppl:s47–8. https://doi.org/10.1016/S0140-6736(02)11819-8 PMID:12504502.
27. Programme on Disease Control in Humanitarian Emergencies, Communicable Diseases Cluster. Communicable diseases following natural disasters: Risk assessment and priority interventions. WHO; 2006. https://preparecenter.org/wp-content/sites/default/files/cd_disasters_26_06.pdf.
28. Piarroux R, Barrais R, Faucher B, Haus R, Piarroux M, Gaudart J, et al. Understanding the cholera epidemic, Haiti. Emerg Infect Dis. 2011 Jul;17(7):1161–8. https://doi.org/10.3201/eid1707.110059 PMID:21762567.
29. Pun SB. Understanding the cholera epidemic, Haiti. Emerg Infect Dis. 2011 Nov;17(11):2178-9; author reply 2179-80. https://doi.org/10.3201/eid1711.110981 PMID:22204043.
30. The Sphere Project. Humanitarian Charter and Minimum Standards in Humanitarian Response. 2011. https://spherestandards.org/wp-content/uploads/2018/06/Sphere_Handbook_2011_English.pdf.
31. Rajabali A, Moin O, Ansari AS, Khanani MR, Ali SH. Communicable disease among displaced Afghans: refuge without shelter. Nat Rev Microbiol. 2009 Aug;7(8):609–14. https://doi.org/10.1038/nrmicro2176 PMID:19609262.
32. World Health Organization. Outbreak surveillance and response in humanitarian emergencies. 2012. https://www.who.int/publications-detail-redirect/outbreak-surveillance-and-response-in-humanitarian-emergencies-who-guidelines-for-ewarn-implementation.
33. Médecins Sans Frontières. Management of a cholera epidemic. https://medicalguidelines.msf.org/en/viewport/CHOL/english/management-of-a-cholera-epidemic-23444438.html?language_content_entity=en.
34. WHO Health Emergencies Program. WHO's electronic early warning, alert, and response system in emergencies: EWARS-in-a-box. World Health Organization. https://cdn.who.int/media/docs/default-source/emergency-preparedness/who-s-ewars-in-a-box-general-features.pdf?sfvrsn=d89b8610_1.
35. Santa-Olalla P, Gayer M, Magloire R, Barrais R, Valenciano M, Aramburu C, et al. Implementation of an alert and response system in Haiti during the early stage of the response to the cholera epidemic. Am J Trop Med Hyg. 2013 Oct;89(4):688–97. https://doi.org/10.4269/ajtmh.13-0267 PMID:24106196.
36. Bui L. Social media, rumors, and hurricane warning systems in Puerto Rico. 2019. https://scholarspace.manoa.hawaii.edu/server/api/core/bitstreams/93674e28-fa67-490f-a862-2a38ebe5fdeb/content.
37. Ahmed K, Altaf MD, Dureab F. Electronic infectious disease surveillance system during humanitarian crises in Yemen. Online J Public Health Inform. 2014 Apr;6(1):e134. https://doi.org/10.5210/ojphi.v6i1.5083.
38. Dureab F, Ismail O, Müller O, Jahn A. Cholera outbreak in Yemen: timeliness of reporting and response in the national electronic disease early warning system. Acta Inform Med. 2019 Jun;27(2):85–8. https://doi.org/10.5455/aim.2019.27.85-88 PMID:31452564.
39. Ahmed K, Bukhari MA, Altaf MD, Lugala PC, Popal GR, Abouzeid A, et al. Development and implementation of electronic disease early warning systems for optimal disease surveillance and response during humanitarian crisis and Ebola outbreak in Yemen, Somalia, Liberia and Pakistan. Online J Public Health Inform. 2019 Sep;11(2):e11. https://doi.org/10.5210/ojphi.v11i2.10157 PMID:31632605.
40. Mayad M, Alyusfi R, Assabri A, Khader Y. An electronic disease early warning system in Sana'a Governorate, Yemen: evaluation study. JMIR Public Health Surveill. 2019 Nov;5(4):e14295. https://doi.org/10.2196/14295 PMID:31742559.
41. Bolu O, Nnadi C, Damisa E, Braka F, Siddique A, Archer WR, et al. Progress toward poliomyelitis eradication – Nigeria, January-December 2017. MMWR Morb Mortal Wkly Rep. 2018 Mar;67(8):253–6. https://doi.org/10.15585/mmwr.mm6708a5 PMID:29494568.

42. Gwenzi W. Wastewater, waste, and water-based epidemiology (WWW-BE): a novel hypothesis and decision-support tool to unravel COVID-19 in low-income settings? Sci Total Environ. 2022 Feb;806(Pt 3):150680. https://doi.org/10.1016/j.scitotenv.2021.150680 PMID:34599955.
43. Abuzerr S, Zinsser K, Assan A. Implementation challenges of an integrated One Health surveillance system in humanitarian settings: a qualitative study in Palestine. SAGE Open Med. 2021 Sep;9:20503121211043038. https://doi.org/10.1177/20503121211043038 PMID:34504706.
44. Mala P, Abubakar A, Takeuchi A, Buliva E, Husain F, Malik MR, et al. Structure, function and performance of Early Warning Alert and Response Network (EWARN) in emergencies in the Eastern Mediterranean Region. Int J Infect Dis. 2021 Apr;105:194–8. https://doi.org/10.1016/j.ijid.2021.02.002 PMID:33556613.
45. Ramesh A, Blanchet K, Ensink JH, Roberts B. Evidence on the effectiveness of Water, Sanitation, and Hygiene (WASH) interventions on health outcomes in humanitarian crises: a systematic review. PLoS One. 2015 Sep;10(9):e0124688. https://doi.org/10.1371/journal.pone.0124688 PMID:26398228.
46. Allen J, Lantagne D, Leandre Joseph M, Yates T. WASH interventions in disease outbreak response. Feinstein International Center, Oxfam, UKAID; 2017. https://policy-practice.oxfam.org/resources/wash-interventions-in-disease-outbreak-response-620202/.
47. Yates T, Vijcic J, Joseph DM, Lantagne DD. Impact of WASH interventions during disease outbreaks in humanitarian emergencies: a systematic review protocol. Humanitarian Evidence Programme; 2014. https://oxfamilibrary.openrepository.com/bitstream/handle/10546/605152/rr-impact-wash-disease-outbreaks-130416-en.pdf?sequence=1&isAllowed=y.
48. Sphere. Sphere Standards Interactive Handbook – Companion standards (MERS,MISMA,CPMS,CAMP,HIS,LEGS,INEE). https://handbook.spherestandards.org/.
49. Helou M, Van Berlaer G, Yammine K. Factors influencing the occurrence of infectious disease outbreaks in Lebanon since the Syrian crisis. Pathog Glob Health. 2022 Feb;116(1):13–21. https://doi.org/10.1080/20477724.2021.1957192 PMID:34313580.
50. Melenotte C, Brouqui P, Botelho-Nevers E. Severe measles, vitamin A deficiency, and the Roma community in Europe. Emerg Infect Dis. 2012 Sep;18(9):1537–9. https://doi.org/10.3201/eid1809.111701 PMID:22932125.
51. Qirbi N, Ismail SA. Ongoing threat of a large-scale measles outbreak in Yemen. Lancet Glob Health. 2016 Jul;4(7):e451. https://doi.org/10.1016/S2214-109X(16)30070-5 PMID:27340001.
52. Pothiawala S. Food and shelter standards in humanitarian action. Turk J Emerg Med. 2016 Mar;15 Suppl 1:34–9. https://doi.org/10.5505/1304.7361.2015.98360 PMID:27437530.
53. WHO. Vaccination in acute humanitarian emergencies: a framework for decision making. 2017. https://apps.who.int/iris/bitstream/handle/10665/255575/WHO-IVB-17.03-eng.pdf?sequence=1&isAllowed=y.
54. Rull M, Masson S, Peyraud N, Simonelli M, Ventura A, Dorion C, et al. The new WHO decision-making framework on vaccine use in acute humanitarian emergencies: MSF experience in Minkaman, South Sudan. Confl Health. 2018 Mar;12(1):11. https://doi.org/10.1186/s13031-018-0147-z PMID:29599819.
55. Close RM, Pearson C, Cohn J. Vaccine-preventable disease and the under-utilization of immunizations in complex humanitarian emergencies. Vaccine. 2016 Sep;34(39):4649–55. https://doi.org/10.1016/j.vaccine.2016.08.025 PMID:27527818.
56. Leach K, Checchi F. The utilisation of vaccines in humanitarian crises, 2015-2019: a review of practice. Vaccine. 2022 May;40(21):2970–8. https://doi.org/10.1016/j.vaccine.2022.03.034 PMID:35341644.
57. Lam E, McCarthy A, Brennan M. Vaccine-preventable diseases in humanitarian emergencies among refugee and internally-displaced populations. Hum Vaccin Immunother. 2015;11(11):2627–36. https://doi.org/10.1080/21645515.2015.1096457 PMID:26406333.
58. Keddy KH, Sooka A, Parsons MB, Njanpop-Lafourcade BM, Fitchet K, Smith AM. Diagnosis of Vibrio cholerae O1 infection in Africa. J Infect Dis. 2013 Nov;208 Suppl 1:S23–31. https://doi.org/10.1093/infdis/jit196 PMID:24101641.
59. Spiegel P, Ratnayake R, Hellman N, Ververs M, Ngwa M, Wise PH, et al. Responding to epidemics in large-scale humanitarian crises: a case study of the cholera response in Yemen, 2016-2018. BMJ Glob Health. 2019 Jul;4(4):e001709. https://doi.org/10.1136/bmjgh-2019-001709 PMID:31406596.
60. Bellos A, Mulholland K, O'Brien KL, Qazi SA, Gayer M, Checchi F. The burden of acute respiratory infections in crisis-affected populations: a systematic review. Confl Health. 2010 Feb;4(1):3. https://doi.org/10.1186/1752-1505-4-3 PMID:20181220.

61. Singh JA. Humanitarian access to unapproved interventions in public health emergencies of international concern. PLoS Med. 2015 Feb;12(2):e1001793. https://doi.org/10.1371/journal.pmed.1001793 PMID:25710504.
62. Polonsky JA, Ivey M, Mazhar MK, Rahman Z, le Polain de Waroux O, Karo B, et al. Epidemiological, clinical, and public health response characteristics of a large outbreak of diphtheria among the Rohingya population in Cox's Bazar, Bangladesh, 2017 to 2019: A retrospective study. PLoS Med. 2021 Apr;18(4):e1003587. https://doi.org/10.1371/journal.pmed.1003587 PMID:33793554.
63. Shortage of cholera vaccines leads to temporary suspension of two-dose strategy, as cases rise worldwide. https://www.who.int/news/item/19-10-2022-shortage-of-cholera-vaccines-leads-to-temporary-suspension-of-two-dose-strategy--as-cases-rise-worldwide.

CHAPTER 16

MODELLING TO INFORM STRATEGY

by Louisa Sun, Gabriel Leung, and Alex R. Cook

The application of mathematical modelling to the dynamics of infectious disease outbreaks has been pivotal over the past five decades. The significance of such modelling escalated during the COVID-19 pandemic, influencing political decisions and shaping public discourse. Infectious disease models enhance our understanding of epidemiology and disease dynamics, predict transmission rates and patterns, and aid in evaluating public health interventions. Despite their utility, models cannot fully encapsulate the complexities of real-world scenarios, which are influenced by dynamic social behaviours and policy changes. This chapter explains the key model parameters and epidemiological indices fundamental to infectious disease modelling, such as the basic reproduction number R_0 and the effective reproduction number R_t. These indices predict disease trajectories, inform vaccination strategies, and guide public health responses.

The chapter also discusses the implications of symptom profiles, infectivity, incubation periods, disease severity, test positivity, and vaccine efficacy on modelling efforts. Furthermore, it underscores the importance of collaborative efforts between modellers and public health officials to ensure the accuracy and applicability of models in diverse contexts. Ultimately, infectious disease models are invaluable tools for forecasting disease spread and severity, guiding critical healthcare resources, and informing policy decisions to mitigate the impact of outbreaks.

INTRODUCTION

The use of mathematical modelling to study the dynamics of infectious disease outbreaks has grown in importance over the past 50 years (1) and has been applied successfully in epidemics such as pandemic influenza (2–4), HIV/AIDS (5–7), Ebola (8–10), and malaria (11–12), as well as large epizootics such as foot and mouth disease (13–15). Modelling became even more prominent over the course of the COVID-19 pandemic, with results making their way into political decisions and public discourse (16–18). Infectious disease models aid our understanding of the epidemiology of disease and disease dynamics, may predict transmission rates and patterns during outbreaks, and inform critical decisions on outbreak response and public health strategies, by helping test the effectiveness of different policy options for controlling the outbreak (1,19–20).

Models also act as a lens to interpret epidemic indicators, and the marriage of model and data may change our understanding of the processes underlying the epidemic. However, while infectious disease models have been demonstrated to be potentially useful in managing outbreaks, none can perfectly predict or capture the complexity of real-life scenarios (21–23) which are constantly evolving and are influenced by a multitude of interlinking factors. Changing policies and social behaviour, in particular, are difficult to adequately characterise (24–27). The performance of infectious disease models is also dependent on the validity of input parameters or other indicators of the epidemic. The truism "garbage in, garbage out" is salient, for no matter how sophisticated the model, if key inputs are inaccurate, so too will be the outputs (21–22,24).

This chapter will not discuss the technicalities of building and validating models, or the capacity and capability issues linked to modelling. These are important and deserve a fuller treatment (such as those presented by Vynnycky and White (28) and Diekmann and Heesterbeek (29)). Working from the assumption that modelling know-how and technical capabilities (such as a suitably powerful compute framework) are available, this chapter discusses some of the more important model parameters and epidemiological indices that are common building blocks in infectious disease modelling. These are summarised in **Table 16.1**.

Epidemiological parameter/index	Main practical applications for outbreak response/planning	Notes
Basic reproduction number, R_0	• Predicts epidemiologic trajectory and pattern of disease spread • Determines vaccination coverage and amount of control needed to curtail spread	Does not vary over the course of the outbreak, but may vary from place to place
Effective reproduction number, R_t	• Aids ongoing public health strategies and policy decisions, based on the estimation of degree to which interventions need to be introduced to reduce disease transmission	Inherently time-varying in response to changes in immunity, policies, and social response
Symptom profile	• Understanding the impacts of different proportions of symptomatic, asymptomatic, or pre-symptomatic infections on progression of the epidemic curve	May change over time as different population subgroups are infected, and potentially as new variants emerge
Infectivity	• Implications on effectiveness of control interventions • Decisions on the frequency and timing of testing	Should not change over the course of the epidemic, though may vary substantially over the course of infection, unless in the case of new variants with sufficiently different viral properties
Incubation period distribution	• Predicts disease transmission and trajectories of spread • Implications on outbreak control	Inherently non-time varying, unless in the case of new variants
Disease severity	• Important for healthcare system capacity/hospital resource planning and allocation to ensure the ability to manage severe cases	Usually does not change over time, unless in the case of new variants. However, this may appear to vary as different patient populations get infected

Epidemiological parameter/index	Main practical applications for outbreak response/planning	Notes
Test positivity	• Directly and indirectly informs areas needing adaptation in ongoing outbreak control and public health response strategies • May signal the presence of cryptic chains of infection	Needs details of who is getting tested to compare between health systems, since routine testing of people not suspected to be infected will yield different rates to testing of contacts or people with symptoms
Vaccine efficacy	• Estimates the effectiveness of vaccination strategies • Enhances the robustness of vaccine efficacy trials by capturing the uncertainties of evolving disease transmission during shorter trial durations	Changes over time since vaccination, and may vary for different levels of severity (e.g., protecting more against severe illness than against infection)

Table 16.1: Important model parameters and epidemiological indices that are common building blocks in infectious disease modelling

TRANSMISSIBILITY OF THE PATHOGEN

The basic reproduction number, or ratio, R_0—which is often misleadingly called the basic reproduction "rate", despite being unitless—is one of the more fundamental characteristics of the outbreak potential of a pathogen in a population. Its theoretical definition is the average number of secondary cases created by a typical infectious individual in an otherwise fully susceptible population, and it quantifies the transmission potential of an infectious pathogen, though over time, the realised transmissibility will usually fall (29–31).

There are several reasons why R_0 is so critical to our understanding of an epidemic. First, it can be used to calculate the proportion F of the population that will be infected by the end of one unmitigated wave of transmission using the relationship $F = 1-\exp(-R_0 F)$. Being able to estimate this early in the wave sets the expectations for the rest of the wave. Second, it determines by how much measures such as non-pharmaceutical interventions need to reduce transmission in order to curb epidemic growth. For instance, if $R_0=3$, transmissibility needs to be reduced by 67 per cent to stop outbreaks. Third, it contributes to determining the speed of the epidemic (alongside the generation time distribution or the serial interval). It is thus useful for obtaining initial predictions of short-term epidemic growth, to inform rapid decisions on bed capacity and other healthcare system response planning. Fourth, it tells us the proportion of the population needed to be infected to reach herd immunity ($1-1/R_0$)—the point at which equipoise is reached between recovery of those currently infected and the infection of susceptible individuals, beyond which the epidemic wanes—either due to immunity-conferring infection or vaccination.

Although it is one of the most fundamental parameters used in infectious disease modelling, it is rarely amenable to direct measurement, for it is affected by social factors that may vary between and within populations, and change over time, such as the intensity of social contacts and the social network structure (31–32). In addition, as immunity builds in the population, or as measures to control spread are implemented, the inherent transmissibility becomes increasingly obfuscated, making it harder to estimate R_0. Methods of estimation include using contact tracing to identify the distribution of secondary cases and taking advantage of the period of exponential growth at the beginning of the epidemic to derive the growth rate, whence the basic reproduction number can be obtained (33–34). There may be substantial variation in estimates from different locations or times due to social and cultural differences in each setting, in addition to differences in inferential approaches.

Many estimation methods are applicable only in the early days of spread, and thus there can be considerable uncertainty of the theoretical R_0 for long-established pathogens once immunity has been established and in the presence of exogenous factors such as non-pharmaceutical interventions or vaccination campaigns. Often, however, it is of interest to determine the extent to which dynamic, exogenous factors are influencing current transmissibility—factors such as changing population immunity or susceptibility, transmission settings, and mobility of the population (1,31).

The effective reproduction number, or R_t, is essentially the dynamic analogue of R_0. It represents the ongoing, actual transmissibility of the pathogen among the remaining susceptible population. Unlike R_0, R_t is inherently time-varying and is also affected by external factors such as population immunity that has been built up through infection or vaccination or both, and other public health measures that have been implemented. When R_t falls to unity, the transmission wave crests, and when it falls further, the case numbers fall. Because both reproduction ratios are compounded over time in determining the number of cases, what may seem to be small fluctuations in R_t can result in a substantial change in case numbers, as was seen during the COVID-19 pandemic when some countries saw resurgences after relatively modest changes in policies that tipped R_t above the threshold of one (**See R_t and COVID-19 cases in Thailand and the U.K.**).

Contact tracing provides the necessary data to accurately estimate the number of people each case infects, and with that, the changing real-time reproduction number. When contact tracing data are unavailable, the seminal method of estimating R_t, proposed by Wallinga and Teunis in 2004 (35), can be used instead. The method combines a timeseries of diagnosed cases with an estimate of the serial interval distribution. Modern extensions of the Wallinga and Teunis method improve the precision of the resulting estimates and include EpiEstim by Cori et al., EpiFilter by Parag, EpiInvert by Alvarez et al., and EpiRegress by Jin et al. (36–39). One substantial challenge that emerged during COVID-19 in low-incidence settings is that R_t estimation becomes very uncertain, and hence less informative, when case numbers are low, such as during periods of strict border controls or lockdowns. Measures and methods to pool information (such as EpiFilter or EpiRegress) may be needed in such situations. Another issue is that not all these methodologies work well when a large proportion of cases originate elsewhere.

It is natural to hope that the effect of changes in response measures could be measured through changes observed in R_t. However, if several responses are changing at the same time, teasing out the effects of each individual element may be challenging (40–41). Doing so may require synthesising evidence from different settings.

R_t and COVID-19 cases in Thailand and the U.K.

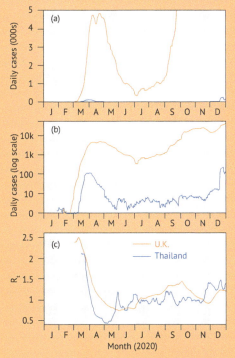

To illustrate how small differences in the effective reproduction number, R_t, impact the dynamics of an outbreak, we compare the situation in two similarly sized countries with drastically different experiences of COVID-19 in 2020.

In Thailand, after autochthonous cases rose substantially in March, a state of emergency was declared (26 March) followed by a curfew (3 April). Panel (c) shows these brought R_t quickly below 1 (at which point the wave peaked—see panel (b)). As cases fell to very low levels, once measures were gradually relaxed from mid-May, few local cases were detected until December.

In the U.K., over the course of March, measures were gradually imposed, such as closures of schools and public venues (20 March), followed by a stay-at-home order (26 March). Panel (c) shows that these measures did not cause R_t to fall by as much as in Thailand. Combined with the higher number of cases in the U.K. at the time control measures were introduced, this meant that when measures were relaxed from May onwards, there was still a substantial amount of infection in the community. Thus, when R_t rose above 1 in July, the absolute number of cases grew markedly (in comparison to Thailand, despite the similar R_t values), necessitating further restrictions and lockdowns.

The difference between these R_t trajectories led to the U.K. having 250,000 confirmed cases over 2020, while Thailand had fewer than 7,000.

a) Smoothed daily reported cases of COVID-19 in Thailand and the U.K., 2020. The Thai numbers hug the *x*-axis. The U.K. cases rise to over 40,000 in December (not shown to allow the Thai data to be seen).
b) As above, but on a logarithmic scale.
c) Estimated effective reproduction number.
(Data from Our World in Data)

THE OVERALL DISEASE PROFILE

It is vital in the early stages of an outbreak to gather as much information as possible about typical symptom profile and how symptoms progress during the course of the disease, and consequently, to collect data on the overall distribution of symptom severity amongst those infected. The overall symptom profile can appear to change with time as different populations and patient subgroups become infected—for instance, if care homes experience clusters (42–43)—or as different prophylactic and early therapeutic drugs are developed and used.

Symptomology may even vary by geographical location or country. For example, Kadirvelu et al. collected an online symptom survey from 190 different countries (44) and found that COVID-19 symptoms varied globally. This survey revealed that, for example, headache was reported more commonly in Brazil and Mexico, but rarely in India. The many differences unearthed in this study could be due to differences in the age ranges of patients with COVID-19 and the survey responders, and could be correlated with the presence of chronic diseases such as asthma and diabetes which have different epidemiology in different settings.

Symptom profile can also change as the pathogen mutates and circulating variants change, as was seen with COVID-19. The most common symptoms of the Omicron subvariants are headache, runny nose, fatigue, and sore throat, as compared to the different profile seen with the earlier Delta variant which causes more high temperatures, loss of taste and smell, and persistent cough (45). Such differences may lead to changes in the ascertainment rate, making indices of severity hard to interpret.

It should therefore be remembered that not all positive or infected cases are symptomatic, and that although it is challenging to determine the true number of asymptomatic cases in any disease, alternative testing methods must be tried to obtain an estimate of this (24,46). This is especially needed if those who are not symptomatic are infectious.

The implications of asymptomatic or pre-symptomatic infection are twofold. Firstly, if asymptomatic, pauci-symptomatic, or pre-symptomatic infections are involved in transmission, the outbreak is harder to contain (47). Models that do not account for these aspects of transmission may, therefore, be overly optimistic about the ability to control the outbreak. Secondly, having a larger proportion of the case population being asymptomatic, all else equal, means that the epidemic curve would have progressed further than models will have predicted if such infections are ignored.

Asymptomatic cases may or may not have the same contagiousness as symptomatic cases, and they may or may not contribute towards protective immunity. Modellers will make assumptions about these factors in their models. Although accurate and complete data collection is essential in developing a reliable model, infectious disease models still may vary in their inputs and assumptions. Two models that use the same data may differ in their outcome estimates.

As the host moves from initial exposure to the pathogen to full recovery from infection, the potential for infectivity rises and falls alongside the development and resolution of symptoms. The dynamics of infectivity have implications for control, such as the duration of quarantine to be recommended and the effectiveness of different frequencies of testing. The degree to which infectivity predates symptom onset is key to whether the outbreak can be contained: compare the limited outbreak of SARS-CoV-1, for which infectivity is high later in the disease, with the pandemic caused by SARS-CoV-2 (48), for which people are infectious before knowing they are infected. Infectivity can be estimated through surrogate clinical and laboratory measures at certain times in the disease course (49–50). For example, the reverse transcription-polymerase chain reaction (RT-PCR) cycle threshold (Ct) value represents the number of amplifications required during the PCR run for the viral RNA in the test sample to be detected. For COVID-19, the Ct value could therefore be used as an estimate of the viral load. Although it is understood these laboratory values or markers typically cannot be generalised to all cases and exceptions to the rule are almost always found, they can offer crude predictions of infectiousness when clinically correlated, and with the understanding of test limitations. Infectivity can potentially also be estimated through the distribution of serial intervals, though the signal is obfuscated by randomness in the incubation period distribution.

Representing the concept of 'infectivity' in models is, however, complicated significantly when changes to real-life factors influencing opportunities for disease transmission are made. These may not be amenable to modelling. For example, there can be widely varying person-to-person contact and exposure patterns between those infected and those susceptible at different time points in the outbreak (51–52). This is partly contributed by natural human behaviour and social interaction patterns during the different phases of the outbreak (26), but also in part directly controlled by changes in movement restrictions, social distancing requirements, school and workplace closures, quarantine policies, and the imposition and duration of isolation for positive cases (34). Changes in these dynamic factors cannot always be well anticipated, or even fully understood, and therefore incorporated in the model.

The length of the incubation period distribution impacts the pace of the epidemic and has implications for outbreak control. Although strictly speaking not classified an infectious disease modelling activity, mathematical and statistical calculations can initially help determine the incubation period of an infectious disease during the earlier stages of an outbreak. This is frequently done by using parametric models or extrapolating specific data from an observed time of exposure, which usually requires concurrently collecting detailed contact tracing data or mapping case travel history. However, the specific point of exposure is not always obvious, and contact tracing is not always possible to do well, as it requires big investments of manpower, time, and resources (53–55) **(See Chapter 11, Contact tracing)**. Nonetheless, several scientific teams were able to use travel history and estimated times of points of exposure, as well as other diagnoses and hospital admission data, to successfully analyse the incubation period range of SARS-CoV-2 during the COVID-19 pandemic (55–56).

In turn, the incubation period plays a role as an important model parametric which has been shown to directly influence the ability to predict disease transmission and trajectories of spread, given that the exposed population to which it is modelled on remains the same. For example, Kahn et al. described different spatiotemporal patterns of disease spread for Ebola, which has a longer incubation period than, say, cholera (57). For diseases with longer incubation periods, infected individuals have the opportunity to move further from the source during their incubation period, and this negatively impacts the predictability of spread and increases the potential for more long-range transmission (58). Importantly, the variability in the incubation period distribution also needs to be quantified. Longer-tailed incubation periods also challenge the effectiveness of border quarantine measures: either a degree of porosity must be accepted, or quarantine lengths extended, for example that which occurred in China for long stretches during the COVID-19 pandemic (59).

Delays in reporting, either because of delays in health seeking after onset or getting laboratory confirmation of infection, are a separate matter from the incubation period, but they function similarly to make the data available to build models and gauge epidemic dynamics always slightly out-of-date (58).

THE SEVERITY OF INFECTIONS

One of the most important uses of infectious disease modelling for planners of the healthcare system is its use for predicting the numbers of severe cases expected to consume hospital resources (60–62). Disease severity can seem highly discrepant when reported from different settings, populations, regions, or countries. This is particularly the case during the earlier phases of an outbreak. Data collection may be incomplete due to the lack of understanding of disease properties, or erratic and patchy due to immature data systems, or it may lag behind real-time developments due to the delays in communication and publication (63–64). Severity data may also be subject to differences in definition in varied settings. For instance, if all cases of disease are isolated in a hospital in one jurisdiction while another hospitalises only those in clinical need, the case-hospitalisation rates will be so different that comparison is pointless. Another phenomenon that must be understood is the inherently complex interplay between the severity of an outbreak and the rapidly changing transmission dynamics as various interventions and control measures are continuously implemented and modified, which may be in an unpredictable and haphazard way, especially in the regions hardest hit and struggling to regain control (1).

Other reasons for underestimation or under-reporting of disease severity include gaps in surveillance systems and poor definitions of clinical severity. A severely overwhelmed healthcare system may well under-report as it cannot keep track of cases or deaths across all healthcare institutions, which must include long-term care facilities or nursing homes. Conversely, there can be a large overestimation if reports are over-inclusive of other comorbidities leading to hospital admission, or if mortality reporting is undiscerning of cause of death for patients with an incidental positive test. Both these scenarios can pose great obstacles to ongoing evaluation and predictions of the outbreak and its true impacts. For example, the severity of the 2009 H1N1 influenza A epidemic in Mexico was grossly overestimated (65–66) and the 2014 Ebola outbreak modelling proved challenging for the opposite reason (67).

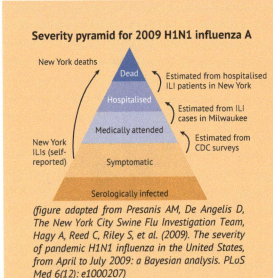

Severity pyramid for 2009 H1N1 influenza A

In the early months of the 2009 H1N1 influenza A pandemic, there was considerable uncertainty on how severe the new virus was because patients who were severely ill were much more likely to be identified. Presanis et al. used Bayesian methods to estimate the severity pyramid (as left) to estimate the proportion of cases at one level of the pyramid reaching a higher level. This allowed information to be synthesised from disparate sources to give a holistic overview of what transpired to be a mild pandemic.

(figure adapted from Presanis AM, De Angelis D, The New York City Swine Flu Investigation Team, Hagy A, Reed C, Riley S, et al. (2009). The severity of pandemic H1N1 influenza in the United States, from April to July 2009: a Bayesian analysis. PLoS Med 6(12): e1000207)

Nonetheless, despite these challenges, modelling is still a valuable and necessary tool. It is needed to forecast the impact of disease severity and guide vital policy decisions, allocate health system resources, and adapt responses. This can be especially applicable during seasonal outbreaks or repeated cycles of outbreak resurgence, as more data become available. Presanis et al. (68) described an approach by fusing data from different subpopulations to obtain an estimated *severity pyramid* which stratifies the risk of progression to a higher disease severity level, thereby depicting the proportion of cases reaching each severity level. The first step was real-time disease reporting and notification, followed by monitoring hospital admissions to estimate hospitalisation and intensive care unit (ICU)-admission rates for cases presenting at various healthcare settings, and then calculating mortality rates for the hospitalised subgroup of patients. Subsequently, using serologic studies to estimate the proportion of population infected, it is possible to extrapolate the infection fatality ratio and the overall case fatality ratio (69).

Another caveat to note is that the model may assume that new cases will fall into the same risk pool, whereas in reality, severity can differ substantially for different patient subpopulations due to age or other significant comorbidities. During an infectious disease outbreak, it is important to determine which population subgroups are at higher risk of severe outcomes. Overall absolute counts of severe cases often do not mean much without accounting for age, yet many repositories of data, even in outbreaks in the "big data" era, do not stratify by age or other major risk factors such as gender or ethnicity. Model outputs referring to case severity should therefore aim to be as granular as possible and distinguish between levels of age-specific severity. Apparent changes in severity can signal changes in the ascertainment rates of mild cases, though this relationship is confounded by genuine changes in infection severity rates due to the emergence of new variants or the build-up of immunity in the population.

Beyond predicting hospital admission rates, it is important to also monitor the proportion of patients who require higher levels of care and monitoring, and therefore require a higher healthcare worker-to-patient ratio, non-invasive or invasive ventilation, or ICU care. All these considerations are critical for hospitals and healthcare systems to prepare, allocate, or redistribute resources to meet ongoing patient care needs. Additionally, it is important to understand the clinical disease course and time-relations with regard to surges in case numbers, so that resources are not suddenly overwhelmed from exponential epidemic growths and lags from infection to clinical severity presentations.

Another important aspect of healthcare resources planning which can be aided by modelling is pharmacological therapeutics. As pandemic influenza continues to be a concern as a potential global public health threat, it is important to be able to estimate appropriate doses of drugs to stockpile for the treatment of active infections as well as pre- or post-exposure prophylaxis (70–71). Additionally, as drugs may be available in very different quantities in different regions and countries, modelling drug effectiveness and understanding the impacts of timing of initiation on disease trajectory can also be very useful guides for optimising therapeutic guideline recommendations (72).

Testing and diagnoses

During any outbreak, it is vital to be able to accurately estimate and monitor trends in infection prevalence to best inform public health response strategies. However, test protocols are often designed for positive case diagnosis and management rather than assessing the current

Frequent testing with a low sensitivity test to control COVID-19

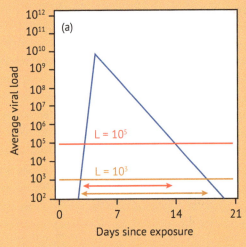
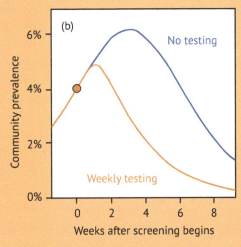

a) Average viral load against time since exposure, and windows in which the virus can be identified for different limits of detection (L).

b) Impact of weekly testing of 75 per cent of the population using a low sensitivity test followed by patient isolation on population-level epidemic dynamics in an agent-based model.

(figure adapted from Larremore DB, Wilder B, Lester E, Shehata S, Burke JM, Hay JA, Tambe M, Mina MJ, Parker R. Test sensitivity is secondary to frequency and turnaround time for COVID-19 screening. Sci Adv. 2021 Jan 1;7(1):eabd5393)

The wide deployment of low-cost, self-administered, but lower sensitivity tests, such as RATs, during the COVID-19 pandemic led to questions about how useful they would be when used broadly in the community or in workplaces. Larremore et al. assessed the impact of using frequent tests with modest sensitivity but immediate results by developing a model of the natural history of infection and the ability of the tests to detect infection, which fed into a transmission dynamic model which assessed the effect of using frequent testing at scale. It is important to have a realistic depiction of the timelines at an individual level if the population-level dynamics are to be characterised adequately.

epidemiology. While test positivity may sound like a simple concept, it is well known that a positive test may not reflect acute infection status. For example, in the case of prolonged viral shedding in patients infected with the SARS-CoV-2 virus (73), a positive test result may not always signify an actual risk of transmission to others. In addition, it is also important to understand that reported case numbers from test positivity only reflect the known proportion of patients diagnosed amongst those who received a test, rather than reflecting the true infection rate of the entire population.

There are many considerations in choosing the type of test to use for a particular disease. It is also critical to understand the purpose of testing, whether it be for diagnostic confirmation of positive cases, or for population prevalence studies. For example, the range of lower sensitivities of certain point-of-care rapid antigen test (RAT) assays may cause more false negative results, as has been seen with COVID-19 and dengue RAT kits (74–75). Still, they are essential tools for mass testing, especially in difficult to reach geographical areas with scarce medical resources. While serology tests are almost never used for diagnosing acute disease, and although they can be a useful tool in trying to determine seroprevalence, there are many challenges and biases in determining standardised positive cut-offs across different populations (76–77). Further considerations include ease of administration or mass reproducibility of testing methods to reflect an accurate measurement that is up-to-date and reliably represents the true infection prevalence of the population.

In infectious disease modelling, it is critical to report how infected cases are being identified. For instance, if mass or routine testing of asymptomatic individuals is being conducted, the test positivity rate would be expected to be much lower than if testing is only of symptomatic individuals presenting to the healthcare system. It is also important to know when these cases are being identified, especially in relation to quarantine periods and the timing and source of infection. This information is necessary for statistics, such as the number of tests per case found, to be interpretable. Gauging the true number of infections or infection prevalence in the majority of cases cannot be oversimplified and correlated with reported test positivity alone.

To estimate the true proportion of infections, several methods have been used, with inherent advantages and disadvantages. Representative population sampling is time and resource consuming, and even the best designs are inherently biased and constrained by various practical and cost limitations. Extrapolation to the entire population will never be precise. Mass testing for an entire population, or specific population subgroups or occupations, has also been conducted. However, in few settings is this sustainable in the long-term, nor is it easily repeated throughout several waves of an outbreak. Despite the challenges with inexactitude of test positivity rates, infectious disease modelling can improve estimations of infection prevalence and seroprevalence by combining test positivity rates with other key indices such as case counts and known viral load kinetics corresponding to disease trajectory (78–79).

PROTECTION CONFERRED BY VACCINATION

Vaccines have been one of the most indispensable tools for mitigating (e.g., influenza, COVID-19), eliminating (e.g., Ebola, polio, tetanus, measles), and eradicating (e.g., smallpox) infectious diseases. However, the COVID-19 pandemic served to highlight and magnify the complexities and intricacies involved in measuring vaccine effectiveness and efficacy. Vaccine efficacy trials face difficulties due to the uncertainties created by the inherently evolving nature of pathogen properties and the resulting ever-changing epidemiology trends of infectious disease outbreaks (80). Measurements of vaccine efficacy are further greatly challenged by different transmission dynamics in different populations and the occasionally short duration of trials (which prevents estimation of the degree of waning and may make vaccines look more effective than they eventually will be). A similar issue arises if the strain circulating during a trial does not match the strain that dominates once mass vaccination begins. A further complication is that the typical design of comparing a vaccine to a placebo makes comparisons between vaccines difficult. Infectious disease modelling can be useful in enhancing the robustness of vaccine efficacy trials by capturing the abovementioned uncertainties of evolving disease transmission (81–82) and extrapolating the effect in small groups for short durations of time to the population level.

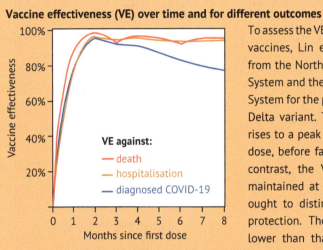

Vaccine effectiveness of mRNA-1273 (by Moderna) against diagnosed COVID-19, hospitalisation, and death, over time

(adapted from Lin DY, Gu Y, Wheeler B, Young H, Holloway S, Sunny SK, Moore Z, Zeng D. Effectiveness of COVID-19 vaccines over a 9-month period in North Carolina. N Engl J Med. 2022 Mar 10;386(10):933-941)

To assess the VE of several widely used COVID-19 vaccines, Lin et al. extracted and linked data from the North Carolina COVID-19 Surveillance System and the COVID-19 Vaccine Management System for the period until the emergence of the Delta variant. The VE for diagnosed COVID-19 rises to a peak about two months after the first dose, before falling over the next half year. In contrast, the VE against severe outcomes is maintained at a high level. Therefore, models ought to distinguish these different forms of protection. The VE against infection may be lower than that against diagnosed COVID-19 if there is differential under-ascertainment of breakthrough infections.

HOW DOES MODELLING WORK DURING OUTBREAKS?

Leaders in government, policy, public health, and various healthcare and industry sectors are constantly confronted with complex and fast-changing scenarios, often with competing needs and priorities. Decisions made on policy and strategy must be scientific and evidence-based to ensure maximal, equitable benefits to populations and communities. It is also imperative that the model be adapted and applied appropriately to different stages of the outbreak, incorporating the impact of interventions and other control strategies as best as possible as the outbreak progresses. Apart from the fundamental technical aspects of infectious disease modelling to support integrated public health response, there are two additional vital aspects required to successfully bridge theory with implementation, and to ensure that modelling outputs, predictions, and frameworks are used best to guide truly meaningful decisions for public health and outbreak response (1,19,83–84).

Firstly, infectious disease modellers cannot work alone. They need up-to-date, accurate, and comprehensive real-world data. This requires the concerted effort of a team of epidemiologists, infection control personnel, laboratory technicians, healthcare workers, hospital operations and logisticians, and other scientific researchers to establish a tight collaborative network. It is also essential to have at least the basic required IT infrastructure and working data systems and software.

Secondly, while the generic structure of infectious disease models can be applied flexibly, it is important to be aware that there is not a single model that can be fully generalised to different geographical locations, host populations, and policy context. The accuracy or robustness of the model will vary (sometimes widely) depending on fundamental inputs such as source data used for model parameters and uncontrollable or unpredictable factors affecting the efficacy of the interventions applied. It is therefore imperative that both infectious disease modellers (including epidemiologists) and policymakers achieve a good and clear two-way communication early on to clearly establish the use-case for the model, and what concerns or questions it should be designed to address. This requires effort from both parties to establish mutual trust and develop long-term collaboration platforms, networks, and relationships. It is equally critical for policymakers to understand the appropriate applications of model outputs and the inherent uncertainties involved, as it is for modellers to recognise and appreciate which aspects of modelling are most relevant to current public health situations, tailor the model to fit contextual needs, and express assumptions and limitations in an open manner (20,81–85).

Many model applications which have successfully influenced strategy in the past, such as in malaria vector control, HIV prevention and treatment, and measles and rubella vaccinations, have been found to amplify these two aspects (86).

CONCLUSION

This chapter discusses the key parameters of infectious disease models that analyse and predict disease transmission and dynamics. Increasingly, these models are used to make sense of the epidemiology of an emerging outbreak and to explore the various response measures that can control, or at least mitigate, the outbreak during its different stages. This helps policymakers and public health leaders make evidence-based policy decisions which achieve the ultimate goal of reducing the morbidity of an outbreak and its social and economic impact.

REFERENCES:

1. Heesterbeek H, Anderson RM, Andreasen V, Bansal S, De Angelis D, Dye C, et al.; Isaac Newton Institute IDD Collaboration. Modeling infectious disease dynamics in the complex landscape of global health. Science. 2015 Mar;347(6227):aaa4339. https://doi.org/10.1126/science.aaa4339 PMID:25766240.
2. Colizza V, Barrat A, Barthelemy M, Valleron AJ, Vespignani A. Modeling the worldwide spread of pandemic influenza: baseline case and containment interventions. PLoS Med. 2007 Jan;4(1):e13. https://doi.org/10.1371/journal.pmed.0040013 PMID:17253899.
3. Fisman D; Pandemic Influenza Outbreak Research Modelling Team (Pan-InfORM). Modelling an influenza pandemic: A guide for the perplexed. CMAJ. 2009 Aug;181(3-4):171–3. https://doi.org/10.1503/cmaj.090885 PMID:19620267.
4. Nsoesie EO, Brownstein JS, Ramakrishnan N, Marathe MV. A systematic review of studies on forecasting the dynamics of influenza outbreaks. Influenza Other Respir Viruses. 2014 May;8(3):309–16. https://doi.org/10.1111/irv.12226 PMID:24373466.
5. Moore JR, Donnell DJ, Boily MC, Mitchell KM, Delany-Moretlwe S, Bekker LG, et al. Model-based predictions of HIV incidence among African women using HIV risk behaviors and community-level data on male HIV prevalence and viral suppression. J Acquir Immune Defic Syndr. 2020 Dec;85(4):423–9. https://doi.org/10.1097/QAI.0000000000002481 PMID:33136739.
6. Sun X, Nishiura H, Xiao Y. Modeling methods for estimating HIV incidence: a mathematical review. Theor Biol Med Model. 2020 Jan;17(1):1. https://doi.org/10.1186/s12976-019-0118-0 PMID:31964392.

7. Bhat R, Sudhakar K, Kurien T, Rao AS. Strengthening India's response to HIV/AIDS epidemic through strategic planning, innovative financing, and mathematical modeling: key achievements over the last 3 decades. J Indian Inst Sci. 2022;102(2):791–809. https://doi.org/10.1007/s41745-022-00331-y PMID:36093271.

8. Merler S, Ajelli M, Fumanelli L, Gomes MF, Piontti AP, Rossi L, et al. Spatiotemporal spread of the 2014 outbreak of Ebola virus disease in Liberia and the effectiveness of non-pharmaceutical interventions: a computational modelling analysis. Lancet Infect Dis. 2015 Feb;15(2):204–11. https://doi.org/10.1016/S1473-3099(14)71074-6 PMID:25575618.

9. Meltzer MI, Santibanez S, Fischer LS, Merlin TL, Adhikari BB, Atkins CY, et al. Modeling in real time during the ebola response. MMWR Suppl. 2016 Jul;65(3):85–9. https://doi.org/10.15585/mmwr.su6503a12 PMID:27387097.

10. Ajelli M, Zhang Q, Sun K, Merler S, Fumanelli L, Chowell G, et al. The RAPIDD Ebola forecasting challenge: model description and synthetic data generation. Epidemics. 2018 Mar;22:3–12. https://doi.org/10.1016/j.epidem.2017.09.001 PMID:28951016.

11. Mandal S, Sarkar RR, Sinha S. Mathematical models of malaria—a review. Malar J. 2011 Jul;10(1):202. https://doi.org/10.1186/1475-2875-10-202 PMID:21777413.

12. Amadi M, Shcherbacheva A, Haario H. Agent-based modelling of complex factors impacting malaria prevalence. Malar J. 2021 Apr;20(1):185. https://doi.org/10.1186/s12936-021-03721-2 PMID:33858432.

13. Santos DV, Silva GS, Weber EJ, Hasenack H, Groff FH, Todeschini B, et al. Identification of foot and mouth disease risk areas using a multi-criteria analysis approach. PLoS One. 2017 May;12(5):e0178464. https://doi.org/10.1371/journal.pone.0178464 PMID:28552973.

14. Pomeroy LW, Bansal S, Tildesley M, Moreno-Torres KI, Moritz M, Xiao N, et al. Data-driven models of foot-and-mouth disease dynamics: a review. Transbound Emerg Dis. 2017 Jun;64(3):716–28. https://doi.org/10.1111/tbed.12437 PMID:26576514.

15. Firestone SM, Hayama Y, Bradhurst R, Yamamoto T, Tsutsui T, Stevenson MA. Reconstructing foot-and-mouth disease outbreaks: a methods comparison of transmission network models. Sci Rep. 2019 Mar;9(1):4809. https://doi.org/10.1038/s41598-019-41103-6 PMID:30886211.

16. Aguas R, White L, Hupert N, Shretta R, Pan-Ngum W, Celhay O, et al.; CoMo Consortium. Modelling the COVID-19 pandemic in context: an international participatory approach [Erratum in: BMJ Glob Health. 2021 Feb;6] [2]. BMJ Glob Health. 2020 Dec;5(12):e003126. https://doi.org/10.1136/bmjgh-2020-003126 PMID:33361188.

17. Kucharski AJ, Russell TW, Diamond C, Liu Y, Edmunds J, Funk S, et al.; Centre for Mathematical Modelling of Infectious Diseases COVID-19 working group. Early dynamics of transmission and control of COVID-19: a mathematical modelling study. Lancet Infect Dis. 2020 May;20(5):553–8. https://doi.org/10.1016/S1473-3099(20)30144-4 PMID:32171059.

18. Wu JT, Leung K, Leung GM. Nowcasting and forecasting the potential domestic and international spread of the 2019-nCoV outbreak originating in Wuhan, China: a modelling study. Lancet. 2020 Feb;395(10225):689–97. https://doi.org/10.1016/S0140-6736(20)30260-9 PMID:32014114.

19. Van Kerkhove MD, Ferguson NM. Epidemic and intervention modelling—a scientific rationale for policy decisions? Lessons from the 2009 influenza pandemic. Bull World Health Organ. 2012 Apr;90(4):306–10. https://doi.org/10.2471/BLT.11.097949 PMID:22511828.

20. Knight GM, Dharan NJ, Fox GJ, Stennis N, Zwerling A, Khurana R, et al. Bridging the gap between evidence and policy for infectious diseases: how models can aid public health decision-making. Int J Infect Dis. 2016 Jan;42:17–23. https://doi.org/10.1016/j.ijid.2015.10.024 PMID:26546234.

21. James LP, Salomon JA, Buckee CO, Menzies NA. The use and misuse of mathematical modeling for infectious disease policymaking: lessons for the COVID-19 pandemic. Med Decis Making. 2021 May;41(4):379–85. https://doi.org/10.1177/0272989X21990391 PMID:33535889.

22. Nixon K, Jindal S, Parker F, Reich NG, Ghobadi K, Lee EC, et al. An evaluation of prospective COVID-19 modelling studies in the USA: from data to science translation. Lancet Digit Health. 2022 Oct;4(10):e738–47. https://doi.org/10.1016/S2589-7500(22)00148-0 PMID:36150782.

23. Kringos D, Carinci F, Barbazza E, Bos V, Gilmore K, Groene O, et al.; HealthPros Network. Managing COVID-19 within and across health systems: why we need performance intelligence to coordinate a global response. Health Res Policy Syst. 2020 Jul;18(1):80. https://doi.org/10.1186/s12961-020-00593-x PMID:32664985.

24. Holmdahl I, Buckee C. Wrong but useful - what Covid-19 epidemiologic models can and cannot tell us. N Engl J Med. 2020 Jul;383(4):303–5. https://doi.org/10.1056/NEJMp2016822 PMID:32412711.

25. Funk S, Salathé M, Jansen VA. Modelling the influence of human behaviour on the spread of infectious diseases: a review. J R Soc Interface. 2010 Sep;7(50):1247–56. https://doi.org/10.1098/rsif.2010.0142 PMID:20504800.

26. Funk S, Bansal S, Bauch CT, Eames KT, Edmunds WJ, Galvani AP, et al. Nine challenges in incorporating the dynamics of behaviour in infectious diseases models. Epidemics. 2015 Mar;10:21–5. https://doi.org/10.1016/j.epidem.2014.09.005 PMID:25843377.

27. Keeling MJ, Rohani P. Modeling infectious diseases in humans and animals. Princeton University Press; 2007.

28. Vynnycky E, White RG. An introduction to infectious disease modelling. Oxford University Press; 2010.

29. Diekmann O, Heesterbeek JA. Wiley series in mathematical and computational biology. Wiley; Chichester, UK: 2000. Mathematical epidemiology of infectious diseases: model building, analysis and interpretation.

30. Heffernan JM, Smith RJ, Wahl LM. Perspectives on the basic reproductive ratio. J R Soc Interface. 2005 Sep;2(4):281–93. https://doi.org/10.1098/rsif.2005.0042 PMID:16849186.

31. Delamater PL, Street EJ, Leslie TF, Yang YT, Jacobsen KH. Complexity of the basic reproduction number (R0). Emerg Infect Dis. 2019 Jan;25(1):1–4. https://doi.org/10.3201/eid2501.171901 PMID:30560777.

32. Ridenhour B, Kowalik JM, Shay DK. Unraveling R0: considerations for public health applications. Am J Public Health. 2014 Feb;104(2):e32–41. https://doi.org/10.2105/AJPH.2013.301704 PMID:24328646.

33. Wallinga J, Lipsitch M. How generation intervals shape the relationship between growth rates and reproductive numbers. Proc Biol Sci. 2007 Feb;274(1609):599–604. https://doi.org/10.1098/rspb.2006.3754 PMID:17476782.

34. Griffin JT, Garske T, Ghani AC, Clarke PS. Joint estimation of the basic reproduction number and generation time parameters for infectious disease outbreaks. Biostatistics. 2011 Apr;12(2):303–12. https://doi.org/10.1093/biostatistics/kxq058 PMID:20858771.

35. Wallinga J, Teunis P. Different epidemic curves for severe acute respiratory syndrome reveal similar impacts of control measures. Am J Epidemiol. 2004 Sep;160(6):509–16. https://doi.org/10.1093/aje/kwh255 PMID:15353409.

36. Cori A, Ferguson NM, Fraser C, Cauchemez S. A new framework and software to estimate time-varying reproduction numbers during epidemics. Am J Epidemiol. 2013 Nov;178(9):1505–12. https://doi.org/10.1093/aje/kwt133 PMID:24043437.

37. Parag KV. Improved estimation of time-varying reproduction numbers at low case incidence and between epidemic waves. PLOS Comput Biol. 2021 Sep;17(9):e1009347. https://doi.org/10.1371/journal.pcbi.1009347 PMID:34492011.

38. Alvarez L, Colom M, Morel JD, Morel JM. Computing the daily reproduction number of COVID-19 by inverting the renewal equation using a variational technique. Proc Natl Acad Sci USA. 2021 Dec;118(50):e210511211. https://doi.org/10.1073/pnas.2105112118 PMID:34876517.

39. Jin S, Dickens BL, Lim JT, Cook AR. EpiRegress: A method to estimate and predict the time-varying effective reproduction number. Viruses. 2022 Jul;14(7):1576. https://doi.org/10.3390/v14071576 PMID:35891556.

40. Lim JS, Cho SI, Ryu S, Pak SI. Interpretation of the basic and effective reproduction number. J Prev Med Public Health. 2020 Nov;53(6):405–8. https://doi.org/10.3961/jpmph.20.288 PMID:33296580.

41. Ozaki J, Shida Y, Takayasu H, Takayasu M. Direct modelling from GPS data reveals daily-activity-dependency of effective reproduction number in COVID-19 pandemic. Sci Rep. 2022 Oct;12(1):17888. https://doi.org/10.1038/s41598-022-22420-9 PMID:36284166.

42. Childs A, Zullo AR, Joyce NR, McConeghy KW, van Aalst R, Moyo P, et al. The burden of respiratory infections among older adults in long-term care: a systematic review. BMC Geriatr. 2019 Aug;19(1):210. https://doi.org/10.1186/s12877-019-1236-6 PMID:31382895.

43. Arons MM, Hatfield KM, Reddy SC, Kimball A, James A, Jacobs JR, et al.; Public Health–Seattle and King County and CDC COVID-19 Investigation Team. Presymptomatic SARS-CoV-2 infections and transmission in a skilled nursing facility. N Engl J Med. 2020 May;382(22):2081–90. https://doi.org/10.1056/NEJMoa2008457 PMID:32329971.

44. Kadirvelu B, Burcea G, Quint JK, Costelloe CE, Faisal AA. Variation in global COVID-19 symptoms by geography and by chronic disease: a global survey using the COVID-19 Symptom Mapper. EClinicalMedicine. 2022 Mar;45:101317. https://doi.org/10.1016/j.eclinm.2022.101317 PMID:35265823.

45. ZOE Health Study [Internet]. ZOE COVID Study. [cited 2022 Nov 9]. https://covid-webflow.joinzoe.com/.

46. Fraser C, Riley S, Anderson RM, Ferguson NM. Factors that make an infectious disease outbreak controllable. Proc Natl Acad Sci USA. 2004 Apr;101(16):6146–51. https://doi.org/10.1073/pnas.0307506101 PMID:15071187.

47. Johansson MA, Quandelacy TM, Kada S, Prasad PV, Steele M, Brooks JT, et al. SARS-CoV-2 transmission from people without COVID-19 symptoms [Erratum in: JAMA Netw Open. 2021 Feb 1;4] [2] [:e211383]. JAMA Netw Open. 2021 Jan;4(1):e2035057. https://doi.org/10.1001/jamanetworkopen.2020.35057 PMID:33410879.

48. Wei WE, Li Z, Chiew CJ, Yong SE, Toh MP, Lee VJ. Presymptomatic transmission of SARS-CoV-2 - Singapore, January 23-March 16, 2020. MMWR Morb Mortal Wkly Rep. 2020 Apr;69(14):411–5. https://doi.org/10.15585/mmwr.mm6914e1 PMID:32271722.

49. La Scola B, Le Bideau M, Andreani J, Hoang VT, Grimaldier C, Colson P, et al. Viral RNA load as determined by cell culture as a management tool for discharge of SARS-CoV-2 patients from infectious disease wards. Eur J Clin Microbiol Infect Dis. 2020 Jun;39(6):1059–61. https://doi.org/10.1007/s10096-020-03913-9 PMID:32342252.

50. Singanayagam A, Patel M, Charlett A, Lopez Bernal J, Saliba V, Ellis J, et al. Duration of infectiousness and correlation with RT-PCR cycle threshold values in cases of COVID-19, England, January to May 2020 [Erratum in: Euro Surveill. 2021 Feb;26] [7]. Euro Surveill. 2020 Aug;25(32):2001483. https://doi.org/10.2807/1560-7917.ES.2020.25.32.2001483 PMID:32794447.

51. Lloyd-Smith JO, Schreiber SJ, Kopp PE, Getz WM. Superspreading and the effect of individual variation on disease emergence. Nature. 2005 Nov;438(7066):355–9. https://doi.org/10.1038/nature04153 PMID:16292310.

52. Elie B, Selinger C, Alizon S. The source of individual heterogeneity shapes infectious disease outbreaks. Proc Biol Sci. 2022 May 11;289(1974):20220232. https://doi.org/10.1098/rspb.2022.0232.

53. Nishiura H. Early efforts in modeling the incubation period of infectious diseases with an acute course of illness. Emerg Themes Epidemiol. 2007 May;4(1):2. https://doi.org/10.1186/1742-7622-4-2 PMID:17466070.

54. Dhouib W, Maatoug J, Ayouni I, Zammit N, Ghammem R, Fredj SB, et al. The incubation period during the pandemic of COVID-19: a systematic review and meta-analysis. Syst Rev. 2021 Apr;10(1):101. https://doi.org/10.1186/s13643-021-01648-y PMID:33832511.

55. Backer JA, Klinkenberg D, Wallinga J. Incubation period of 2019 novel coronavirus (2019-nCoV) infections among travellers from Wuhan, China, 20-28 January 2020. Euro Surveill. 2020 Feb;25(5):2000062. https://doi.org/10.2807/1560-7917.ES.2020.25.5.2000062 PMID:32046819.

56. Linton NM, Kobayashi T, Yang Y, Hayashi K, Akhmetzhanov AR, Jung SM, et al. Incubation period and other epidemiological characteristics of 2019 novel coronavirus infections with right truncation: a statistical analysis of publicly available case data. J Clin Med. 2020 Feb;9(2):538. https://doi.org/10.3390/jcm9020538 PMID:32079150.

57. Kahn R, Peak CM, Fernández-Gracia J, Hill A, Jambai A, Ganda L, et al. Incubation periods impact the spatial predictability of cholera and Ebola outbreaks in Sierra Leone. Proc Natl Acad Sci USA. 2020 Mar;117(9):5067–73. https://doi.org/10.1073/pnas.1913052117 PMID:32054785.

58. Soltanolkottabi M, Ben-Arieh D, Wu CH. Game theoretic modeling of infectious disease transmission with delayed emergence of symptoms. Games (Basel). 2020 Apr;11(2):20. https://doi.org/10.3390/g11020020.

59. Why is China's quarantine so long and does science back it up? South China Morning Post. (2021, November 25). https://www.scmp.com/news/china/science/article/3156796/quarantine-china-why-so-long-and-does-science-back-it.

60. Garcia-Vicuña D, Esparza L, Mallor F. Hospital preparedness during epidemics using simulation: the case of COVID-19. Cent Eur J Oper Res. 2022;30(1):213–49. https://doi.org/10.1007/s10100-021-00779-w PMID:34602855.

61. Watson SK, Rudge JW, Coker R. Health systems' "surge capacity": state of the art and priorities for future research. Milbank Q. 2013 Mar;91(1):78–122. https://doi.org/10.1111/milq.12003 PMID:23488712.

62. Fattahi M, Keyvanshokooh E, Kannan D, Govindan K. Resource planning strategies for healthcare systems during a pandemic. Eur J Oper Res. 2023 Jan;304(1):192–206. https://doi.org/10.1016/j.ejor.2022.01.023 PMID:35068665.

63. Gardner L, Ratcliff J, Dong E, Katz A. A need for open public data standards and sharing in light of COVID-19. Lancet Infect Dis. 2021 Apr;21(4):e80. https://doi.org/10.1016/S1473-3099(20)30635-6 PMID:32791042.

64. Jewell NP, Lewnard JA, Jewell BL. Caution warranted: using the Institute for Health metrics and evaluation model for predicting the course of the COVID-19 pandemic. Ann Intern Med. 2020 Aug;173(3):226–7. https://doi.org/10.7326/M20-1565 PMID:32289150.

65. Charu V, Chowell G, Palacio Mejia LS, Echevarría-Zuno S, Borja-Aburto VH, Simonsen L, et al. Mortality burden of the A/H1N1 pandemic in Mexico: a comparison of deaths and years of life lost to seasonal influenza. Clin Infect Dis. 2011 Nov;53(10):985–93. https://doi.org/10.1093/cid/cir644 PMID:21976464.

66. Fraser C, Donnelly CA, Cauchemez S, Hanage WP, Van Kerkhove MD, Hollingsworth TD, et al.; WHO Rapid Pandemic Assessment Collaboration. Pandemic potential of a strain of influenza A (H1N1): early findings. Science. 2009 Jun;324(5934):1557–61. https://doi.org/10.1126/science.1176062 PMID:19433588.

67. Aylward B, Barboza P, Bawo L, Bertherat E, Bilivogui P, Blake I, et al.; WHO Ebola Response Team. Ebola virus disease in West Africa—the first 9 months of the epidemic and forward projections. N Engl J Med. 2014 Oct;371(16):1481–95. https://doi.org/10.1056/NEJMoa1411100 PMID:25244186.

68. Presanis AM, Lipsitch M, Hagy A, Reed C, Riley S, Cooper B, et al.; Daniela De Angelis; Swine Flu Investigation Team, New York City Department of Health and Mental Hygiene. The severity of pandemic H1N1 influenza in the United States, April - July 2009. PLoS Curr. 2009 Sep;1:RRN1042. PMID:20029614.

69. Brazeau NF, Verity R, Jenks S, Fu H, Whittaker C, Winskill P, et al. Estimating the COVID-19 infection fatality ratio accounting for seroreversion using statistical modelling. Commun Med (Lond). 2022 May;2(1):54. https://doi.org/10.1038/s43856-022-00106-7 PMID:35603270.

70. Kim S, Bin Seo Y, Lee J, Kim YS, Jung E. Estimation of optimal antiviral stockpile for a novel influenza pandemic. J Infect Public Health. 2022 Jul;15(7):720–5. https://doi.org/10.1016/j.jiph.2022.05.012 PMID:35667304.

71. Greer AL, Schanzer D. Using a dynamic model to consider optimal antiviral stockpile size in the face of pandemic influenza uncertainty. PLoS One. 2013 Jun;8(6):e67253. https://doi.org/10.1371/journal.pone.0067253 PMID:23805303.

72. Whittaker C, Watson OJ, Alvarez-Moreno C, Angkasekwinai N, Boonyasiri A, Carlos Triana L, et al. Understanding the potential impact of different drug properties on severe acute respiratory syndrome coronavirus 2 (SARS-CoV-2) transmission and disease burden: a modelling analysis. Clin Infect Dis. 2022 Aug;75(1):e224–33. https://doi.org/10.1093/cid/ciab837 PMID:34549260.

73. Long H, Zhao J, Zeng HL, Lu QB, Fang LQ, Wang Q, et al. Prolonged viral shedding of SARS-CoV-2 and related factors in symptomatic COVID-19 patients: a prospective study. BMC Infect Dis. 2021 Dec;21(1):1282. https://doi.org/10.1186/s12879-021-07002-w PMID:34961470.

74. Guglielmi G. Fast coronavirus tests: what they can and can't do. Nature. 2020 Sep;585(7826):496–8. https://doi.org/10.1038/d41586-020-02661-2 PMID:32939084.

75. Mahajan R, Nair M, Saldanha AM, Harshana A, Pereira AL, Basu N, et al. Diagnostic accuracy of commercially available immunochromatographic rapid tests for diagnosis of dengue in India. J Vector Borne Dis. 2021;58(2):159–64. https://doi.org/10.4103/0972-9062.321747 PMID:35074951.

76. Chan Y, Fornace K, Wu L, Arnold BF, Priest JW, Martin DL, et al. Determining seropositivity-A review of approaches to define population seroprevalence when using multiplex bead assays to assess burden of tropical diseases. PLoS Negl Trop Dis. 2021 Jun;15(6):e0009457. https://doi.org/10.1371/journal.pntd.0009457 PMID:34181665.

77. McConnell D, Hickey C, Bargary N, Trela-Larsen L, Walsh C, Barry M, et al. Understanding the challenges and uncertainties of seroprevalence studies for SARS-CoV-2. Int J Environ Res Public Health. 2021 Apr;18(9):4640. https://doi.org/10.3390/ijerph18094640 PMID:33925518.

78. Chiu WA, Ndeffo-Mbah ML. Using test positivity and reported case rates to estimate state-level COVID-19 prevalence and seroprevalence in the United States. PLOS Comput Biol. 2021 Sep;17(9):e1009374. https://doi.org/10.1371/journal.pcbi.1009374 PMID:34491990.

79. Hay JA, Kennedy-Shaffer L, Kanjilal S, Lennon NJ, Gabriel SB, Lipsitch M, et al. Estimating epidemiologic dynamics from cross-sectional viral load distributions. Science. 2021 Jul;373(6552):eabh0635. https://doi.org/10.1126/science.abh0635 PMID:34083451.

80. Madewell ZJ, Dean NE, Berlin JA, Coplan PM, Davis KJ, Struchiner CJ, et al. Challenges of evaluating and modelling vaccination in emerging infectious diseases. Epidemics. 2021 Dec;37:100506. https://doi.org/10.1016/j.epidem.2021.100506 PMID:34628108.

81. Madewell ZJ, Pastore Y Piontti A, Zhang Q, Burton N, Yang Y, Longini IM, et al. Using simulated infectious disease outbreaks to inform site selection and sample size for individually randomized vaccine trials during an ongoing epidemic. Clin Trials. 2021 Oct;18(5):630–8. https://doi.org/10.1177/17407745211028898 PMID:34218667.

82. Andrews MA, Bauch CT. The impacts of simultaneous disease intervention decisions on epidemic outcomes. J Theor Biol. 2016 Apr;395:1–10. https://doi.org/10.1016/j.jtbi.2016.01.027 PMID:26829313.

83. Kretzschmar M. Disease modeling for public health: added value, challenges, and institutional constraints. J Public Health Policy. 2020 Mar;41(1):39–51. https://doi.org/10.1057/s41271-019-00206-0 PMID:31780754.

84. Metcalf CJ, Edmunds WJ, Lessler J. Six challenges in modelling for public health policy. Epidemics. 2015 Mar;10:93–6. https://doi.org/10.1016/j.epidem.2014.08.008 PMID:25843392.

85. Driedger SM, Cooper EJ, Moghadas SM. Developing model-based public health policy through knowledge translation: the need for a 'Communities of Practice'. Public Health. 2014 Jun;128(6):561–7. https://doi.org/10.1016/j.puhe.2013.10.009 PMID:24461909.

86. Becker AD, Grantz KH, Hegde ST, Bérubé S, Cummings DAT, Wesolowski A. Development and dissemination of infectious disease dynamic transmission models during the COVID-19 pandemic: what can we learn from other pathogens and how can we move forward? Lancet Digit Health. 2021 Jan;3(1):e41-e50.

CHAPTER 17

INTEGRATED OUTBREAK ANALYTICS (IOA)

by Simone E. Carter and Pascale Lissouba

Integrated outbreak analytics (IOA) is an emerging practice that brings together a multidisciplinary team under a health ministry to look for locally-based solutions to public health problems. This chapter will focus on the IOA approach in public health emergencies, though IOA teams may also support a ministry of health (MoH) or response actors working on recurrent public health concerns such as malnutrition or measles. In an emergency, this team seeks to better understand disease dynamics and its impact on communities, to create a more accountable, appropriate, and effective response.

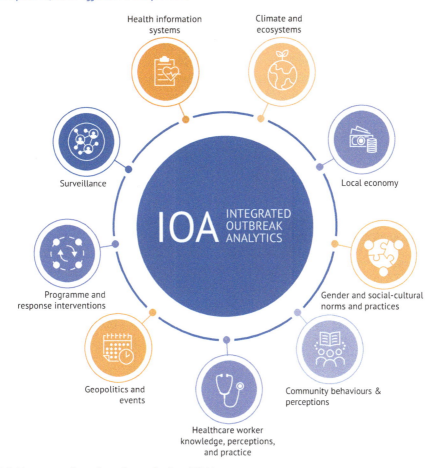

Figure 17.1: Integrated outbreak analytics (IOA)

INTRODUCTION

The IOA approach is to bring together individuals from different organisations and specialisations including epidemiology (descriptive and analytic), the social and behavioural sciences, data sciences (including modelling), and animal and environmental science. IOA teams bring together data from surveillance, laboratory work, vaccination programmes, infection prevention and control (IPC) and other programmes, health information systems (HIS), community and healthcare workers (HCWs), and political, economic, and environmental events (all informed by explicitly presented information on social context and gender norms). IOA goes beyond mixed methods work and seeks to bring different stakeholders and expertise together, seeing how different types of data (routine or specifically sought) can be used together.

A large-scale outbreak will demand a full-time IOA team. Though the ways IOA is implemented will vary by country, context, and public health concern, the principles of collaborative work from multiple disciplines (1), capacity building, and evidence use are consistent in all applications of IOA.

Objectives of IOA

- To drive comprehensive, accountable, and effective public health and clinical strategies for outbreak management and control
- To produce data from multiple disciplinary perspectives that can rapidly and systematically inform operational decisions
- To drive a holistic understanding of public health dynamics, and highlight the impacts of both the outbreak and response control interventions
- To advance local- and national-level mechanisms and methods for relevant, useful, and rapid evidence generation
- To build, strengthen, and scale local, subnational, and national capacity to conduct IOA

THE EMERGENCE OF IOA

IOA grew organically from outbreak responders identifying a need to develop operational and "field"-based solutions. It became formalised during the 2018–2020 Ebola virus disease (EBOD) outbreak in the east of the Democratic Republic of the Congo (DRC). The approach is increasingly being mainstreamed in a variety of contexts.

Following lessons learned from the 2014–2015 EBOD outbreak (2) and the subsequent 2015–2016 Zika outbreak, DRC 2018–2020 Ebola response actors (MoH and international partners) made significant investments to improve analytics from routine surveillance, clinical care, social and behavioural sciences, and other outbreak response data (3). In the first months of the 10th EBOD outbreak in 2018, a team of data scientists and epidemiologists were rapidly deployed to support the DRC MoH, setting up an "Epidemiological Cell" (Epi Cell) to conduct outbreak analytics (4), including visualisation and analysis of key surveillance and outbreak data. While this information was critical to identifying where to invest response efforts, it did not explain the factors influencing the outbreak dynamics, missing factors such as:

- access and availability of services prior to and during the outbreak

- use of healthcare services and factors influencing use
- pre-existing socioeconomic conditions, including gender norms which may influence exposure and healthcare seeking behaviour

To fill these data gaps, the Social Sciences Analytics Cell (CASS) was set up to complement the information provided by the Epi Cell.

In 2018, Epi Cell data were largely provided by surveillance and case management response (5). Data included the number of cases, broken down by age and sex by location and over time. The data also provided information on delays in seeking treatment, analyses regarding signals and alerts, and modelling to estimate outbreak risks.

In February 2019, the CASS was formalised under the DRC MoH response structure. It developed Terms of Reference (ToR) to systematise mixed methods data in support and contribution to the Epi Cell and all response pillars. In March 2019, the CASS and Epi Cell operated as one unit (CASS-Epi Cell, subsequently simplified as the Cell), regularly reviewing the outbreak situation and identifying questions requiring integrated analyses. To support this, additional data sources (and the disciplinary expertise to analyse them) were brought into the Cell including:
- systematic survey data from households and HCWs on perceptions and behaviours associated with disease transmission and impacts of the response on different groups within communities
- programme data from other pillars, including IPC data and risk communication and community engagement (RCCE)
- HIS data to identify trends in healthcare service use by location over time
- tracking of public events such as national elections, attacks on communities, newly introduced free healthcare policies, and programmatic changes by location

As the Cell added data sources and associated disciplines and actors, IOA (3) was created. It was conceived as a process which starts when the different actors look at the outbreak context, identify trigger questions, and agree on how best to understand and answer the questions. For a look at the flow of IOA from trigger questions to data collection and recommendations, see the example of CASS-Epi analysis below.

Following data collection and analysis, discussions among individuals yield participative analysis, a key process within IOA. The analysis is continued among multiple partners and levels to reinforce the use of evidence and co-development of actions at multiple levels (e.g., local, provincial, national) and among different partners (e.g., MoH, non-governmental organisations [NGOs], pillar or cluster, etc.). See **Figure 17.2** for an illustration of the process flow of an IOA.

IOA beyond Ebola and beyond the DRC

IOA has since been applied in other outbreaks. The first Cell became the Cellule d'Analyse Intégrée (Integrated Analytics Cell) or CAI and has supported the MoH to use IOA in the DRC looking at a broad range of health emergencies including recurrent outbreaks and public health concerns such as malnutrition and gender-based violence (6–12).

The IOA Cell has also been replicated in many countries facing outbreaks including Guinea, Ghana, Republic of Congo (13), Uganda, and Haiti, and is increasingly being recognised as invaluable for strategy in a variety of contexts.

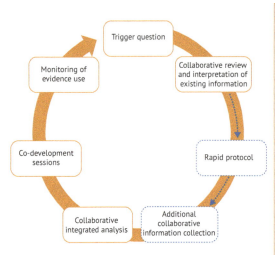

The IOA process usually starts with a specific trigger question raised by stakeholders and decision-makers involved in the outbreak. The origin of the question can vary widely depending on the specific situation. Possible triggers include epidemiological shift, a notable trend, or a request for investigation from a pillar.

Short **TOR** may be rapidly developed and approved by all involved stakeholders, describing the objective, methods, and expected outputs.

Passive data **from various sources are collected and reviewed**. This allows the multidisciplinary team to collaboratively identify which information is missing and to agree on next steps.

Where evidence gaps are identified, all stakeholders collaborate to identify and develop **relevant** reactive data collection and management methods and tools. This may require the development of a collaborative rapid protocol.

If needed, additional data/information is rapidly collected and will be incorporated into a **collaborative and possibly iterative** integrated analysis produced by the multidisciplinary team.

The results are presented to all stakeholders, fostering a common understanding and interpretation of the situation and leading to the co-development of actionable and timebound recommendations.

These recommendations are monitored for implementation and impact.

 THE IOA PROCESS IS FLEXIBLE.

Reviewing and interpreting existing information often requires contacting and engaging with stakeholders who may already be collecting additional information.

Depending on the IOA structure and stakeholder agreements, a **TOR** or similar document may eliminate the need for a rapid protocol when gathering additional information, unless new authority approval or engagement is required. If local health authorities raise the trigger question and the process involves collaborative efforts supporting that authority, a rapid protocol may not be necessary.

However, if additional information is needed, a rapid protocol (or similar document) may be written to state how, who, where, when, and why this information will be collected, and how it relates to the trigger question.

Figure 17.2: The IOA process

Case study 1: EBOD in the DRC at end 2018

In the first months of the EBOD outbreak in the DRC towards the end of 2018, certain healthcare facilities continued to have many cases of EBOD while daily updates were showing low levels of signals of suspected Ebola cases. The CASS teams organised sessions with healthcare facility workers using barrier (and enabler) analyses to understand the factors contributing to the low levels of signals. Barriers identified included:
- logistics (e.g., access to communication devices)
- accessibility and security issues preventing a response to signals
- failed identification of symptoms

The CASS teams presented findings to the MoH response coordination, as well as to the NGOs working in the healthcare facilities, so that adapted interventions and strategies could be developed. Although access to the location remained challenging, telephone credit was provided as well as motorbikes to act on signals by bringing sick patients into town promptly.

> **Case study 2: The DRC – a surge in EBOD cases among children in 2019**
>
> In 2019, there was a surge in cases of children under five years infected by EBOD. The Cell agreed that data from families of cases, healthcare facilities, and HCWs, as well as data from Infection Prevention and Control-Water, Sanitation, and Hygiene (IPC-WASH) teams would be required to fully understand the situation.
>
> Illness narratives and verbal autopsies were undertaken with parents and HCWs to better understand the factors associated with infection, focusing on behaviours and events during their exposure period. Analyses found that though parents were quick to take their children to healthcare facilities, both HCWs and parents were unable to cite the most common EBOD symptoms.
>
> Analyses of HIS data also found that since the provision of free healthcare during the outbreak, there had been an increase (up to threefold in some facilities) in healthcare services use, specifically among children under five years of age. However, reports showed that less than half of these facilities had received IPC support. The narratives from many HCWs and patients reported a lack of good IPC practice.
>
> The Cell was able to conduct transmission chain analyses based on these factors and found that children were likely infecting each other within healthcare facilities. This collaborative work led to changes in training for surveillance, IPC, and RCCE pillars.

KEY IOA PRINCIPLES

The following **eight key principles** form the backbone of the IOA approach:

Integrated, holistic: Data from multiple disciplines are used to understand dynamic factors influencing transmission and control dynamics, as well as the broader impacts of outbreaks.

Contextual, localised: The impact of outbreaks is to be understood at ground level, allowing for recommendations that are tailored to local communities.

Country-owned: In-country IOA teams should primarily involve national and subnational experts, supported by external partners and, as necessary, deployed international experts, but always based on equitable partnerships with local actors. All recommendations are co-developed with the MoH and partners (NGOs, communities, etc.).

Evidence-based: IOA first seeks to understand what data already exist. Further investigative efforts are determined with stakeholders and include systems allowing monitoring of the use of evidence over time by public health response actors.

Operationally relevant: Aims to produce trustworthy data for rapid operational decisions whilst minimising negative impacts to communities.

Data transparent: Where country-specific data protection policies allow, evidence and data are open source and accessible.

Partnership first: Collaborative multisectoral approach working under a unified Cell-like structure in conjunction with MoH. This approach seeks to reduce duplication.

Capacity strengthening: Outcomes and plans should always aim to support MoH and other key stakeholders' capacity to conduct IOA.

IOA STEP APPROACH

Whether working in a large-scale outbreak or on a long-term public health concern (like malnutrition), teams working on IOA start with a trigger question. The answers to the trigger question need to inform the public health response.

A trigger question may come from health officials observing surveillance data (for example, *"why are there spikes in measles in a health zone among children in the past month?"*) or from HIS data (*"why has there been a drop in post-natal services use in one health zone?"*). A sector or pillar could observe spikes in polio in one location, a WASH cluster could ask about drivers of diarrhoea in one city. Local government could ask about impacts from a change in context (*"what are the health impacts of the recent volcanic eruption?"*).

Following agreement on trigger questions, terms of reference and scope should quickly be developed by the team and relevant stakeholders (e.g., MoH at the local level, cluster or pillar or group raising the question). It is critical that the data users agree that the methods and data sources proposed will be sufficient to inform programming.

Existing data are collated and reviewed, then analysed each by their own specialists and disciplines. New data are collected based on agreed needs and methods. Analysed data are brought together and considered by the IOA team. The results are then presented to the evidence users (adapted versions and presentations depending on the audience) and recommendations are co-developed for action. This process is demonstrated in **Figure 17.2**, and see the example of CASS-Epi analysis.

Example of CASS-Epi analysis to respond to a trigger question on nosocomial infection (NI) rates in the DRC (November 2019 10th Ebola outbreak)

Trigger question

What factors are contributing to NI?

- Question raised by rates of NI in a particular health zone or by IPC-WASH pillars

Pro-active data collection (creation of datasets)

Systematic HCW surveys to understand:

- sampling different categories of HCWs
- HCW-perceived capacity to detect a case, prevent NI, and what information, materials, and support are required
- HCW-perceived roles and capacity to apply trainings received
- HCW knowledge and identification of risks within facilities and communities

Reactive data collection

- barrier analysis with HCWs in areas specifically identified as having high rates of NI (possible to also compare with neighbouring health area with low rates of NI)
- participative methods (e.g., interviews, mapping, barrier analysis) with HCWs to understand perceived causes, contributors

Additional data required from multiple disciplines and actors to understand the situation

IPC-WASH data
- number of kits provided by location (and healthcare facility type)
- types of trainings provided to different types of HCWs

Surveillance data
- number of NI by location over time

Events data
- any information on access to facilities/communication on disease
- free healthcare services policies

HIS data
- monitoring changes in healthcare facility use

How results will be used
- prioritise areas for training of HCWs
- develop HCW training based on HCW recommendations for how best to stop NI
- develop distribution priorities based on NI data and HCW survey data

IOA AS A MULTIDISCIPLINARY APPROACH

In each public health context and case, data included are collected from and analysed by multiple disciplines, actors, and sources. Data sources may include:
- surveillance
- HIS data (e.g., routine healthcare services use, vaccination, or malnutrition rates)
- programmes data (e.g., vaccination data, IPC-WASH interventions, cash transfers)
- community data (e.g., prevention or risk behaviour, perceptions and understanding of a disease, or impacts of outbreak or response interventions)(14)
- HCW data (e.g., perceived capacity to detect or prevent disease, or understand impacts of outbreak and/or response on services use)
- documented events (e.g., border closures, ruptures in vaccination stock)
- gender and social norms (e.g., who is responsible for prevention, caring for sick, or decision-making for healthcare services use and/or vaccination)
- socioeconomic data which could explain factors influencing health risks and realities

These data sources, as relevant to understanding the dynamics of polio cases in the DRC in 2022, are presented in **Figure 17.3**.

Although each data source and piece of information should be collected and analysed by a specialist in that field, a multidisciplinary team can improve the quality and use of data. For example, social scientists developing surveys to understand behavioural risks of HCWs which could contribute to NI should help IPC specialists to know what questions need to be asked to identify risks. Data scientists developing models to understand transmission risks may improve their codes for analysis by examining data by specific sex, age, or location categories identified from the social sciences surveys.

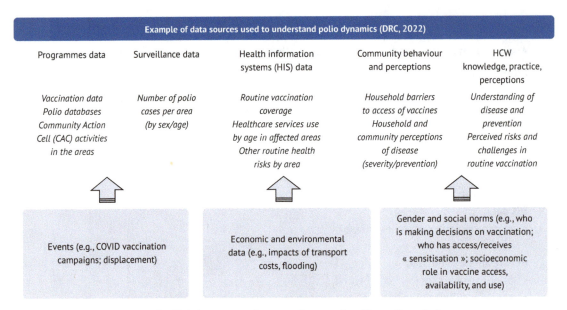

Figure 17.3: Data sources in IOA (an example to understand polio outbreaks)

APPROACHES TO IOA

IOA has been instituted using four different approaches depending on the context.

1. **"Analytics Cell" response unit set up for large/high-risk outbreaks**

   This situation is where the IOA system was first developed, as outlined above for Ebola. The IOA approach is deployed in a response structure where multiple stakeholders work together under the MoH, for example, an incident management system (IMS) (15), with various organisations sending specific information to the IOA. The Cell works collaboratively to see how their data can be utilised, first collecting and reviewing pre-existing data to develop an evidence-based response plan, and then working with the response coordination to identify gaps in information. The Cell will regularly meet, reviewing the daily epidemiological trends to guide outbreak response strategy.

2. **IOA for longer term, recurrent, or endemic public health situations**

   The IOA approach may be used outside of a formal Cell. A trigger may arise (an increase in measles cases, or drop in vaccination rates in a particular location) and IOA will first review all existing data (HIS, surveillance, existing interventions, and bringing in additional data on socioeconomic situations, events [displacement, natural disasters, or conflict]. Based on this, first analysis information needs to better explain the trend will be identified. Methods will be developed based on the information required. The process is done from onset with local stakeholders.

   Depending on information needs, appropriate methods for data collection will be agreed. Tools would be developed with partners to ensure agreement to inform decision-making. Data will be collected and analysed at the outbreak location, with presentations aimed to explain the many factors involved and to develop an approach directly with partners.

3. **IOA supporting early warning of public health concerns (e.g., vaccine preventable outbreaks)**

   IOA can be used to complement efforts upon the early warning of vaccine preventable outbreaks of disease (16). Data sources that might trigger the IOA process in such cases include HIS data, early warning alert and response systems (EWARS), community, and other data. Information to understand if there were any vaccine supply issues (e.g., programmes data) or occurrence of events, such as conflict or heavy rains, which could limit community access to routine vaccination services, could be quickly collected. Local level researchers could collect qualitative data from communities and HCWs in that area to understand the potential factors. Sociocultural factors regarding vaccination (family decision-makers, access to information about vaccination and healthcare facilities) would also be considered.

4. **IOA in emergency response teams for more holistic and integrated data use during outbreak investigations**

    Investigations by a MoH emergency response team alerted to an outbreak can be improved using IOA. Examples here include the use of IOA in alerts around Marburg fever in Ghana in 2022 and plague in the DRC in 2021. This would mean looking at pre-existing healthcare services usage, vaccination rates, or other health issues in the area, thus identifying any recent changes prior to the alert. Questions should be raised as to any events which may have occurred triggering or increasing the risk of the outbreak such as extreme rain or an insecurity which may force families into precarious living conditions. Programmes data could indicate a drop in recent humanitarian services provision which could contribute to health behaviour, risks, or outcomes. Finally, the investigation team should be supported to collect community data and understand who in households is responsible for caring for the sick, and who makes decisions on expenditure, notably for prevention. Information from HCWs can understand their capacity to detect the disease for early treatment and prevention of NIs.

TRACKING THE USE OF IOA EVIDENCE

A key principle of IOA is the use of evidence. IOA teams require a trigger question that ensures evidence generation can result in evidence use. This is not only done to track evidence use but is also a process to ensure best evidence use. Tools to monitor the use of evidence should be applied by disease, location, sector/actor, disease, and over time. In addition, tracking should also consider the collaborative effort to advise (e.g., local health actor, cluster or pillar, NGO) as well as by the type of recommendation (e.g., programmatic, strategic, advocacy based) as highlighted in **Table 17.1**.

Category	Type of influence	Example
Programme intervention	Influence shifts in daily or routine programming	• Vaccination campaigns are re-organised on weekends to better respond to community availability and improve uptake • Community dialogue sessions organised to work with men who are identified as less informed about disease prevention
Strategic	Influence new programmes or interventions are developed	• Water network constructed to address recurrent WASH-related outbreaks • Mosquito net distribution campaign organised to mitigate risks identified from the misunderstanding of Ebola-like symptoms

Category	Type of influence	Example
Advocacy	Influence new strategies and response plans are drafted	• Funding proposal drafted based on evidence to scale up long-term investment to address outbreak risks based on evidence

Table 17.1: Categories of co-developed recommendations which can be tracked

What should an IOA monitoring tool record?

The IOA monitoring tool should record the recommendation, how it responds to IOA findings, and what specific actions will be taken to contribute to the recommendation. For each action, the following information should be documented and tracked:
- study question
- location
- sector (e.g., WASH/nutrition)
- type of actor responsible (NGO, MoH, civil society)
- individual responsible (name/contact)
- agreed timelines to complete the action
- requirements for action (e.g., funding, advocacy)
- agreed indicators to demonstrate the action has been completed
- reasons for delay
- narrative process for implementation

In addition, an IOA monitoring tool could include data on:
- who benefits from the action (e.g., women, children)
- the category of action (e.g., programme activity, strategic, or advocacy)
- if, following the action, an evaluation to measure impact has been developed

CONCLUSION

Following the success of integrated analytics for Ebola, COVID, and recurrent outbreaks in the DRC, the DRC MoH decided to invest in national capacity and set up a full-time IOA Cell (the CAI) under the National Institute for Public Health as a fixed, sustainable unit. The approach is being adopted in other countries. IOA has grown from a niche approach for EBOD in the DRC to become an essential pillar of outbreak response in many countries in Africa. Used in the response to a variety of infectious disease outbreaks, it is increasingly used to tackle non-infectious public health concerns. It is an increasingly acknowledged system to inform strategy and to understand and predict the effectiveness and acceptance of health interventions.

REFERENCES:

1. Choi BC, Pak AW. Multidisciplinarity, interdisciplinarity and transdisciplinarity in health research, services, education and policy: 1. Definitions, objectives, and evidence of effectiveness. Clin Invest Med. 2006 Dec;29(6):351–64. PMID:17330451.
2. Bardosh KL, de Vries DH, Abramowitz S, Thorlie A, Cremers L, Kinsman J, et al. Integrating the social sciences in epidemic preparedness and response: a strategic framework to strengthen capacities and improve global health security. Global Health. 2020 Dec;16(1):120. https://doi.org/10.1186/s12992-020-00652-6 PMID:33380341.

3. Carter SE, Ahuka-Mundeke S, Pfaffmann Zambruni J, Navarro Colorado C, van Kleef E, Lissouba P, et al. How to improve outbreak response: a case study of integrated outbreak analytics from Ebola in Eastern Democratic Republic of the Congo. BMJ Glob Health. 2021 Aug;6(8):e006736. https://doi.org/10.1136/bmjgh-2021-006736 PMID:34413078.

4. Polonsky JA, Baidjoe A, Kamvar ZN, et al. Outbreak analytics: a developing data science for informing the response to emerging pathogens. Philos Trans R Soc Lond B Biol Sci. 2019;374(1776):20180276. https://doi.org/10.1098/rstb.2018.0276.

5. Mobula LM, Samaha H, Yao M, Gueye AS, Diallo B, Umutoni C, et al. Recommendations for the COVID-19 response at the national level based on lessons learned from the Ebola virus disease outbreak in the Democratic Republic of the Congo. Am J Trop Med Hyg. 2020 Jul;103(1):12–7. https://doi.org/10.4269/ajtmh.20-0256 PMID:32431285.

6. Carter SE, Gobat N, Pfaffmann Zambruni J, Bedford J, van Kleef E, Jombart T, et al. What questions we should be asking about COVID-19 in humanitarian settings: perspectives from the Social Sciences Analysis Cell in the Democratic Republic of the Congo. BMJ Glob Health. 2020 Sep;5(9):e003607. https://doi.org/10.1136/bmjgh-2020-003607 PMID:32948618.

7. Carter S, Moncrieff IS, Akilimali PZ, Kazadi DM, Grépin KA. Understanding the broader impacts of COVID-19 on women and girls in the DRC through integrated outbreak analytics to reinforce evidence for rapid operational decision-making. Anthropol Action. 2022;29(1):47–59. https://doi.org/10.3167/aia.2022.290106.

8. Integrated analyses of the determinants of child nutritional status: Manono and Kabalo health zones, Tanganyika province, DRC - Report n° 1 - Democratic Republic of the Congo | ReliefWeb. Published September 9, 2022. Accessed February 2, 2023. https://reliefweb.int/report/democratic-republic-congo/integrated-analyses-determinants-child-nutritional-status-manono-and-kabalo-health-zones-tanganyika-province-drc-report-ndeg-1.

9. Stark L, Meinhart M, Vahedi L, Carter SE, Roesch E, Scott Moncrieff I, et al. The syndemic of COVID-19 and gender-based violence in humanitarian settings: leveraging lessons from Ebola in the Democratic Republic of Congo. BMJ Glob Health. 2020 Nov;5(11):e004194. https://doi.org/10.1136/bmjgh-2020-004194 PMID:33208316.

10. Community dynamics around the plague outbreak. Published August 23, 2021. Accessed February 2, 2023. https://www.unicef.org/drcongo/en/node/3121.

11. Integrated Analytics Cell. Integrated Analyses of factors contributing to cholera outbreaks - Kalemie, Nyemba and Moba health zones, Tanganyika Province, DRC - Democratic Republic of the Congo | ReliefWeb. Published October 18, 2022. Accessed February 2, 2023. https://reliefweb.int/report/democratic-republic-congo/integrated-analytics-cell-integrated-analyses-factors-contributing-cholera-outbreaks-kalemie-nyemba-and-moba-health-zones-tanganyika-province-drc.

12. Integrated analyses of barriers and opportunities for access to polio vaccination services - Democratic Republic of the Congo | ReliefWeb. Published December 21, 2022. Accessed February 2, 2023. https://reliefweb.int/report/democratic-republic-congo/integrated-analyses-barriers-and-opportunities-access-polio-vaccination-services.

13. Analyse intégrée des facteurs limitant le recours à la vaccination contre la Covid-19 au Congo, avril 2022 - Democratic Republic of the Congo | ReliefWeb. Published May 25, 2022. Accessed February 2, 2023. https://reliefweb.int/report/democratic-republic-congo/analyse-integree-des-facteurs-limitant-le-recours-la-vaccination-contre-la-covid-19-au-congo-avril-2022.

14. Field Exchange Issue IO. 2 April 2022 - World | ReliefWeb. Published May 5, 2022. Accessed February 2, 2023. https://reliefweb.int/report/world/ioa-field-exchange-issue-2-april-2022.

15. Emergency response framework (ERF), 2nd edition. Accessed February 2, 2023. https://www.who.int/publications-detail-redirect/9789241512299.

16. IOA Field Exchange Volume 4, September 2022 - World | ReliefWeb. Published September 29, 2022. Accessed February 2, 2023. https://reliefweb.int/report/world/ioa-field-exchange-volume-4-september-2022.

CHAPTER 18

RESEARCH TO INFORM PRACTICE

by Thomas A. J. Rowland, David Paterson, and Mo Yin

Over recent decades, it has become increasingly common for scientific research to be conducted during outbreaks of severe and emerging infectious diseases, contributing not only to knowledge enabling a better future response but changing practice in real time. This has made research more immediately relevant to practice in outbreak responses. This chapter describes how research can be conducted and used in such challenging outbreak settings.

As an emergency progresses, it is likely that requests for collaboration by external researchers will increase and this requires planning and management. Individuals considering research in an outbreak setting must consider the physical, human, and financial resources needed, and factor in ethical, cultural, and legal matters. The results of research must be disseminated through various routes to ensure important findings reach implementers and influence future policy. Post-outbreak research should be maintained utilising infrastructure and relationships established as part of preparation for a future emergency.

INTRODUCTION: PRE-PLANNING RESEARCH

Historically, research on viral haemorrhagic fevers and other severe emerging and re-emerging diseases has been conducted during outbreaks, yielding significant insights. However, these studies were often hastily assembled amidst the urgency of an outbreak with makeshift or less-than-ideal designs. Consequently, the findings were sometimes partial and potentially skewed or biased. Despite this, in the absence of more reliable data, these early and possibly flawed conclusions sometimes remained influential.

Moreover, even when the requisite investigations were agreed upon, the process of setting up the study—securing ethical approvals, sourcing necessary equipment, medications, diagnostics, and vaccines, and assembling a qualified team—often took so long that the outbreak was too far advanced for the initiation and satisfactory completion of the research.

A major advance in recent years has been the concept of pre-planning of studies and clinical trials for more robust and reliable data. However, it has become evident that even with prior planning and approvals, there remains the potential for substantial delays. This was observed during the 2009 influenza pandemic when it proved impossible to implement certain important, approved studies across subsequent waves. Additionally, when outbreaks are very extensive or transcend national borders, more coordination is needed to ensure that studies can be implemented where and when appropriate, and that the data will be consistent for merging into meaningful, interpretable results. The importance of such prior planning and coordination was made especially clear during the West Africa Ebola epidemic of 2014–2016 and was underscored by the experiences of the COVID-19 pandemic.

Research conducted during outbreaks must be a formalised process to generate reliable data to allow us to learn from an outbreak and apply this knowledge to improve our management in real time and in the future. This chapter is aimed at practitioners and other responders who are trying to understand how to engage with research and suggests solutions to problems that may arise. It will address the "what, who, how, and with what", specifically considering tensions that can arise between researchers and operational stakeholders. Common research questions are discussed, providing examples of epidemiological, anthropological, and clinical questions that researchers can investigate prospectively during an outbreak response.

WHY IS RESEARCH IN OUTBREAKS IMPORTANT?

Research in outbreaks involves the process of finding answers to emergent questions. When an outbreak begins, there are many knowledge gaps including potentially the causative pathogen and its origin, mechanisms of transmission, the at-risk population, clinical features, treatments, and public health or pharmaceutical control measures (1). Social science research can elucidate the cultural context and drivers of behaviours and provide insights into local acceptability of control measures and behaviours that might be protective (**See Chapter 17, Integrated outbreak analytics**). Such basic research questions are essential for outbreak control.

Often, when research is discussed, we usually only consider the professional researchers trying to draw generalisable conclusions. The U.S. Federal Code distinguishes "public health activities" to describe and understand the event in order to design effective control measures which are not subject to research regulations, from "research" which is subject to those constraints, though the conceptual boundary between these categories is blurred (2). The dichotomy may have arisen from suspicion surrounding the motives of research derived from past abuses, as an attempt to protect the enquiries essential to outbreak management. Many people involved in outbreak control perform both types of research, but it is useful to highlight the dichotomy that sometimes exists between practitioners/responders and researchers as this can lead to tensions and interfere with efficient epidemic control.

Much important research to be performed in outbreaks centres not on scientific questions, but on improving the quality and delivery of the response (i.e., operational and logistical challenges). The designing and monitoring of a forecasting model to support supply chain management for a steady and appropriate provision of essentials is a form of research. Other "response-enabling" research can relate to optimising information technology and communication systems, and assessing new processes, technologies, systems, or equipment.

THE RESEARCH AND OUTBREAK RESPONSE INTERFACE

An effective outbreak response requires both operational and research components. Unfortunately, there has historically been tension due to perceived (or real) differences in the interests, incentives, and perspectives of the respective stakeholders. These differences can be reinforced by varying legal and regulatory environments. Understanding the sources of this tension can improve cooperation and ultimately lead to better outcomes. In many cases it may be best to acknowledge the differences and tackle the issues head-on.

While both practitioners' and researchers' fundamental aim is to save lives and improve disease control, in practice, motivations and deliverables may differ. For example, the practitioner is incentivised to stop an outbreak as quickly as possible while the researcher will aim to increase knowledge via peer-reviewed publications. Research may not benefit involved communities at the time but will be useful for future events. High-profile discoveries can be essential for career advancement, the reputation of the researcher's home institution, and to access future research funding.

The tension in roles can spill over into questions of attribution of authorship of published studies. Much outbreak research involves the contribution of other responders and practitioners working in the event who may not be involved in designing the methodology or analysing the results. There are no universally accepted guidelines for qualification for authorship on a research paper. While it is generally agreed anyone who makes a substantial contribution to the work described should be included as an author, it is often left to the research team itself to decide who is included, and in what order. To avoid resentment and disputes which might interfere with cohesive and coordinated outbreak control, explicit discussions concerning roles and potential inclusion in authorship should begin early in the research.

The unusually intense burden of work during an outbreak response also amplifies these structural tensions. Operational stakeholders may see involvement in time-consuming research that may not directly benefit the response as a challenge to efficient operations. Healthcare workers (HCWs) may see research as a distraction from their clinical duties, and indeed, as bringing additional unwelcomed work.

The wholly legitimate concern that the research should not interfere with essential outbreak control activities entails that projects should only be permitted on questions deemed central to managing the current or future outbreaks, or to the prevention and control of the disease more broadly. A process for research prioritisation and selection within the overall outbreak management strategy will be essential to prevent the response leadership from being overwhelmed by competing requests.

The roles and responsibilities of all staff involved in a study must be clear, with advance consultation, agreement, and understanding reached with the teams and staff involved in the outbreak investigation, to avoid unintentional interference or confusion. The requirement to communicate the importance of the studies goes alongside the mandate for selection of the most important research questions. The leaders of the response should assist in this articulation.

It may not always be easy for the public to readily distinguish between research and response, and tensions can arise where public perceptions of research influence the willingness to engage with outbreak control measures. Populations affected by outbreaks are often frightened by the disease itself, disturbed by the disruption the response entails, and may mistrust authority, sometimes with good reason. The populations most affected by severe emerging infectious diseases are sometimes also those with historical reasons to be distrustful of research and are aware of the history of international researchers conducting unethical pharmaceutical trials. The fear of losing public confidence can lead practitioners and response leaders to disengage with research. However, successful research can improve populations' relationships with practitioners.

Researchers must be transparent with the local community about the difference between the research and outbreak control activities. For example, people providing biological samples for research purposes should understand that such samples were not taken to guide their individual care and that they may not receive individualised results. Confusion over such issues has caused anxiety and mistrust in past responses. If they are to receive results, the time frame should be explicit. Any intentions of researchers concerning the subsequent use of any such samples, or of other data gathered (e.g., by questionnaires), should be explained to research subjects, as outlined in the information and consent process described in the research proposal.

Legal complexities vary considerably between practitioners and researchers. Formal research is regulated by governments, with standards set by international agreements, national laws, and ethics assessments, and requires strict processes designed to protect participants, as well as the integrity and quality of the data. Processes to review proposed studies must be rigorous and careful, but they cannot follow the slow pace of conventional research review in an outbreak where lives are imminently at risk and the highest imperative is to understand and curtail the event. To prevent the obstruction of a timely, fundamental understanding of the outbreak, there is often a pragmatic distinction drawn between research conducted solely to describe and achieve rapid control of the current outbreak and research that is more generalisable to future disease control. For example, questionnaires or data compiled to elucidate who has been infected identify contacts who may have been exposed or establish that the risk factors for infection are not generally considered to require formal ethical approval. On the other hand, a study to test a new drug does require such review. The boundaries between the basic outbreak investigation and additional research may not always be distinct, and many people involved in the control of an outbreak perform work which contributes to both objectives. Flexible systems to provide urgent, appropriate review of proposed research should be prepared early or in advance to function within the compressed timeframes presented by an outbreak.

IMPORTANT RESEARCH IN AN OUTBREAK

The questions that need to be answered at the start of an outbreak usually evolve considerably with time. Understanding the common research questions and when they are likely to be relevant will help streamline the changes in research focus.

Epidemiological

Following identification of the pathogen or syndrome, the most important research questions for outbreak control practitioners in the earliest stages involve characterising the affected and at-risk populations, and the means and ease of transmission. These are usually addressed by the initial outbreak response team and, for some diseases, many of the factors may already be known (**See Chapter 10, Field epidemiology**). More extensive research will be required in the case of a novel pathogen, a sporadic and/or less-researched pathogen, or an existing pathogen presenting out of its usual geographical range or in an unusual way.

Once the pathogen has been identified and characterised, tracking the strains/variants longitudinally should be undertaken as the outbreak evolves. This is particularly relevant for viral pathogens, as exemplified by SARS-CoV-2, but can also be important for other pathogens, for example, outbreaks caused by drug-resistant bacteria. Emerging variants may present with different clinical syndromes, have altered susceptibility to existing treatments or vaccine-induced immunity, result in altered sensitivity of available diagnostics, or display different transmission characteristics. Current capacities for understanding the molecular epidemiology of outbreaks illustrate how one research tool, genomic analysis, has shifted to being considered a fundamental part of understanding transmission dynamics in real time during outbreak responses, as well as elucidating other key features of disease severity and impact (**See Chapter 21, Genomics**).

Understanding transmission dynamics raises several subsidiary research questions including, but not restricted to:
- the role of alternative routes of transmission
- the relative importance of each route
- the number of people typically infected following exposure to an index case (attack rate) in different contexts
- the possibility of "superspreading events" indicating a requirement for specific, adapted, case detection, and disease control measures
- the life cycle of the vector, if one or more, are implicated
- the interactions of the population with the vector(s) and how these can be altered
- the period of infectivity of a case and mechanisms of transmission over the course of the illness
- the infectivity of an asymptomatic infected individual
- the most effective prevention measures

Such research requires the engagement of experts in epidemiology, social sciences, and laboratory sciences, together with the datasets they bring.

Natural history
Outcomes are improved by understanding the acquisition of infection, clinical features, their evolution through the illness, immune response, pathology, and the range of outcomes in the affected population. Some of the fundamental questions concern:
- why and how are people exposed?
- why do only some acquire infection?
- why do some infected people develop disease?
- why do some people develop more severe disease?
- why are some people apparently more infectious to others, and does this change over the course of the disease? How might this affect the routes of transmission and other transmission dynamics?

HCWs comprise one group usually requiring early attention. Often, outbreaks are heralded by HCW infections and the subsequent amplification of the outbreak through nosocomial transmission (**See Chapter 26, IPC**). The urgent research questions relevant to HCWs are often focused on identifying the types of exposures which may increase the likelihood of acquiring infection and understanding the conditions enhancing their potential infectiousness to others. Such data can be rapidly applied to the selection of protective measures and equipment. The identification of other groups at high risk of disease acquisition through, for example, occupational, geographical, or social reasons, can also enable the identification of protective measures.

Behavioural science
Essential to any outbreak response is the understanding of the views, cultural practices, beliefs, and drivers of behaviour of the affected community. These will both shape the way

in which the pathogen interacts with the community and how the community responds to the measures to control the outbreak. Research which generates an understanding of beliefs, practices, and behaviours, and how they may or may not be alterable, will inform disease control strategy. Behavioural science researchers (including social anthropologists), community-based leaders, and risk communication and community engagement (RCCE) experts will be amongst the necessary multidisciplinary team to drive such efforts (**See Chapter 17, Integrated outbreak analytics; See Chapter 33, RCCE**). In addition, their expertise is also required to encourage acceptance and participation in proposed research, communicating concerns both ways to better align the community and the researchers around the research.

> **Changing burial practices to prevent Ebola virus disease (EBOD) infections in West Africa**
>
> The corpses of those who die from EBOD remain infectious after death, and unprotected touching of the corpse of a deceased person can lead to transmission. During the 2014–2016 EBOD outbreak in West Africa, customary death rites, including the washing of the body by family, were a major source of transmission (3–5). This was rapidly identified by outbreak control teams, and guidance derived from earlier Central African outbreaks was issued that emphasised "safe burial" by specialised burial teams, with non-compliance sanctioned. Despite this, unsafe burial practices continued in some cases, partly due to the burial teams being overwhelmed with cases. Behavioural scientists were employed to investigate the causes of this non-compliance through surveys and interviews. Eventually, new "safe and dignified" burial guidelines were adopted that emphasised much greater involvement of families and religious and cultural leaders, a point which had been demonstrated effective in earlier outbreaks. More safe burials were conducted, cutting off a major mode of transmission and slowing the outbreak. These lessons were relearned to a similar effect in the later 2019–2020 EBOD outbreak in the Democratic Republic of the Congo.

Environmental studies

We have insufficient knowledge of the drivers and precipitating factors for sporadic outbreaks of severe emergent diseases. Sometimes, the animal or other environmental reservoirs and factors contributing to disease emergence and spillover into humans are unknown, or only partially known. When environmental studies are indicated, they should be undertaken with consideration of the impact of seasonal or other fluctuating factors. Preparation by international and national actors for the rapid implementation of relevant studies is an essential enabler of outbreak research. The Quadripartite (World Health Organization [WHO], Food and Agriculture Organization [FAO], World Organisation for Animal Health [WOAH], and United Nations Environment Programme [UNEP]) has an important role in such preparedness, as do many other academic and public/animal health alliances and institutions.

Measuring the effect of interventions

Where control interventions are unproven for a particular disease or in a particular population, their effectiveness should be assessed and monitored. Researchers must balance the need to provide as much protection as possible to the community affected by the outbreak with the desire to identify the most effective interventions. Such interventions may involve treatments, vaccines, or other public health, behavioural, or non-pharmaceutical control measures. The most valid test of effectiveness is usually a randomised trial, which, if properly configured, also tends to be the most generalisable. Adaptive clinical trials may be suitable for outbreaks as they are designed to factor in emergent findings and deliver useful results more efficiently (**See Chapter 27, Research for therapeutics**). However, randomised trials may not always be possible, appropriate, or acceptable. The approach employed will depend on the nature of the disease or the compound or device to be evaluated and the context of the outbreak. The need to evaluate interventions with the highest likelihood of utility means that there must be consideration of access to a sufficient number of cases to deliver a meaningful result, which may entail prioritisation if there are several potential candidates.

Assessing new diagnostic tools

Many common and outbreak-prone infectious diseases have an initial presentation of non-specific symptoms and signs. Accurate and early identification of those infected enables treatment and infection prevention and control (IPC) protocols to be initiated. Identifying those who have been infected in the past can help in understanding the extent of immunity and transmission patterns. However, many severe, emerging and re-emerging, outbreak-prone diseases do not have diagnostics validated for field use across the range of needs.

New diagnostic tests require research to evaluate their performance in field conditions, whether designed as a rapid screening test or a more specific confirmatory test (**See Chapter 20, Diagnostics**). Many factors can influence the performance of a diagnostic assay in real-world settings, including temperature, humidity, complexity of the instructions, the nature and quality of the sample, skill of the operator, and the presence of other infections or biological factors. Diagnostic tests are usually regulated by the same government agency that approves new medications. If it is expected that a test will have widespread use for clinical or public health purposes, regulators should be engaged early to ensure that the methods used and data collected for evaluation are acceptable, and that the correct comparators and performance expectations are agreed upon, along with any necessary collaborations. National or international regulators may fast-track their usual processes and grant "emergency use authorisations" that will confer legitimacy to newly developed tests and speed their adoption by clinicians and public health actors (6).

ESTABLISHING RESEARCH TEAMS AND MANAGING OFFERS OF RESEARCH ASSISTANCE

The process of identifying the most essential topics to be studied and generating specific research questions must involve discussions with local communities and other local and national researchers, as well as any international expert groups or agencies which may become involved. This co-creation is to ensure the pertinence of the research questions to be explored, the acceptability of the studies, and the establishment of collaborations which will not only improve national capacity for future research but also the international expertise base. The diversity of researchers involved in the response to a large outbreak widens the range of research that may be conducted. However, care should be taken to ensure complementarity, rather than duplication or competitiveness which can threaten the prospect of meaningful findings, destroy trust, and challenge overall outbreak management.

At the start of an outbreak, any research that is conducted is likely to be conducted by those who are already nearby. Outbreaks that start in hard-to-reach communities may not receive external support until they increase in size and perceived significance. However, initial responders and local public health authorities may already have relationships with researchers, in-country or from abroad, especially in situations concerning particular pathogens.

As an outbreak becomes larger, or if a high consequence pathogen is involved, national authorities may request assistance or international researchers with a special interest in the disease may offer assistance. Some of the latter will be from research groups with a special focus on the pathogen causing the outbreak, or who have developed an experimental diagnostic, therapeutic, or vaccine candidate to be evaluated and must take advantage of every opportunity to investigate it in the field. Other researchers may have a more general interest. Some individuals offering assistance may not be scientifically trained but may be motivated by other beliefs or the prospect of commercial advantage.

National authorities and the WHO usually take a lead role in agreeing and facilitating the research team(s) judged most appropriate to the situation. National authorities may wish to manage the arrival and deployment of international teams to prevent unnecessary duplication and prevent patients and initial responders from being overwhelmed by ongoing negotiation over "access to patients" (7–8). Ideally, a nationally approved process will be created to agree on the essential research needs and the national and international parties or collaborations to be involved. The WHO and other international agencies or alliances often support such process definition and can assist in the complex areas of identifying appropriate expertise, activating existing collaborations, interacting with the pharmaceutical and biotechnology sector, and coordinating procurement and associated global regulatory functions connected to research. The WHO R&D Blueprint promotes the rapid activation of research and development during outbreaks and epidemics to accelerate the availability of effective diagnostics assays, medicines, and vaccines (9). The Blueprint has developed concepts of prepared trial designs to be implemented by multiple countries and sites during overlapping or sequential events to ensure the compilation of sufficient, robust data.

Ensuring that useful research is facilitated without interfering with the outbreak response is difficult. The management of research offers and requests for data will depend on the coordination of the response to the outbreak. Some national governments and the WHO will create a process for researchers to access data generated from the outbreak response. Systems can also be established to limit the number of researchers in a particular area to avoid multiple studies overburdening practitioners and patients or performing multiple underpowered studies in the available patient pool without generating conclusive results.

The creation of national research programmes allows for more effective research

A key priority following the emergence of SARS-CoV-2 was the rapid identification of effective pharmaceutical treatments (3,10). Hundreds of clinical trials were initiated but, despite most investigating the same treatments, they were individually too small to determine effectiveness. In contrast, the U.K. government required public hospitals interested in testing COVID-19 treatments

> to participate in the Randomised Evaluation of COVID-19 Therapy (RECOVERY) trial, rather than creating their own, smaller trials. This ensured that frontline clinicians were not faced with requests to complete multiple enrolment questionnaires for diverse trials and concurrently turned the RECOVERY trial into the largest such trial in the world. This approach paid off when the RECOVERY trial was the first to identify an effective treatment, dexamethasone, which was quickly incorporated into clinical guidelines globally (11–12).

The arrival of well-resourced international researchers can also undermine local leadership of the research effort and skew the selection of research priorities. Early leadership at the national level from the appropriate government ministries or other bodies, such as the national academy of sciences, can help minimise this tendency. Most large international donors are aware of the dangers of undermining national leadership.

SUPPORTING THE IMPLEMENTATION OF OUTBREAK RESEARCH

Effective research in an outbreak relies on quickly assembling the necessary scientific infrastructure, often in an area with minimal existing facilities, while addressing ethical and legal issues and ensuring results are rapidly disseminated to practitioners.

Physical, human, and financial resources

Outbreaks often occur in communities that are hard to reach and have poor infrastructure. This makes it difficult to establish the physical infrastructure for research, such as offices, meeting rooms, accommodation, and laboratories, particularly when these spaces are already in high demand by outbreak practitioners. Laboratory facilities will be in demand to provide diagnostic and clinical services and may not have the space to accommodate researchers. Building new facilities requires transporting the necessary equipment and identifying local construction teams. Once a laboratory is established, consumables will need to be regularly replenished. New, more mobile, technologies may reduce some of the older customary infrastructure requirements (e.g., for molecular assays and genomic sequencing). Care should be taken to not draw resources away from the outbreak response, although the increased demand for equipment may lead to more efficient procurement if coordinated.

When an outbreak occurs in an established or developed setting where research already exists, then it may be possible to benefit by adapting the existing research capabilities toward the requirements of the new health emergency. There were many examples of scientists and existing research infrastructure pivoting from normal work to support the COVID-19 research response. As part of their epidemic preparedness planning, countries could consider mapping their existing research infrastructure to consider how this capacity could be flexibly adapted to contribute to a future epidemic response.

Even with research priorities and pre-existing resources pivoting towards a major outbreak threat, additional financial resources will be needed and may come from national, international, public, and private funders, and international agencies.

> **Research prioritisation and funding during a health emergency**
>
> The Global Research Collaboration for Infectious Disease Preparedness (GloPID-R), a coalition of research funders, aims to improve research preparedness for infectious disease outbreaks through improved coordination amongst funders. Improving research preparedness and therefore, the research response, entails the development of systematic approaches for the prioritisation of research. GloPID-R has been developing a process for prioritisation, and other work has been recently published proposing to scope and describe past and existing approaches to research prioritisation in events. The focusing of resources and the sequencing of activities, which an efficient prioritisation process would encourage, would streamline the development of the most essential disease control interventions and reduce diffuse and unproductive research. The WHO R&D Disease Roadmaps provides a framework for the prioritisation and sequencing of work on each nominated priority pathogen during and between outbreaks. Research prioritisation approaches and roadmaps must also ensure continued focus on sustaining the continuing interepidemic science and R&D work.

Data and sample sharing

Access to the pathogen is essential for research. However, the number of requests for this can be overwhelming. There are legal restrictions for the transfer of pathogens across international borders, while the sharing of clinical samples may require consent from the national authorities, and in some cases, from the patient through the informed consent process. The WHO may, on request of countries, facilitate the sharing of samples to its networks of international reference laboratories. Both the WHO and these laboratories have developed policies to equitably manage the sharing of patient samples and data and may be able to provide advice to responders and health authorities with these requests (13–14). Other international laboratory collaborations may have processes and protocols for sample sharing which could be employed to support countries in specific areas of research relevant to outbreaks.

Data and sample sharing should be managed according to national laws and international legal and normative frameworks. Research funders and other relevant authorities should require research grantees to provide and adhere to a data management and dissemination plan and, where relevant, a sample sharing plan in accordance with these, as required by the nature of the research. The WHO has recommended policies for data sharing during and around outbreaks, with the goal of rapid acceleration and expansion of knowledge, available to all, to improve health outcomes and disease prevention and control strategies. Emerging approaches to "open data" and "open science" are particularly relevant to outbreak research responses, including, and perhaps, especially, in low- or middle-income countries.

> **Nagoya Protocol of the Convention on Biological Diversity**
>
> The Nagoya Protocol on Access to Genetic Resources and the Fair and Equitable Sharing of Benefits Arising from their Utilization is a supplementary agreement to the Convention on

> Biological Diversity (CBD), an international treaty amongst 193 countries (15–16). The Protocol covers genetic resources and the traditional knowledge associated with them. Its purpose is to establish legal certainty and clarity concerning fair and non-arbitrary rules for access to genetic resources and for sharing the benefits generated by their exploitation. While it aims to create conditions which promote research contributing to biodiversity conservation and sustainable use by establishing mutually agreed terms of sharing, it also recognises that due regard must be given to present or imminent emergencies that threaten human, animal, or plant health. Whilst the rules and considerations for biological samples are fully addressed, the detailed management of digital sequence information under the Nagoya Protocol is still under consideration by the States Party to the CBD.

Dissemination of results

Agreements on research to be conducted during an outbreak should provide clarity on the roles of participants, including the organisation of communications with target audiences, and with an equitable publications plan. This also includes ensuring agreement among all involved research contributors, institutions, and governments.

Significant results of research must be communicated in an appropriate format to policymakers and practitioners for implementation. Until recently, most research focused on publication in specialised scientific journals. The disadvantages of this include that the target audience is already familiar with the research field, leading to jargon and unexplained scientific concepts. Many journals now require inclusion of a non-technical summary of the nature of the study, the key findings, and the potential impact of the research within the published paper. However, the publication process, including peer review, is typically slow and access may require subscription. Some research funders now demand that publications resulting from their funding be made openly available, even if the selected journal normally operates a paywall. Specific provision for charges levied by journals for open access should be incorporated into the budgets for research grants. However, this does not affect the speed at which research findings will appear.

To overcome the limitations of publishing in journals, researchers have found more informal mechanisms to disseminate their results. Over the last decade, and particularly during the COVID-19 pandemic, researchers published their articles on preprint servers such as BioRxiv. There are many such preprint outlets which publish papers which have not yet been peer reviewed, or are in the process of peer review, rounds of which can be followed on the server in some platforms (e.g., f1000). These are free to access and allow research to be quickly disseminated. However, articles in this early stage have not been peer reviewed or subjected to editorial processes; as such, a reader must balance the speed to share with the integrity bypassed (17). For several major epidemics since 2003, representatives from national governments, science funders, and public health agencies, and editors of leading journals, have been signatory to declarations that all findings should be shared openly and as early as possible (taking into account the need to ensure quality). Editors have agreed that prior sharing of results important for immediate public health policy will not prejudice their decision to accept the eventual scientific publication. This was an important advance but is also limited to a small selection of public health emergencies. Efforts should continue to expand this practice generically to all public health emergencies.

Apart from scientific publication and the direct, urgent, communication of results, the dissemination of research findings in a variety of printed and discussion fora, adapted to the needs of various target audiences, should be planned and performed. The target audiences include policymakers and other relevant authorities, the population in the outbreak area, practitioners, and other sectors which intersected with the outbreak control or were impacted by the outbreak (e.g., transport, commerce, environment, agriculture, and the communities involved in the research). This dissemination plan should be considered an integral part of the research outcome, funded and evaluated as a fundamental aspect of the research proposal, and monitored as part of the funder's research oversight.

Legal and ethical considerations

The precise legal and ethical considerations will depend on jurisdiction and context. Major areas of concern for researchers include the regulations and normative standards governing research on human subjects, animals, or the environment, and the rules surrounding data access and sharing.

Research conducted on humans is often regulated or managed by referencing international codes, usually with some reference to the Nuremberg code and Declaration of Helsinki which were initially agreed upon in response to the unethical human experimentation undertaken by the Nazis during World War II and other events (10). Generic international ethical guidance on research involving human subjects in outbreaks has been prepared by the Council for International Organizations of Medical Sciences (CIOMS) (18). The WHO has developed much more contextualised guidance and standards for research in outbreaks, as well as provided ethical review of specific research in which the WHO is directly involved (19). For a more detailed explanation of the ethics of research, one needs to consider the regulations that highlight the importance of informed consent of participants, avoidance of harm, and scientifically valid questions and methods (**See Chapter 5, Ethics**). In most countries, adherence to regulations and standards is monitored by research ethics committees (also known as institutional review boards) which may require modifications to research proposals before approval, and, when necessary, during the progress of the research. This review process normally takes weeks or months, but many countries have designed expedited processes for research review during outbreaks; the development of such accelerated processes in advance of outbreaks, in readiness for rapid action, is recommended. During certain previous outbreaks in low- and middle-income countries, a few researchers from high-income countries erroneously assumed that the processes for ethics review did not exist, and/or that the urgency of the resolution of unanswered questions justified ad hoc studies, without reviewed protocols or approvals. This is never the case. If there is doubt about the nature of the relevant ethical review process, advice should be explicitly sought from the national authorities, or the WHO.

Much of the data collected for research in outbreaks will contain sensitive personal information such as medical records and demographic details which are subject to national and international data protection laws, with strict penalties for inappropriate disclosure. Expert advice should be sought about the constraints on sharing such data internationally, as some data protection regimens have exemptions to permit easier sharing of data in a public health emergency, usually mediated by the government (20–21). Anonymised data is somewhat easier to share than identifiable data, so removing the identifiable information in any dataset can make it easier to share for research purposes. However, researchers recently demonstrated weaknesses in anonymisation, allowing discoverability of identifiable features. As such, increased attention to the quality of anonymisation methods is warranted.

RESEARCH IN THE POST-OUTBREAK PHASE

Large outbreaks often spark investment in research infrastructure, and the development of productive relationships between practitioners and researchers and between local and international researchers and their institutions. However, at the conclusion of the acute phase of an outbreak response, the interest and funding required to maintain these connections may disappear. The final data collected during an outbreak offers analytical capacity which may contain important insights for the management of future outbreaks. Research infrastructure such as laboratories and equipment can be repurposed for local needs, but this requires training and funding of staff and consumables.

Samples collected during the outbreak may be of ongoing research interest but are not infrequently transferred to HICs where international research teams are based. This may be due to biosecurity or practical reasons, but inevitably removes key sources of data which are of continuing local interest and relevance and could be used to maintain and extend local research capacity. Maintaining productive research collaborations is beneficial for all parties in the longer term and allows for the identification and exploration of underlying questions which could not have been addressed during the outbreak. However, achieving this requires convincing the government, the private sector, and philanthropic funders of these benefits once the immediate emergency (and their attention) has subsided. New technologies and methods which may have been introduced during the outbreak can be merged with those previously employed and become part of the new standard for research and public health investigations.

Existing datasets will also likely remain of considerable research interest and should be curated and maintained. Efforts should be made to develop policies and processes to make them available to legitimate researchers. Larger institutions and international agencies may have a role in creating data repositories or knowledge observatories. Consideration should be given to how best to preserve biological samples for future investigation, possibly through some form of biobanking.

Sierra Leone – The U.K. Ebola virus biobank

As part of its response to the 2014–2016 EBOD outbreak in Sierra Leone, Public Health England (PHE), the main public health agency of the U.K., conducted thousands of laboratory tests for the Ebola virus. In 2015, with the approval of the Sierra Leone government and the Ministry of Health and Sanitation in Sierra Leone (MOHS), the PHE biobank was created (22). A total of 9,955 samples and their associated data were transferred to the U.K. and a joint governance group was formed with representatives from Sierra Leone, the U.K., and other interested parties, funded by the Wellcome Trust. The biobank is accessible to all researchers who must first obtain ethical approval from their local ethics committee and the Sierra Leone national ethics committee. Access to the biobank is intended to be equitable between researchers from developed countries and low- and middle-income countries and must serve both a global public good and the people of Sierra Leone (23).

CONCLUSION

Research in outbreaks and epidemics is key to the process of developing reliable evidence to improve the management of infectious disease emergencies. When managed well, practitioners and responders can work closely with national and international researchers to develop robust evidence that can be rapidly disseminated and directly improve the response to an outbreak, often in real time. Effective research brings together people with the right mix of skills, local and technical knowledge, appropriate physical infrastructure, and high-quality data, while working within the relevant ethical and legal frameworks. Consultation and information exchange with the local community and all relevant authorities should be performed prior to the commencement of research, and regularly while it is being performed. Feedback to the local community should be the norm when results and findings are available. The rapid and widespread dissemination of results is essential to ensure the findings are quickly put into practice. Planning is required for the further exploitation of data generated and the management of clinical or environmental samples, including storage and onward use. As the emergency ends, research infrastructure built during the response, often at great expense, should be adapted to "business as usual" and long-term funding acquired to ensure that it is applied for the benefit of future local and international scientific capacity.

REFERENCES:

1. Snider DE Jr, Stroup DF. Defining research when it comes to public health. Public Health Rep. 1997; 112(1):29–32. PMID:9018284.
2. The Common Rule. CFR vol. 45 (2018). https://www.hhs.gov/ohrp/regulations-and-policy/regulations/45-cfr-46/revised-common-rule-regulatory-text/index.html.
3. Alirol E, Kuesel AC, Guraiib MM, de la Fuente-Núñez V, Saxena A, Gomes MF. Ethics review of studies during public health emergencies - the experience of the WHO ethics review committee during the Ebola virus disease epidemic. BMC Med Ethics. 2017 Jun;18(1):43. https://doi.org/10.1186/s12910-017-0201-1 PMID:28651650.
4. Manguvo A, Mafuvadze B. The impact of traditional and religious practices on the spread of Ebola in West Africa: time for a strategic shift. Pan Afr Med J. 2015 Oct;22(Suppl 1 Suppl 1):9. https://doi.org/10.11604/pamj.supp.2015.22.1.6190 PMID:26779300.
5. Richards P, Amara J, Ferme MC, Kamara P, Mokuwa E, Sheriff AI, et al. Social pathways for Ebola virus disease in rural Sierra Leone, and some implications for containment. PLoS Negl Trop Dis. 2015 Apr;9(4):e0003567. https://doi.org/10.1371/journal.pntd.0003567 PMID:25886400.
6. World Health Organization. Diagnostics laboratory emergency use listing [Internet]. https://www.who.int/teams/regulation-prequalification/eul.
7. Science in emergencies: UK lessons from Ebola: Second report of session 2015-16 [Internet]. London, UK. https://publications.parliament.uk/pa/cm201516/cmselect/cmsctech/469/46902.htm.
8. Gelinas L, Lynch HF, Bierer BE, Cohen IG. When clinical trials compete: prioritising study recruitment. J Med Ethics. 2017 Dec;43(12):803–9. https://doi.org/10.1136/medethics-2016-103680 PMID:28108613.

9. World Health Organization. Background to the WHO R&D Blueprint pathogens. https://www.who.int/observatories/global-observatory-on-health-research-and-development/analyses-and-syntheses/who-r-d-blueprint/background.
10. Nuffield Council on Bioethics. Research in global health emergencies. Nuffield Council on Bioethics; 2020 Jan.
11. HM Government. Technical report on the COVID-19 pandemic in the UK. https://www.gov.uk/government/publications/technical-report-on-the-covid-19-pandemic-in-the-uk (2023).
12. Horby P, Lim WS, Emberson JR, Mafham M, Bell JL, Linsell L, et al.; RECOVERY Collaborative Group. Dexamethasone in hospitalized patients with Covid-19. N Engl J Med. 2021 Feb;384(8):693–704. https://doi.org/10.1056/NEJMoa2021436 PMID:32678530.
13. Measles and Rubella Laboratory Network. https://www.who.int/europe/initiatives/measles-and-rubella-laboratory-network.
14. Virus sharing. https://www.who.int/initiatives/global-influenza-surveillance-and-response-system/virus-sharing.
15. Nagoya Protocol on Access to Genetic Resources and the Fair and Equitable Sharing of Benefits Arising from their Utilization to the Convention on Biological Diversity.
16. What is the Nagoya Protocol? Imperial College London. https://www.imperial.ac.uk/research-and-innovation/support-for-staff/research-office/what-is-the-nagoya-protocol/.
17. Bagdasarian N, Cross GB, Fisher D. Rapid publications risk the integrity of science in the era of COVID-19. BMC Med. 2020 Jun;18(1):192. https://doi.org/10.1186/s12916-020-01650-6 PMID:32586327.
18. Council for International Organizations of Medical Sciences (CIOMS); 2016. International Ethical Guidelines for Health-related Research involving Humans.
19. WHO Working Group on Ethics & COVID-19. Ethical standards for research during public health emergencies: distilling existing guidance to support COVID-19 R&D. World Health Organization.
20. Regulation (EU) 2016/679 of the European Parliament and of the Council of 27 April 2016 on the protection of natural persons with regard to the processing of personal data and on the free movement of such data, and repealing Directive 95/46/EC (General Data Protection Regulation). Vol. OJ L 119/1. 2016.
21. The Health Service (Control of Patient Information) Regulations. Vol. SI 2002/1438. 2002.
22. Hannigan B, Whitworth J, Carroll M, Roberts A, Bruce C, Samba T, et al. The Ministry of Health and Sanitation, Sierra Leone - Public Health England (MOHS-PHE) Ebola Biobank. Wellcome Open Res. 2019 Oct;4:115. https://doi.org/10.12688/wellcomeopenres.15279.2 PMID:31544157.
23. Committee on Clinical Trials During the 2014-2015 Ebola Outbreak, Board on Global Health, Board on Health Sciences Policy, Health and Medicine Division, & National Academies of Sciences, Engineering, and Medicine. Integrating clinical research into epidemic response: the Ebola experience. 24739 (National Academies Press, 2017). https://doi.org/10.17226/24739.

CHAPTER 19

ESTABLISHING LABORATORY CAPACITY

by Rosanna W. Peeling, Noah Takah Fongwen, and Amadou Sall

The delivery of laboratory services at each level of a healthcare system requires investment in a robust infrastructure with appropriate technology, human resources, and quality management. Data connectivity linking the results of laboratory, community, and home-based testing to public health programmes allows timely reporting for diseases of public health importance and outbreak alerts. Interoperability and harmonisation of the different data systems used by diagnostic companies, national and regional public health systems, and global surveillance systems are urgently needed. Building surge testing capacity, with equitable access to diagnostics, is essential to improving global health security. Sustainability of laboratory capacity for infectious disease emergency preparedness and effective response will require diverse partnerships and long-term commitment of resources to keep the world's population safe.

INTRODUCTION

The laboratory plays a critical role in patient management and control of infectious disease transmission. However, laboratories remain undervalued and underinvested in many countries, often leading to a breakdown of the public health response in times of infectious disease emergencies. On 16 March 2020, when the Director-General of the World Health Organization (WHO) officially declared COVID-19 a pandemic, he urged countries to "test, test and test" (1). He said testing, isolation, and contact tracing should be the backbone of the global pandemic response. The role of the laboratory as a critical pillar of the public health system in preparedness and response to infectious disease emergencies has never been clearer, and yet it appears that many countries have slept through repeated alarms calling for building laboratory capacity to improve surveillance and outbreak response to infectious disease emergencies (2–4).

Laboratories within a healthcare system provide microbiology, biochemistry, and haematology services to support clinical diagnosis and enable patient care. In the mid-2000s, laboratory medicine in Africa was described as a barrier to effective healthcare and that laboratory services had become the "Achilles heel" of global efforts to manage infectious diseases and antimicrobial resistance (5–6). In 2008, the WHO issued the Maputo Declaration to advocate for building laboratory capacity and developed the Stepwise Laboratory Improvement Process Towards Accreditation (SLIPTA) and the Strengthening Laboratory Management Toward Accreditation (SLMTA) to assist laboratories in setting up a phased process for laboratory capacity building with quality indicators and an ultimate goal of attaining international accreditation such as ISO 15189 (7–8).

There was steady albeit slow progress, mainly due to limited appreciation of the value of laboratory services and the lack of consistent funding (9–10). In the last two decades, countries celebrated dramatic improved access to diagnostic services through the widespread introduction of rapid tests, especially for HIV and malaria. The flipside of that celebration was a steady decline in the political will to invest in a robust, sustainable laboratory infrastructure for public health, particularly in low- and middle-income countries. In 2015–2016, as the Ebola virus disease outbreaks were coming under control in West Africa, the Commission on a Global Health Risk Framework for the Future made 26 recommendations, ten of which were directed at "reinforcing national public health capabilities and infrastructure such as disease surveillance systems and laboratory networks" (3,11). As potential pandemics pose major threats not only to health but also the global economy and security, the Commission advocated for greater investments in countering infectious diseases. This chapter examines the role of the laboratory in infectious disease emergency preparedness and response and proposes considerations for improving national laboratory capacity. This is needed in the context of diverse health system infrastructures, human and economic resources available, rapidly evolving diagnostic and digital technologies, and increasing public health needs.

THE ROLE OF THE LABORATORY IN INFECTIOUS DISEASE EMERGENCY PREPAREDNESS AND RESPONSE

Investing in a robust laboratory infrastructure starts with recognising the many critical roles that laboratories play in preparedness and response to infectious disease emergencies (**Figures 19.1a and 19.1b**).

In an infectious disease emergency, the laboratory plays a critical role in identifying the cause of the outbreak and confirming suspect cases. In the early phase of an outbreak, before drugs and vaccines are available, rapid case detection and confirmation to enable the implementation of public health measures are the only means of interrupting disease transmission in a population.

In the case of a novel pathogen, the initial clinical case definition may be incomplete. Testing as many suspect cases as possible in the early days of an outbreak, the laboratory plays an important role in refining the clinical case definition as more symptoms and signs are being recognised as part of the clinical presentation (12). This is important not only for improving patient management but also to provide a standardised case definition for reporting to ensure the accuracy of case counts.

The laboratory also has a major role in evaluating the performance and operational characteristics of tests to ensure that they are fit for purpose (**See Chapter 20, Diagnostics**). When community testing is introduced, the laboratory plays an important role in providing training to community health workers, ensuring biosafety and monitoring the quality of tests and testing.

Although there is limited time during an infectious disease emergency to conduct research to accrue evidence for policy, the laboratory should be involved in several important areas of research. Testing of different populations enables the identification of vulnerable populations such as infants, pregnant women, and the elderly. Research to determine modes and dynamics of transmission is critically important to inform disease control strategies (**See Chapter 18, Research to inform practice**). During the COVID-19 pandemic, when tests were used to screen asymptomatic individuals at high risk of both acquiring and transmitting

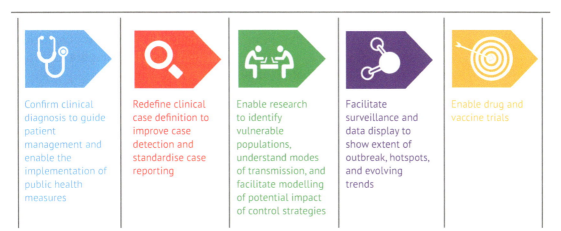

Figure 19.1a: The role of the laboratory in infectious disease emergency response

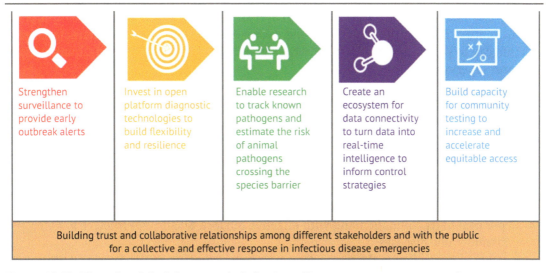

Figure 19.1b: The role of the laboratory in infectious disease emergency preparedness

infection (e.g., healthcare and essential workers), laboratories participated in research on the effectiveness of different screening strategies to maximise the prevention of transmission, protect the vulnerable, and save lives. The laboratory also plays an important role in drug and vaccine trials **(See Chapter 27, Research for therapeutics)**. Finally, testing provides data for modelling to predict trends and estimate the potential impact of different policy scenarios **(See Chapter 16, Modelling to inform strategy)**.

As therapeutics and vaccines become available, testing becomes less of a priority, and there is limited reporting from community-based and self-testing. The laboratory should then consider switching to wastewater surveillance to monitor the pathogen load in communities (13–14). Laboratories with the capacity to perform genomic sequencing can track the evolution of variants as the pandemic evolves (15–17) **(See Chapter 21, Genomics)**.

In times between infectious disease emergencies, laboratories play an important role in surveillance to provide early alerts of potential infectious disease outbreaks. This is also the time to conduct research on novel tools, such as open platform and genomic sequencing technologies, to allow maximum flexibility to detect new and re-emerging pathogens of epidemic potential. Research to track the genetic evolution of pathogens of epidemic potential may provide predictions for early warnings of potential outbreaks.

The recent convergence of diagnostic and digitising technologies has allowed countries to build and fine-tune ecosystems for data connectivity so that findings from all levels of the health system can be collated and turned into real-time intelligence to provide early alerts and inform control strategies (18–20). Building capacity for anonymising and collating data for display on dashboards is important to allow laboratories to communicate their results in a transparent manner to different stakeholders and the public.

Equitable access to life-saving commodities, including diagnostics, is an important element of an effective emergency response (21). A 2022 report from the Lancet Commission on Diagnostics found that 47 per cent of the world's population has limited or no access to diagnostic services, including imaging (22). Building capacity for community-based testing, such as pharmacy-based testing, allows for more equitable access to testing and the source of extra capacity and resilience needed in the health system response during emergencies. It is the responsibility of laboratories to evaluate the performance and operational characteristics of tests that can be performed outside of laboratory settings and provide training, quality assurance, and supervision (23).

BUILDING LABORATORY CAPACITY: THE ONE HEALTH CONCEPT

Heymann et al (2015) proposed that a resilient health system to stop naturally occurring outbreaks of infectious disease should have the same attributes as one needed to prevent, detect, and respond to the deliberate use of a biological agent (2). These attributes include:
- a national biosecurity system to ensure that especially dangerous pathogens are secured with biosafety and biosecurity best practices in place
- a nationwide laboratory network with a specimen referral system reaching at least 80 per cent of its population and with effective modern diagnostics in place to detect epidemic-prone diseases
- a timely biosurveillance electronic reporting system meeting WHO, World Organisation for Animal Health (OIE), and the Food and Agriculture Organization (FAO) requirements

The One Health concept has become increasingly important for public health emergencies in recognition of the complex interconnections between people, animals, and their shared environment. For years, the monitoring of influenza strains causing illness in birds and poultry and their potential to cross the species barrier into humans was undertaken as research in high-income countries. In recent years, zoonotic diseases with spillover have occurred with increasing frequency, and building laboratory capacity for the global surveillance of infectious diseases of epidemic potential has become a high priority (**See Chapter 13, One Health**).

BUILDING CORE LABORATORY CAPACITY

Laboratories involved in emergency response have three separate but interrelated functions of providing diagnostic testing, surveillance, and research, supported by a range of enabling functions as shown in **Figure 19.2**. Diagnostic services should encompass the disciplines of microbiology, biochemistry, and haematology to ensure the full range of services needed for case detection and patient management. Imaging and scanners should also be available for clinical decision support. For surveillance, a network of surveillance sites should be selected based on population density, epidemiologic data, and history of outbreaks. A sampling framework should be developed to instruct the sites who to sample, how often, and what specimens to collect (**See Chapter 9, Surveillance**). Testing can be performed either at the surveillance site or specimens can be collected and sent to a central laboratory for processing. For research, the laboratory should evaluate the performance of novel technologies and determine whether they are fit for purpose and at what level of the healthcare system they should be deployed, and use implementation science to determine how testing can be scaled up rapidly in the event of an emergency.

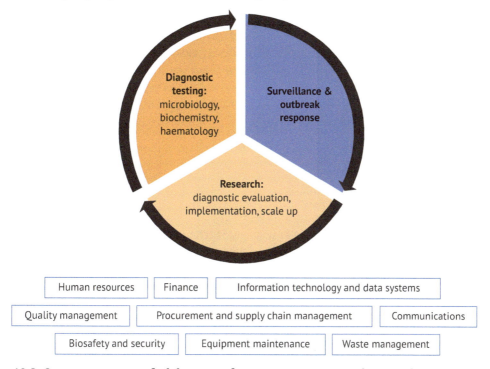

Figure 19.2: Core components of a laboratory for emergency preparedness and response

EMBEDDING A LABORATORY INFRASTRUCTURE WITHIN A HEALTHCARE SYSTEM

Ideally, countries should embed the laboratory infrastructure as the backbone of a healthcare system. At the core of every laboratory infrastructure is the national reference laboratory that provides oversight to all laboratory services within the healthcare system. There are a range of options for building up a laboratory infrastructure under the national reference laboratory. Major considerations are whether to build a centralised or decentralised laboratory system.

Centralised vs decentralised laboratory systems

The choice of establishing a centralised laboratory system with a robust specimen transport network compared to a decentralised laboratory system containing laboratories with different competencies at every level of the healthcare system depends on the resources available, geographic topology, and how the healthcare system is organised.

A centralised laboratory system is less costly than a decentralised system and is easier to organise and operate. However, depending on the robustness and efficiency of the specimen transport network, the turnover time for returning results for patient management may be longer. Having to arrange for a follow-up visit for patients to obtain their testing results and receive treatment also adds stress to already overburdened healthcare systems.

On the other hand, a decentralised laboratory system consists of a tiered laboratory system with appropriate technologies, human resources, connectivity, and quality management at every level. This system has the benefit of providing on-site testing for a majority of the population, increasing the efficiency of the healthcare system and avoiding delays to care. However, this type of system is more expensive to operate, and training, supply chain management, providing quality assurance to laboratories, and point-of-care (POC) testing sites at all levels of the healthcare system can be an enormous challenge.

To address the inequities of access to testing during the COVID-19 pandemic, some countries, such as Brazil, passed a law to allow testing in pharmacies (24). Over 100 countries developed policies to allow self-testing at home (25). The rapid expansion of testing outside of the laboratory system adds to the resilience of the health system in public health emergencies and can become an extension of a tiered laboratory system.

Figure 19.3 shows how a tiered laboratory system can work. The national laboratory at the pinnacle of the laboratory system has the responsibility of providing quality assurance and training to laboratories at all levels, including community-based testing sites. Research, including genomic sequencing, is also performed at the top-level laboratories on specimens collected from surveillance sites at different levels of the healthcare system with the aim of identifying and tracking pathogens and the evolution of variants that may pose public health risks. The top-tier laboratories should have personnel with advanced training in informatics and computational biology to analyse and interpret genomic data. The amount of research decreases with each level of the laboratory system, and at the care and community level, the laboratory should be mainly concerned with provision of the most common diagnostic services.

In practical terms, countries can establish a list of priority diseases of epidemic potential in collaboration with other countries in the region and use the recommendations of the 2008 Maputo Declaration (7) to:
- review and agree on a list of supplies and tests needed at each level of an integrated tiered laboratory network
- develop a consensus to guide the standardisation of laboratory equipment at each level of the laboratory network

- develop a consensus on key considerations to guide maintenance and service contracts for equipment at various levels of the laboratory network
- develop resilience in terms of technological competence and capacity (traditional vs high-tech solutions and mobile laboratories)

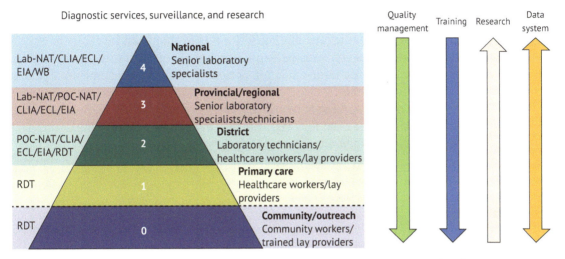

Examples of diagnostic technologies available at different tiers of the healthcare system: CLIA: chemiluminescence immunoassay; ECL: electrochemiluminescence immunoassay; EIA: enzyme immunoassay; Lab-NAT: laboratory-based nucleic acid testing; POC-NAT: nucleic acid testing at point-of-care; RDT: rapid diagnostic test; WB: Western blot

Figure 19.3: A tiered laboratory system for emergency preparedness and response (adapted from WHO HIV testing guidelines)
The arrows represent the direction of the effort, with quality management and training provided by more sophisticated centres. Research needs come from community centres and the data system implemented across the whole system.

Laboratory quality management

Quality assurance is a cornerstone of effective healthcare delivery and public health response (26–27). This is especially important when POC testing is needed to interrupt the chain of transmission within communities (28). In the event of an outbreak, failure to identify pathogens correctly can have catastrophic consequences, as a delay in determining the true cause of infection can lead to inadequate or the implementation of incorrect disease control measures. A well-functioning laboratory system must include a functional quality management programme to ensure the accuracy of data for patient management and to inform disease control strategies. Laboratory quality management systems ensure quality in three phases:
- the pre-analytical phase of ensuring appropriate specimen collection, labelling, transport, and storage
- the analytical phase of ensuring the right test is being used and recording the results
- the post-analytic phase of accurate reporting and interpretation and ensuring that the results reach the provider in a timely manner for patient care

Laboratory test results are only as good as the specimens collected for the test. If errors are made in the pre-analytical phase, no matter how good the laboratory is, the results will not be of use to patients or for public health.

Quality management of testing, which includes external and internal quality assessment, refers to all procedures used to monitor the quality of tests and testing in the laboratory. External quality assessment (EQA) involves interlaboratory comparison using proficiency panels, while internal quality assessment schemes involve retesting routine samples to identify discrepancies within a laboratory. EQA can provide information on weaknesses in the quality of the test used and the competency of the staff performing the test. There are different EQA programmes for different pathogens but subscriptions to them can be costly as access to well-characterised samples is a challenge. The quality management of laboratory systems should be built or optimised during inter-epidemic periods so that they become an essential component of any laboratory system.

Countries should develop biobanking networks for pathogens of public health importance. Well-characterised samples can be used for diagnostic test evaluation and EQA (29). Countries can also utilise the quality management systems they developed for HIV and malaria rapid tests as templates to build capacity for the quality management of tests for diseases of public health importance (28,30).

Data connectivity and data sharing

The convergence of digitisation, information technology, artificial intelligence, and machine learning has enabled disease control programmes to turn data into intelligence to enable timely public health response. During the COVID-19 pandemic, global, regional, national, and local websites displayed daily COVID-19 case counts, deaths, and trends to inform and mobilise effective public health measures to interrupt the chain of transmission in communities. Data sharing provided a power tool for galvanising all parties during the pandemic. The Organisation for Economic Co-operation and Development (OECD) has identified transparency, communication, and trust as important elements of data systems (31).

The adoption of technologies for the digitisation and connectivity of epidemiologic and testing data has made it possible to have close to real-time tracking of an outbreak allowing real-time data to be translated into intelligence to inform disease control strategies. Digitising testing results and having the infrastructure for data connectivity, once thought of as "nice to have", are now essential for the surveillance of diseases of epidemic potential and other communicable and non-communicable diseases.

The ability to digitise laboratory and rapid POC test results can standardise the reading and interpretation of results. Test data can be linked to proficiency testing to ensure testing quality, reducing interpretation and transcription errors. Remote monitoring of POC instrument functionality and utilisation through connectivity allows programmes to optimise instrument placement, algorithm adoption, and supply management. Alerts can be built into the system to raise the alarm at unusual trends such as outbreaks.

However, to realise the full potential of data connectivity, the global health community needs to propose models for protecting intellectual property to foster innovation and safeguard data security and confidentiality. There are currently diverse data systems used by diagnostic companies for reporting test results, making automated data acquisition of testing results and reporting to national and regional public health systems difficult. The harmonisation and interoperability of different data systems is urgently needed.

As part of epidemic preparedness, laboratory information systems must be extended to include data from community- and home-based testing and linked to public health programmes, allowing timely data analysis to identify hotspots and unusual trends and inform control strategies.

Communication

The laboratory should also be able to communicate testing results and provide interpretations of the findings in clear public health messages. Building reliable and sustained channels of communication with different stakeholders and engendering trust take time and are not easily done during emergencies. The use of dashboards for data display is useful for identifying outbreak trends and hotspots and providing transparent means of communications to relevant stakeholders and the public for a more effective and collaborative response. During an outbreak, there should be regular briefings on laboratory findings and their relevance to public health policy for both public health programmes and the public.

There is often a delicate balance between the need for socioeconomic recovery and restrictions due to public health measures. Transparency of testing data can help all stakeholders understand the public health response needed.

BUILDING SURGE CAPACITY AND RESILIENCE

During the COVID-19 pandemic, all countries, regardless of their income level, experienced challenges associated with the scale-up of COVID-19 testing to meet the demand for molecular or nucleic acid amplification testing (32). Surge capacity requires increased testing volume with quality-assured results and the timely return of test results so that public health measures can be implemented without delay. However, laboratory-based molecular testing requires sophisticated instruments, expensive reagents, and advanced technical competency to prevent false-positive results due to contamination. In recent years, there has been a proliferation of sample-in-answer-out molecular tests that can be performed at the POC, requiring only a few minutes of hands-on time and minimal training. However, their availability is limited by the speed of manufacturing of both the instrument and cartridges.

A longer term solution for resilience is to adopt more open or flexible diagnostic testing platforms that are not specifically designed for the detection of a single pathogen or condition. Open platforms include thermocyclers that can perform nucleic acid amplification tests, such as polymerase chain reaction (PCR), or technologies for isothermal amplifications such as the loop-mediated isothermal amplification (LAMP) or recombinase polymerase amplification (RPA) assays (33–34). They require more training compared to the "plug and play" format of POC molecular platforms, but can be used with different reagent mixes that are commercially available or can be developed *de novo* in a laboratory for the detection of any pathogen. Having all laboratory staff cross-trained on these open platform technologies allows the laboratory to be more responsive to new or re-emerging pathogens.

Another means of scaling up testing capacity during the COVID-19 pandemic was to combine molecular testing with rapid antigen testing. When it became clear that infected but asymptomatic individuals with COVID-19 could also transmit infection, governments realised that scaling up molecular testing for population-wide screening was going to be challenging. The availability of single-use disposable rapid antigen tests (RATs), which could be manufactured in the millions per month, made scaling up testing possible, as these tests could be performed with minimal training. Users could follow video instructions accessible online. Even though RATs are not as sensitive as molecular tests, they can be used to detect individuals with high viral loads who are at risk of transmitting their infection to others in the community (35). Those who were symptomatic but tested negative with the RAT were then tested by molecular tests. This algorithm eased the demand on molecular testing and sped up time to results. Widespread testing in community-based clinics, pharmacies, and at home, followed by self-isolation or quarantine, became an effective public health response. The laboratory should play a role in resolving these issues as part of their responsibility during inter-epidemic periods.

The deployment of mobile laboratories with state-of-the-art equipment was shown to be useful in conducting on-site investigations of outbreaks of dengue and Ebola virus disease (36–37). During the tenth outbreak of Ebola virus disease in the Democratic Republic of the Congo in 2018–2020, the Institut National de Recherche Biomédicale strategically positioned 13 field laboratories with dedicated equipment to quickly detect cases as the outbreak evolved. The laboratories were operated by national staff who quickly trained local persons to work and manage future outbreaks. These laboratories analysed ≈230,000 Ebola diagnostic samples under stringent biosafety measures, documentation, and database management standards. Three types of mobile laboratories were deployed:
- basic laboratories for confirming clinical diagnosis and providing patient management support such as chemistry and haematology
- standard mobile laboratories for diagnosis and monitoring viral load and conducting survivor follow-up
- advanced laboratories to track transmission patterns through genomic sequencing

These laboratories were very useful for outbreak response and investigation to allow test results to be available in a timely manner. This meant real-time guidance for public health decision-making through diagnosis and genomic sequencing. However, there were also problems with security threats that delayed or impeded the deployment and supervision of activities, sample handling, and staff movement. Logistics to ensure a continuing supply of reagents and consumables and the deployment of trained personnel were also challenging. Waste management was an enormous problem as biomedical waste cannot be left on site. During this outbreak, tons of biomedical waste had to be airlifted to a proper place for incineration and disposal.

During the COVID-19 pandemic, the Institut Pasteur Dakar (IPD) in Senegal used a mobile laboratory truck (MLT) to provide testing to areas with poor or non-existent health infrastructure (38). The IPD MLT provided high-complexity infectious disease testing to Touba, the second largest city in the country. As a result, test results that had taken up to several days were available to clinicians in just 24 hours. The MLT provides rapid, real-time laboratory services for rural and remote areas without electrical power and could also be deployed at international/domestic airports, borders, and mass gatherings for surveillance and increased access to testing.

Finally, it must be remembered that it is not enough to just build surge laboratory capacity for a more effective response to infectious disease emergencies. This effort must be accompanied by health system resilience to handle the increased demand on health services (39).

> **Building surge testing capacity during the COVID-19 pandemic**
>
> A systematic review revealed that countries used different strategies to scale up testing during the pandemic (32). Some countries set up temporary testing centres, but finding qualified technologists and ensuring quality assurance for these temporary testing centres was challenging. Some countries called on staff from academic and research laboratories to help, but these laboratories were not set up for high throughput testing and were not linked into a system for the timely reporting of results to inform public health action. Countries such as Brazil passed legislation to allow pharmacies to sell tests and perform testing. Since there are 88,000 pharmacies in Brazil, surge testing capacity, quality assured by trained professionals, was achieved. Countries without robust laboratory systems or access to rapid tests had significantly lower testing rates for the identification of COVID-19 cases to enable public health measures compared with countries with robust laboratory systems.

ESTABLISHING A LABORATORY NETWORK AS PART OF A PUBLIC HEALTH SYSTEM OR INFRASTRUCTURE

To be responsive in an infectious disease emergency, the laboratory needs to interact with public health authorities on many fronts, starting with an agreement on a list of priority diseases of epidemic potential for the country and the region. There should be well-established channels for laboratories to communicate their testing results and research findings in the context of epidemiologic data so that appropriate public health measures can be implemented to slow or prevent transmission. The laboratory needs to evaluate different types of tests and how they should be used at different stages of an emergency (12). The laboratory should be communicating with all stakeholders, including the public, on the need for testing and what tests should be used for the right patient at the right time. Building long-term working relationships to engender trust with all stakeholders for a more equitable and collaborative response is an important priority during inter-epidemic periods.

Sustainability

A global effort to build robust laboratory capacity for public health is an urgent priority because in a closely connected global community, we are only as safe as the most fragile state. Any country lacking testing capacity to detect cases enables an outbreak to spread rapidly to neighbouring countries. Justifying continual investments in building laboratory capacity for cooperative research and infectious disease surveillance is essential but not straightforward (40). Time and time again, funding to build laboratory capacity for surveillance and research is available during and after a major outbreak, with the purchase of equipment and training of laboratory staff to perform testing. However, since donor funding is usually time-limited and government funding is constantly subject to competing priorities, the ability of the laboratory to continue to maintain equipment, procure reagents and consumables, and ensure staff competencies for surveillance may gradually be eroded to the point where only syndromic surveillance, such as for influenza-like illness, is maintained, leaving countries with inadequate laboratory capacity to respond to the next infectious disease emergency.

> **Sustainable laboratory systems for surveillance and outbreak response in Africa**
>
> There have been tremendous efforts at strengthening laboratory capacity after each outbreak but investments to sustain that capacity beyond donor aid and time-limited grants are essential. Lessons from the Ebola outbreak in West Africa led to the implementation of a multi-year capacity building programme that integrated training and mentorship on biorisk management, quality management, molecular and serological diagnostics, and facility engineering. The result of the effort is a Guinean-run and maintained facility with a demonstrated capacity for performing disease surveillance, outbreak response, and diagnostics for infectious diseases including Guinean's priority diseases and pathogens that represent major threats to global health security (41). Similar programmes need to be implemented in other regions (42–43). Long-term partnerships, such as the collaboration of the U.S. Centers for Disease Control and Prevention (U.S. CDC) with the Kenyan Medical Research Institute (KEMRI), are excellent examples of what is needed to ensure sustainability (44–45).
>
> Since 2017, the Africa CDC has established a Regional Integrated Surveillance and Laboratory Network (RISLNET) to coordinate and integrate all public health laboratory, surveillance, and emergency response assets, including public health data, to effectively support the prevention, rapid detection, and response to current and emerging public health threats within its geographic regions of Africa. RISLNET facilitates close networking among many stakeholders for the development and implementation of regionally appropriate plans for antimicrobial resistance, pandemic preparedness, and rapid response. It promotes partnerships and collaboration on public health research, training, knowledge exchange, and experience sharing at the regional level in Africa.

CONCLUSION

It is often said that pandemics do not create new problems, they merely make us face problems that we have long ignored. Poor access to laboratory services is one such problem that has been raised as the Achilles' heel of global health since 2006, and yet, the COVID-19 pandemic has shown that much more remains to be done. Building laboratory and diagnostic capacity through sustained partnerships and networks and the rapid adoption of technological advances to strengthen data connectivity should enable countries to have a state-of-the-art diagnostic system that serves as a pillar of the healthcare system to increase health system efficiency, decrease costs, and save lives and livelihoods in the next infectious disease emergency.

REFERENCES:

1. World Health Organization. Director general's opening remarks at the March 16 2020 media briefing. https://www.who.int/director-general/speeches/detail/who-director-general-s-opening-remarks-at-the-media-briefing-on-covid-19---16-march-2020.
2. Heymann DL, Chen L, Takemi K, Fidler DP, Tappero JW, Thomas MJ, et al. Global health security: the wider lessons from the west African Ebola virus disease epidemic. Lancet. 2015 May;385(9980):1884–901. https://doi.org/10.1016/S0140-6736(15)60858-3 PMID:25987157.
3. Sands P, Mundaca-Shah C, Dzau VJ. The neglected dimension of global security – A framework for countering infectious disease crises. N Engl J Med. 2016 Mar;374(13):1281–7. https://doi.org/10.1056/NEJMsr1600236 PMID:26761419.

4. Boodman C, Heymann DL, Peeling RW. Inadequate diagnostic capacity for monkeypox-sleeping through the alarm again. Lancet Infect Dis. 2023 Feb;23(2):140-141. https://doi.org/10.1016/S1473-3099(22)00744-7 PMID:36402145.

5. Petti CA, Polage CR, Quinn TC, Ronald AR, Sande MA. Laboratory medicine in Africa: a barrier to effective health care. Clin Infect Dis. 2006 Feb;42(3):377–82. https://doi.org/10.1086/499363 PMID:16392084.

6. Berkelman R, Cassell G, Specter S, Hamburg M, Klugman K. The "Achilles heel" of global efforts to combat infectious diseases. Clin Infect Dis. 2006 May;42(10):1503–4. https://doi.org/10.1086/504494 PMID:16619171.

7. World Health Organization's Regional Office for Africa. The Maputo declaration on strengthening of laboratory systems. 2008. https://www.who.int/publications/m/item/the-maputo-declaration-on-strengthening-of-laboratory-systems.

8. Yao K, Maruta T, Luman ET, Nkengasong JN. The SLMTA programme: transforming the laboratory landscape in developing countries. Afr J Lab Med. 2014;3(3):194. https://doi.org/10.4102/ajlm.v3i2.194 PMID:26752335.

9. Masanza MM, Nqobile N, Mukanga D, Gitta SN. Laboratory capacity building for the International Health Regulations (IHR[2005]) in resource-poor countries: the experience of the African Field Epidemiology Network (AFENET). BMC Public Health. 2010 Dec 3;10 Suppl 1(Suppl 1):S8. https://doi.org/10.1186/1471-2458-10-S1-S8 PMID:21143830.

10. Parsons LM, Somoskovi A, Lee E, Paramasivan CN, Schneidman M, Birx D, et al. Global health: integrating national laboratory health systems and services in resource-limited settings. Afr J Lab Med. 2012 Jun;1(1):11. https://doi.org/10.4102/ajlm.v1i1.11 PMID:29062731.

11. Peter T, Keita MS, Nkengasong J. Building laboratory capacity to combat disease outbreaks in Africa. Afr J Lab Med. 2016 Oct;5(3):579. https://doi.org/10.4102/ajlm.v5i3.579 PMID:28879145.

12. Peeling RW, Heymann DL, Teo YY, Garcia PJ. Diagnostics for COVID-19: moving from pandemic response to control. Lancet. 2022 Feb;399(10326):757–68. https://doi.org/10.1016/S0140-6736(21)02346-1 PMID:34942102.

13. Safford HR, Shapiro K, Bischel HN. Opinion: wastewater analysis can be a powerful public health tool-if it's done sensibly. Proc Natl Acad Sci USA. 2022 Feb;119(6):e2119600119. https://doi.org/10.1073/pnas.2119600119 PMID:35115406.

14. Daughton CG. Wastewater surveillance for population-wide Covid-19: the present and future. Sci Total Environ. 2020 Sep;736:139631. https://doi.org/10.1016/j.scitotenv.2020.139631 PMID:32474280.

15. Wilkinson E, Giovanetti M, Tegally H, San JE, Lessells R, Cuadros D, et al. A year of genomic surveillance reveals how the SARS-CoV-2 pandemic unfolded in Africa. Science. 2021 Oct;374(6566):423–31. https://doi.org/10.1126/science.abj4336 PMID:34672751.

16. Telenti A, Arvin A, Corey L, Corti D, Diamond MS, García-Sastre A, et al. After the pandemic: perspectives on the future trajectory of COVID-19. Nature. 2021 Aug;596(7873):495–504. https://doi.org/10.1038/s41586-021-03792-w PMID:34237771.

17. Khoury MJ, Holt KE. The impact of genomics on precision public health: beyond the pandemic. Genome Med. 2021 Apr;13(1):67. https://doi.org/10.1186/s13073-021-00886-y PMID:33892793.

18. Gous N, Boeras DI, Cheng B, Takle J, Cunningham B, Peeling RW. The impact of digital technologies on point-of-care diagnostics in resource-limited settings. Expert Rev Mol Diagn. 2018 Apr;18(4):385–97. https://doi.org/10.1080/14737159.2018.1460205 PMID:29658382.

19. Cheng B, Cunningham B, Boeras DI, Mafaune P, Simbi R, Peeling RW. Data connectivity: a critical tool for external quality assessment. Afr J Lab Med. 2016 Oct 17;5(2):535. https://doi.org/10.4102/ajlm.v5i2.535 PMID:28879129.

20. Wood CS, Thomas MR, Budd J, Mashamba-Thompson TP, Herbst K, Pillay D, et al. Taking connected mobile-health diagnostics of infectious diseases to the field. Nature. 2019 Feb;566(7745):467–74. https://doi.org/10.1038/s41586-019-0956-2 PMID:30814711.

21. Kavanagh MM, Erondu NA, Tomori O, Dzau VJ, Okiro EA, Maleche A, et al. Access to lifesaving medical resources for African countries: COVID-19 testing and response, ethics, and politics. Lancet. 2020 May;395(10238):1735–8. https://doi.org/10.1016/S0140-6736(20)31093-X PMID:32386564.

22. Fleming KA, Horton S, Wilson ML, Atun R, DeStigter K, Flanigan J, et al. The Lancet Commission on diagnostics: transforming access to diagnostics. Lancet. 2021 Nov;398(10315):1997–2050. https://www.thelancet.com/commissions/diagnostics https://doi.org/10.1016/S0140-6736(21)00673-5 PMID:34626542.

23. Boeras DI, Nkengasong JN, Peeling RW. Implementation science: the laboratory as a command centre. Curr Opin HIV AIDS. 2017 Mar;12(2):171–4. https://doi.org/10.1097/COH.0000000000000349 PMID:28079592.

24. Agência Nacional de Vigilância Sanitária – Anvisa. Brazilian Health Regulatory Agency. https://www.gov.br/anvisa/pt-br/english.

25. World Health Organization. New FAO-OIE-UNEP-WHO platform to tackle human, animal and environmental health challenges. https://www.who.int/europe/news/item/22-11-2021-new-fao-oie-unep-who-platform-to-tackle-human-animal-and-environmental-health-challenges.

26. Public Health England. UK Standards for Microbiology Investigations. Quality assurance in the diagnostic infection laboratory. Quality Guidance | Q 2 | Issue no: 8 | Issue date: 23.07.21 | Page: 1 of 23.

27. Mantke OD, Corman VM, Taddei F, McCulloch E, Niemeyer D, Grumiro L, et al. Importance of external quality assessment for SARS-CoV-2 antigen detection during the COVID-19 pandemic. J Clin Virol. 2022 Sep;154:105222. https://doi.org/10.1016/j.jcv.2022.105222 PMID:35797940.

28. Fonjungo PN, Osmanov S, Kuritsky J, Ndihokubwayo JB, Bachanas P, Peeling RW, et al. Ensuring quality: a key consideration in scaling-up HIV-related point-of-care testing programs. AIDS. 2016 May;30(8):1317–23. https://doi.org/10.1097/QAD.0000000000001031 PMID:26807969.

29. Peeling RW, Boeras D, Wilder-Smith A, Sall A, Nkengasong J. Need for sustainable biobanking networks for COVID-19 and other diseases of epidemic potential. Lancet Infect Dis. 2020 Oct;20(10):e268–73. https://doi.org/10.1016/S1473-3099(20)30461-8 PMID:32717208.

30. World Health Organization. Joint WHO-CDC Conference on Laboratory Quality Systems, Lyon, April 2008--joint statement and recommendations. Wkly Epidemiol Rec. 2008 Aug 8;83(32):285-7. English, French. PMID:18689005.

31. Organization for Economic Co-operation and Development. Open Government Data Project. https://www.oecd.org/gov/digital-government/open-government-data.htm.

32. Muttamba W, O'Hare BA, Saxena V, Bbuye M, Tyagi P, Ramsay A, et al. A systematic review of strategies adopted to scale up COVID-19 testing in low-, middle- and high-income countries. BMJ Open. 2022 Nov;12(11):e060838. https://doi.org/10.1136/bmjopen-2022-060838 PMID:36396316.

33. Inaba M, Higashimoto Y, Toyama Y, Horiguchi T, Hibino M, Iwata M, et al. Diagnostic accuracy of LAMP versus PCR over the course of SARS-CoV-2 infection. Int J Infect Dis. 2021 Jun;107:195–200. https://doi.org/10.1016/j.ijid.2021.04.018 PMID:33862213.

34. Davi SD, Kissenkötter J, Faye M, Böhlken-Fascher S, Stahl-Hennig C, Faye O, et al. Recombinase polymerase amplification assay for rapid detection of Monkeypox virus. Diagn Microbiol Infect Dis. 2019 Sep;95(1):41–5. https://doi.org/10.1016/j.diagmicrobio.2019.03.015 PMID:31126795.

35. Esso L, Epée E, Bilounga C, Abah A, Hamadou A, Dibongue E, et al. Cameroon's bold response to the COVID-19 pandemic during the first and second waves. Lancet Infect Dis. 2021 Aug;21(8):1064–5. https://doi.org/10.1016/S1473-3099(21)00388-1 PMID:34331876.

36. Dieng I, Diarra M, Diagne MM, Faye M, Dior Ndione MH, Ba Y, et al. Field deployment of a mobile biosafety laboratory reveals the co-circulation of dengue viruses serotype 1 and serotype 2 in Louga City, Senegal, 2017. J Trop Med. 2021 Mar;2021:8817987. https://doi.org/10.1155/2021/8817987 PMID:33868410.

37. Mukadi-Bamuleka D, Ahuka-Mundeke S, Ariën KK. Ebola virus: DRC field laboratories' rapid response. Nature. 2022 Apr;604(7905):246. https://doi.org/10.1038/d41586-022-01005-6 PMID:35414664.

38. Fall A, Dieng I, Touré CT, Mhamadi M, Sadio BD, Ndione MH, et al. Institut Pasteur Dakar Mobile Lab: part of the solution to tackle COVID pandemic in Senegal, a model to be exploited. COVID. 2022;2(10):1509–17. https://doi.org/10.3390/covid2100108.

39. Haldane V, De Foo C, Abdalla SM, Jung AS, Tan M, Wu S, et al. Health systems resilience in managing the COVID-19 pandemic: lessons from 28 countries. Nat Med. 2021 Jun;27(6):964–80. https://doi.org/10.1038/s41591-021-01381-y PMID:34002090.

40. Yeh KB, Parekh FK, Tabynov K, Tabynov K, Hewson R, Fair JM, et al. Operationalizing cooperative research for infectious disease surveillance: lessons learned and ways forward. Front Public Health. 2021 Sep;9:659695. https://doi.org/10.3389/fpubh.2021.659695 PMID:34568249.

41. Ndjomou J, Shearrer S, Karlstrand B, Asbun C, Coble J, Alam JS, et al. Sustainable laboratory capacity building after the 2014 Ebola outbreak in the Republic of Guinea. Front Public Health. 2021 Jun;9:659504. https://doi.org/10.3389/fpubh.2021.659504 PMID:34178918.

42. Njukeng PA, Njumkeng C, Ntongowa C, Abdulaziz M. Strengthening laboratory networks in the Central Africa region: a milestone for epidemic preparedness and response. Afr J Lab Med. 2022 May;11(1):1492. https://doi.org/10.4102/ajlm.v11i1.1492 PMID:35747554.

43. Idubor OI, Kobayashi M, Ndegwa L, Okeyo M, Galgalo T, Kalani R, et al. Improving detection and response to respiratory events - Kenya, April 2016-April 2020. MMWR Morb Mortal Wkly Rep. 2020 May;69(18):540–4. https://doi.org/10.15585/mmwr.mm6918a2 PMID:32379727.

44. Njelesani J, Dacombe R, Palmer T, Smith H, Koudou B, Bockarie M, et al. A systematic approach to capacity strengthening of laboratory systems for control of neglected tropical diseases in Ghana, Kenya, Malawi and Sri Lanka. PLoS Negl Trop Dis. 2014 Mar;8(3):e2736. https://doi.org/10.1371/journal.pntd.0002736 PMID:24603407.

45. Hunsperger E, Juma B, Onyango C, Ochieng JB, Omballa V, Fields BS, et al.; CDC and KEMRI Laboratory and Epidemiology Team. Building laboratory capacity to detect and characterize pathogens of public and global health security concern in Kenya. BMC Public Health. 2019 May;19(S3 Suppl 3):477. https://doi.org/10.1186/s12889-019-6770-9 PMID:32326916.

CHAPTER 20

EVALUATING AND IMPLEMENTING NEW DIAGNOSTICS

by Devy Emperador, Camille Escadafal, and Daniel G. Bausch

Accurate diagnostics are key for surveillance and response to epidemics and pandemics. However, especially in these urgent and challenging settings, many diagnostic tests may come to the market without extensive evaluation. Their accuracy may not be assured. Furthermore, mutation of a given pathogen during and between outbreaks may call into question the accuracy of diagnostic assays previously evaluated and confirmed.

We aim to introduce technologies used for identifying outbreak-prone infectious diseases, and highlight key considerations for the evaluation of the accuracy of diagnostics for outbreak-prone pathogens (especially during epidemics and pandemics), key challenges in diagnostic test implementation during an epidemic, and emerging or future challenges and opportunities for the rapid development, evaluation, and implementation of diagnostics during outbreaks.

INTRODUCTION

Diagnostic tests are essential tools for detecting and identifying infectious diseases. They allow healthcare professionals to make accurate diagnoses and implement appropriate treatments, epidemiologists to track disease spread, and public health authorities to enact informed and evidence-based policies. They are of critical importance in outbreak management.

Evaluating the performance of diagnostic tests during an outbreak is essential to ensure their accuracy and reliability. The identification of SARS-CoV-2, a novel virus that emerged in January 2020, resulted in the rapid development of diagnostics and other medical countermeasures, with the first diagnostic tests available within weeks. Subsequently, diagnostic tests played a crucial role in managing the pandemic, identifying infected individuals, tracking the spread of the disease, and detecting new and potentially more transmissible and/or pathogenic virus variants. However, the unprecedented demand for testing and rapid influx of a multitude of diagnostic tests into the market highlighted the need for new processes of evaluation of diagnostics to ensure their accuracy.

Similarly, the 2022 emergence of mpox in countries around the world emphasised the importance of evaluating diagnostic tests for outbreak management. Prior to 2022, mpox outbreaks occurred, albeit sporadically, in Central and West Africa. The lack of diagnostic capacity to support the surveillance and management of mpox only became an issue when the disease spread to high-income countries.

In this chapter, we highlight key considerations for evaluating and implementing new diagnostics for emerging infectious diseases, as well as discuss the challenges and opportunities for improving diagnostic response in future epidemics and pandemics. Ultimately, we aim to show the importance of diagnostic testing for outbreak management and the need for continued investment and innovation to ensure future preparedness and response.

CONSIDERATIONS FOR ASSESSING DIAGNOSTIC TEST PERFORMANCE

Most emerging and outbreak-prone diseases, such as Ebola virus disease (EBOD), COVID-19, or mpox, initially present as non-specific clinical syndromes, and are difficult to distinguish on clinical grounds from other more common diseases. Rapid confirmation through a diagnostic test is imperative. Diagnostic assays may target the infecting pathogen itself or the immune response to it (**Figure 20.1**) using several different technologies and platforms (**Table 20.1**). In addition to common platforms that have been in use for decades or more, many new and innovative diagnostic approaches are on the horizon, with the potential to enhance diagnostics for both endemic and epidemic-prone diseases worldwide. These include next-generation technologies for genomic sequencing, clustered regularly interspaced short palindromic repeats (CRISPR)-based diagnostics, and wearable and home-use tools, which all potentially benefit from the application of artificial intelligence, machine learning, and advanced digital connectivity (1).

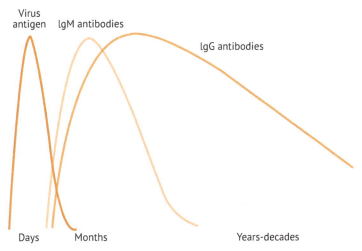

Figure 20.1: Typical dynamics of virus replication and antibody responses after an acute infection, providing a framework for different types of biomarkers to be detected at different stages of disease

Technology type	Characteristics	Test format	Suitability for field setting*
Culture	• Isolate and identify pathogen of interest (bacterial, viral, parasitic, or fungal) • High sensitivity and specificity • Remains gold standard for detection of many diseases • May require sophisticated equipment to conduct	• Virus cell culture • Bacteria culture in medium	• Virus culture: - • Bacteria culture: + / ++

Technology type	Characteristics	Test format	Suitability for field setting*
Molecular	• Detection of pathogen nucleic acid (DNA or RNA) • High sensitivity • Considered gold standard, especially for pathogens that are difficult to grow • May require sophisticated equipment to conduct	• PCR • LAMP • CRISPR • Sequencing	• PCR: + / ++ • LAMP: ++ • CRISPR: + • Sequencing: + / ++
Immunoassays	• Detection of pathogen antigen or host antibodies • Antibody detection useful for identifying recent or past infection; may not always be useful for clinical diagnosis • Antigen detection useful for direct detection of pathogen of interest	• ELISA • LFA • Luminex	• ELISA: + • LFA: +++ • Luminex: + / ++
Microscopy	• Direct detection of pathogen of interest • Gold standard for certain pathogens • Viral detection – requires sophisticated equipment to conduct	• Light microscopy • Electron microscopy	• Light microscopy: ++ / +++ • Electron microscopy: -

*- not suitable, + less suitable, ++ moderately suitable, +++ highly suitable.
CRISPR, clustered regularly interspaced short palindromic repeats; ELISA, enzyme linked immunosorbent assay; LAMP, loop-mediated isothermal amplification; LFA, lateral flow assay; PCR, polymerase chain reaction

Table 20.1: Main diagnostic technologies for infectious diseases and examples of their use

The choice of which technology to employ is based on several considerations, including intended use (e.g., identification of acute cases versus previous exposure), test performance (e.g., sensitivity and specificity), cost and availability of resources (e.g., laboratory equipment, reagents, disposables), staff time and training, and biosafety and biosecurity levels. Timing of collection and choice of sample type should be based on the kinetics of the pathogen, immune response for the given disease, and presence of the pathogen in different body compartments/fluids, as well as risk and acceptability for the participants and healthcare workers taking the sample. Data for many outbreak-prone pathogens may be scarce. This is especially true for novel pathogens such as SARS-CoV-2 (at least when the virus first emerged), as well as rarer, less-studied pathogens like the monkeypox and Zika viruses. As a result of this limited knowledge, early decisions regarding diagnostic tests may need to be adaptively adjusted as the outbreak progresses.

Regardless of the technology type or diagnostic platform, understanding how well a test detects the pathogen of interest is key to selecting and implementing the appropriate tool for outbreak response and disease surveillance. Ideally, performance data would be readily available for all potential diagnostics in laboratory as well as field settings. However, as noted above, these data are often not available in the early phases of an outbreak, and therefore, systems for the rapid implementation of studies on diagnostic test performance are critical.

> **Availability of EBOD diagnostics after the 2013-2016 West Africa epidemic**
>
> At the onset of the 2013-2016 EBOD epidemic in West Africa, most laboratories responding to the outbreak relied on in-house polymerase chain reaction (PCR) assays. While these were faster to develop, it became challenging to ensure comparable results between the different tests. The establishment of the processes of Emergency Use Authorization by the U.S. Food and Drug Administration (U.S. FDA) and Emergency Use Listing by the World Health Organization (WHO) in 2014 incentivised the development and availability of commercial diagnostics. By 2016, 10 PCR and four rapid diagnostic tests (RDTs) were approved by the U.S. FDA or WHO. However, only two of the 14 approved tests were used routinely during a subsequent EBOD outbreak in the Democratic Republic of the Congo in 2018 (2). What happened?
>
> Although potentially devastating when they occur, outbreaks of most emerging infectious diseases (e.g., EBOD) remain rare, unpredictable, and relatively small, requiring small volumes of diagnostic tests compared to other more common and widespread diseases. Consequently, research and development for such outbreak-prone diseases often pose a high financial risk to test developers. Even when assays have been developed and have regulatory approval, there are often long lead times for test developers to produce them at scale, which can cause delays in testing at the onset of an outbreak. Furthermore, when emergency authorisation reviews stopped after the West Africa EBOD outbreak, there were limited avenues for new tests to be evaluated. To ensure the availability of diagnostics for future EBOD outbreaks, countries and the global health community must make investments in diagnostic preparedness, possibly including pre-payment of a set volume of tests, distribution processes, and the ability to identify an avenue for evaluating and approving new tests.

The diagnostic test to be evaluated is commonly called the *index test*. Diagnostic accuracy studies aim to quantify how well the index test performs in the population of interest by evaluating the accuracy of the test in discriminating between people with or without the target disease or condition (3–4) (**See Chapter 10, Field epidemiology**). The main characteristics defining the performance of a test are its ***clinical sensitivity***, the probability that a person with the target disease will test positive, and ***clinical specificity***, the probability that an uninfected person without the target disease will test negative. In addition, the analytical specificity of a test, or its cross-reactivity, is important, referring to its ability to differentiate between the target pathogen and other pathogens causing a similar syndrome. Sensitivity and specificity of the index test are normally determined by comparing it against a *reference* or *gold standard* test, which is used to identify samples from persons who are truly infected or uninfected, and usually tabulated in a 2 x 2 table (**Table 20.2a-d**). Procuring well-characterised samples for which confidence is high that they either contain or do not contain the biomarker (i.e., the indicator measured and interpreted to give a test result), ideally along a range of concentrations, is essential to assess test performance.

		Reference standard test		Total
		Positive	Negative	
Index test	Positive	TP	FP	TP + FP
	Negative	FN	TN	FN + TN
	Total	TP + FN	FP + TN	

TP, true positive; FP, false positive; FN, false negative; TN, true negative
- Test sensitivity = 100 x TP/(TP+FN)
- Test specificity = 100 x TN/(FP+TN)
- Positive predictive value (PPV) = 100 x TP/(TP+FP)
- Negative predictive value (NPV) = 100 x TN/(FN+TN)

Table 20.2a: The 2 x 2 table to evaluate test performance

		Reference standard test		Total
		Positive	Negative	
Index test	Positive	9	99	108
	Negative	1	891	892
		10	990	1000

- Test sensitivity = 90%
- Test specificity = 90%
- Positive predictive value (PPV) = 8%
- Negative predictive value (NPV) = 99.9%

Table 20.2b: Example 1: Disease prevalence = 1%

		Reference standard test		Total
		Positive	Negative	
Index test	Positive	90	90	180
	Negative	10	810	820
		100	900	1000

- Test sensitivity = 90%
- Test specificity = 90%
- Positive predictive value (PPV) = 50%
- Negative predictive value (NPV) = 98.8%

Table 20.2c: Example 2: Disease prevalence = 10%

		Reference standard test		Total
		Positive	Negative	
Index test	Positive	180	80	260
	Negative	20	720	740
		200	800	1000

- Test sensitivity = 90%
- Test specificity = 90%
- Positive predictive value (PPV) = 69%
- Negative predictive value (NPV) = 97%

Table 20.2d: Example 3: Disease prevalence = 20%

If a prospective study was conducted, the ***positive predictive value*** (PPV, the probability that a positive result indicates the presence of disease) and ***negative predictive value*** (NPV, the probability that a negative result indicates the absence of disease) can be calculated. Unlike sensitivity and specificity, which are inherent values of the test, PPV and NPV are affected by disease prevalence.

There are standard guidelines and information on best practices for the evaluation of diagnostic tests for use in clinical laboratories (5–7). Below we discuss some key considerations for designing a study to evaluate diagnostic test accuracy in the challenging context of an epidemic or pandemic.

Defining evaluation objectives through key use cases

A *use case* is a description of all the ways that an end user wants to use a system, in this instance, a diagnostic test. Before any evaluation planning, there must be agreement on the key use cases for the test. Although primarily used in test development (8), an understanding of the various testing use cases and priorities during an epidemic or pandemic is needed to identify the appropriate diagnostic tool to implement. Broadly, the main diagnostic use cases for a pathogen include screening, triage, diagnosis, confirmation, and surveillance (**Table 20.3**). Detailed use cases for each of these can be developed through consideration of the population for testing, where and how testing will occur, who will conduct the test, and what the clinical action and/or response will be once the results are available, including, for instance, sample or patient referral or implementation of vector control or vaccination campaigns (8–9). A review of the current literature on the appropriate biomarker for detection is important to develop the evaluation study—a task which is challenging for previously unknown pathogens.

Consider the following use cases that are common circumstances for the deployment of diagnostic tests for outbreak-prone pathogens:
- Screening or triaging symptomatic persons who present to a healthcare facility
- Distinguishing infected from non-infected individuals in a large population, regardless of whether they are symptomatic or asymptomatic

In the first situation, a test with high sensitivity will be required to identify the highest proportion of truly infected persons in order to initiate treatment and prevention measures, such as patient isolation. In the second situation, if the infection is rare, or to support contact tracing or the identification of outbreak hotspots in the community, high specificity will be required. Otherwise, a high proportion of those who test positive will not actually have the infection (i.e., a false positive).

	Diagnostic use case			
	Triage	**Diagnosis**	**Confirmation**	**Surveillance**
Intended use	Determine if an individual has a reasonable likelihood of a current COVID-19 infection, warranting temporary isolation pending confirmatory testing	Diagnose an individual with a SARS-CoV-2 infection	Confirm that an individual is currently infected with SARS-CoV-2 after triage testing	Monitor population to obtain early indications of a COVID-19 outbreak
Use setting	• Community • Health clinic • Hospital lab	• Clinic • Hospital lab	• Hospital lab • Reference lab	• Community • Health centre • Clinic/hospital lab • Reference lab
Sample type	• Nasal swab • Nasopharyngeal swab	• Nasal swab • Nasopharyngeal swab	• Nasal swab • Nasopharyngeal swab	• Nasal swab • Nasopharyngeal swab • Blood • Waste water
User training	Low	Medium – High	High	Medium – High
Technology types/ platforms	• LFA (Ag)	• LFA (Ag) • POC MDx • MDx	• MDx • Sequencing	• LFA (Ag, Ab) • ELISA (Ag, Ab) • POC MDx • MDx • Sequencing

Ab, antibody; Ag, antigen; LFA, lateral flow assay; MDx, molecular diagnostic; POC, point-of-care

Table 20.3: COVID-19 diagnostic use cases

The development of COVID-19 diagnostics serves as a clear example of consideration of the use case. At the beginning of the pandemic, the utility of detecting the SARS-CoV-2 antigen for the diagnosis of symptomatic persons was unclear. Antigen-based RDTs were being developed, and the question of how they would perform compared to molecular detection was key. Given that many countries were experiencing delays in reporting of results or had limited access to testing (10), the advantages of RDTs (e.g., ease of use, rapid results) would help improve the rapid identification of persons with COVID-19.

Identifying the appropriate study design

Diagnostic evaluation studies may be either prospective or retrospective in design, each with their own advantages and disadvantages (**Table 20.4**). In a prospective study, persons suspected of having the target condition are consecutively enrolled and tested using the index and reference tests. If a small proportion of those tested are likely to be positive, a practical study approach is to first test all subjects using the reference standard, and then test only the positives and a random sample of negatives using the index tests. In a retrospective study, the index and reference tests are applied to previously collected and stored specimens. Although more rapid compared to a prospective study design, results from retrospective studies may lead to bias and the overestimation of diagnostic accuracy when, for example, stored samples come from only the sickest and healthiest subjects, who might have extremely high or low pathogen burdens, respectively. Specificity can be affected when negative samples come from a group that may not be indicative of the study population, for example, samples from healthy individuals with different exposure status, or which exclude individuals with similar symptoms as the pathogen of interest but caused by pathogens co-circulating in the region.

	Prospective design	**Retrospective design**
Advantages	• Better defined participant sample and clinical • Implement standardised methods for sample collection and testing	• Convenient – samples already available • Faster to set up and complete • Usually less expensive to conduct
Disadvantages	• Longer length of time to set up and conduct • Sensitive to changes in disease incidence • Usually more expensive to conduct	• Specimen quality may be affected by storage • Clinical information might be limited or unavailable • Informed consent for additional testing may not be available

Table 20.4: Advantages and disadvantages of prospective versus retrospective test evaluation studies

Regardless of study design, it is important to ensure an adequate sample size to accurately estimate test sensitivity and specificity. Sample size calculations should consider the anticipated sensitivity or specificity of the test, disease prevalence among the study population, and other statistical considerations (11). The anticipated performance of a test is an important parameter; ways of determining this include following the figures set in Target Product Profiles (TPPs) for the diagnostic test (**See What is a TPP?**) or, if a TPP has not been developed, estimating the minimal acceptable performance based on the use case. For example, a diagnostic test will usually require higher accuracy for case confirmation than for triage, given that you want to ensure the detection of the specific pathogen. In this case, the sample size for the evaluation study would need to be greater in order to include a sufficient number of positive cases.

> **What is a TPP?**
>
> A TPP is a strategic document that summarises the key characteristics of a new or innovative product to address an unmet clinical need. In the TPP, key features (e.g., use case, user requirements, storage requirements, price) and performance specifications are identified in advance to ensure that the final desired product is considered throughout all stages of development. Global TPPs have been developed for diagnostics to address outbreak-prone pathogens, including the SARS-CoV-2, Ebola, and Zika viruses. Although there is no strict methodology to develop a TPP, the development of TPPs for diagnostics for the aforementioned viruses included incorporating data from systematic literature reviews and consensus building of criteria from experts and stakeholders.
>
> For COVID-19, four priority TPPs were drafted to:
> - identify suspected COVID-19 cases at point-of-care
> - diagnose and confirm suspected COVID-19 cases for moderate- or high-volume testing
> - identify prior SARS-CoV-2 infection at point-of-care
> - identify prior SARS-CoV-2 infection for moderate- or high-volume testing
>
> Each TPP will describe acceptable and desirable criteria and will be different depending on the use case. For example, acceptable and desirable test sensitivity for the first TPP is set at ⩾80 per cent and ⩾90 per cent, respectively, while for the second TPP it is ⩾95 per cent and ⩾98 per cent, respectively.
>
> Examples of available TPPs for outbreak diseases include:
> - Ebola TPP: https://journals.plos.org/plosntds/article?id=10.1371/journal.pntd.0003734
> - Zika TPP: https://www.who.int/publications/m/item/target-product-profiles-for-better-diagnostic-tests-for-zika-virus-infection
> - SARS-CoV-2 TPP: https://www.who.int/publications/m/item/covid-19-target-product-profiles-for-priority-diagnostics-to-support-response-to-the-covid-19-pandemic-v.0.1
> - Mpox TPP: https://www.who.int/publications/i/item/9789240076464
> - Cholera TPP: https://www.gtfcc.org/resources/target-product-profile-for-a-rapid-diagnostic-test-for-surveillance-of-cholera-outbreaks/

Identifying the appropriate reference standard

Inherent to assessing the performance of an index test is selection of the appropriate comparator—ideally a well-established, well-characterised, and widely accepted reference standard. Some reference standards are well established, such as PCR testing for the Ebola virus. At times, the reference standard may comprise a combination of multiple different tests, or both laboratory and clinical criteria, such as for severe dengue fever. However, in many cases, and especially for newly emerged and rarely seen pathogens (e.g., leptospirosis), there is no defined reference standard or the reference standard is difficult to implement in the field (e.g., virus cell culture). In these cases, composite reference standards may be used, in which disease positive and negative are based on two reference test results.

Quality assurance and monitoring

Quality assurance should be incorporated into all studies. Testing sites and study conduct should be compliant with Good Clinical Practice (GCP) and Good Clinical Laboratory Practice (GCLP), especially when conducting prospective studies (7,12–13). Minimum requirements to ensure compliance include:
- proper documentation to capture study results (e.g., reference and index test results, participant clinical information)
- training personnel on GCP, GCLP, and relevant processes to conduct evaluations
- up-to-date standard operating procedures that describe all activities related to diagnostic evaluation studies

While quality assurance and monitoring plans may take time to set up, establishing these processes early guarantees the rapid availability of performance results that are high quality and reliable.

Quality assurance and monitoring are even more important when tests are rolled out for use in the field. In the laboratory, personnel can ensure quality results in various ways, including the inclusion and monitoring of internal controls, measuring differences in results between test operators, and conducting verification studies when new testers, equipment, or lots are introduced. When tests are rolled out at multiple sites, implementing an external quality assessment programme or activity is important to assess technical capacity and ensure consistent results (14). With external quality assessment, testing sites can benchmark their results to a panel of known positive and negative samples and assist with identifying areas of improvement within the testing site.

CONSIDERATIONS FOR TEST PROCUREMENT

Previously identified use cases are key to support test implementation since the use case will also describe the intended healthcare level for implementation and any potential changes in the current testing algorithm, especially if the diagnostic test is meant to replace or add to current practice and guidelines. For example, many were eager to use antibody rapid tests to confirm immunity to SARS-CoV-2 post-vaccination or post-infection (15). However, since the correlates of protection for COVID-19 were unknown and are not necessarily based on antibody titre alone, this was not an appropriate use case (16). Consequently, the WHO guidance is that antibody rapid tests be used mainly for disease surveillance (17). For any country wishing to implement a particular test, the feasibility and sustainability of the supply chain, including reagents and consumables (including any required cold chain/cold storage), as well as equipment and its maintenance/services—sustainability and feasibility in that country will also be a critical consideration as to which test/test types are suitable.

ACKNOWLEDGING THE ROLE OF DIAGNOSTICS EVALUATION

Advances have been made in the last few years to improve the availability and rollout of diagnostics during health emergencies. Lessons from the response to the 2013-2016 EBOD outbreak in West Africa resulted in the development of the WHO R&D Blueprint (18). With its mission including support for the development, evaluation, and rollout of diagnostics for outbreak-prone diseases, as well as those yet to emerge (commonly termed "Disease X"), the R&D Blueprint framework provided critical support for the laboratory and diagnostic response to the COVID-19 pandemic. This included increased collaboration between academia and industry, and increased acceptance and demand for diagnostics from governments. Nevertheless, challenges remain to optimally evaluate and implement tests during an epidemic or pandemic (**Table 20.5**).

Challenge	Possible solutions
Access to well-characterised clinical samples (including complete clinical data) and reference materials	• Ownership of samples and related clinical data must be clearly defined prior to any clinical study • Find mechanisms that can ensure ownership of samples by local study sites but also allow conditional access to selected external partners for test evaluation purposes • Ongoing efforts at the regional and international levels to define sample ownership and access through the implementation of virtual biobanks and biobanking networks • Online catalogue of all available reference and control materials for various outbreak-prone pathogens
Achieve a study's objectives in the context of ever-changing positivity rates	• Work with a network of partners with agreements already in place so evaluation plans can shift from one site to another • Integrate adaptive clinical study designs during protocol development and study implementation
Ensure high-quality clinical trial data across all partners involved	• Implement a network of study sites ahead of any health emergencies that may arise to ensure common practices are performed to a high standard. Such a network should include scientists, experts, and key opinion leaders who work in the fields of outbreak-prone diseases, clinical trial conduct, and ethical and regulatory frameworks of different geographical areas
Delay from key actors (e.g., laboratories, clinical partners, ethics boards) to draft and approve study protocols to initiate activities	• Implement partner agreements and a network of study sites ahead of health emergencies that may arise to ensure rapid and smooth reaction and scale-up (administrative, regulatory and ethics considerations, logistics, laboratory capacity, human resources, etc.) • Develop generic and adaptive protocols that have already been reviewed by key actors and require minimal input to be implemented in a timely manner • Develop "emergency mode" processes that can be activated in the case of a health emergency (e.g., WHO Emergency Use Authorization list) • Provide sufficient resources, especially staff, to enable timely completion of review processes
Unwillingness of the study population to participate in a study due to the stigma linked to the disease or fear of negative impact on employment	• Integration of engagement with local communities in the first stages of the clinical study (**See Chapter 33, RCCE**)

Challenge	Possible solutions
Ensure the availability of quality diagnostics after an acute health emergency	• Promote the development and availability of regional manufacturing sites • Streamline guidance on appropriate tools for response • Maintain database of upcoming and available diagnostic technologies

Table 20.5: Challenges and possible solutions to improve diagnostic availability and rollout for outbreak pathogens

Conducting test evaluations during outbreaks is especially challenging as resources and trained staff are already engaged in response activities. Furthermore, evaluation sites must have experience, as well as previous training in GCP and GCLP, with appropriate external monitoring, which may be especially challenging during epidemics.

To ensure impartiality of any study analysis and interpretation of results, test evaluations should be conducted independently. Maintaining impartiality may be challenging while simultaneously maintaining a relationship with private partners that are key for future test development. Tests should be purchased (not provided for free by manufacturers), with test manufacturers having no oversight regarding study design, implementation, data analysis, or publication of results. Given that rapid and transparent access to study results is critical to response, data from diagnostic evaluation studies should be readily submitted and available to the scientific community through open-access platforms such as the WHO COVID-19 Data Repository (19) or FIND's pathogen Test Directories (20).

The willingness of subjects to enrol in test evaluations during outbreaks can be compromised by possible stigma from being diagnosed with the disease, or even from undergoing testing. This was observed in West Africa during the 2013-2016 EBOD outbreak and during the COVID-19 pandemic in certain countries and communities where social stigma associated with the disease played a role in deterring many from accessing testing (21). Study participants may also be reluctant to be tested when a positive result may lead to limitations on movement and potentially hamper income. Early and transparent community engagement to allow for full understanding and buy-in to the research is essential and can potentially improve the uptake of new tests and ensure that the rollout of accurate diagnostics has maximum benefit to the community. The integration of social and behavioural science research into the evaluation study may provide feedback to enhance understanding between the researchers and participants, helping to elicit the most successful approaches for all concerned.

Timing is a crucial and highly constraining factor when conducting prospective evaluation studies. Testing must occur at a time and place where transmission and test positivity rates are sufficiently high to achieve adequate sample size and interpretable results. This has been especially challenging during the COVID-19 pandemic, in which waves of transmission varied in intensity across countries and regions. Rapid mobilisation is often hindered by lengthy procedures required to launch a clinical evaluation, including reaching an agreement on a study protocol, establishing and training a study team, importation of tests (including both regulatory approval and transport logistics), and Ethics Committee approval (**See Chapter 18, Research to inform practice**).

Success requires a significant investment in preparedness to respond rapidly when the time comes. Like the initiatives for the evaluation of vaccines and therapeutics for outbreak-prone diseases (22), the availability of generic protocols for diagnostic evaluations and the establishment of test evaluation networks that can either be disease agnostic or adapted to a new pathogen would be beneficial. A diagnostic test evaluation network could build on similar principles. For example, the International Severe Acute Respiratory and emerging Infection Consortium (ISARIC) is a clinical research network that rapidly updated existing protocols and case report forms to evaluate mpox treatments in the U.K. once the outbreak of mpox was identified in the country (23). Another good example is the newly established PANTHER network (Pandemic Preparedness Platform for Health and Emerging Infections Response), which aims to provide a flexible clinical research platform response for outbreak-prone pathogens such as Lassa and monkeypox viruses in Africa (24). These protocols could be agreed on by the international community and local ethics committees to allow rapid activation once an outbreak is confirmed (25).

Similarly, the COVID-19 pandemic has highlighted the inadequate emergency capability among current processes at multiple healthcare levels, from clinics and laboratories to local, regional, and global public health responders, as well as regulatory bodies. Implementing standard operating procedures and a more streamlined process that can be activated once an epidemic or pandemic is declared would allow for a timelier response. An example of this was the development and activation of an emergency use authorisation process that allowed for medical countermeasures to be rapidly reviewed and temporarily approved for use during the 2013–2016 EBOD epidemic in West Africa (**See Availability of EBOD diagnostics**) (26). This mechanism was subsequently activated for the Zika virus epidemic and COVID-19 pandemic, providing a crucial avenue for assessing and approving quality diagnostics as other regulatory agencies followed suit (**See FIND evaluation of SARS-CoV-2 diagnostics**). The development of "global emergency standards" (27) that harmonise key activities is a crucial next step to rapidly initiate test evaluations, ensure collaboration, and harmonise results to support diagnostic roll-out for outbreaks.

FIND evaluation of SARS-CoV-2 diagnostics

FIND is a global non-profit organisation connecting countries and communities, funders, decision-makers, healthcare providers, and developers to spur diagnostic innovation and make testing an integral part of sustainable, resilient health systems. Throughout the COVID-19 pandemic, there was a large influx of commercial COVID-19 diagnostic tests advertised. To keep track of the changes in the diagnostic landscape, FIND developed a directory of COVID-19 tests (28). As most available performance data were directly from manufacturers, there was a need for independent clinical evaluation data. FIND emitted several calls for Expressions of Interest to identify SARS-CoV-2 diagnostic tests to be included in the evaluation studies. Tests were selected based on supplier-reported analytical and clinical performance, sample type, ease of use, supplier manufacturing and distribution capacity, price, and regulatory status. From March 2020, FIND conducted clinical performance evaluations in collaboration with a network of 20 clinical partner sites throughout the Americas, Europe, Africa, and Asia.

> By early 2021, clinical performance results obtained through retrospective studies of 24 molecular and 51 antibody assays were published on the FIND website (29). By December 2022, 55 prospective evaluation studies were conducted to provide performance data on 36 antigen RDTs. Performance results were highly variable among test types and across evaluation sites. Learning from this experience, FIND and partners intend to continue to develop resources, such as protocol templates and test network sites, that can be rapidly activated and implemented when outbreaks occur.

Another key gap identified during the COVID-19 pandemic that hindered the rollout of diagnostics was access to samples and reference materials for development and evaluation. Well-characterised clinical samples are fundamental to high-quality product evaluation studies. However, accessing samples can be challenging, since these need to be appropriately collected and linked to full clinical and epidemiologic data to fully inform the study analysis. Ethical approval is often required to use such samples, but this may vary depending on the country of ownership and the country of the organisation(s) doing the study. Ownership of samples must be clearly defined before any evaluation, and agreement among the diverse partners involved can sometimes be delicate. It is important to find mechanisms that can ensure ownership of samples to local study sites but also allow conditional access to selected qualified external partners for diagnostic evaluation or development purposes. Indeed, work is ongoing at the regional and international levels to define sample ownership and access through the implementation of virtual biobanks and biobanking networks (30–31), as well as developing and providing reference materials for use for test development and evaluation of key outbreak-prone pathogens (32).

Perhaps most importantly, there must be agreements on the sharing of benefits of the partners contributing to the evaluation, perhaps akin to the Nagoya Protocol on Access and Benefit-sharing which regulates access to genetic resources and the fair and equitable sharing of benefits arising from their utilisation (33). Despite a diagnostic test demonstrating promising performance results, it often remains challenging to ensure continuous availability of the test during and after the outbreak. The market for outbreak-prone diseases is small and unpredictable which discourages commercial test developers from investing sustainably in this field (**See Availability of EBOD diagnostics**). Mechanisms to incentivise and support manufacturers to maintain the availability and affordability of much-needed tests are required, as is creative thinking regarding sustainable economic models. This includes:
- investments in the development and evaluation of novel diagnostic platforms suitable for decentralised settings to aid in the detection of multiple outbreak-prone pathogens
- investments in scaled, regional manufacturing, particularly in low- and middle-income countries, where many infectious disease outbreaks occur
- collaborative efforts to allow for access to biological materials (e.g., antibodies, antigens, and well-characterised samples) to accelerate the development and evaluation of diagnostic tools
- agreements on technology transfer and intellectual property

> **Mpox 2022 outbreak and diagnostics equity**
>
> Mpox is a zoonotic viral disease endemic in parts of Africa. However, from January 2022 through March 2023, over 85,000 cases and 100 deaths were reported in 110 countries, the vast majority being high-income countries outside of the African continent, propagated almost exclusively by human-to-human transmission (34). As the disease started to affect multiple high-income countries, it gained much more attention, spurring research and the rapid development of commercial diagnostics. However, there was limited data on test performance, posing a barrier to implementation.
>
> Molecular testing is the gold standard assay for monkeypox virus detection since it is highly sensitive and specific. However, relying only on molecular testing can be costly and requires a strong healthcare infrastructure, including laboratories with the appropriate equipment and trained staff, which may not be available, especially when cases occur in remote settings. Many lower income countries would greatly benefit from an approach using simpler, cheaper, and more rapid tests (e.g., lateral flow assays) that would allow local testing. However, there is to date little effort in the research and development of rapid testing platforms for mpox, nor evaluation of the products that do exist. To address this gap, FIND is working to evaluate existing rapid tests, collaborating with partners in the U.K., Central African Republic, and Democratic Republic of the Congo.
>
> The increased global attention has had a positive impact on the research and development of diagnostics to curtail the multi-country mpox epidemic. However, as the mpox outbreak wanes in many high-income countries, there is a risk that the global interest in research and development and funding for this disease will wane as well—a reminder that we must continually advocate for equitable access to diagnostics to reach all populations in need (25).

CONCLUSION

The COVID-19 pandemic highlighted the critical need for more rapid responses for emerging and re-emerging disease outbreaks. Although molecular tests such as PCR were rapidly available and granted emergency use authorisation within two months of the WHO declaration of a public health emergency of international concern (**Figure 20.2**), there remained challenges in access to a broader range of rapid, quality diagnostic results worldwide, with RDTs being available only eight months after the declaration.

At the 2021 meeting of the G7 countries hosted by the U.K., an ambitious goal was introduced to improve response to future pandemic threats using lessons learned from COVID-19 and previous epidemics—the 100 Days Mission. The initial response is crucial to changing the course of an outbreak, and ideally, preventing it from becoming a pandemic. The overall aim of the 100 Days Mission is to provide safe, effective, and affordable rapid diagnostics, therapeutics, and vaccines within the first 100 days of the declaration of a major infectious disease event. Whether through the 100 Days Mission or other mechanisms, a concerted shift towards preparedness is required to meet the diagnostic goals of the 100 Days Mission. As disease outbreaks continue to occur throughout the world, it is imperative that researchers, laboratorians, and the global health community can rapidly evaluate diagnostic tools at the onset of their establishment, reducing the chances of deploying poorly performing diagnostics that can impede disease control.

Evaluating and Implementing New Diagnostics

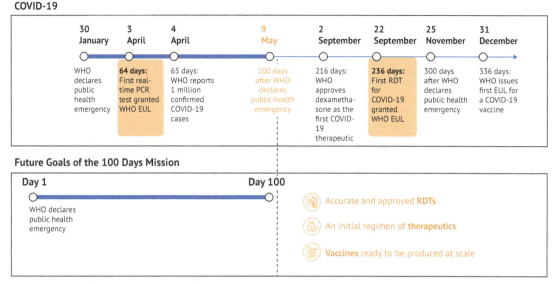

Figure 20.2: Timeline of diagnostic response to COVID-19 and the future goals of the 100 Days Mission

Lastly, as for all matters of health, which is a human right, we must advocate for universal health coverage and global equity in access to diagnostics, as well as other medical countermeasures (**Figure 20.3**). When evaluating and implementing new diagnostic tests for emerging diseases, all countries and populations affected should be considered equally, with their specific needs and local context, so that solutions provided can address the needs of all concerned (**See Mpox 2022 outbreak**).

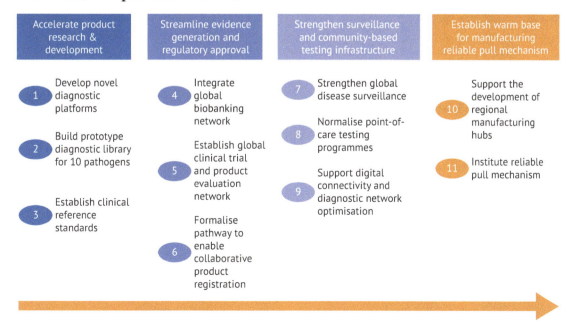

Figure 20.3: Advocacy for evidence-based policy, equitable access, and universal health coverage

REFERENCES:

1. Hoppe A, Vessiere A, Bausch DG. Leveraging COVID-19 diagnostics to confront both epidemic and endemic diseases. In: Evaluating a Pandemic [Internet]. WORLD SCIENTIFIC; 2023. p. 47–66. https://doi.org/10.1142/9789811262821_0004.
2. Cnops L, De Smet B, Mbala-Kingebeni P, van Griensven J, Ahuka-Mundeke S, Ariën KK. Where are the Ebola diagnostics from last time? [Internet]. Nature. 2019 Jan;565(7740):419–21. https://doi.org/10.1038/d41586-019-00212-y PMID:30670861.
3. Umemneku Chikere CM, Wilson K, Graziadio S, Vale L, Allen AJ. Diagnostic test evaluation methodology: a systematic review of methods employed to evaluate diagnostic tests in the absence of gold standard - An update. PLoS One. 2019 Oct;14(10):e0223832. https://doi.org/10.1371/journal.pone.0223832 PMID:31603953.
4. Šimundić AM. Measures of diagnostic accuracy: basic definitions. EJIFCC. 2009 Jan;19(4):203–11. PMID:27683318.
5. Public Health England; UK Standards for Microbiology Investigations. Evaluations, validations and verifications of diagnostic tests [Internet]. https://assets.publishing.service.gov.uk/government/uploads/system/uploads/attachment_data/file/601969/Q_1i5.pdf; 2017.
6. OIE. Principles and methods of validation of diagnostic assays for infectious diseases. In: Manual of Diagnostc Tests for Aquatic Animals. 2019.
7. Banoo S, Bell D, Bossuyt P, Herring A, Mabey D, Poole F, et al.; TDR Diagnostics Evaluation Expert Panel. Evaluation of diagnostic tests for infectious diseases: general principles. Nat Rev Microbiol. 2006 Dec;4(12 Suppl):S20–32. https://doi.org/10.1038/nrmicro1570 PMID:17366684.
8. Halteres SARS-CoV-2 Use Case Tables | Halteres Associates [Internet]. https://halteresassociates.com/halteres-sars-cov-2-use-case-tables/.
9. FIND. SARS-CoV-2 diagnostic use cases [Internet]. https://www.finddx.org/dx-use-cases/.
10. Banatvala J. COVID-19 testing delays and pathology services in the UK. Lancet. 2020 Jun;395(10240):1831. https://doi.org/10.1016/S0140-6736(20)31037-0 PMID:32473100.
11. Hajian-Tilaki K. Sample size estimation in diagnostic test studies of biomedical informatics. J Biomed Inform. 2014 Apr;48:193–204. https://doi.org/10.1016/j.jbi.2014.02.013 PMID:24582925.
12. Vijayananthan A, Nawawi O. The importance of Good Clinical Practice guidelines and its role in clinical trials. Biij. 2008 Jan;4(1):e5. https://doi.org/10.2349/biij.4.1.e5 PMID:21614316.
13. Ezzelle J, Rodriguez-Chavez IR, Darden JM, Stirewalt M, Kunwar N, Hitchcock R, et al. Guidelines on good clinical laboratory practice: bridging operations between research and clinical research laboratories. J Pharm Biomed Anal. 2008 Jan;46(1):18–29. https://doi.org/10.1016/j.jpba.2007.10.010 PMID:18037599.
14. Ellerbrok H, Jacobsen S, Patel P, Rieger T, Eickmann M, Becker S, et al. External quality assessment study for ebolavirus PCR-diagnostic promotes international preparedness during the 2014 - 2016 Ebola outbreak in West Africa. PLoS Negl Trop Dis. 2017 May;11(5):e0005570. https://doi.org/10.1371/journal.pntd.0005570 PMID:28459810.
15. Fox T, Geppert J, Dinnes J, Scandrett K, Bigio J, Sulis G, et al. Antibody tests for identification of current and past infection with SARSCoV2. Cochrane Database of Systematic Reviews. 2022;(11).
16. Bausch D, Hampton L, Perkins M, Saville M. COVID-19: why we can't use antibody tests to show that vaccines are working | Gavi, the Vaccine Alliance [Internet]. https://www.gavi.org/vaccineswork/covid-19-why-we-cant-use-antibody-tests-show-vaccines-are-working; 2021.
17. WHO. Diagnostic testing for SARS-CoV-2 [Internet]. https://www.who.int/publications-detail-redirect/diagnostic-testing-for-sars-cov-2; 2020.
18. Mehand MS, Al-Shorbaji F, Millett P, Murgue B. The WHO R&D Blueprint: 2018 review of emerging infectious diseases requiring urgent research and development efforts. Antiviral Res. 2018 Nov;159:63–7. https://doi.org/10.1016/j.antiviral.2018.09.009 PMID:30261226.
19. FIND. COVID-19 Data Repository [Internet]. https://www.openicpsr.org/openicpsr/covid19.
20. FIND. DxConnect test directories [Internet]. https://www.finddx.org/tools-and-resources/dxconnect/test-directories/.
21. WHO. Good participatory practice guidelines for trials of emerging (and re-emerging) pathogens that are likely to cause severe outbreaks in the near future and for which few or no medical countermeasures exist (GPP-EP) [Internet]. https://www.who.int/publications/m/item/good-participatory-practice-guidelines-for-trials-of-emerging-(and-re-emerging)-pathogens-that-are-likely-to-cause-severe-outbreaks-in-the-near-future-and-for-which-few-or-no-medical-countermeasures-exist-(gpp-ep).

22. Bausch DG, Sprecher AG, Jeffs B, Boumandouki P. Treatment of Marburg and Ebola hemorrhagic fevers: a strategy for testing new drugs and vaccines under outbreak conditions. Antiviral Res. 2008 Apr;78(1):150–61. https://doi.org/10.1016/j.antiviral.2008.01.152 PMID:18336927.
23. Monkeypox Response [Internet]. https://isaric.org/research/monkeypox-response/.
24. PANTHER - Home [Internet]. https://pantherhealth.org/.
25. Adetifa I, Muyembe JJ, Bausch DG, Heymann DL. Mpox neglect and the smallpox niche: a problem for Africa, a problem for the world. The Lancet [Internet]. 2023 May 2; https://www.sciencedirect.com/science/article/pii/S0140673623005883 https://doi.org/10.1016/S0140-6736(23)00588-3.
26. World Health Organization. WHO Emergency Use Assessment and Listing for Ebola Virus Disease IVDs PUBLIC REPORT Product: OraQuick® Ebola Rapid Antigen Test Kit. World Health Organization; Report No.: EA 0023-021-00.
27. Pollock NR, Wonderly B. Evaluating novel diagnostics in an outbreak setting: lessons learned from Ebola. Kraft CS, editor. Journal of Clinical Microbiology. 2017 May;55(5):1255–61.
28. FIND COVID-19 Test directory. https://www.finddx.org/tools-and-resources/dxconnect/test-directories/covid-19-test-directory/.
29. FIND evaluations of SARS-CoV-2 assays. https://www.finddx.org/covid-19/find-evaluations-of-sars-cov-2-assays/.
30. FIND. FIND VBD - Index [Internet]. https://vbd.finddx.org/.
31. Africa CDC. Establishment of a biobanking network as a sustainable mechanism to accelerate development and evaluation of diagnostic tests in Africa. Africa CDC; 2020 Sep.
32. Mattiuzzo G, Bentley EM, Page M. The role of reference materials in the research and development of diagnostic tools and treatments for haemorrhagic fever viruses. Viruses. 2019 Aug;11(9):781. https://doi.org/10.3390/v11090781 PMID:31450611.
33. Convention on Biological Diversity. Nagoya protocol on access to genetic resources and the fair and equitable sharing of benefits arising from their utilization to the convention on biological diversity [Internet]. Montreal: https://www.cbd.int/abs/; 2011.
34. World Health Organization (WHO). 2022-23 Mpox (Monkeypox) Outbreak: Global Trends.2023. https://worldhealthorg.shinyapps.io/mpx_global/.

CHAPTER 21

PATHOGEN GENOMICS FOR SURVEILLANCE AND OUTBREAK INVESTIGATIONS

by Tze-Minn Mak, Marc Stegger, Kåre Mølbak, and Sebastian Maurer-Stroh

Advances in sequencing technology have enabled whole genome sequencing of microorganisms, allowing their rapid identification and characterisation and measure of relatedness to the highest resolution possible. This facilitates the tracking of pathogen evolution and spread, as well as the identification of variants of interest or concern. Pathogen genomics came into the spotlight with the COVID-19 pandemic. The unprecedented, close to real-time collection of SARS-CoV-2 whole genome sequences spurred rapid diagnostic development and informed outbreak response and surveillance strategies. This chapter provides an overview of the technical processes of sequencing and discusses the value and limitations of pathogen genomics in surveillance and outbreak response.

INTRODUCTION: PATHOGEN CHARACTERISATION IN THE ERA OF NEXT-GENERATION SEQUENCING

The characterisation of microorganisms using a variety of methods (**Table 21.1**) has been a cornerstone in outbreak investigations since the early days of modern microbiology (**Figure 21.1**). Of these, sequence-based genotyping methods, which are based on sequencing of one (gene sequencing) or more genomic targets (multi-locus sequence typing), or of whole genomes (whole genome sequencing [WGS]), have the advantage of being highly reproducible. In particular, the discriminatory power of WGS using next-generation sequencing (NGS) technologies has demonstrated utility in surveillance and outbreak investigation (**Figures 21.2 and 21.3**) and is the focus of this chapter. For this reason, WGS has been successfully applied on a wide range of pathogens including respiratory tract pathogens (1) and vaccine preventable diseases (2), vector-borne pathogens (3–4), blood- and sexually-transmitted pathogens (5–7), and nosocomial infections (8–9), as well as zoonotic (10) and food- and waterborne diseases (11–13), with different applications in infection control (**Table 21.2**).

The rapid advancements in NGS and big data are currently introducing profound changes in methods for outbreak investigations, with many phenotyping methods becoming obsolete or recommended only in certain situations. Currently, the shift towards WGS for pathogen characterisation is seen at an unprecedented scale as innovations in sequencing technology have coincided with several prominent outbreaks. At the same time, the promotion and practice of transparent and equitable data sharing has encouraged greater collaboration between public health institutions and academia, resulting in a synergistic cycle of bioinformatics development and further genome sequence data sharing. This is reflected by the number of sequences made available in more recent outbreaks (**Figure 21.1**).

Phenotypic methods

Definition: Methods used to characterise microbes by observable traits
Examples:
- *Morphological characterisation*: Microbial classification based on observable microscopic features or morphology in various culture media.
- *Serotyping*: A way of grouping microbes based on their surface antigens or other molecules using specific antibodies.
- *Biotyping*: The identification of microbes based on their reaction to biochemical tests.
- *Phage typing*: A method of identifying bacterial strains based on their differential susceptibility to bacteriophages.

Genotypic methods

Definition: Methods used to characterise microbes based on genetic variability at one or more specific sites (i.e., loci) in the genome
Examples:
- *Non-sequence-based genotyping methods*: DNA-banding-pattern-based methods that compare the electrophoretic profiles of restriction-enzyme-cut genomes or polymerase chain reaction (PCR)-amplified genes from various strains (e.g., Pulsed Field Gel Electrophoresis [PFGE] and Multiple Locus Variable-number Tandem Repeat Analysis [MLVA] for bacteria).
- *Sequenced-based genotyping methods*: Grouping of strains by *in silico* identification of genetic variability at one (e.g., specific gene sequencing) or more sites (e.g., Multi-Locus-Sequence Typing [MLST] for bacteria) or across the whole genome (WGS).

*Not all methods apply to all kinds of microbes. For example, identifying viruses tends to rely on genotypic methods.

Table 21.1: Overview of methods for microbial characterisation

During the COVID-19 pandemic, the rapid sharing of high-quality genome sequences proved critical for various response measures including confirming a novel coronavirus and developing and evaluating diagnostic tests and vaccines. Further, the democratisation of WGS capabilities to low- and middle-income countries during the pandemic enabled the sharing of more geographically representative sequences, allowing for the identification and risk assessment of viral variants, and providing insights into global genomic epidemiology of SARS-CoV-2 (14). The role of pathogen genomics has since been recognised as a game-changer in pandemic response, with the World Health Organization (WHO) formally convening a 10-year global genomic surveillance strategy for pathogens with pandemic and epidemic potential (15).

SEQUENCING AS A MEASURE OF RELATEDNESS

Sequencing is a laboratory method used to determine the order of nucleotides that make up the genetic content of an organism. By comparing mutations in the genomes of causative pathogens, as well as identifying acquisition and loss of genetic elements, sequencing enables the understanding of genomic plasticity and has been applied for several purposes.

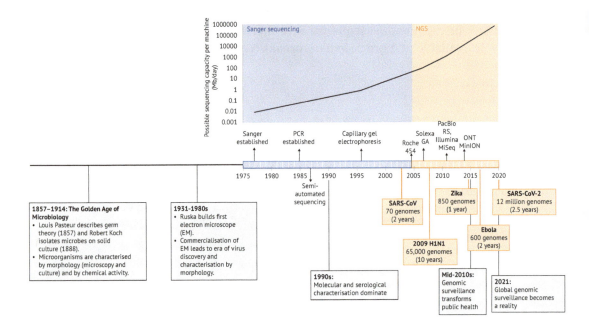

Figure 21.1: Key milestones and trends in pathogen characterisation (grey boxes), with the shift towards WGS coinciding with the introduction of NGS technology

The line graph shows the increase in possible sequencing capacity per machine coinciding with the major developments in sequencing. An exponential rise in sequencing capacity is seen with the launch of key second- (Roche 454, Solexa GA, and Illumina MiSeq) and third-generation sequencers (PacBio RS and Oxford Nanopore Technologies [ONT] MinION). As NGS technology became more widely available and accessible, more whole genome sequences were made publicly accessible from surveillance programmes as well as during the outbreaks of the 21st century, with real-time global genomic surveillance becoming a reality during the COVID-19 pandemic. Approximate total number of species-specific whole genome sequences available on public databases hosted by the National Center for Biotechnology Information (NCBI) and GISAID Data Science Initiative (as of September 2022) is shown in the orange boxes.

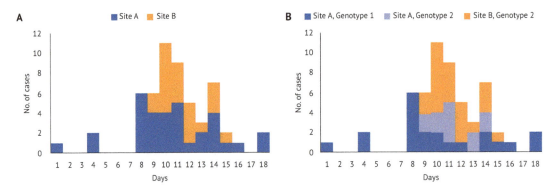

Figure 21.2: WGS improves outbreak reconstruction

(A) An epidemic curve without further pathogen characterisation. From the shape of the curve, it may be inferred that the outbreak was due to a single introduction followed by propagated transmission from Site A to Site B.
(B) The addition of genotyping data shows two genotypes co-circulating in Site A with potential propagated transmission of genotype 2 to Site B.

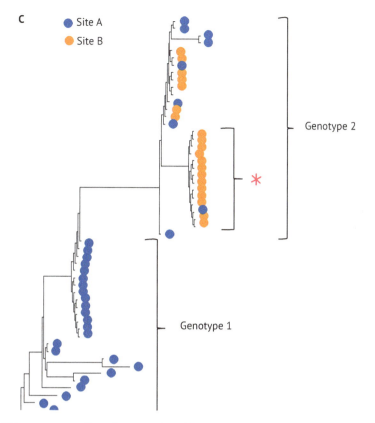

Figure 21.3: WGS improves outbreak reconstruction
(C) Phylogenetic analysis using WGS data provides the highest resolution, where diversity of co-circulating strains is now observed in site A. Introduction from Site A to Site B is likely due to multiple introduction events. Additionally, a single introduction followed by propagated spread in a subset of cases, as indicated by *, is observed and further investigation into this subset of cases may reveal a common exposure.

Pathogen	Utility of genomics and public health outcome
HIV	Relied on the deep sequencing ability of NGS to reconstruct HIV transmission networks, thus directing public health interventions (6).
Yellow fever virus	WGS was used to demonstrate that an outbreak of yellow fever in Brazil was caused by repeated sylvatic spillover events and not urban transmission. Since sylvatic transmission involves different mosquito species, the study informed targeted vector control strategies (4).
Candida auris	WGS of patient and environmental fungal isolates was used to identify contaminated equipment as the source of nosocomial infections (16).
Ebola virus	Used WGS to demonstrate the potential for sexual transmission of Ebola virus from persistently infected asymptomatic individuals. This led to changes in WHO guidelines, with a recommendation made for semen testing (17–18).

Pathogen	Utility of genomics and public health outcome
Lujo virus	Early application of WGS for discovering a novel virus causing an outbreak of haemorrhagic fever. The discovery led to the development of diagnostics for further investigation into the reservoir, geographic distribution, and pathogenicity of Lujo viruses (19).
Salmonella	Demonstrated the ability to infer MLST from WGS data as a replacement to traditional serotyping methods for surveillance of *Salmonella*, leading to more efficient workflows (20).
Escherichia coli	Used WGS in a prospective manner to characterise the novel Shiga toxin-producing entero-aggregative *Escherichia coli* O104:H4 strain during an outbreak. This study demonstrated that virulence factors can be reliably inferred from WGS data and led to the development of specific diagnostics used to confirm fenugreek sprouts as the source. Using comparative genomics, the study also proposed an evolutionary model for the emergence of this hybrid strain (21).
Anthrax	Proof-of-concept example for rapid forensic investigation of biothreat agents using third-generation NGS in a high-containment laboratory setting (22).

Table 21.2: Examples highlighting the utility of WGS in public health

Sequencing has been widely used for outbreak reconstruction, complementing contact tracing efforts. While contact tracing involves interviewing infected individuals to determine the time of disease onset as well as potential sources of exposure and forward transmission **(See Chapter 11, Contact tracing)**, sequencing to track infections does not rely on self-reported behaviour, which is sometimes useful. Since pathogens accumulate mutations as they replicate within a host, pathogen sequences obtained from epidemiologically-related cases are expected to share greater sequence similarity compared to unrelated cases. Mutations can therefore be used as "markers" to infer spatio-temporal transmission events. These inferred relationships (phylogenies) are often visualised as phylogenetic trees **(Figure 21.4)**.

SEQUENCING FOR PHENOTYPIC ASSESSMENT

Other than marker mutations to track relatedness, the identification of phenotypic mutations (i.e., those that confer traits that may increase virulence or pathogenicity) is important for risk assessment and mitigation strategies. Advancements in computational approaches to sequence data and protein structural dynamics allow an understanding of whether mutations have had any effect on viral protein conformation which may lead to changes in their interaction with therapeutic drugs or with host proteins (e.g., increased binding affinity to host receptors or potential immune escape). Combined with metadata (e.g., surveillance data on person, place, and time), emerging phenotypic mutations predicted to be of concern can be prioritised for further experimental validation. Additional clinical metadata such as disease severity, treatment, or vaccination history are also critical for risk assessment of mutations' relevant advantageous phenotypic change **(See Phenotypic inference for risk assessment)**.

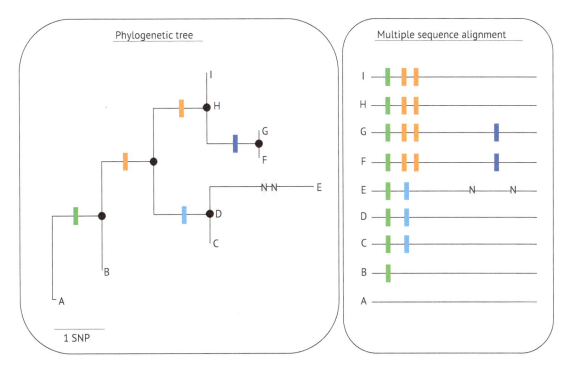

Figure 21.4: Phylogenetic tree
A phylogenetic tree (left) built based on a multiple sequence alignment (right) for sequences A to I. The phylogenetic tree depicts the relationship between sequences based on shared mutations (coloured rectangles). Phylogenetic trees are typically rooted to a known ancestral sequence (in this case, A). Sequences that have been sampled (A to I) form the tips of the tree, whereas the nodes (inlay black circles) are inferred hypothetical common ancestors connecting the tips back to the root. Branches connect the tips to nodes, where branch lengths usually correspond to the number of mutations (i.e., single nucleotide polymorphisms [SNPs]). Mutations shared by more sequences (e.g., in green) occur nearer to the root, while more recently occurring mutations occur closer to the tips, where descendants from a branch share the same mutation. As branch lengths correspond to the number of mutations, missing data from incomplete sequences (e.g., sequence E, with two gaps in sequence denoted as "N") will appear as longer branch lengths.

ENABLING TECHNOLOGIES: SEQUENCING

Prior to 2005, Sanger sequencing was used mainly for gene sequencing. In many instances, gene sequencing provided sufficient accuracy in characterising outbreak clusters, or at least allowed the identification of non-related specimens. However, Sanger is limited to homologous fragments of DNA (typically up to 1000bp) and requires several overlapping PCR reactions to complete larger genes or whole pathogen genomes. The finite amount of clinical specimens constrained the practical application of WGS by Sanger to cases with residual specimens after diagnostic use, smaller pathogens, or those amenable to isolation. WGS by Sanger sequencing was therefore largely confined to the documentation of small numbers of archetypical strains from each outbreak. Sequencing capacity was limited and real-time genomic surveillance was not feasible.

In contrast, second-generation NGS sequencers generate billions of nucleotide sequences during each run, where each genome is sequenced multiple times in small random fragments. There are several NGS technologies available, each differing in chemistries, read length, and accuracy (reviewed elsewhere) (23–24). Despite these differences, the workflows are generally similar (**See NGS sequencing strategies**).

The initial impetus for the adoption of NGS within public health was driven by larger pathogens, such as bacteria, where a plethora of other, often laborious, techniques was needed to identify pathogens, their serotypes, virulence factors, antimicrobial resistance profiles, and genotypes. For example, despite currently having a higher cost per isolate, routine WGS of *Salmonella* was no more expensive than existing typing methods due to the amount of information provided and the potential of added public health benefit (25). WGS provides a single unified test, where resolution of strain discrimination is increased and importantly, information on antimicrobial resistance and virulence factors can be extracted *in silico*.

For viruses, factors including the increased usage of antivirals targeting multiple genes necessitated the surveillance of more viral genes and NGS became a practical choice. Further, the promise of increased resolution for transmission investigation and the need to evaluate whole genomes for pandemic risk assessment of zoonotic viruses or to evaluate recombination events (26) collectively propelled the transition towards NGS.

Long-read third-generation NGS further increased the capability to complete genomes that were difficult to resolve by short-read sequencers such as those with areas of multiple sequence repeats. The pocket-sized long-read MinION sequencer has also enabled sequencing to reach remote sites and was important during the Ebola virus disease (27) and Zika (28) outbreaks. This development was also driven by its low initial setup costs that are diminishing compared to the more established second- and even other third-generation NGS machinery. Controlled and powered through a laptop, this technology has the potential for scalability in mobile laboratories (**See Chapter 19, Laboratory capacity**), and is now a standard piece of equipment in many rapid response mobile laboratories (RRMLs) alongside molecular and serological testing capabilities.

NGS sequencing strategies

As shown in **Figure 21.5**, each sequencing run comprises two key components: laboratory procedures and computational sequence analyses.

Several sequencing strategies have been designed and can be used across sequencing platforms. The most direct approach is simply loading total extracted nucleic acid into the sequencer and then computationally determining which microbes are present and at what proportions. This method is referred to as metagenomics or shotgun sequencing and is a powerful, unbiased approach to identify all microbes according to taxonomic assignment. The ability to perform metagenomics directly on clinical specimens makes it particularly useful for novel pathogens which are not detected by regular diagnostic workflows, or for pathogens that are not easily cultivable in a laboratory setting. However, causative pathogens may be present in low volumes, and the overwhelming presence of genetic material from host and commensal microorganisms in clinical samples sequesters much of the sequencing capacity away from the intended target. In such runs, host and commensal reads typically constitute >99 per cent of reads. As a result, the multiplexing potential (i.e., the number of samples included per sequence run) is often compromised to increase the detection and coverage of the causative pathogen. Nevertheless, whole genome pathogen coverage is not guaranteed and has been described as a "needle-in-a-haystack" endeavour.

Several approaches have been developed to enrich for pathogen sequences prior to sequencing (29–31). For example, if the causative pathogen is already known, whole genome tiled amplification may be performed prior to sequencing (27,32). This strategy is highly reproducible and has been the main enabler behind most of the SARS-CoV-2 genomes collected to date. An advantage of this method is that genome coverage remains high even if novel variants emerge and can be quickly modified to improve areas of drop-off due to individual primer mismatches (33). This strategy greatly increases sensitivity, enabling whole genomes to be retrieved from samples with low viral loads.

For bacteria, WGS is usually performed on isolates from traditional cultures. However, the increasing use of culture-independent diagnostics tests (CIDTs) in clinical laboratories is a challenge for this approach. CIDTs, including PCR-based methods, offer fast test results. However, an isolate for WGS will only be available if the laboratory undertakes a culture of the material that was positive by the CIDT, and this requires commitment and resources. Further technological development may resolve this issue.

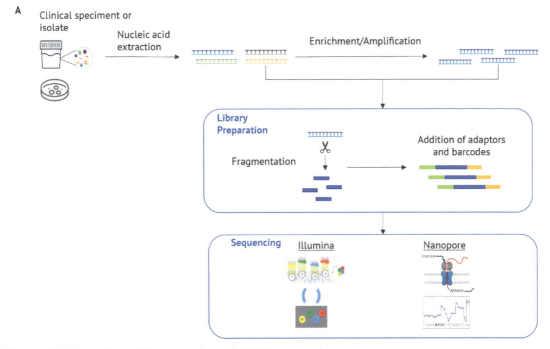

Figure 21.5: Overview of key steps in each WGS sequencing run

Overview of key steps in each WGS sequencing run, which consists of (A) laboratory procedures and (B) computational steps (below). (A) Once nucleic acid is extracted from a clinical specimen or isolate, it can be either used directly (metagenomics) or enriched for a particular target using PCR or baiting approaches. For second-generation sequencing, DNA is first mechanically or enzymatically fragmented to smaller fragments, followed by the addition of adaptors to the terminal ends of each fragment. This allows the DNA to bind to sequencing flow cells, where actual sequencing reactions take place (illustrated example: Illumina). As several samples can be sequenced in parallel, unique molecular barcodes are also added to the ends of each DNA fragment to allow them to be computationally differentiated from one another at the end of the sequencing reaction. For third-generation long-read sequencing, adaptor and barcodes are added directly to the terminal ends of template DNA prior to the sequencing reaction, without fragmentation (illustrated example: Nanopore). Eventually, captured sequencing signals are converted into raw sequencing reads.

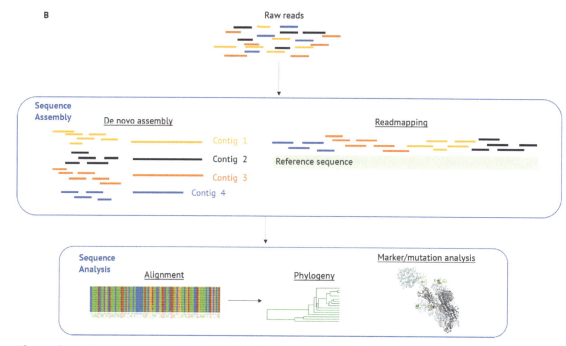

Figure 21.6: Key computational steps in each WGS sequencing run
Raw sequencing reads from the NGS machines are computationally converted into final sequences by one or two sequence assembly methods. In de novo assembly, sequencing reads are pieced together based on their overlapping terminal ends, while read mapping involves aligning raw reads to a known reference sequence. The assembled sequence is a consensus sequence of all aligned reads and represents the most frequently occurring nucleotide at each position. This sequence can be compared to other sequences to study evolutionary relationships and to identify the presence of mutations compared to known reference sequences. Further structural modelling may be performed to visualise the effects of these mutations in a three-dimensional protein structure.

GENOMIC EPIDEMIOLOGY FOR SURVEILLANCE AND OUTBREAK INVESTIGATION

A common goal for prospective genomic surveillance is the early identification of outbreaks. With the improved resolution at which clusters can be delineated from one another with WGS data, public health practitioners can distinguish new introduction events from prolonged endemic transmission and work out how each contributes to disease incidence in various settings. When integrated with syndromic surveillance, sequencing can also enable the detection of novel pathogens serving either to confirm an outbreak or to provide initial evidence that an outbreak is underway.

Once an outbreak is putatively identified, intense sampling of cases and suspected sources is necessary to provide confidence in analysis. Where possible, it is also necessary to include a representative reference set both to support and refute hypotheses. Importantly, findings must be backed by sound epidemiologic information. While rapid communication is useful, scientific rigour cannot be compromised and in emergency situations, coordinated scientific communication translates more effectively to response by relevant authorities rather than limited piecemeal studies.

Genomics for real-time surveillance for foodborne pathogens

National molecular surveillance networks, such as PulseNet in the U.S., have been very effective in the early detection of foodborne outbreaks. Using PFGE (**Table 21.1**), it was estimated that PulseNet prevents an estimated 270,000 cases of foodborne bacterial illnesses annually. With the promise of greater discriminatory power, PulseNet began its transition towards adopting WGS in 2013. Early adoption of WGS on listeria surveillance proved promising, with a >30 per cent increase in outbreak detection and a fourfold increase in linking cases to a food source (34). This expanded ability to detect and resolve outbreaks was also observed for other common foodborne pathogens such as *Salmonella* and *Escherichia coli*, where WGS uncovered more cases and potential food sources compared to genotyping methods (12–13).

2010 Haiti cholera outbreak: lessons from the early application of genomics for outbreak investigations

In October 2010, nine months after a catastrophic earthquake caused widespread damage to infrastructure and sanitation systems, an outbreak of cholera erupted in Haiti resulting in significant mortality. As Haiti had not reported cholera for decades, speculation that cholera was introduced by the United Nations (UN) staff deployed from cholera-endemic countries led to riots which disrupted relief efforts.

Initial PFGE patterns of the Haiti outbreak strains already supported a single foreign source followed by propagated spread (35). Three early comparative genomic studies supported this conclusion; however, when considered individually, source attribution was disputed as the investigations included relatively small numbers of isolates and lacked full representation of contemporaneous circulating references from all cholera-endemic regions. Crucially, one of the studies compellingly pinpointed Nepal as a source but lacked other geographic references (36). The other two had included a limited number of geographically diverse references and included similarities to South Asian strains (37–38). In recognising the limitations of available references, one of the studies rightfully called for large-scale studies of both outbreak cases and circulating references (38).

Nevertheless, the collective lines of evidence corroborated with epidemiological findings including unsanitary conditions at the UN camp, the coincidence of the outbreak with the arrival of the troops from Nepal, and spatio-temporal emergence of early outbreak clusters (39), ultimately leading to the UN's acknowledgement of its role in the epidemic (40).

Similarly, the ability of phylogenetics to uncover possible zoonotic sources relies on the available reference sequences from suspected animal reservoirs, food sources, or the environment, underscoring again the importance of One Health surveillance (10,41).

If the disease is widespread in the community, phylogenetics is also useful in institutional settings, allowing public health officials to discern between propagated transmission and multiple sources from the community. Infection control measures can be tailored to the transmission dynamics (42–46).

When propagated transmission is sustained in the community, the ability to distinguish transmission networks facilitates the identification of pathogen or human factors associated with larger clusters, providing an opportunity to mitigate (6–7,47). In the case of chronic infectious diseases such as tuberculosis, the high rates of asymptomatic or undiagnosed cases and long incubation periods obscure transmission links by epidemiology alone. The integration of genomics has improved the ability to demarcate transmission clusters and identify possible "superspreaders" to be prioritised for contact tracing. The ability of WGS to distinguish between the relapse of latent infection or reinfection may be used to evaluate past therapeutic interventions (47–48). Another example is the within-host variation observed with long-term infection with *Pseudomonas* in cystic fibrosis patients or the carriage diversity in *Staphylococcus aureus* that limits the potential identification of patient-to-patient transmissions (49–50).

When genomic surveillance is applied to international travellers, the capacity to characterise viruses is extended globally. Such efforts may identify outbreaks in countries where there had been little detection, though the politics of how to act on such knowledge is complex. For example, the diagnostic testing of travel-associated cases uncovered a hidden Zika outbreak in Cuba, and the application of genomic sequencing uncovered insights into the timing, sources of introduction, and delayed establishment of Zika virus in Cuba, thereby providing an explanation for the outbreak occurring a year after the main Zika outbreaks in neighbouring islands (51). Sequencing of travel-associated mpox cases prior to the current 2022 global outbreak provided the phylogenetic link to more ancestral zoonotic strains (52–53). Metagenomics has also been successfully applied to travel surveillance by investigating human waste storage tanks from international flights to depict the circulation and influx of antimicrobial resistance genes and other human pathogens from different world regions (54). The full potential of genomic travel surveillance was not realised during the COVID-19 pandemic, despite both high- and low-income countries massively sequencing imported cases and making them publicly available. Among the reasons could be a fear of travel bans, and a lack of prior frameworks for appropriate metadata tracking (including sampling strategy) or tagging onto genomes. Travel sequencing is useful for understanding the disease in a broader sense, but the time lags involved means it often provides little immediate practical help in deciding on travel-related public health measures.

While sequencing provides a measure of relatedness, several factors can affect the accuracy of epidemiological inferences. Firstly, inference is intrinsically dependent on the pathogen mutation rate and can be dramatically affected by genetic recombination. For example, when a novel pathogen from a single source first emerges into a population and has not yet diverged sufficiently, sequencing will not help. In this scenario, all samples appear clonal and point to a continuous common source, and contact tracing remains the only way to resolve such cases.

Secondly, the consensus sequence represents the most frequently occurring nucleotide at each position of the genome at the time of sample collection and is a snapshot summary of pathogen diversity. It does not fully reflect the extent and dynamics of intra-host diversity nor the diversity that is transferred during the point of transmission to the next susceptible host. This means that while related cases are expected to have similar sequences, identical sequences do not automatically indicate that cases form part of the same transmission chain.

Likewise, linked cases may differ by small numbers of nucleotides due to the selection of a subset of intra-host diversity at the point of sampling.

Thirdly, sampling strategy is crucial for accurate analysis. When sampling is opportunistic rather than probabilistic, uncertainty and biases can affect the accuracy of epidemiological estimates (55).

These uncertainties underscore the importance of integrating phylogenetic interpretation with all available epidemiological data and careful communication of findings and limitations (56).

Performing WGS on a discrete dataset (e.g., from a single outbreak) does not pose the same challenges as implementing WGS as a routine microbiology service for public health surveillance. Challenges include translating WGS results into a useable format for laboratory reporting, clinical case management, and outbreak investigation, as well as meeting the requirement to communicate that information in an understandable and universal language for clinical and public health action (57).

PHENOTYPIC INFERENCE FOR RISK ASSESSMENT

The ability of WGS to define pathogens beyond the species and subtype level down to the identification of phenotypic mutations enables more granular attribution of risk and burden of disease. Prior to the COVID-19 pandemic, genomic surveillance of antimicrobial resistance and of several vaccine preventable diseases was already ongoing for the purpose of identifying the burden of circulating phenotypic mutations to evaluate existing intervention strategies.

For example, national influenza centres (NICs) across the globe collect a subset of influenza isolates and submit them to designated collaborating centres (WHO CCs) for antigenic characterisation as part of the biannual vaccine composition review process. Many countries have begun adopting a "WGS-first" screening approach to make more comprehensive and informed decisions on sample selection for virus isolation and submission, ensuring more accurate representation of circulating diversity and the inclusion of strain samples with potentially phenotypic mutations (e.g., from severely ill or recently vaccinated individuals). Additionally, strains with mutations that result in changes in glycosylation patterns at the receptor binding domain could lead to immune escape and should be submitted for further evaluation in the vaccine review process.

In addition to seasonal influenza, pandemic influenza remains a perennial threat, with numerous cases of human infection of avian influenza reported yearly. With few instances of suspected human-to-human transmissions (58–59), these spillover events were largely due to direct or close contact with infected poultry. However, studies demonstrated that only five mutations in an avian influenza H5N1 isolate, or four in an experimental recombinant, might be sufficient for transmission between mammals (60–61). These mutations have also been individually detected in naturally occurring avian and human H5 influenza viruses (62), raising concerns that progressive adaptation enabling human infection can occur, prompting the proposed use of genetic sequences for relative pandemic risk assignment to prioritise prevention or response measures (63).

To differentiate phenotypic mutations from marker mutations, the inspection of several different factors is required. These include structural location, potential alterations in receptor, antibody, or drug binding affinity, effect on protein stability or virus replication, and co-occurrence with other mutations, as well as frequency and distribution of occurrence.

Online tools that compare query sequences with references and highlight phenotypically or epidemiologically candidate mutations are particularly useful for such analysis. For example, GISAID offers the accompaniment tools such as FluSurver and CoVsurver for influenza and SARS-CoV-2, respectively. In addition to identifying candidate mutations, these tools evaluate the geographical and temporal distribution of each listed mutation, provide 3D structural mapping, and link to available literature. The tools have been successfully used to identify more appropriate candidates for further experimental evaluation (64–66).

For bacterial surveillance, phenotypic mutations leading to host- and environment-adaptation, virulence, and drug-resistance are often located on mobile genetic elements which comprise part of the accessory genome that in many cases, defines the pathogenicity or success of the pathogens. This aspect of detecting signatures of genomic variation is a key part of surveillance but is most often organism specific.

RAPID SHARING OF GENOMIC DATA

As exemplified during the COVID-19 pandemic, timely sharing of genomic data by as many countries as possible is critical for accurate geographical and temporal representation of disease epidemiology. Such information has enabled policymakers to identify which variants are present or emerging, where they circulate, assess if they present a greater risk, and define which groups are most susceptible to these risks (14).

While numerous repositories containing genomic data exist (**Table 21.3**), a shift towards the ability to integrate complex datasets, incorporating One Health and clinical and epidemiological data, is important to answer the above questions. The rapid inclusion of such information with genomic data will help frame observations such as the emergence of new variants or antimicrobial resistance profiles.

Further, ethical issues such as data governance and security, and ensuring the privacy and non-exploitation of marginalised or indigenous populations, must be addressed while navigating issues relating to trust and geopolitical sensitivities. If good stewardship requires safeguarding data, how can public health agencies and data sharing platforms strike a balance between protecting data owners without hampering research progress (67)? As mentioned in the WHO's guiding principles, the sharing of genomic data should be "as open as possible and as closed as necessary", with the decision on whether to share based on the data generator's wish to retain their ownership rights (68). Publicly accessible platforms may allow anonymity, while others require verified user access.

Much success in the rapid COVID-19 genomics response has been attributed to GISAID that has become the main source of SARS-CoV-2 genomic and related metadata (69–70). GISAID's ability to respond to real-time genomic surveillance stemmed from pre-existing collaborations with global public health laboratories through a longstanding partnership within the WHO's Global Influenza Surveillance and Response System (GISRS) (14,71). While GISAID data is free to use and is publicly available, it requires user identification and protects the ownership rights of sequence contributors by ensuring all users abide by the same conditions on the use of data, requiring acknowledgement for example, in publications.

In addition to its unique data governance, GISAID continually responded to the needs of its users throughout the pandemic by providing options for high-throughput data submissions, maintaining high quality data standards through sequence review and annotation performed by a global curation team, as well as providing tools and data packages to empower equitable data utilisation by all registered users. GISAID's model is thus well positioned to serve as a blueprint for other priority pathogens.

Name	Website	Description
International Nucleotide Sequence Database Collaboration	• NCBI Genbank https://www.ncbi.nlm.nih.gov/genbank/ • DNA DataBank of Japan (DDBJ) https://www.ddbj.nig.ac.jp/index-e.html • European Nucleotide Archive (ENA) www.ebi.ac.uk/ena/browser/home	General genetic sequence database comprising public domain sequences (anonymously usable with no acknowledgment required). Incomplete coverage of priority pathogens compared to GISAID.
Bacterial and Viral Bioinformatics Resource Center	https://www.bv-brc.org	Information system integrating tools based on the above public domain genetic sequences and features of bacteria, archea, and virus families containing human pathogens.
GISAID	https://gisaid.org	Real-time pathogen surveillance data science platform governed by data access agreement (free public access with user credentials). Hosts genomic and related metadata of priority pathogens (currently influenza, SARS-CoV-2, monkeypox, arboviruses, and respiratory syncytial virus [RSV]) and provides tools for analysis.
EnteroBase	https://enterobase.warwick.ac.uk	Database for analysing and visualising genomic variation within enteric bacteria.

Table 21.3: Examples of genome sequence repositories

CONCLUSION

COVID-19 has led to significant investments to increase raw sequencing capability and capacity worldwide, with several initiatives providing training and bioinformatics support. Efforts must now shift towards sustaining capacity and improving capabilities in low- and middle-income countries for improved preparedness (14), including the development and regulation of quality assurance (72–75). Sequencing capacities and assets need to become 'pathogen agnostic' (as opposed to remaining in vertical disease-specific programmes) and be integrated into collaborative (genomic) surveillance systems so that they are sustained at a suitable level between outbreaks/pandemics and can pivot easily to new pathogens as they emerge.

As surveillance needs constantly evolve according to the changing circumstances of public health events, the objective of genomic surveillance should be scalable according to phases of preparedness, response, and recovery (15). This includes the need to define the optimal degree of sampling, which may be achieved by modelling various datasets from many parts of the world.

Additionally, dialogue between multiple stakeholders is necessary to ensure appropriate use, balancing between maximising public health benefit while ensuring sustainability. Critically, the push towards genomic surveillance should focus on complementing existing surveillance outcomes and should not draw resources away from other essential functions (15).

The realisation of real-time genomics during COVID-19 was a success story of a globally concerted push towards more equitable access to novel health technology and the timely sharing of data based on trust. This achievement has led to a unified recognition of the role of pathogen genomics for public health purposes, providing an impetus for continued collaboration and the broader application of genomics to address public health needs.

REFERENCES:

1. Ghedin E, Sengamalay NA, Shumway M, Zaborsky J, Feldblyum T, Subbu V, et al. Large-scale sequencing of human influenza reveals the dynamic nature of viral genome evolution. Nature [Internet]. 2005 Oct;437(7062):1162–6. https://doi.org/10.1038/nature04239 PMID:16208317.
2. Martin J, Burns CC, Jorba J, Shulman LM, Macadam A, Klapsa D, et al. Genetic characterization of novel oral polio vaccine type 2 viruses during initial use phase under emergency use listing — Worldwide, March–October 2021. MMWR Morb Mortal Wkly Rep [Internet]. 2022 Jun 17;71(24):786–90. https://doi.org/10.15585/mmwr.mm7124a2 PMID:35709073.
3. Sun H, Binder RA, Dickens B, de Sessions PF, Rabaa MA, Ho EXP, et al. Viral genome-based Zika virus transmission dynamics in a paediatric cohort during the 2016 Nicaragua epidemic. eBioMedicine [Internet]. 2021 Oct;72:103596. https://doi.org/10.1016/j.ebiom.2021.103596 PMID:34627081.
4. Faria NR, Kraemer MUG, Hill SC, Goes de Jesus J, Aguiar RS, Iani FCM, et al. Genomic and epidemiological monitoring of yellow fever virus transmission potential. Science [Internet]. 2018 Aug 31;361(6405):894–9. https://doi.org/10.1126/science.aat7115 PMID:30139911.
5. Osnes MN, Didelot X, Korne-Elenbaas J de, Alfsnes K, Brynildsrud OB, Syversen G, et al. Sudden emergence of a Neisseria gonorrhoeae clade with reduced susceptibility to extended-spectrum cephalosporins, Norway. Microbial Genomics [Internet]. 2020 Dec 1;6(12). https://doi.org/10.1099/mgen.0.000480 PMID:33200978.
6. Ratmann O, Grabowski MK, Hall M, Golubchik T, Wymant C, Abeler-Dörner L, et al. Inferring HIV-1 transmission networks and sources of epidemic spread in Africa with deep-sequence phylogenetic analysis. Nat Commun [Internet]. 2019 Mar 29;10(1). https://doi.org/10.1038/s41467-019-09139-4 PMID:30926780.
7. Gibson KM, Jair K, Castel AD, Bendall ML, Wilbourn B, Jordan JA, et al. A cross-sectional study to characterize local HIV-1 dynamics in Washington, DC using next-generation sequencing. Sci Rep [Internet]. 2020 Feb 6;10(1). http://dx.doi.org/10.1038/s41598-020-58410-y PMID: 32029767.
8. Sherry NL, Lane CR, Kwong JC, Schultz M, Sait M, Stevens K, et al. Genomics for molecular epidemiology and detecting transmission of carbapenemase-producing *Enterobacterales* in Victoria, Australia, 2012 to 2016. Diekema DJ, editor. J Clin Microbiol [Internet]. 2019 Sep;57(9). https://doi.org/10.1128/JCM.00573-19 PMID: 31315956.
9. Zhu Y, Zembower TR, Metzger KE, Lei Z, Green SJ, Qi C. Investigation of respiratory syncytial virus outbreak on an adult stem cell transplant unit by use of whole-genome sequencing. Diekema DJ, editor. J Clin Microbiol [Internet]. 2017 Oct;55(10):2956–63. https://doi.org/10.1128/JCM.00360-17. PMID: 28747373.
10. Kafetzopoulou LE, Pullan ST, Lemey P, Suchard MA, Ehichioya DU, Pahlmann M, et al. Metagenomic sequencing at the epicenter of the Nigeria 2018 Lassa fever outbreak. Science [Internet]. 2019 Jan 4;363(6422):74–7. https://doi.org/10.1126/science.aau9343 PMID: 30606844.
11. Zhang Z, Liu D, Li S, Zhang Z, Hou J, Wang D, et al. Imported human norovirus in travelers, Shanghai port, China 2018: an epidemiological and whole genome sequencing study. Travel Medicine and Infectious Disease [Internet]. 2021 Sep;43:102140. https://doi.org/10.1016/j.tmaid.2021.102140 PMID: 34271206.
12. Sarno E, Pezzutto D, Rossi M, Liebana E, Rizzi V. A review of significant European foodborne outbreaks in the last decade. Journal of Food Protection [Internet]. 2021 Dec;84(12):2059–70. https://doi.org/10.4315/JFP-21-096 PMID: 34197583.

13. Stevens EL, Carleton HA, Beal J, Tillman GE, Lindsey RL, Lauer AC, et al. Use of whole genome sequencing by the federal interagency collaboration for genomics for food and feed safety in the United States. Journal of Food Protection [Internet]. 2022 May;85(5):755–72. https://doi.org/10.4315/JFP-21-437 PMID: 35259246.

14. Brito AF, Semenova E, Dudas G, Hassler GW, Kalinich CC, Kraemer MUG, et al. Global disparities in SARS-CoV-2 genomic surveillance. Nat Commun [Internet]. 2022 Nov 16;13(1). https://doi.org/10.1038/s41467-022-33713-y PMID: 36385137.

15. Carter L, Yu MA, Sacks J, Barnadas C, Pereyaslov D, Cognat S, et al. Global genomic surveillance strategy for pathogens with pandemic and epidemic potential 2022–2032. Bull World Health Organ [Internet]. 2022 Apr 1;100(04):239–239A. https://doi.org/10.2471/BLT.22.288220 PMID: 35386562.

16. Eyre DW, Sheppard AE, Madder H, Moir I, Moroney R, Quan TP, et al. A *Candida auris* outbreak and its control in an intensive care setting. N Engl J Med [Internet]. 2018 Oct 4;379(14):1322–31. https://doi.org/10.1056/NEJMoa1714373 PMID: 30281988.

17. Mate SE, Kugelman JR, Nyenswah TG, Ladner JT, Wiley MR, Cordier-Lassalle T, et al. Molecular evidence of sexual transmission of Ebola virus. N Engl J Med [Internet]. 2015 Dec 17;373(25):2448–54. https://doi.org/10.1056/NEJMoa1509773 PMID: 26465384.

18. Butler D. What first case of sexually transmitted Ebola means for public health. Nature [Internet]. 2015 Oct 16. https://doi.org/10.1038/nature.2015.18584.

19. Briese T, Paweska JT, McMullan LK, Hutchison SK, Street C, Palacios G, et al. Genetic detection and characterization of Lujo virus, a new hemorrhagic fever–associated arenavirus from Southern Africa. Buchmeier MJ, editor. PLoS Pathog [Internet]. 2009 May 29;5(5):e1000455. https://doi.org/10.1371/journal.ppat.1000455 PMID: 19478873.

20. Ashton PM, Nair S, Peters TM, Bale JA, Powell DG, Painset A, et al. Identification of *Salmonella* for public health surveillance using whole genome sequencing. PeerJ [Internet]. 2016 Apr 5;4:e1752. https://doi.org/10.7717/peerj.1752 PMID: 27069781.

21. Mellmann A, Harmsen D, Cummings CA, Zentz EB, Leopold SR, Rico A, et al. Prospective genomic characterization of the German enterohemorrhagic Escherichia coli O104:H4 outbreak by rapid next generation sequencing technology. Ahmed N, editor. PLoS ONE [Internet]. 2011 Jul 20;6(7):e22751. https://doi.org/10.1371/journal.pone.0022751 PMID: 21799941.

22. McLaughlin HP, Bugrysheva JV, Conley AB, Gulvik CA, Cherney B, Kolton CB, et al. Rapid nanopore whole-genome sequencing for anthrax emergency preparedness. Emerg Infect Dis [Internet]. 2020 Feb;26(2):358–61. https://doi.org/10.3201/eid2602.191351 PMID: 31961318.

23. Morey M, Fernández-Marmiesse A, Castiñeiras D, Fraga JM, Couce ML, Cocho JA. A glimpse into past, present, and future DNA sequencing. Molecular Genetics and Metabolism [Internet]. 2013 Sep;110(1-2):3–24. https://doi.org/10.1016/j.ymgme.2013.04.024 PMID: 23742747.

24. Hu T, Chitnis N, Monos D, Dinh A. Next-generation sequencing technologies: an overview. Human Immunology [Internet]. 2021 Nov;82(11):801–11. https://doi.org/10.1016/j.humimm.2021.02.012 PMID: 33745759.

25. Ford L, Glass K, Williamson DA, Sintchenko V, Robson JMB, Lancsar E, et al. Cost of whole genome sequencing for non-typhoidal Salmonella enterica. Mossong J, editor. PLoS ONE [Internet]. 2021 Mar 19;16(3):e0248561. https://doi.org/10.1371/journal.pone.0248561 PMID: 33739986.

26. Stelzl E, Haas B, Bauer B, Zhang S, Fiss EH, Hillman G, et al. First identification of a recombinant form of hepatitis C virus in Austrian patients by full-genome next generation sequencing. Wedemeyer H, editor. PLoS ONE [Internet]. 2017 Jul 25;12(7):e0181273. https://doi.org/10.1371/journal.pone.0181273 PMID: 28742818.

27. Quick J, Loman NJ, Duraffour S, Simpson JT, Severi E, Cowley L, et al. Real-time, portable genome sequencing for Ebola surveillance. Nature [Internet]. 2016 Feb;530(7589):228–32. https://doi.org/10.1038/nature16996 PMID: 26840485.

28. de Jesus JG, Giovanetti M, Rodrigues Faria N, Alcantara LCJ. Acute vector-borne viral infection: Zika and MinION surveillance. Riley LW, Blanton RE, editors. Microbiol Spectr [Internet]. 2019 Jul 19;7(4). https://doi.org/10.1128/microbiolspec.AME-0008-2019 PMID: 31400093.

29. Bowden KE, Joseph SJ, Cartee JC, Ziklo N, Danavall D, Raphael BH, et al. Whole-genome enrichment and sequencing of Chlamydia trachomatis directly from patient clinical vaginal and rectal swabs. Rasmussen AL, editor. mSphere [Internet]. 2021 Apr 28;6(2). https://doi.org/10.1128/mSphere.01302-20 PMID: 33658279.

30. Singanallur NB, Anderson DE, Sessions OM, Kamaraj US, Bowden TR, Horsington J, et al. Probe capture enrichment next-generation sequencing of complete foot-and-mouth disease virus genomes in clinical samples.

Journal of Virological Methods [Internet]. 2019 Oct;272:113703. https://doi.org/10.1016/j.jviromet.2019.113703 PMID: 31336142.

31. Munyuza C, Ji H, Lee ER. Probe capture enrichment methods for HIV and HCV genome sequencing and drug resistance genotyping. Pathogens [Internet]. 2022 Jun 16;11(6):693. https://doi.org/10.3390/pathogens11060693 PMID: 35745547.

32. Quick J, Grubaugh ND, Pullan ST, Claro IM, Smith AD, Gangavarapu K, et al. Multiplex PCR method for MinION and Illumina sequencing of Zika and other virus genomes directly from clinical samples. Nat Protoc [Internet]. 2017 May 24;12(6):1261–76. https://doi.org/10.1038/nprot.2017.066 PMID: 28538739.

33. Lambisia AW, Mohammed KS, Makori TO, Ndwiga L, Mburu MW, Morobe JM, et al. Optimization of the SARS-CoV-2 ARTIC network V4 primers and whole genome sequencing protocol. Front Med [Internet]. 2022 Feb 17;9. https://doi.org/10.3389/fmed.2022.836728 PMID: 35252269.

34. Ribot EM, Freeman M, Hise KB, Gerner-Smidt P. PulseNet: entering the age of next-generation sequencing. Foodborne Pathogens and Disease [Internet]. 2019 Jul;16(7):451–6. https://doi.org/10.1089/fpd.2019.2634 PMID: 31241352.

35. Centers for Disease Control and Prevention (CDC). Update: cholera outbreak --- Haiti, 2010. MMWR Morb Mortal Wkly Rep. 2010 Nov;59(45):1473–9.

36. Hendriksen RS, Price LB, Schupp JM, Gillece JD, Kaas RS, Engelthaler DM, et al. Population genetics of Vibrio cholerae from Nepal in 2010: evidence on the origin of the Haitian outbreak. Relman D, editor. mBio [Internet]. 2011 Sep;2(4). https://doi.org/10.1128/mBio.00157-11 PMID: 21862630.

37. Chin CS, Sorenson J, Harris JB, Robins WP, Charles RC, Jean-Charles RR, et al. The origin of the Haitian cholera outbreak strain. N Engl J Med [Internet]. 2011 Jan 6;364(1):33–42. https://doi.org/10.1056/NEJMoa1012928 PMID: 21142692.

38. Reimer A, Domselaar G, Stroika S, Walker M, Kent H, Tarr C, et al. Comparative genomics of Vibrio cholerae from Haiti, Asia, and Africa. Emerg Infect Dis [Internet]. 2011 Nov;17(11). https://doi.org/10.3201/eid1711.110794 PMID: 22099115.

39. Frerichs RR, Keim PS, Barrais R, Piarroux R. Nepalese origin of cholera epidemic in Haiti. Clinical Microbiology and Infection [Internet]. 2012 Jun;18(6):E158–63. https://doi.org/10.1111/j.1469-0691.2012.03841.x PMID: 22510219.

40. Gibbons N, Pham P, Vinck P. The United Nations material assistance to survivors of cholera in Haiti: consulting survivors and rebuilding trust. PLoS Curr [Internet]. 2017. https://doi.org/10.1371/currents.dis.1b01af244fe3d76d6a7013e2f1e3944d PMID: 29188126.

41. Andersen KG, Rambaut A, Lipkin WI, Holmes EC, Garry RF. The proximal origin of SARS-CoV-2. Nat Med [Internet]. 2020 Mar 17;26(4):450–2. https://doi.org/10.1038/s41591-020-0820-9 PMID: 32284615.

42. Borges V, Isidro J, Macedo F, Neves J, Silva L, Paiva M, et al. Nosocomial outbreak of SARS-CoV-2 in a "Non-COVID-19" hospital ward: virus genome sequencing as a key tool to understand cryptic transmission. Viruses [Internet]. 2021 Apr 1;13(4):604. https://doi.org/10.3390/v13040604 PMID: 33916205.

43. Valley-Omar Z, Nindo F, Mudau M, Hsiao M, Martin DP. Phylogenetic exploration of nosocomial transmission chains of 2009 Influenza A/H1N1 among children admitted at Red Cross War Memorial Children's Hospital, Cape Town, South Africa in 2011. Khudyakov YE, editor. PLoS ONE [Internet]. 2015 Nov 13;10(11):e0141744. https://doi.org/10.1371/journal.pone.0141744 PMID: 26565994.

44. Lim W-Y, Tan GSE, Htun HL, Phua HP, Kyaw WM, Guo H, et al. First nosocomial cluster of COVID-19 due to the Delta variant in a major acute care hospital in Singapore: investigations and outbreak response. Journal of Hospital Infection [Internet]. 2022 Apr;122:27–34. https://doi.org/10.1016/j.jhin.2021.12.011 PMID: 34942201.

45. Piazza A, Principe L, Comandatore F, Perini M, Meroni E, Mattioni Marchetti V, et al. Whole-genome sequencing investigation of a large nosocomial outbreak caused by ST131 H30Rx KPC-producing Escherichia coli in Italy. Antibiotics [Internet]. 2021 Jun 15;10(6):718. https://doi.org/10.3390/antibiotics10060718 PMID: 34203731.

46. Pérez-Lago L, Martínez-Lozano H, Pajares-Díaz JA, Díaz-Gómez A, Machado M, Sola-Campoy PJ, et al. Overlapping of independent SARS-CoV-2 nosocomial transmissions in a complex outbreak. Imperiale MJ, editor. mSphere [Internet]. 2021 Aug 25;6(4). https://doi.org/10.1128/mSphere.00389-21 PMID: 34346709.

47. Gardy JL, Johnston JC, Sui SJH, Cook VJ, Shah L, Brodkin E, et al. Whole-genome sequencing and social-network analysis of a tuberculosis outbreak. N Engl J Med [Internet]. 2011 Feb 24;364(8):730–9. https://doi.org/10.1056/NEJMoa1003176 PMID: 21345102.

48. Guthrie JL, Strudwick L, Roberts B, Allen M, McFadzen J, Roth D, et al. Comparison of routine field epidemiology and whole genome sequencing to identify tuberculosis transmission in a remote setting. Epidemiol Infect [Internet]. 2020;148. https://doi.org/10.1017/S0950268820000072 PMID: 32014080.
49. Hall MD, Holden MT, Srisomang P, Mahavanakul W, Wuthiekanun V, Limmathurotsakul D, et al. Improved characterisation of MRSA transmission using within-host bacterial sequence diversity. eLife [Internet]. 2019 Oct 8;8. https://doi.org/10.7554/eLife.46402 PMID: 31591959.
50. Paterson GK, Harrison EM, Murray GGR, Welch JJ, Warland JH, Holden MTG, et al. Capturing the cloud of diversity reveals complexity and heterogeneity of MRSA carriage, infection and transmission. Nat Commun [Internet]. 2015 Mar 27;6(1). https://doi.org/10.1038/ncomms7560 PMID: 25814293.
51. Grubaugh ND, Saraf S, Gangavarapu K, Watts A, Tan AL, Oidtman RJ, et al. Travel surveillance and genomics uncover a hidden Zika outbreak during the waning epidemic. Cell [Internet]. 2019 Aug;178(5):1057–1071.e11. https://doi.org/10.1016/j.cell.2019.07.018 PMID: 31442400.
52. Mauldin MR, McCollum AM, Nakazawa YJ, Mandra A, Whitehouse ER, Davidson W, et al. Exportation of monkeypox virus from the African continent. The Journal of Infectious Diseases [Internet]. 2020 Sep 3;225(8):1367–76. https://doi.org/10.1093/infdis/jiaa559 PMID: 32880628.
53. Happi C, Adetifa I, Mbala P, Njouom R, Nakoune E, Happi A, et al. Urgent need for a non-discriminatory and non-stigmatizing nomenclature for monkeypox virus. PLoS Biol [Internet]. 2022 Aug 23;20(8):e3001769. https://doi.org/10.1371/journal.pbio.3001769 PMID: 35998195.
54. Nordahl Petersen T, Rasmussen S, Hasman H, Carøe C, Bælum J, Charlotte Schultz A, et al. Meta-genomic analysis of toilet waste from long distance flights; a step towards global surveillance of infectious diseases and antimicrobial resistance. Sci Rep [Internet]. 2015 Jul 10;5(1). https://doi.org/10.1038/srep11444 PMID: 26161690.
55. Inward RPD, Parag KV, Faria NR. Using multiple sampling strategies to estimate SARS-CoV-2 epidemiological parameters from genomic sequencing data. Nat Commun [Internet]. 2022 Sep 23;13(1). https://doi.org/10.1038/s41467-022-32812-0 PMID: 36151084.
56. Villabona-Arenas ChJ, Hanage WP, Tully DC. Phylogenetic interpretation during outbreaks requires caution. Nat Microbiol [Internet]. 2020 May 19;5(7):876–7. https://doi.org/10.1038/s41564-020-0738-5 PMID: 32427978.
57. Chattaway MA, Dallman TJ, Larkin L, Nair S, McCormick J, Mikhail A, et al. The transformation of reference microbiology methods and surveillance for Salmonella with the use of whole genome sequencing in England and Wales. Front Public Health [Internet]. 2019 Nov 21;7. https://doi.org/10.3389/fpubh.2019.00317 PMID: 31824904.
58. Ungchusak K, Auewarakul P, Dowell SF, Kitphati R, Auwanit W, Puthavathana P, et al. Probable person-to-person transmission of avian influenza A (H5N1). N Engl J Med [Internet]. 2005 Jan 27;352(4):333–40. https://doi.org/10.1056/NEJMoa044021 PMID: 15668219.
59. Qi X, Qian Y-H, Bao C-J, Guo X-L, Cui L-B, Tang F-Y, et al. Probable person to person transmission of novel avian influenza A (H7N9) virus in Eastern China, 2013: epidemiological investigation. BMJ [Internet]. 2013 Aug 6;347(aug06 2):f4752–2. https://doi.org/10.1136/bmj.f4752 PMID: 23920350.
60. Herfst S, Schrauwen EJA, Linster M, Chutinimitkul S, de Wit E, Munster VJ, et al. Airborne transmission of influenza A/H5N1 virus between ferrets. Science [Internet]. 2012 Jun 22;336(6088):1534–41. https://doi.org/10.1126/science.1213362 PMID: 22723413.
61. Imai M, Watanabe T, Hatta M, Das SC, Ozawa M, Shinya K, et al. Experimental adaptation of an influenza H5 HA confers respiratory droplet transmission to a reassortant H5 HA/H1N1 virus in ferrets. Nature [Internet]. 2012 May 2;486(7403):420–8. https://doi.org/10.1038/nature10831 PMID: 22722205.
62. Russell CA, Fonville JM, Brown AEX, Burke DF, Smith DL, James SL, et al. The potential for respiratory droplet–transmissible A/H5N1 influenza virus to evolve in a mammalian host. Science [Internet]. 2012 Jun 22;336(6088):1541–7. https://doi.org/10.1126/science.1222526 PMID: 22723414.
63. Lipsitch M, Barclay W, Raman R, Russell CJ, Belser JA, Cobey S, et al. Viral factors in influenza pandemic risk assessment. eLife [Internet]. 2016 Nov 11;5. https://doi.org/10.7554/eLife.18491 PMID: 27834632.
64. Maurer-Stroh S, Li Y, Bastien N, Gunalan V, Lee RTC, Eisenhaber F, et al. Potential human adaptation mutation of influenza A(H5N1) virus, Canada. Emerg Infect Dis [Internet]. 2014 Sep;20(9):1580–2. https://doi.org/10.3201/eid2009.140240 PMID: 25153690.
65. Cotter CR, Jin H, Chen Z. A single amino acid in the stalk region of the H1N1pdm influenza virus HA protein affects viral fusion, stability and infectivity. Pekosz A, editor. PLoS Pathog [Internet]. 2014 Jan 2;10(1):e1003831. https://doi.org/10.1371/journal.ppat.1003831 PMID: 24391498.

66. Mou K, Mukhtar F, Khan MT, Darwish DB, Peng S, Muhammad S, et al. Emerging mutations in Nsp1 of SARS-CoV-2 and their effect on the structural stability. Pathogens [Internet]. 2021 Oct 6;10(10):1285. https://doi.org/10.3390/pathogens10101285 PMID: 34684233.
67. Van Noorden R. Scientists call for fully open sharing of coronavirus genome data. Nature [Internet]. 2021 Feb 3;590(7845):195–6. https://doi.org/10.1038/d41586-021-00305-7 PMID: 33542487.
68. WHO guiding principles for pathogen genome data sharing [cited 2023 Apr 10]. https://www.who.int/publications/i/item/9789240061743.
69. Swaminathan S. The WHO's chief scientist on a year of loss and learning. Nature [Internet]. 2020 Dec 17;588(7839):583–5. https://doi.org/10.1038/d41586-020-03556-y PMID: 33335314.
70. Khare S, Gurry C, Freitas L, B Schultz M, Bach G, Diallo A, et al. GISAID's role in pandemic response. China CDC Weekly [Internet]. 2021;3(49):1049–51. https://doi.org/10.46234/ccdcw2021.255 PMID: 34934514.
71. GISRS laid the foundation for protection through collaboration [cited 2022 Nov 22]. https://www.who.int/news/item/29-07-2022-gisrs-laid-the-foundation-for-protection-through-collaboration.
72. Kostkova P. Disease surveillance data sharing for public health: the next ethical frontiers. Life Sci Soc Policy [Internet]. 2018 Jul 4;14(1). https://doi.org/10.1186/s40504-018-0078-x PMID: 29971516.
73. Jackson C, Gardy JL, Shadiloo HC, Silva DS. Trust and the ethical challenges in the use of whole genome sequencing for tuberculosis surveillance: a qualitative study of stakeholder perspectives. BMC Med Ethics [Internet]. 2019 Jul 4;20(1). https://doi.org/10.1186/s12910-019-0380-z PMID: 31272443.
74. Grad YH, Lipsitch M. Epidemiologic data and pathogen genome sequences: a powerful synergy for public health. Genome Biol [Internet]. 2014 Nov;15(11). https://doi.org/10.1186/s13059-014-0538-4 PMID: 25418119.
75. Haring RC, Blanchard JW, Korchmaros JD, Lund JR, Haozous EA, Raphaelito J, et al. Empowering equitable data use partnerships and indigenous data sovereignties amid pandemic genomics. Front Public Health [Internet]. 2021 Nov 11;9. https://doi.org/10.3389/fpubh.2021.742467 PMID: 34858924.

CHAPTER 22

CLINICAL CARE IN CHALLENGING SETTINGS

by Sean Wu Jiawei, Lubaba Shahrin, and Robert Fowler

Infectious disease emergencies strain even the best-resourced health systems, threatening the ability to provide high quality clinical care. During an outbreak, a strategic approach is needed to maintain and build on the pillars that ensure the best clinical outcomes. These include the optimisation of supportive care, continuous monitoring of processes and outcomes, real-time data sharing, flexible protocols that can evolve with surges in health demand, and the adoption of new research findings. While managing an extraordinary event, health systems must maintain their essential services, including those that are not outbreak related.

INTRODUCTION

Providing the best clinical care during outbreaks is challenging for all health systems. Regardless of baseline resources, most healthcare systems function within limited reserves. A major outbreak increases clinical demands for the disease itself, but the knock-on effects can interfere with other acute medical care requirements and disrupt primary and preventative care, amplifying the negative effects of an outbreak for many years after the event. There may exist gaps in knowledge, especially for new and emerging pathogens, and treatment strategies must rapidly evolve through observation of clinical patterns, research, and therapeutic trials.

Past outbreaks and pandemics demonstrate that health systems and clinicians often focus on the *unique* features of new and emerging pathogens in order to build case definitions, provide pathogen-specific treatments, and reduce transmission. Although this focus on differences is important in differentiating between endemic and new pathogens, it is also important to highlight the similarities between a new disease and well-known conditions. Failure to do so can lead to an under-appreciation of pre-existing evidence-based treatments in favour of those that are new, untested, and potentially harmful (1). It is therefore critical to simultaneously provide the best clinical care based on applying pre-existing knowledge *and* conduct research needed to evolve the evidence base. By providing good care, healthcare systems maintain the trust of patients and populations. This allows for patients' continued engagement with healthcare workers (HCWs) and the outbreak response.

Best supportive care improves individual patient outcomes that in turn support public trust and improve adherence to treatment recommendations and appropriate health-seeking behaviour. Maintaining trust is especially important in the early stages of a disease outbreak with high morbidity and mortality. For example, in Ebola virus disease (EBOD) outbreaks, when the case fatality rate is high and with family and friends unaware of the care received, people may choose to not present for treatment. Anger and violence towards hospitals, treatment centres, and public health officials have been observed in relation to AIDS, Ebola, and COVID-19 responses (2). This lack of trust can lead to ineffective public health interventions, allowing transmission to continue (3). The provision of best available care in these circumstances provides the rare opportunity for clinical care to directly influence the effectiveness of a public health response.

This chapter will focus on the challenges and importance of establishing best clinical care across all health systems during outbreaks and pandemics (**Figure 22.1**). A successful approach will:
- emphasise best supportive care
- discuss how health systems can adapt to surges in demand
- highlight the importance of maintaining essential health services
- describe how real-time research and knowledge are essential to patient care
- utilise research to ensure the best use of new therapeutics

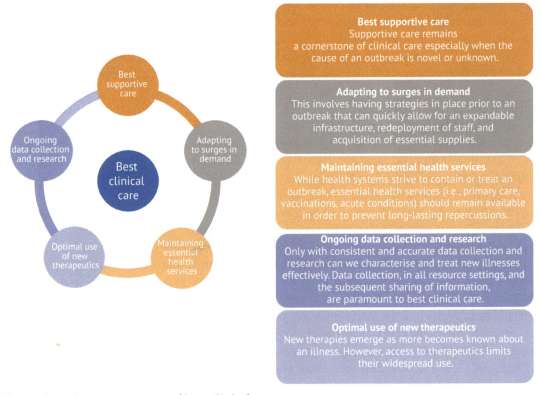

Figure 22.1: Core components of best clinical care

BEST SUPPORTIVE CARE

At the onset of outbreaks for new and emerging infections, there is a dearth of knowledge about effective and/or direct-acting medical treatments. Instead of focusing on the unknown, the approach should be first to provide the best supportive clinical care and generalise evidence-based management strategies to the emerging disease. Best supportive care, even without direct-acting antivirals, remains the standard of care for many viral diseases. Similarly, for many critical illnesses where a specific aetiology is unclear, supporting organ dysfunction with oxygen, invasive ventilation, intravenous fluids, and dialysis, among others, improves survival. When there are so many unknowns in an outbreak, reducing the variation in supportive care protocols will allow an earlier interpretation and establishment of best practice.

The importance of best supportive care has been demonstrated in contemporary outbreaks. During the polio epidemics, bulbar and respiratory polio commonly led to ventilation failure and death before tracheostomy and positive pressure ventilation were introduced (4). Prior to 2014, case weighted mortality during Ebola outbreaks was approximately 67 per cent (5). However, with the introduction of supportive care and improved clinical experience, mortality in Africa fell to 39.5 per cent across the entire outbreak (6–7).

> **West African Ebola outbreak: supportive care results in a sharp decline in mortality**
>
> Best supportive care reduced the case fatality rates of patients infected with ebolavirus from 70 per cent to 39.5 per cent. Less than six months after the implementation of supportive care strategies based on increasing clinical experience, mortality rates in one treatment centre in Sierra Leone reduced from 47.7 per cent in September to 23.5 per cent by December 2014 (8).
>
> Best supportive care measures comprised consistent monitoring of vital signs including oxygen saturation, diagnostic laboratory testing of haematology, electrolytes, renal, hepatic, coagulation function, and acid-base balance, and rapid diagnostic testing for malaria (6). Treatments typically consisted of reversal of hypovolaemia with intravenous crystalloids, electrolyte replenishment, reversal of non-anion gap acidaemia due to diarrhoea and renal dysfunction, correction of vitamin K-dependent coagulopathy, treatment of malaria, and empiric prophylaxis or treatment of bacterial infections.
>
> These specific supportive care measures were subsequently incorporated into international guidelines and have been temporally associated with markedly reduced Ebola mortality (6). In better supported clinical settings such as in Europe and North America, the mortality rate for Ebola is even lower, at 18.5 per cent (7).

During the early COVID-19 pandemic in 2020, the mortality rate of critically ill patients with COVID-19 was 62 per cent. Over time, the mortality rate fell globally to approximately 37 per cent and was even lower in certain high-resource countries (8–10). This pattern was also observed during EBOD outbreaks. A prominent feature of early discussions on the treatment of COVID-19 both in the scientific literature and the lay press was on the possible novel elements of the clinical syndrome (e.g., inflammation, coagulation, oxygenation, and ventilation mechanics) as opposed to focusing on the commonalities with other respiratory illnesses. This resulted in the use of non-evidence-based treatment. Treatment variability across the world led to a plethora of early low-quality observational studies and trials that were unable to define the best evidence base in valid fashion (1). A unified implementation of best supportive care with concurrent rapid characterisation of the illness through good quality research, such as generalisable observational studies and large randomised clinical trials, would have saved many lives (10–12).

ONGOING DATA COLLECTION AND RESEARCH

In situations of high uncertainty, characterising the illness by understanding patient characteristics, the natural history of the disease, complications, outcomes, and the efficacy of proposed treatments helps guide future strategies and resource management. When outbreaks are overwhelming clinical capacity, there may be limited personnel to carry out data collection. A tiered data collection protocol based on resources available may help circumvent this on a collective scale (**Figure 22.2**). At the most basic tier, all centres should prioritise the collection of essential information (i.e., outlined in the T0 or T1 forms from the World Health Organization [WHO], as well as long-term follow-up data if possible) (13). The T0 and T1 forms—which include important questions on the time, place, person, and clinical variables—help investigators understand the source of an outbreak and its mode of transmission, propose initial control measures, and perform rapid risk assessments.

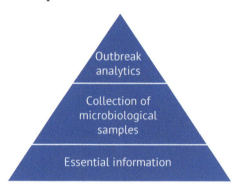

Figure 22.2: Tiered data collection during an outbreak

Data collection often takes a backseat during the onset of an outbreak. However, collecting essential information, such as is outlined in the WHO T0 and/or T1 case investigation forms, is the first step in characterising and subsequently managing new infections. Centres with more abundant resources can also collect microbiological samples and take part in analytics (**See Chapter 17, Integrated outbreak analytics**).

With the rapid expansion of internet access and vast improvements in data storage, sharing information collected by healthcare centres around the world has never been easier. This evolution of technology allows professionals on the ground to share, discuss, and analyse information in real time. The recent COVID-19 pandemic is the best example of how knowledge sharing platforms can help improve clinical care. The speed at which data was shared—through peer-reviewed publications, preprints, online databases, or social media—and the quantity of data shared was unprecedented.

Best practice guidelines

Best practice guidelines are defined as "statements that include recommendations intended to optimise patient care that are informed by a systematic review of evidence and an assessment of the benefits and harms of alternative care options" (14). Such guidelines are established by recognised authorities such as the WHO, the European Centre for Disease Prevention and Control (ECDC), the International Society for Infectious Diseases (ISID), the U.S. Centers for Disease Control and Prevention (U.S. CDC), and other national authorities globally.

When the pathogen causing the outbreak is well known, best practice guidelines informing clinical care as well as infection control strategies are readily accessible. Examples include Ebola, influenza, and measles which are described in multiple open access WHO publications (15–17). Commonalities across these publications include the description of the clinical syndrome with proposed case definitions, diagnostic assays, clinical management recommendations with mention of pathogen-specific therapeutics if available, and infection prevention and control (IPC) strategies.

Guidelines are not universal and must be adapted to the local context. In resource-limited settings, guidelines that emphasise the use of single rooms, one-to-one clinical care, and expensive disinfection protocols are often impractical and unrealistic. In order to remedy this, guidelines that prioritise and stratify interventions based on effectiveness, resource requirements, and cost-effectiveness will help governments, hospitals, and healthcare providers align guidance with local best possible practices (18).

When the outbreak-causing pathogen is new and evidence is sparse, guidelines do not exist. However, COVID-19 has demonstrated that a "living guideline" can be rapidly developed and updated as the evidence base grows. On 27 May 2020, just five months after identification of the outbreak, the WHO published its first interim clinical management guidance (19).

MANAGING SURGE

The COVID-19 pandemic has highlighted that maintaining the same levels of clinical care in an emergency can be challenging and sometimes impossible. The following reorganisations may be effective in resource-constrained settings.

Triaging patients to prioritise care

This process is created based on the best available data on the case definition of a disease during an outbreak and aims to separate patients based on illness severity and likelihood of infection. Successful triage prioritises emergency care, improves early detection rates, can reduce the case fatality of critically ill patients, and limits the spread of infection in the hospital (20–21).

Creating a zoning system in the hospital

Establishing separate wards for suspected or confirmed cases during an outbreak is necessary when managing a highly contagious disease. Dedicated, specifically trained teams of healthcare providers using appropriate personal protective equipment (PPE) can be deployed to specific settings. Defining dedicated zones can minimise transmission and allow critical expertise to develop with the application of well-practised work processes. Healthcare systems can focus resources and enable continuous learning for dedicated staff involved in outbreak care.

Referral mechanism

Elective procedures or services can be referred to a designated specialised facility. For instance, antenatal checks, obstetric emergencies, and cardiovascular and cerebrovascular emergencies are essential services that need dedicated facilities or zones separate from the outbreak handling zone. Non-urgent or elective procedures may be postponed to allow redeployment of resources (e.g., healthcare staff, clinical care logistics, and hospital beds) for immediate needs.

Feasible diagnostic approaches

Radiologic and laboratory diagnostic procedures from dedicated facilities often become challenging during an outbreak. During the COVID-19 pandemic, high-resolution computed tomography (CT) was recommended in some jurisdictions to assess the severity of lung injury and the need for mechanical ventilation. However, some limited resource settings could not initially use existing infrastructure for COVID-19 patients due to IPC concerns. Similarly, during EBOD outbreaks, makeshift laboratories and point-of-care testing were introduced to lessen the burden on general diagnostic laboratory functions.

In order to respond to surges in healthcare demand, health systems must also be able to train and re-deploy HCWs efficiently. Protocols pre-established to reskill workers can help systems respond to evolving challenges. Emphasis should be placed on reskilling staff from local centres as they understand the local context and culture, allowing for easy integration into their temporary roles. However, a lack of workers may make it necessary to recruit from other regions (22). There are several mechanisms to achieve this including the Global Outbreak Alert and Response Network (GOARN), support from multilateral governmental- and WHO-facilitated clinical responses such as the African Union, the WHO Emerging Diseases Clinical Assessment and Response Network (EDCARN), and myriad international non-governmental organisations (23).

Dhaka 2018: managing surge in cases of acute watery diarrhoea in a major outbreak

The International Centre for Diarrhoeal Disease Research, Bangladesh (icddr,b) treats more than 150,000 cases of diarrhoea annually, including two seasonal peaks. In 2018, one peak saw almost 30,000 patients with diarrhoea, with over 1,000 cases per day. The average duration of hospital stay of 11 hours and mortality rates remained similar compared to non-peak times. There were just 13 deaths. Success can largely be attributed to:

- the ability to quickly strengthen hospital capacity by creating make-shift wards within tents, hiring temporary previously trained staff from a pre-selected pool, and increasing stockpiles of medication
- the rapid identification of pathogens which allowed for risk stratification and rapid implementation of life-saving treatments (e.g., the need for antibiotics and/or the need to further stockpile intravenous [IV] fluids)
- a surveillance and monitoring system that helped predict future cases through data obtained on sociodemographic characteristics, water, sanitation, hygiene practices, microbiology, clinical care, and patient outcomes
- engagement with government health partners to improve sanitation practices by using this data. The research was able to not only inform patient care, but also uncover practices outside the hospital that led to an increased risk of diarrhoeal disease. The data subsequently informed regionwide infection control strategies with an emphasis on hygiene and sanitation.

It was estimated that over 17,000 deaths were possibly averted (24).

ENSURING ADEQUATE CARE FOR ALL MEDICAL CONDITIONS

As highlighted earlier in this chapter, an overemphasis on the outbreak pathogen can come at the expense of care for patients afflicted by the more usual illnesses (**See Chapter 23, Essential services**). This was especially true during the early phases of the COVID-19 pandemic where overwhelmed healthcare systems cancelled scheduled procedures and discouraged admissions to hospital for fear of a pandemic wave. This, coupled with a reluctance of people to present to hospitals for fear of acquiring COVID-19, led to significant delays in definitive care for conditions requiring urgent intervention (e.g., myocardial ischaemia and stroke). Medical and surgical care for acute and chronic conditions, primary care in the community, and preventative care (e.g., vaccinations, prenatal care, screening programmes) were all interrupted. The consequences of this lapse in holistic care only became evident later. Ultimately, these challenges led to an increase in preventable morbidity and mortality across the population and is one explanation for the excess mortality—above what could be predicted by COVID-19 alone—observed in many countries. The rates of antimicrobial resistance and hospital-acquired infections also rose during the recent pandemic, re-emphasising the importance of adhering to good antimicrobial stewardship and infection control practices. Maintaining an appropriate balance of outbreak- and non-outbreak-related medical care is critical in the provision of optimal care (25–26).

BEST USE OF THERAPEUTICS

Therapeutics in outbreaks take many forms including vaccinations, antimicrobials, convalescent plasma, and monoclonal antibodies, among others. Vaccines play a central role in controlling outbreaks; however, the development of vaccines is historically a slow process requiring multiple phases of testing for safety and immunogenicity followed by regulatory approval. Even after approval, vaccine unavailability due to either limited stocks or difficulties in maintaining a cold chain or administering vaccines often prevents immediate widespread use (**See Chapter 28, Vaccine development**). During the COVID-19 pandemic, the process by which vaccines were developed, approved, distributed, and administered was considerably streamlined. Approval of the first vaccine was less than one year into the pandemic (27).

For viral-mediated disease transmission, the development of effective antivirals requires a comprehensive understanding of the molecular processes of the virus and usually requires several decades of study. However, drug repurposing studies—studying new indications for old drugs—can be faster and might lead to treatments in an ongoing outbreak (28). Remdesivir, originally developed for EBOD, and nirmatrelvir/ritonavir, originally developed for Venezuelan equine encephalitis virus, were repurposed and approved for COVID-19 (28). However, drug repurposing should not undermine basic research agendas or create shortages of essential drugs for other patients (**See Chapter 27, Research for therapeutics**).

As more people are exposed to and recover from infection, convalescent plasma, which provides passive immunity in naïve individuals, becomes a viable therapeutic candidate. However, producing convalescent plasma is expensive and requires specialised technology not usually available in low- and middle-income settings. Using the example of the COVID-19 pandemic, donors with high titres of SARS-CoV-2 antibodies were identified to undergo plasmapheresis. The resulting blood products were screened for infectious agents, stored at temperatures below 6°C, and finally administered. The expiration period was five days at normal refrigeration temperature and one year at −18°C, highlighting the challenges with its use (24). While convalescent plasma may be a generalisable candidate therapy across many new and emerging infectious illnesses, there is still limited evidence of efficacy in any viral illness, emphasising the importance of rigorous evaluation in clinical trials (24).

Monoclonal antibodies (mAbs) bind target antigens and facilitate the recruitment of immune cells to neutralise pathogens. They have been used with some promise in respiratory syncytial virus (RSV), human immunodeficiency virus (HIV), EBOD, *Clostridium difficile* infections, and most recently, were found to be definitively effective for COVID-19. Within 16 months of the pandemic, six mAbs were developed and received emergency use authorisation (EUA). The dynamic COVID-19 pandemic has also highlighted the importance of the specificity of mAbs to the variants for which they were developed. As new SARS-CoV-2 variants arose, early mAbs were often found to be less effective (29).

OTHER ENABLERS OF BEST CLINICAL CARE
Ensuring safe working environments
A critical element of providing best care during an outbreak or pandemic is to ensure a safe clinical environment for patients and a safe working environment for HCWs. If patients and their families perceive that the healthcare environment is not safe, whether from hospital transmission of infections, illness unintentionally induced by interaction with the healthcare system, or a lack of security, they may choose to avoid healthcare facilities. This phenomenon was observed during the EBOD outbreaks. This was in part due to a lack of early understanding of transmission, inadequate PPE, and a dearth of experience in relevant IPC practices. In some healthcare settings, a low threshold for admission unnecessarily exposed patients to nosocomial spread. Nosocomial transmission to HCWs further leads to worker absenteeism and reduces the delivery of effective care (30). Developing targeted occupational health policies for staff safety and reviewing investment in occupational health are important parts of preparedness to deliver high quality clinical care (**See Chapter 26, IPC; See Chapter 31, Mental health**).

Telehealth
Embracing telehealth can reduce transmission while enabling essential healthcare services. During the COVID-19 pandemic, there was a widespread adoption of telehealth services across different disciplines. Telemedicine in outpatient consults is the most common and arguably the most successful example (31). Beyond outpatient consults, there was an evolution of virtual care used in both non-COVID-19 and COVID-19 settings. Patients with neurological disease, including stroke and Parkinson's disease, and chronic pulmonary conditions received telerehabilitation (31). Telemonitoring was used successfully in the management of many diseases such as diabetes, hypertension, and heart failure (32). Virtual wards, where patients who traditionally require hospitalisation receive hospital-level care at home, were piloted successfully (33). Tele-critical consultations even emerged as a way to improve access to specialists while reducing transmission (34). Telemedicine, together with home delivery systems, was also used in the remote diagnosis and management of COVID-19 infections (35). The COVID-19 pandemic highlighted the diverse uses of telemedicine and the real-world benefits, including its ability to transcend geographical boundaries, offload hospital burden, reduce transmission while providing care, and conserve PPE (36).

CONCLUSION

Providing the best possible clinical care during outbreaks and pandemics is challenging. HCW infections and even deaths resulting from workplace transmission are well documented. They are arguably the major reason why the best clinical care may not be provided during an infectious disease emergency. Beyond this fear and risk, HCWs are under great physical and psychological stress. This is compounded by an almost invariable unmet demand in many other resources realised by health systems. However, the best clinical care can be provided if health systems, and particularly hospitals, are ready with the understanding of the importance of good supportive care, a safe environment, and a capacity to evolve in all aspects as the outbreak progresses. The provision of safe and effective care to patients, in addition to creating safe and supportive working environments for healthcare teams, helps ensure that patients, health workers, and the population have confidence in the outbreak response. An awareness of the potential impact on primary, preventative, and secondary to quaternary care for usual acute and chronic conditions can help abate excess mortality in the broadest sense.

REFERENCES:

1. Ho M, Tadrous M, Iacono A, Suda K, Gomes T. Outpatient purchasing patterns of hydroxychloroquine and ivermectin in the USA and Canada during the COVID-19 pandemic: an interrupted time series analysis from 2016 to 2021. J Antimicrob Chemother. 2022 Dec;78(1):242–51. https://doi.org/10.1093/jac/dkac382 PMID:36374569.
2. Ratcliffe R. Arsonists attack Ebola clinics in DRC as climate of distrust grows. The Guardian (2019).
3. Lamontagne F, Clément C, Fletcher T, Jacob ST, Fischer WA 2nd, Fowler RA. Doing today's work superbly well—treating Ebola with current tools. N Engl J Med. 2014 Oct;371(17):1565–6. https://doi.org/10.1056/NEJMp1411310 PMID:25251518.
4. Wunsch H. The outbreak that invented intensive care. Nature. 2020 Apr; https://doi.org/10.1038/d41586-020-01019-y PMID:32246120.
5. World Health Organization. Therapeutics for Ebola virus disease. https://www.who.int/publications-detail-redirect/9789240055742.
6. Mbonye AK, Wamala JF, Nanyunja M, Opio A, Makumbi I, Aceng JR. Ebola viral hemorrhagic disease outbreak in West Africa-lessons from Uganda. Afr Health Sci. 2014 Sep;14(3):495–501. https://doi.org/10.4314/ahs.v14i3.1 PMID:25352864.
7. Centers for Disease Control and Prevention. 2014–2016 Ebola outbreak in West Africa | History | Ebola (Ebola Virus Disease). https://www.cdc.gov/vhf/ebola/history/2014-2016-outbreak/index.html (2020).
8. Yang X, Yu Y, Xu J, Shu H, Xia J, Liu H, et al. Clinical course and outcomes of critically ill patients with SARS-CoV-2 pneumonia in Wuhan, China: a single-centered, retrospective, observational study. Lancet Respir Med. 2020 May;8(5):475–81. https://doi.org/10.1016/S2213-2600(20)30079-5 PMID:32105632.
9. Docherty AB, Harrison EM, Green CA, Hardwick HE, Pius R, Norman L, et al.; ISARIC4C investigators. Features of 20 133 UK patients in hospital with covid-19 using the ISARIC WHO Clinical Characterisation Protocol: prospective observational cohort study. BMJ. 2020 May;369(m):m1985. https://doi.org/10.1136/bmj.m1985 PMID:32444460.
10. Group IC, et al. ISARIC COVID-19 Clinical Data Report issued: 27 March 2022. 2020.07.17.20155218 Preprint at https://doi.org/10.1101/2020.07.17.20155218. (2022).
11. RECOVERY Collaborative Group; Horby P, Lim WS, Emberson JR, Mafham M, Bell JL, Linsell L, et al. Dexamethasone in hospitalized patients with Covid-19. N Engl J Med. 2021 Feb 25;384(8):693–704. https://doi.org/10.1056/NEJMoa2021436 PMID:32678530.
12. WHO Solidarity Trial Consortium; Pan H, Peto R, Henao-Restrepo AM, Preziosi MP, Sathiyamoorthy V, Abdool Karim Q, et al. Repurposed antiviral drugs for Covid-19 - interim WHO Solidarity Trial results. N Engl J Med. 2021 Feb 11;384(6):497–511. https://doi.org/10.1056/NEJMoa2023184 PMID:33264556.
13. Perrocheau A, Brindle H, Roberts C, Murthy S, Shetty S, Martin AI, et al.; "Minimum Variables for Outbreak Investigation Working Group of the WHO Outbreak Toolkit project". Data collection for outbreak investigations: process for defining a minimal data set using a Delphi approach. BMC Public Health. 2021 Dec;21(1):2269. https://doi.org/10.1186/s12889-021-12206-5 PMID:34895199.

14. Panteli D, Legido-Quigley H, Reichebner C, et al. Clinical Practice Guidelines as a quality strategy. In: Busse R, Klazinga N, Panteli D, et al., editors. Improving healthcare quality in Europe: characteristics, effectiveness and implementation of different strategies [Internet]. Copenhagen (Denmark): European Observatory on Health Systems and Policies; 2019. (Health Policy Series, No. 53.) 9. https://www.ncbi.nlm.nih.gov/books/NBK549283/.
15. World Health Organization. Interim infection prevention and control guidance for care of patients with suspected or confirmed filovirus haemorrhagic fever in health-care settings, with focus on Ebola. https://www.who.int/publications/i/item/WHO-HIS-SDS-2014.4-Rev.1.
16. World Health Organization. Guidelines for the clinical management of severe illness from influenza virus infections. 2022. https://www.who.int/publications/i/item/9789240040816.
17. World Health Organization. Guide for clinical case management and infection prevention and control during a measles outbreak. 2020. https://www.who.int/publications/i/item/9789240002869.
18. Maaløe N, Ørtved AM, Sørensen JB, Sequeira Dmello B, van den Akker T, Kujabi ML, et al. The injustice of unfit clinical practice guidelines in low-resource realities. Lancet Glob Health. 2021 Jun;9(6):e875–9. https://doi.org/10.1016/S2214-109X(21)00059-0 PMID:33765437.
19. Clinical management of COVID-19: Living guideline, 13 January 2023. https://www.who.int/publications-detail-redirect/WHO-2019-nCoV-clinical-2023.1.
20. Mitchell R, Fang W, Tee QW, O'Reilly G, Romero L, Mitchell R, Bornstein S, Cameron P. Systematic review: what is the impact of triage implementation on clinical outcomes and process measures in low- and middle-income country emergency departments? Acad Emerg Med. 2024 Feb;31(2):164-182. https://doi.org/10.1111/acem.14815 PMID:37803524.
21. Karat AS, Gregg M, Barton HE, Calderon M, Ellis J, Falconer J, Govender I, Harris RC, Tlali M, Moore DAJ, Fielding KL. Evidence for the use of triage, respiratory isolation, and effective treatment to reduce the transmission of Mycobacterium tuberculosis in healthcare settings: a systematic review. Clin Infect Dis. 2021 Jan 23;72(1):155-172. https://doi.org/10.1093/cid/ciaa720 PMID:32502258.
22. Shahrin L, Parvin I, Sarmin M, Abbassi NA, Ackhter MM, Alam T, et al. In-person training on COVID-19 case management and infection prevention and control: evaluation of healthcare professionals in Bangladesh. PLoS One. 2022 Oct;17(10):e0273809. https://doi.org/10.1371/journal.pone.0273809 PMID:36201257.
23. World Health Organization. Classification and minimum standards for emergency medical teams. 2021. https://www.who.int/publications/i/item/9789240029330.
24. Jorda A, Kussmann M, Kolenchery N, Siller-Matula JM, Zeitlinger M, Jilma B, et al. Convalescent plasma treatment in patients with Covid-19: a systematic review and meta-analysis. Front Immunol. 2022 Feb;13:817829. https://doi.org/10.3389/fimmu.2022.817829 PMID:35197981.
25. Centers for Disease Control and Prevention. COVID-19: U.S. impact on antimicrobial resistance, special report 2022. https://stacks.cdc.gov/view/cdc/119025.
26. Sands KE, Blanchard EJ, Fraker S, Korwek K, Cuffe M. Health care-associated infections among hospitalized patients with COVID-19, March 2020-March 2022. JAMA Netw Open. 2023 Apr 3;6(4):e238059. https://doi.org/10.1001/jamanetworkopen.2023.8059 PMID:37052918.
27. Bok K, Sitar S, Graham BS, Mascola JR. Accelerated COVID-19 vaccine development: milestones, lessons, and prospects. Immunity. 2021 Aug;54(8):1636–51. https://doi.org/10.1016/j.immuni.2021.07.017 PMID:34348117.
28. von Delft A, Hall MD, Kwong AD, Purcell LA, Saikatendu KS, Schmitz U, et al. Accelerating antiviral drug discovery: lessons from COVID-19. Nat Rev Drug Discov. 2023 Jul;22(7):585–603. https://doi.org/10.1038/s41573-023-00692-8 PMID:37173515.
29. Corti D, Purcell LA, Snell G, Veesler D. Tackling COVID-19 with neutralizing monoclonal antibodies. Cell. 2021 Jun;184(12):3086–108. https://doi.org/10.1016/j.cell.2021.05.005 PMID:34087172.
30. Alshutwi SS. 'Senior nursing students and interns' concerns and willingness to treat patients with COVID-19: a strategy to expand national nursing workforce during the COVID-19 pandemic. Risk Manag Healthc Policy. 2021 Jan;14:39–48. https://doi.org/10.2147/RMHP.S279569 PMID:33447108.
31. Bokolo Anthony Jnr. Use of telemedicine and virtual care for remote treatment in response to COVID-19 pandemic. J Med Syst. 2020 Jun;44(7):132. https://doi.org/10.1007/s10916-020-01596-5 PMID:32542571.
32. Iellamo F, Sposato B, Volterrani M. Telemonitoring for the management of patients with heart failure. Card Fail Rev. 2020 Apr;6:e07. https://doi.org/10.15420/cfr.2019.20 PMID:32377386.

33. Ko SQ, Kumar SK, Jacob J, Hooi BM, Soo M, Nashi N, et al. Technology-enabled virtual ward for COVID management of the elderly and immunocompromised in Singapore: a descriptive cohort. BMC Infect Dis. 2023 Feb;23(1):102. https://doi.org/10.1186/s12879-023-08040-2 PMID:36809977.

34. Dhala A, Sasangohar F, Kash B, Ahmadi N, Masud F. Rapid implementation and innovative applications of a virtual intensive care unit during the COVID-19 pandemic: case study. J Med Internet Res. 2020 Sep;22(9):e20143. https://doi.org/10.2196/20143 PMID:32795997.

35. Liu L, Gu J, Shao F, Liang X, Yue L, Cheng Q, et al. Application and preliminary outcomes of remote diagnosis and treatment during the COVID-19 Outbreak: retrospective cohort study. JMIR Mhealth Uhealth. 2020 Jul;8(7):e19417. https://doi.org/10.2196/19417 PMID:32568722.

36. Ganjali R, Jajroudi M, Kheirdoust A, Darroudi A, Alnattah A. Telemedicine solutions for clinical care delivery during COVID-19 pandemic: a scoping review. Front Public Health. 2022 Jul;10:937207. https://doi.org/10.3389/fpubh.2022.937207 PMID:35937265.

CHAPTER 23

MAINTAINING ESSENTIAL HEALTH AND SOCIAL SERVICES

by Zheng Huan Javier Thng, Simone E. Carter, and William Fischer

In a public health emergency, regular healthcare and social services require specific attention to ensure they are maintained while resources are diverted towards the emergency. Delays in access to care for infectious conditions such as malaria, tuberculosis, and HIV, and non-infectious diseases, including cardiac disease, stroke, and cancers (the prevalence of which does not decrease during public health emergencies), compound preventable morbidity and mortality. A conscious effort is required to maintain acute care, primary care, and preventative and screening programmes.

For vulnerable groups such as children and women, the risk of exploitation, neglect, and abuse increases. Protection services are more important than ever during an infectious disease emergency and will need support and likely, additional resourcing. Schools should only be closed if strongly justified. If inevitable, alternative modes of education should be implemented while ensuring the appropriate infrastructure is in place. It is critical to ensure the availability of these health and social services to uphold the principles of justice and equality.

INTRODUCTION

An infectious disease emergency invariably threatens to disrupt the function of usual healthcare and the delivery of social services. These disruptions may result from overwhelmed health systems, the diversion of resources towards the public health emergency, patient fears of accessing health facilities, and the outbreak control measures themselves. While these disruptions occur in all countries at all income levels, vulnerable communities and individuals are disproportionately affected.

Baseline mortality is the reference level describing the expected number of deaths in a population. Excess mortality occurs in an infectious disease emergency but is invariably greater than the sum of the baseline mortality and deaths from the outbreak disease. This is the result of disruption to emergency and standard medical services.

Disruptions in essential health service delivery during public health emergencies is multifactorial. Diversion of resources and providers during public health emergencies lead some facilities to adopt crisis standards of care, reducing the availability of elective and preventative services for non-emergency conditions (1). Almost 50 per cent of countries surveyed reported clinical staff being redeployed to support the COVID-19 response, with 29 per cent reporting insufficient supply of healthcare providers for essential health service delivery (2). A disproportionate increase in rates of infection and death among healthcare workers during public health emergencies, such as Ebola virus disease (EBOD) and COVID-19, led to human resource shortages that layered on top of an already stressed system. Furthermore, the mental health toll of public health emergency response, such as increased rates of anxiety and depression, impacted the trained workforce (3). On the demand side, fear of nosocomial transmission plays a prominent role in the delay or avoidance of presenting to healthcare settings, as do movement restrictions. Delays in access to care due to reduced public transportation and overcrowding in emergency rooms can further complicate healthcare delivery during public health emergencies.

Social services that protect vulnerable populations and individuals may be discontinued as health systems pivot to focus on the outbreak. The temporary loss of family planning and systems that prevent abuse and exploitation can be somewhat invisible in the short term but result in further widening of inequalities in the longer term.

An awareness of the health and social impacts of not maintaining these pre-existing services is the first step in ensuring their continuation during an infectious disease emergency. Ultimately, building resilience into workflows can help ensure the ability to both respond effectively to public health emergencies as well as maintain essential healthcare services and the delivery of social services.

MAINTENANCE OF ESSENTIAL HEALTH SERVICES
Presentations for non-outbreak conditions

During public health emergencies, access to non-outbreak healthcare is often meaningfully affected. In a survey conducted by the World Health Organization (WHO) in May 2020, more than 90 per cent reported a disruption in essential health service delivery during the COVID-19 pandemic with the greatest impact in low- and middle-income countries (4). Disruptions were reported on both the demand side (due to public hesitancy to present to a healthcare setting for fear of infection) and supply side (due to human and material resource diversion and infection prevention restrictions).

Failing access for routine health emergencies

Studies of patients with myocardial infarctions during the COVID-19 pandemic showed that both admissions and timing of admissions were affected. A study of ST-elevation myocardial infarctions (STEMI) in 141 countries across six continents found that hospital admissions for acute coronary syndrome were reduced by more than 40 per cent (5). Additionally, patients generally presented later than pre-pandemic; there was an increase in the number of patients who presented outside the optimal window for primary percutaneous intervention which resulted in a higher mortality rate, particularly in low- and middle-income countries (5–6).

Obstetric and surgical emergencies were similarly affected. An Israeli study found a significant increase in urgent and acute obstetric interventions in hospitals as a result of delayed presentation. However, maternal and neonatal morbidity were not affected (7).

A study in Turkey found a 25 per cent decrease in surgical admissions, and those who were admitted were categorised as more severe, resulting in an increased proportion that required open intervention. There was also an increase in the treatment rejection rate during the COVID-19 pandemic attributed to an increased risk of nosocomial COVID-19 infection and the restricted visitation policies that accompanied infection prevention measures (8). The 2014–2016 EBOD epidemic had a similar effect in Sierra Leone and Guinea. In Sierra Leone, the epidemic was associated with a 70 per cent decrease in hospital admissions and 50 per cent decline in the number of major surgeries between May and October 2014 (9). In Guinea, child health services were most affected, with substantial decreases in the number of children seen for diarrhoea and acute respiratory infections (up to 60 and 58 per cent, respectively) (10).

Decreasing outpatient visits and the acceptance of telemedicine

Prevention and screening services were even more affected than emergency and inpatient services, with more than 40 per cent reporting limiting community-based care and access to mobile clinics (2). Immunisations were particularly affected with nearly 40 per cent of Gavi-supported countries reporting a decline in routine vaccination coverage due to concerns including movement restrictions and SARS-CoV-2 transmission worries (11). Similarly, pandemic-related disruptions to family planning and contraception services, non-communicable disease management including rehabilitation, and mental and neurological services were similarly affected with high rates of disruption reported by low- and middle-income countries (4).

The number of outpatient visits in the U.S. decreased gradually as the pandemic progressed but occurred concurrently with an increase in telemedicine visits (12). Despite limitations in the ability to conduct a physical examination and in some cases, reduced patient satisfaction with the patient-doctor relationship, telemedicine visits can increase the efficiency of healthcare delivery during public health emergencies (13). The use of telemedicine has declined following the peak of COVID-19 activity, with only its use in psychiatric care currently remaining at pandemic levels (14). Despite its limitations, telemedicine represents a potentially transformative technology that can be used to increase access to healthcare among marginalised and vulnerable populations now and scaled up during public health emergencies to maintain outpatient and preventative care.

Diagnosis and management of chronic conditions

Communicable diseases programmes. The impact of public health emergencies can also be felt by international programmes targeting communicable diseases including tuberculosis, malaria, and HIV, all leading causes of death globally. A decrease in the number of smear-positive tuberculosis cases in Liberia during the 2014–2016 EBOD epidemic resulted in reduced treatment success rates, with 69 per cent success during and 73 per cent after the epidemic compared to 80 per cent before the epidemic (15). Similarly, during the COVID-19 pandemic, a mathematical model conducted by the WHO to study the effects of COVID-19 on tuberculosis management revealed that a 25 per cent reduction in tuberculosis detection for even six months can lead to a 26 per cent increase in tuberculosis deaths, which is a step back to the levels of tuberculosis mortality in 2012 (16). Malaria control was similarly affected during the 2014 EBOD epidemic with 74,000 fewer cases between 1 January to 30 November 2014, compared to the same period in 2013 (17).

	Pre-EBOD (Jan 2013–Mar 2014)	EBOD crisis (Apr 2014–Jun 2015)	Post-EBOD (July–Dec 2015)
Smear-positive tuberculosis (mean no. of cases per quarter)	855	640	568
Treatment success rates	80%	69%	73%

Table 23.1: Cases of smear-positive tuberculosis and treatment success rates before, during, and after the EBOD crisis in Liberia

Likewise, prevention programmes, such as the distribution of insecticide-treated bed nets and prophylactic antimalarial treatments, were also significantly disrupted. Modelling of the impacts of COVID-19 on malaria management suggested that a 25 per cent reduction in insecticide-treated nets and antimalarial drug coverage led to an increase of 240.5 million cases and 520,900 thousand deaths globally (18–19).

Furthermore, reductions in HIV testing in low-, middle-, and high-income countries can have a profound impact on treatment and prevention. A 46 per cent drop in HIV testing in Guinea during the EBOD epidemic is estimated to have led to 713 additional deaths (20–21). HIV testing in the U.S. was reduced by 68–97 per cent during the COVID-19 pandemic and remained low even after lockdown measures were lifted (22). Similarly, reductions in sexually transmitted infection screening likely led to an underdiagnosis of chlamydia and a potentially increased risk of transmission (23).

Reductions in diagnostics due to public health emergencies can lead to delayed treatment and increased mortality. Home testing, introduced during the COVID-19 pandemic and more recently the mpox pandemic, offers a way of overcoming public health emergency-related limitations and maintaining access to diagnostics during emergencies.

Non-communicable diseases. Disruptions in the diagnosis and management of medical conditions are not limited to infectious diseases but can also impact other chronic conditions including diabetes mellitus. The difficulty in seeking non-urgent medical advice and the fear of visiting health services due to the risk of infection are factors that result in reduced follow up. Closure of outpatient facilities, insufficient stocks of personal protective equipment (PPE), and lockdowns are additional challenges that have complicated the diagnosis and management of both infectious and non-communicable diseases (24).

A study in North Carolina, U.S., showed that up to 21 per cent more patients delayed their diabetes care in 2020, compared to a four-year average between 2018 and 2021 (25). Another study in the U.K. showed that over a one-month period in April 2020, there were up to 88 per cent fewer diabetic health checks compared to a ten-year average from 2011 to 2020 (26). Poor glycaemic control in COVID-19 patients is associated with prolonged hospitalisation and an increased mortality rate (27). Therefore, ensuring timely diabetic follow-up can be lifesaving. Poorly controlled diabetes also has long-term irreversible impacts including retinopathy, peripheral neuropathy, and cardiovascular conditions.

Preventative measures for non-outbreak conditions

Vaccinations. Public health emergencies can also increase the vulnerability and susceptibility of a population through reductions in routine vaccination programmes. A 2020 WHO survey revealed significant disruptions to immunisation practices, with an 89 per cent reduction in vaccine demand in the Africa region, 75 per cent in the Americas region, and 73 per cent in the Eastern Mediterranean region, resulting in a 39 per cent reduction in routine immunisation coverage (4). Reductions in diagnostics and surveillance, coupled with supply chain interruptions, movement restrictions, and fears of nosocomial transmission, reduced vaccine coverage and increased susceptibility to preventable infectious diseases.

Elimination goal	Effect of public health emergencies
Achieve a world free of poliomyelitis	**COVID-19** During the COVID-19 pandemic in 2020, there were 959 cases of circulating vaccine-derived poliovirus type 2 (cVDPV2) compared to 2019 when there were 366 cVDPV2 cases (28).
Maternal and neonatal tetanus elimination	**EBOD** A study of African nations during the West African EBOD crisis showed that Liberia had lower tetanus coverage during the outbreak in 2014 (50 per cent) compared to previous years (76 per cent in 2013), and this persisted following the outbreak in 2015 (29).
Measles elimination	**EBOD** A study showed that during the EBOD crisis, there was a significant reduction in children being vaccinated against measles in Liberia and Guinea. The study found that in 2017, even despite mass vaccination campaigns post-EBOD, the vaccination rates did not return to pre-EBOD levels. This corresponds with the finding that the number of confirmed cases in 2017 remains higher than that of the pre-EBOD period (30–31). **COVID-19** A report published by the WHO and UNICEF showed that there was an almost 80 per cent increase in measles cases in January and February 2022 compared to the same period in 2021. The bulk of these cases were from Africa and the Eastern Mediterranean region.

Table 23.2: Public health crises affect vaccination goals

Health screening. Disruption in prevention services and health screening, as reported during COVID-19, can also have a profound impact on cancer screening (32). Decreased cancer screening leads to delays in cancer diagnosis and treatment initiation which are associated with increased mortality and lead to increased demands on healthcare systems, with an increase in patients requiring complex care (33).

Innovations in home diagnostics may help maintain health screening during public health emergencies as faecal immunochemical test (FIT), self-administered Pap smears, and breast self-examinations can effectively detect cancers of the colon, cervix, and breast, respectively (34). The use of FIT in England during the COVID-19 pandemic was effective in triaging for urgent colorectal cancer referrals (35). Therefore, while self-sampling is imperfect, these methods can support cancer screening during public health emergencies.

MAINTENANCE OF ESSENTIAL SOCIAL SERVICES
Education for children and adolescents

Schools are important not just for their role in education but also as a platform for the administration of other important social services such as child protection, mental health, and nutritional services.

During public health emergencies, education can be severely compromised or discontinued. During the recent COVID-19 pandemic, children around the world were affected by school closures. A UNICEF study showed that in Asia, almost 100 per cent of children missed out on schooling during parts of March to May 2020. For some countries such as Bangladesh and the Philippines, these disruptions lasted more than a year (36).

A direct impact of school closure is the associated learning loss. A study in Pakistan by the Brookings Institute showed that without any remediation intervention, three months of school closure for a Grade 3 pupil (Primary 3) will equate to one year of learning loss by Grade 10 (Secondary 4) (37). The long-term negative effects of school closures could be attributed to the lack of practice and reinforcement. Even when students have caught up, additional time might be needed to cover new topics due to the inertia faced by students from the disruption in learning. These compounding effects lead to long-term educational loss that can have ramifications in terms of the attainment of skills and competencies (38).

The impacts are further amplified in vulnerable groups including girls (in some contexts) and children with disabilities. For those living with disabilities, alternative modes of learning, such as distance learning, may be unsuitable and further compromise learning. A report by the Malala Fund showed that during the Ebola outbreak, secondary school-aged girls in the regions of Guinea, Liberia, and Sierra Leone were most likely to drop out as a result of school closures (39).

The decision to close and reopen schools should be decentralised instead of being nation- or state-wide. Each local authority should be given a set of evidence-based guidelines with which they can assess against their local situation. One such resource is the COVID-19 Modelling Consortium Framework by The University of Texas (40). This framework helps decision-makers establish their goals of reopening, what strategies can be reasonably implemented, and how the risks and outcomes can be effectively monitored. Another resource developed for Indonesian schools considered the disease intensity (the proportion of confirmed cases versus close contacts), disease severity (number of intensive care unit patients and deaths), and the impact of the disease on the healthcare system (e.g., cases amongst healthcare workers, bed occupancy, PPE availability) when making an assessment on the appropriateness of reopening schools (41). Intermediary solutions, including staggering the reopening of schools, should also be considered to allow schools to reopen as soon as possible.

Should school closures be inevitable, access to alternative modes of teaching is critical to ensure continuity of education. A common experience across developed countries during the COVID-19 pandemic was distance learning via teleconferencing platforms. These services require good internet accessibility and electronic devices capable of accessing media platforms which are not always available to persons of low socioeconomic status or in different national contexts. Increased infrastructural investments by the state can be considered to ensure remote access to telecommunication services amongst school-going children, as can income-based subsidisation or the provision of personal computing devices.

Next, there will be a need to normalise and establish functional systems for distance learning to ensure a smooth transition to an alternative digital learning platform. To ensure familiarity and functional systems, schools should consider integrating these media platforms and other online teaching aids during face-to-face lessons even during periods without an emergency. Beyond the technical means of conducting these lessons, encouraging the spirit of independent and self-motivated learning, despite extended periods without face-to-face interactions, will be useful. Suggestions of how to promote learning include demonstrating the purpose and usefulness of the content taught, incentivising performance through a reward system, and having one-to-one sessions with students for targeted feedback and socio-emotional support (42).

During school closures, it will also be important to consider the impact on particularly vulnerable groups including those with disabilities. The United Nations (UN) Human Rights Office has come up with guidance that seeks to ensure children with disabilities will not be left behind (43). Some recommendations to ensure equal access include the development of accessible and adapted learning materials, good internet access, and the development of software that is accessible to those with disabilities, which may include providing assistive devices. Other recommendations touch on the need to support and train parents and teachers to enable them to support the child.

Transition to online learning in Uruguay

In Uruguay, every child who enters the public education system is given a computer and can access the internet for free in schools. During the pandemic, schools used an online teaching platform to ensure continuity in learning. This platform has been shown to be an effective mode of teaching and has in fact resulted in an improvement in students' test scores by a 0.2 standard deviation compared to scores prior to the pandemic (42).

Challenges in returning to school in Sierra Leone

Post-EBOD in Sierra Leone, focus group discussions with children described some of the common reasons children were not returning to school (44). Some felt disheartened as they had forgotten what they had learned and had been held back in their educational level. Others shared that their families were no longer able to afford paying their school fees due to the economic impacts of the EBOD pandemic. Children in Sierra Leone also feared that by returning to school, they could catch Ebola, affecting their own health and the health of their families. Lastly, some children shared that after schools closed, the physical infrastructure of the school had fallen into a state of disrepair.

Child protection

Public health emergencies affect children in other ways. Movement restriction during disease outbreaks denies them access to other adults from trusted organisations. This puts children in vulnerable situations including violence at home and forced labour.

With increased mortality in the population, what we may not consider is that these people are often someone's parents or caregivers. During public health emergencies, the rate of orphanhood rises. Often, being orphaned leads to other child protection risks including discrimination, child labour, and sexual exploitation (45). One reason could be the loss of protection and income, forcing these orphans to fill the roles of financial providers to their families.

Child labour increases during public health emergencies. For instance, during the 2014–2015 EBOD crisis, 43 per cent of 216 children studied in Sierra Leone had to work to support their families (44). Children are forced to work during public health emergencies due to various factors:

- out of necessity to provide for one's family after the death or illness of usual providers
- to compensate for the loss of income caused by outbreak control measures
- as a result of school closures – with children having nothing else to do at home, family members could force them to work

Outbreak control measures often force families to stay at home together over long periods, which may lead to family tensions. Add to that the stressors that occur during a period of crisis as well as the loss of income, and this may escalate and children may become victims of abuse (46). During public health emergencies, the lack of access to other trusted adults and organisations means that these abuses may be unidentified and timely intervention therefore not forthcoming. The impact of child abuse may go beyond the immediate physical and/or emotional hurt and include longer term impacts such as the development of psychological illness.

The key to resolving the exploitation and abuse of children is to ensure that child protection services continue to run without interruption. The opening of such services must be prioritised to protect one of the most vulnerable groups in our society. Accessibility to such services must also be considered. The easiest way for a child to seek help would be via schools, which reiterates the importance of keeping schools open through public health emergencies.

Hospitals need to play a role in ensuring the safety of children as well (47). Doctors, nurses, and social workers can undergo training to identify and flag possible child abuse and exploitation. At the same time, posters and other media communication should be displayed in patient-facing locations—including the emergency department and clinics—so that victims are aware of the help available to them.

When such services are disrupted, there is also a need to ensure that children are screened on their return to school. Teachers and other staff should be trained to look out for signs of internalised stigma. This is when a child has accepted negative views of themselves, thereby affecting their sense of self-worth. Left unchecked, this can lead to depression and other long-term psychiatric problems. The Child Attitude Toward Illness Scale (48) and the Internalized Stigma of Mental Illness Scale (49) are assessment tools that can assist teachers with flagging psychological issues.

Since many of these problems arise from issues related to financial hardship, social safety nets are needed, especially during periods of crisis when economic pressures are the greatest.

An adequate social safety net can ensure that each family is able to meet a minimum standard of living without having to resort to the extremes of forcing a child into early employment.

> **Social safety net programmes in Mauritania**
>
> In Mauritania, two programmes exist that aim to reduce child labour due to financial shocks. These are the TEKAVOUL social transfer programme and the ELMAOUNA shock response programme (50) which are supported by the World Bank. On top of the TEKAVOUL programme which provides a consistent source of income to the extremely poor, the ELMAOUNA shock response programme ensures that when faced with 'shocks' (including droughts), families will have additional funds which they can tap into, instead of having to look for alternative sources of income which may include child labour.

Adolescent health services

A UNICEF report showed that during the 2014–2015 EBOD crisis, there was a 25 per cent increase in teenage pregnancy (46). This was a result of various socioeconomic factors, including an increase in transactional sex due to financial pressures, the spending of limited money on more essential items like food instead of contraception, and choosing to have children due to a sense of hopelessness about the future. This hopelessness is often associated with school closures, where girls no longer see a route back to education and employment. Teenage pregnancy can have many adverse consequences. During infectious disease outbreaks, especially in regions with limited healthcare resources, access to medical facilities and appropriate obstetric support may be limited, especially if healthcare systems are overwhelmed with crisis management. This will increase infant and maternal mortality during childbirth. In Kenya, a study reported an increase in the proportion of adolescent maternal deaths, from 6.2 per cent before the COVID-19 pandemic to 10.9 per cent during the pandemic (51). In the long term, teenage pregnancy will also deter or prevent women from continuing to pursue an education even after schools reopen, affecting their future.

Another UNICEF report showed that the impact of COVID-19 on well-being and mental health was disproportionately greater in adolescents, especially young women and those in lower income countries (**See Chapter 31, Mental health**) (52). However, even those in countries with access to mental health services faced challenges in seeking professional help during the COVID-19 pandemic. In the Republic of Ireland, the rate of referrals to mental health services fell by 53 per cent compared to pre-pandemic (53). This can be attributed to school closures resulting in a lack of timely identification of symptoms by teachers and other staff. It can also be a result of containment measures limiting visits of non-urgent conditions to outpatient and hospital emergency services.

Protection for women against domestic violence

During a public health emergency, the reduced safeguards and protection services, as well as increased domestic interaction forced by outbreak control measures, can bring about serious harm to women. This is especially so in countries where gender inequality is already prevalent.

An increase in intimate partner violence may occur during public health emergencies. This occurs for a variety of reasons, many of which are related to outbreak control measures. When governments impose lockdowns, there will be increased exposure to potential perpetrators at home. Furthermore, quarantine measures could increase existing controlling behaviours of perpetrators who abuse others to re-establish a sense of control that they feel has been taken away from them (46). This is also further exacerbated by the economic stressors caused by income losses. Another issue is the reduction in protective services which may be forced to shut or scale down in public health emergencies. The reduced access to medical facilities may also have the side effect of preventing women from obtaining medical proof of their assaults, making their pursuit of justice even more difficult.

Similar to the protection against child abuse and exploitation, gender-based services providing protection and respite to women should be prioritised and granted exemptions from closure. Additionally, women should have easy access to confidential spaces and trusted healthcare workers so they can disclose abuses they are facing and seek assistance and justice. Finally, there is a need to increase communication and awareness of individual rights and the services from which they can seek help, especially during public health emergencies. These messages should be able to reach women who are unable to leave their homes, such as via social media, television, or radio broadcasts.

Family planning services

A WHO survey of health services during the COVID-19 pandemic showed that 68 per cent of the 105 countries surveyed reported disruptions in family planning services (2). More alarmingly, a UN Population Fund report estimated that three months of high-level disruption to such services can lead to 44 million women being unable to use modern contraceptives, resulting in one million additional unintended pregnancies (54). This can have a massive adverse impact on women including disruptions to education and employment, and the creation of new financial issues due to costs associated with raising a child.

Disruptions to family planning services can be caused by containment measures and a reduction in visits to healthcare settings. It can also be worsened by the cessation or reduction of community engagement programmes. Furthermore, supply chain disruptions may also deny women who have sought contraceptives.

To counter the disruptions caused by a public health crisis, telemedicine services can be tapped to minimise disruption to women who seek family planning services. However, in communities without good access to telemedicine, the engagement of community health workers may be needed. These workers help bring services directly to women within their communities so they need not travel to a hospital to seek assistance. These workers can also better adapt to the prevailing restrictions in their region. Other solutions may include providing family planning services in pharmacies. On top of supplying contraceptives, pharmacists and staff may be trained to provide resources and recommendations to those who require additional assistance (55–56).

CONCLUSION

Public health emergencies are inevitable. It is vital to plan well in advance in order to limit the collateral damage that can arise from interruptions to essential services. Preparing to maintain essential services is critical to minimise excess mortality. Policies should be formulated with the most vulnerable of our society in mind. Safe environments with clear and reassuring communication about risks can help maintain health and social services. Scaling back on services may be necessary but must be minimised and specifically favour the vulnerable. Technologic innovations need to be utilised at scale and will also help minimise the indirect harms of an infectious disease emergency.

REFERENCES:

1. Centers for Disease Control and Prevention (CDC). COVID-19: Science Briefs. https://www.cdc.gov/mmwr/volumes/70/wr/mm7046a5.htm.
2. World Health Organization. Pulse survey on continuity of essential health services during the COVID-19 pandemic: interim report. Geneva, Switzerland: World Health Organization; 2020. pp. 1–21.
3. Shaukat N, Ali DM, Razzak J. Physical and mental health impacts of COVID-19 on healthcare workers: a scoping review. Int J Emerg Med. 2020 Jul;13(1):40. https://doi.org/10.1186/s12245-020-00299-5 PMID:32689925.
4. The Independent Panel for Pandemic Preparedness and Response. Impact on Essential Health Services. https://theindependentpanel.org/wp-content/uploads/2021/05/Background-paper-8-Impact-on-Essential-Health.pdf.
5. Pessoa-Amorim G, Camm CF, Gajendragadkar P, De Maria GL, Arsac C, Laroche C, et al. Admission of patients with STEMI since the outbreak of the COVID-19 pandemic: a survey by the European Society of Cardiology. Eur Heart J Qual Care Clin Outcomes. 2020 Jul;6(3):210–6. https://doi.org/10.1093/ehjqcco/qcaa046 PMID:32467968.
6. Chew NW, Ow ZG, Teo VX, Heng RR, Ng CH, Lee CH, et al. The global effect of the COVID-19 pandemic on STEMI care: a systematic review and meta-analysis. Can J Cardiol. 2021 Sep;37(9):1450–9. https://doi.org/10.1016/j.cjca.2021.04.003 PMID:33848599.
7. Kugelman N, Lavie O, Assaf W, Cohen N, Sagi-Dain L, Bardicef M, et al. Changes in the obstetrical emergency department profile during the COVID-19 pandemic. J Matern Fetal Neonatal Med. 2022 Nov;35(21):4116–22. https://doi.org/10.1080/14767058.2020.1847072 PMID:33198540.
8. Göksoy B, Akça MT, Inanç ÖF. The impacts of the COVID-19 outbreak on emergency department visits of surgical patients. Ulus Travma Acil Cerrahi Derg. 2020 Sep;26(5):685–92. https://doi.org/10.14744/etd.2020.67927 PMID:32946100.
9. Bolkan HA, Bash-Taqi DA, Samai M, Gerdin M, von Schreeb J. Ebola and indirect effects on health service function in Sierra Leone. PLoS Curr. 2014 Dec;6:6. https://doi.org/10.1371/currents.outbreaks.0307d588df619f9c9447f8ead5b72b2d PMID:25685617.
10. Barden-O'Fallon J, Barry MA, Brodish P, Hazerjian J. Rapid assessment of Ebola-related implications for reproductive, maternal, newborn and child health service delivery and utilization in Guinea. PLoS Curr. 2015 Aug;7:7. https://doi.org/10.1371/currents.outbreaks.0b0ba06009dd091bc39ddb3c6d7b0826 PMID:26331094.
11. Gavi. COVID-19 Tracking Parameters on Country Impact and Response. Geneva, Switzerland; 2020. pp. 1-32.
12. The Commonwealth Fund. Impact of COVID-19 on Outpatient Visits in 2020: Visits Stable Despite Late Surge. https://www.commonwealthfund.org/publications/2021/feb/impact-covid-19-outpatient-visits-2020-visits-stable-despite-late-surge. Published February 2021.
13. Ftouni R, AlJardali B, Hamdanieh M, Ftouni L, Salem N. Challenges of telemedicine during the COVID-19 pandemic: a systematic review. BMC Med Inform Decis Mak. 2022 Aug;22(1):207. https://doi.org/10.1186/s12911-022-01952-0 PMID:35922817.
14. McCracken CE, Gander JC, McDonald B, Goodrich GK, Tavel HM, Basra S, et al. Impact of COVID-19 on trends in outpatient clinic utilization: a tale of 2 departments. Med Care. 2023 Apr;61(4 Suppl 1):S4–11. https://doi.org/10.1097/MLR.0000000000001812 PMID:36893413.
15. Konwloh PK, Cambell CL, Ade S, Bhat P, Harries AD, Wilkinson E, et al. Influence of Ebola on tuberculosis case finding and treatment outcomes in Liberia. Public Health Action. 2017 Jun;7(1 Suppl 1):S62–9. https://doi.org/10.5588/pha.16.0097 PMID:28744441.
16. World Health Organization. COVID-19: considerations for tuberculosis (TB) care. World Health Organization; 2021 May. Report no.: WHO/2019-nCoV/TB_care/2021.1.

17. Plucinski MM, Guilavogui T, Sidikiba S, Diakité N, Diakité S, Dioubaté M, et al. Effect of the Ebola-virus-disease epidemic on malaria case management in Guinea, 2014: a cross-sectional survey of health facilities. Lancet Infect Dis. 2015 Sep;15(9):1017–23. https://doi.org/10.1016/S1473-3099(15)00061-4 PMID:26116183.

18. Weiss DJ, Bertozzi-Villa A, Rumisha SF, Amratia P, Arambepola R, Battle KE, et al. Indirect effects of the COVID-19 pandemic on malaria intervention coverage, morbidity, and mortality in Africa: a geospatial modelling analysis. Lancet Infect Dis. 2021 Jan;21(1):59–69. https://doi.org/10.1016/S1473-3099(20)30700-3 PMID:32971006.

19. Global Malaria Programme. Tailoring malaria interventions in the COVID-19 response. World Health Organization; 2020 May. Report no.: WHO/UCN/GMP/2020.02.

20. Brolin Ribacke KJ, Saulnier DD, Eriksson A, von Schreeb J. Effects of the West Africa Ebola virus disease on health-care utilization–a systematic review. Front Public Health. 2016 Oct;4:222. https://doi.org/10.3389/fpubh.2016.00222 PMID:27777926.

21. Parpia AS, Ndeffo-Mbah ML, Wenzel NS, Galvani AP. Effects of response to 2014–2015 Ebola outbreak on deaths from malaria, HIV/AIDS, and tuberculosis, West Africa. Emerg Infect Dis. 2016 Mar;22(3):433–41. https://doi.org/10.3201/eid2203.150977 PMID:26886846.

22. Chmielewska B, Barratt I, Townsend R, Kalafat E, van der Meulen J, Gurol-Urganci I, et al. Effects of the COVID-19 pandemic on maternal and perinatal outcomes: a systematic review and meta-analysis. Lancet Glob Health. 2021 Jun;9(6):e759–72. https://doi.org/10.1016/S2214-109X(21)00079-6 PMID:33811827.

23. Chang JJ, Chen Q, Dionne-Odom J, Hechter RC, Bruxvoort KJ. Changes in testing and diagnoses of sexually transmitted infections and HIV during the COVID-19 pandemic. Sex Transm Dis. 2022 Dec;49(12):851–4. https://doi.org/10.1097/OLQ.0000000000001639 PMID:35470350.

24. World Health Organization. The impact of the COVID-19 pandemic on noncommunicable disease resources and services: results of a rapid assessment. Geneva, Switzerland: World Health Organization; 2020. pp. 2–13.

25. Bancks MP, Lin MY, Bertoni A, Futrell WM, Liu Z, Ostasiewski B, et al. Impact of the COVID-19 pandemic on diabetes care among a North Carolina patient population. Clin Diabetes. 2022;40(4):467–76. https://doi.org/10.2337/cd21-0136 PMID:36385975.

26. Carr MJ, Wright AK, Leelarathna L, Thabit H, Milne N, Kanumilli N, et al. Impact of COVID-19 restrictions on diabetes health checks and prescribing for people with type 2 diabetes: a UK-wide cohort study involving 618 161 people in primary care. BMJ Qual Saf. 2022 Jul;31(7):503–14. https://doi.org/10.1136/bmjqs-2021-013613 PMID:34642228.

27. Chander S, Deepak V, Kumari R, Leys L, Wang HY, Mehta P, et al. Glycemic control in critically ill COVID-19 patients: systematic review and meta-analysis. J Clin Med. 2023 Mar;12(7):2555. https://doi.org/10.3390/jcm12072555 PMID:37048638.

28. World Health Organization. Circulating vaccine-derived poliovirus type 2-global update. Dis Outbreak News. 2021.

29. Ridpath AD, Scobie HM, Shibeshi ME, Yakubu A, Zulu F, Raza AA, Masresha B, Tohme R. Progress towards achieving and maintaining maternal and neonatal tetanus elimination in the African region. The Pan African Medical Journal. 2017;27(Suppl 3). https://doi.org/10.11604/pamj.supp.2017.27.3.11783.

30. Delamou A, Ayadi AM, Sidibe S, Delvaux T, Camara BS, Sandouno SD, et al. Effect of Ebola virus disease on maternal and child health services in Guinea: a retrospective observational cohort study. Lancet Glob Health. 2017 Apr;5(4):e448–57. https://doi.org/10.1016/S2214-109X(17)30078-5 PMID:28237252.

31. World Health Organization. Unicef. UNICEF and WHO warn of perfect storm of conditions for measles outbreaks, affecting children [Internet]. https://www.who.int/news/item/27-04-2022-unicef-and-who-warn-of--perfect-storm--of-conditions-for-measles-outbreaks--affecting-children.

32. Cancino RS, Su Z, Mesa R, Tomlinson GE, Wang J. The impact of COVID-19 on cancer screening: challenges and opportunities. JMIR Cancer. 2020 Oct;6(2):e21697. https://doi.org/10.2196/21697 PMID:33027039.

33. Hanna TP, King WD, Thibodeau S, Jalink M, Paulin GA, Harvey-Jones E, O'Sullivan DE, Booth CM, Sullivan R, Aggarwal A. Mortality due to cancer treatment delay: systematic review and meta-analysis. BMJ. 2020 Nov 4;371:m4087. https://doi.org/10.1136/bmj.m4087. PMID:33148535.

34. Luu T. Reduced cancer screening due to lockdowns of the COVID-19 pandemic: reviewing impacts and ways to counteract the impacts. Front Oncol. 2022 Jul;12:955377. https://doi.org/10.3389/fonc.2022.955377 PMID:35965514.

35. Kamel F, Zulfiqar S, Penfold W, Weatherell S, Madani R, Nisar P, et al. The use of the faecal immunochemical test during the COVID-19 pandemic to triage urgent colorectal cancer referrals. Colorectal Dis. 2022 Jun;24(6):727–36. https://doi.org/10.1111/codi.16120 PMID:35297169.

36. UNICEF ROSA, UNICEF EAPRO, UNESCO Bangkok, Cambridge Education. Situation Analysis on the Effects of and Responses to COVID-19 on the Education Sector in Asia. UNICEF; 2021 Oct.

37. Kaffenberger M. Modelling the long-run learning impact of the Covid-19 learning shock: actions to (more than) mitigate loss. Int J Educ Dev. 2021 Mar;81:102326. https://doi.org/10.1016/j.ijedudev.2020.102326 PMID:33716394.

38. Chun HK, Comyn P, Moreno da Fonseca P. Skills development in the time of COVID-19: taking stock of the initial responses in technical and vocational education and training. Geneva: International Labour Office; 2021.

39. Malala Fund. Girls' education and COVID-19: what past shocks can teach us about mitigating the impact of pandemics. Malala Fund; 2020 Apr.

40. Dibner KA, Schweingruber HA, Christakis DA. Reopening K-12 schools during the COVID-19 pandemic: a report from the National Academies of Sciences, Engineering, and Medicine. JAMA. 2020 Sep;324(9):833–4. https://doi.org/10.1001/jama.2020.14745 PMID:32761241.

41. Kristiyanto RY, Chandra L, Hanjaya H, Hakim MS, Nurputra DK. School reopening: evidence-based recommendations during COVID-19 pandemic in Indonesia. Journal of Community Empowerment for Health. 2020;4(1):43–55. https://doi.org/10.22146/jcoemph.57524.

42. Muñoz-Najar A, Gilberto A, Hasan A, Cobo C, Azevedo JP, Akmal M. Remote learning during COVID-19: lessons from today. Principles for tomorrow; 2021. https://doi.org/10.1596/36665.

43. United Nations. COVID-19 and the rights of persons with disabilities: Guidance. UN Human Rights Office of the High Commissioner. 2020 Apr 29.

44. Isabelle Risso-Gill and Leah Finnegan. Children's Ebola Recovery Assessment: Sierra Leone. Save the Children, World Vision International and Plan International, UNICEF; 2015.

45. Peterman A, Potts A, O'Donnell M, Thompson K, Shah N, Oertelt-Prigione S, Van Gelder N. Pandemics and violence against women and children. Washington, DC: Center for Global Development; 2020 Apr 1.

46. Bakrania S, Chávez C, Ipince A, Rocca M, Oliver S, Stansfield C, et al. Impacts of Pandemics and Epidemics on Child Protection: Lessons learned from a rapid review in the context of COVID-19. Innocenti Working Papers, UNICEF Office of Research; 2020 Jul.

47. Garstang J, Debelle G, Anand I, Armstrong J, Botcher E, Chaplin H, et al. Effect of COVID-19 lockdown on child protection medical assessments: a retrospective observational study in Birmingham, UK. BMJ Open. 2020 Sep;10(9):e042867. https://doi.org/10.1136/bmjopen-2020-042867 PMID:32994262.

48. Ramsey RR, Ryan JL, Fedele DA, Mullins LL, Chaney JM, Wagner JL. Child Attitude Toward Illness Scale (CATIS): A systematic review of the literature. Epilepsy Behav. 2016 Jun;59:64–72. https://doi.org/10.1016/j.yebeh.2016.03.026 PMID:27096812.

49. Boyd JE, Adler EP, Otilingam PG, Peters T. Internalized Stigma of Mental Illness (ISMI) scale: a multinational review. Compr Psychiatry. 2014 Jan;55(1):221–31. https://doi.org/10.1016/j.comppsych.2013.06.005 PMID:24060237.

50. Alliance Sahel. An inclusive social protection system in Mauritania. [Internet] 2022 [cited 2022 Nov 30]. https://www.alliance-sahel.org/en/an-inclusive-social-protection-system-in-mauritania/.

51. Shikuku DN, Nyaoke IK, Nyaga LN, Ameh CA. Early indirect impact of COVID-19 pandemic on utilisation and outcomes of reproductive, maternal, newborn, child and adolescent health services in Kenya: a cross-sectional study. Afr J Reprod Health. 2021 Dec;25(6):76–87. PMID:37585823.

52. UNICEF. Impact of COVID-19: adolescent well-being and mental health. Sustainable Development Goals. 2021;(3):1–8.

53. McNicholas F, Kelleher I, Hedderman E, Lynch F, Healy E, Thornton T, et al. Referral patterns for specialist child and adolescent mental health services in the Republic of Ireland during the COVID-19 pandemic compared with 2019 and 2018. BJPsych Open. 2021 May;7(3):e91. https://doi.org/10.1192/bjo.2021.48 PMID:33938419.

54. United Nations Population Fund. Impact of the COVID-19 pandemic on family planning and ending gender-based violence, female genital mutilation and child marriage. Interim Tech Note. 2020 Apr 27;7.

55. Salve S, Raven J, Das P, Srinivasan S, Khaled A, Hayee M, et al. Community health workers and Covid-19: cross-country evidence on their roles, experiences, challenges and adaptive strategies. PLOS Glob Public Health. 2023 Jan;3(1):e0001447. https://doi.org/10.1371/journal.pgph.0001447 PMID:36962877.

56. NHS England. High street pharmacies spot cancers in new NHS early diagnosis drive. NHS England; 2022 Jun. https://www.england.nhs.uk/2022/06/high-street-pharmacies-spot-cancers-in-new-nhs-early-diagnosis-drive/.

CHAPTER 24

CRITICAL CARE IN OUTBREAKS

by Ziwei Liu, Richard Kojan, and William Fischer

Patient-centric supportive critical care represents clinical supportive care for patients with life-threatening illness. Coupled with rapid diagnostics and pathogen-specific treatment, it is an essential aspect of the case management pillar in outbreak response. The goal of critical care is to support organ function, manage complications of existing organ dysfunction, and prevent new organ dysfunction. This requires the right staff, stuff, systems, and space to provide the care that is needed.

INTRODUCTION

Critical care is medical care for patients with life-threatening illness, often with evidence of organ dysfunction or failure requiring organ supportive care. The goal of critical care is to support existing organ function, treat acute organ injury, and prevent further organ failure. This represents the foundation of clinical care for all severely ill patients. This approach is particularly true before an aetiological agent is identified, and continues, coupled with pathogen-specific treatment, once a diagnosis has been confirmed. This chapter reviews the role of critical care during an outbreak of an infectious disease or public health emergency, details the spectrum of critical care using Ebola virus disease (EVD)* caused by the Ebola virus as a case study, introduces strategies for operationalising the provision of critical care during an outbreak, and finally, highlights the role of research to improve both critical care and pathogen-specific treatment to advance the care of patients in an outbreak setting. It should be noted that there is growing inequity in access to medical care—including critical care—across the globe and the result is both a disparity in outcomes and the development of mistrust among underserved populations. These two effects conspire to delay the control of outbreaks.

Case study – part 1

A 30-year-old man was admitted to the Béni Ebola Treatment Unit (ETU) in the Democratic Republic of the Congo (DRC) on 3 May 2019. His journey allows us to understand the role of critical care in outbreaks, the components that constitute critical care, the difference it can make for patients and communities, and how research is essential to improve critical care for future patients and future outbreaks.

Michel has a prior medical history notable only for hypertension. He was not vaccinated against Ebola virus and his symptoms started 10 days prior to presentation, after a family funeral where he performed rites. He developed fever, arthralgia, myalgia, and intense malaise. He first sought care

> from a traditional practitioner, then at a local health centre. On his third visit to a dispensary, he was admitted to hospital, and finally referred to the ETU three days later when EVD was suspected.
>
> His initial physical examination was notable for extreme weakness with signs of dehydration and dry mucosal membranes. The examination revealed no neurological abnormalities. However, his vital parameters were concerning, with a temperature of 39.1°C, blood pressure 105/64 mmHg, heart rate 121 beats per minute, respiratory rate 28 breaths per minute, and oxygen saturation 98 per cent on room air. His blood sugar level at admission was 122 mg/dL (normal range 70–130 mg/dL) or 6.8 mmol/L.

THE ROLE OF CRITICAL CARE IN OUTBREAK RESPONSE

Outbreaks of infectious diseases pose considerable challenges to healthcare facilities, public health experts, healthcare workers (HCWs), and affected communities. By stretching healthcare systems beyond their capacity, recent outbreaks of Ebola virus disease (EBOD) and COVID-19 increased the morbidity and mortality of those infected, as well as among those with other diseases, as healthcare systems become unable to deliver essential health services due to the redeployment of staff and resources. Effective outbreak response encompasses a comprehensive approach to identifying infected individuals, providing the needed care for infected individuals to maximise their chance for survival, tracing contacts of those individuals who may become symptomatic and infectious, engaging with the community to prevent further transmission, and maintaining essential health services delivery to ensure patients with every other illness still have access to treatment and preventative services. The care provided to those who are identified and isolated is one part of this response but it involves a spectrum of activities. This begins with triage and risk assessment and includes the treatment and prevention of organ dysfunction, and research to improve care for the next patient and for the next outbreak. Access to critical care is not universal due to the significant resources required, including experienced staff, critical care equipment (stuff), a systematic strategy of evaluation and management, and a safe place to deliver effective care (often referred to as the 4S's—staff, stuff, system, space) (1). The resulting disparity in access to critical care is a reversible cause of increased morbidity and mortality in both outbreak and non-outbreak settings.

COMPONENTS OF CRITICAL CARE

Triage

Critical care begins with triage—a process of rapidly examining all patients upon arrival to a healthcare facility to stratify patients based on disease severity (2) and risk. Often in outbreak settings, triage is also used to assess how to best allocate limited resources. This was seen globally during COVID-19 where in some contexts, need outstripped the availability of oxygen and/or mechanical ventilation. In the absence of triage, medical care may be provided randomly or on a first come, first served basis rather than through an organised approach consistent with the ethical goals of an allocation framework (3).

Triage can be systematised with protocols which provide a structured decision-making strategy for healthcare providers to quickly identify patients who require immediate critical care and also to ensure equal, equitable, and effective provision of that care. The World

Health Organization (WHO) Emergency Triage Assessment and Treatment (ETAT) triage tool rapidly sorts patients into three categories, including those who require immediate emergency or critical care treatment, those who require rapid assessment and treatment, and those with non-urgent conditions, based on the presence of emergency or priority signs and symptoms (4). The triage protocol follows the ABC framework which prioritises organ systems that would require emergency treatment beginning with the **airway (A)**, followed by **breathing (B)**, **circulation + coma/convulsions (C)**, and **dehydration** (or **disability** in other triage protocols, referring to mental status) **(D)**. The ETAT ABC evaluation takes less than 20 seconds and does not require any additional equipment other than the ability to look, listen, and feel. If a patient has any of the ABC signs, emergency treatment and critical care management should be initiated immediately.

The equipment for vital sign measurement (including a sphygmomanometer and oxygen saturation probes which are extremely helpful to identify hypotension and hypoxia, respectively) should be included as necessary equipment in any critical care setting. Oxygen saturation probes have the added benefit of being able to rapidly measure heart rate without the need for a clock.

Abnormalities identified during triage should prompt immediate treatment followed by close observation to ensure continued clinical improvement in a critical care setting. If assessments of airway, breathing, circulation, coma, and convulsions are all normal, or if emergency treatments have been given for any problem identified, the next evaluation is for severe dehydration (D). Signs and symptoms include lethargy, sunken eyes, or depressed fontanelles in infants, and a skin pinch that takes longer than two seconds to return to its pre-pinch state. It is essential when evaluating for severe dehydration to also evaluate for signs of severe malnutrition and anaemia as this will affect how patients, particularly paediatric patients, are volume resuscitated.

Screening during outbreaks

In addition to triage, screening patients to determine if they meet the case definition of the outbreak disease is a key aspect of care for any patient. This will generally be established at the point of entry to the facility but can be an issue for admission to a critical care setting. Any patient who meets the case definition of the outbreak disease requires infection prevention measures. Patient screening is guided by case definitions which can change even within the same outbreak. Cases are commonly categorised as suspected cases, probable cases, laboratory-confirmed cases, and non-cases (4). The upgrading of suspect case to probable case is usually driven by the evaluation of a suspect case by a clinician.

Case study – part 2

In the previous example, Michel's recent direct contact with a dead body and symptoms met the WHO case definition during an EVD outbreak. This required immediate isolation where diagnostics could be conducted and supportive care provided (5).

> Emergency triage revealed no evidence of airway obstruction but his respiratory rate of 28 was faster than normal. An oxygen saturation of 98 per cent suggests this is not due to hypoxia and might point to increased ventilation to compensate for metabolic acidosis. Additionally, the combination of dry mucous membranes, thirst, tachycardia, fever, and borderline blood pressure is concerning for some degree of dehydration and/or sepsis necessitating volume resuscitation. Collectively, his fever, increased respiratory rate, and heart rate could be consistent with sepsis and were concerning for a patient at high risk of progressing to critical illness. Such a patient needs both treatment to prevent the need for life-sustaining interventions and close monitoring in a critical care setting.

Basic supportive care

Beyond the initial emergency triage, priority signs and symptoms should be assessed to identify individuals who require closer monitoring, given their higher risk of progressing to critical illness. This is particularly important during outbreaks of EBOD, where organ dysfunction has been identified as a modifiable risk factor for mortality (2–3). In an ideal setting, patients with, and at risk for, life-threatening illness would be admitted to an intensive care unit (ICU) or other type of critical care setting. These patients require higher resource life-sustaining interventions including vasopressors, high-flow oxygen or non-invasive ventilation, and mechanical ventilation or extra-corporeal membrane oxygenation (ECMO), measures that necessitate closer monitoring and a higher provider-to-patient ratio. If resources are limited and healthcare settings are designed and staffed to enable close and frequent patient assessments, patients who are at high risk for developing life-threatening illness but do not yet need life-sustaining interventions could be closely monitored in non-critical care settings. This can work as long as patient assessments are structured in a way to quickly identify a patient who is clinically deteriorating.

The evaluation can be aided by checklists or flowcharts. In the case of EVD, the WHO has introduced a daily assessment checklist with nine questions to guide clinicians (6) **(Table 24.1)**. The systematic assessments and regular repeat assessments of all patients are essential to identify patients in need of emergency treatment and modify treatments as the patient's clinical status evolves. Serial assessments include volume status and volume resuscitation, symptom management, vital and other physical signs, and clinical chemistry including electrolytes, haematology, and coagulation parameters. Treatment is directed at co-infections and complications including encephalopathy, seizures, respiratory failure, acute renal failure, anaemia, and/or bleeding. Supportive care includes the administration of supplemental oxygen, anti-emetics, oral or intravenous fluids, and renal replacement therapy (RRT) where appropriate.

Just as triage and regular assessments and re-evaluation of patients help identify individuals in need of critical care, they can also help with de-escalation of care as a patient improves. Although the decision to transfer a patient out of a critical care setting is patient-, provider-, and health system-dependent, patients who display evidence of clinical improvement and those who no longer require life-sustaining interventions nor need more frequent monitoring than every six hours could be considered for transfer out of a critical care setting.

Assessment	Plan

1. Is the patient at high risk of complications?
   a. Airway obstruction or respiratory distress?
   b. Tachypnea (RR >22 or fast for age) or SpO$_2$ <92%?
   c. Shock? Hypotension, weak or rapid pulse, cold extremities, or delayed capillary refill?
   d. Signs of severe dehydration?
   e. Altered mentation or seizure?
   f. Oliguria or anuria, urine output <0.5 (adult)/1.0 mL (child)/kg/hour?
   g. Haemorrhagic manifestations?
   h. Severe hypoglycaemia (glucose <54 mg/dL or <3 mmol/L)?
   i. Severe electrolyte abnormalities?
   j. Severe weakness with inability to ambulate or eat/drink?
	❏ NOT at high risk
	Regular assessment – three times a day
	❏ HIGH risk
	Increased interval of assessments: _____
	❏ Plan: _____

2. Fluid status assessment
   a. Able to drink normally?
   b. Able to drink some but not enough to correct dehydration or meet daily fluid requirements?
   c. Signs of sepsis or shock (HR >90, SBP <100, RR >22). And for child: cold extremities, weak fast pulse, delayed capillary refill >3 sec?
	❏ Continue with oral fluids
	❏ Add maintenance fluids
	❏ Bolus IV fluids: _____ mL

3. Laboratory assessment
   a. Does potassium or magnesium need to be replaced?
   b. Is renal failure present?
      i. If yes, has the patient been adequately fluid resuscitated?
      ii. Is a urinary catheter needed to monitor urine output?
	❏ Replace potassium
	❏ Replace magnesium
	❏ Place a urinary catheter
	❏ Use ultrasound to assess fluid status

4. Severe hypoglycaemia
   a. Evidence of hypoglycaemia (glucose <54 mg/dL or <3 mmol/L)?
      i. If yes, are they symptomatic and require D50 or D10?
      ii. If no, are they able to eat and drink or do they require continuous infusion of D5 or D10?
	❏ Euglycaemic
	❏ D50 (adult) or D10 (child) for symptomatic hypoglycaemia
	❏ D5 or D10 for asymptomatic hypoglycaemia

5. Treatment of potential bacterial co-infections
   a. Is the patient at high risk of co-infections?
      i. If yes, is the patient being treated with ceftriaxone?
      ii. If no, is the patient being treated with cefixime?
   b. Does the patient still need to be treated with antibiotics?
	❏ Ceftriaxone
	❏ Cefixime
	❏ Antibiotics discontinued

6. Treatment of potential malaria
   a. Does the patient have signs of severe malaria?
      i. If yes, is the patient being treated with artesunate?
      ii. If no, is the patient being treated with an antimalarial medication?
   b. Can the antimalarials be stopped due to a negative malaria test?
	❏ Artesunate
	❏ Artesunate-amodiaquine (ASAQ)
	❏ Malaria-negative
	❏ Malaria treatment completed

7. Nutrition
   a. Is the patient able to eat and drink?
      i. If yes, can maintenance fluids be stopped?
	❏ Able to eat and drink
	❏ NOT able to eat and drink and requires maintenance fluids

8. Prevention
   a. Can the IV line be removed?
   b. Can the urinary catheter be removed?
   c. Does the patient require assistance walking or can they walk on their own?
	Remove IV line ❏ Yes ❏ No
	Remove urinary catheter
	❏ Yes ❏ No
	Patient requires assistance walking
	❏ Yes ❏ No

Assessment	Plan
9. Is the patient a pregnant woman? a. Is she having an abortion? Premature birth? Has she had an incomplete abortion? If no, is the foetus viable?	Date of last menstrual period: _____ Echo: _____ Plan: _____
D, dextrose; HR, heart rate; IV, intravenous; RR, respiratory rate; SBP, systolic blood pressure; SpO$_2$, oxygen saturation	

Table 24.1: Daily assessment checklist for patients with EVD
(World Health Organization, reproduced under CC-BY-NC-ND license (6))

Fluid status assessment and treatment

Volume resuscitation is a crucial aspect of critical care to maintain tissue perfusion in patients with hypovolaemia due to dehydration, haemorrhage, sepsis, and/or septic shock. Dehydration is caused by volume loss due to vomiting, diarrhoea, or insensible losses, and typically responds well to volume repletion. In the early stages of dehydration, volume repletion can occur through oral or nasogastric routes, whereas more profound dehydration often requires intravenous resuscitation. Sepsis (7), however, is defined by life-threatening organ dysfunction due to a dysregulated immune response to an infection. It requires both intravenous volume resuscitation and pathogen-specific therapy. Septic shock is a subset of sepsis characterised by persistent hypotension despite adequate fluid resuscitation and evidence of increased lactic acid levels denoting impaired tissue hypoxia, necessitating the use of vasopressor medication to maintain organ perfusion pressure. Central venous catheters (CVCs) and arterial lines are usually required for treatment and monitoring, respectively, though intra-osseous cannulation can be considered for temporary medication administration. As infection, sepsis, and septic shock exist on a spectrum, early recognition and appropriate treatment can prevent progression to more severe disease and death. Patients with sepsis and septic shock require fluid resuscitation that is balanced to maintain tissue perfusion without causing fluid overload. Importantly, the volume and rate of fluid resuscitation should take into account a number of host and disease-related factors including the patient's age, nutritional status, underlying comorbidities, ongoing fluid losses, anaemia, physical examination findings, and the aetiology of infection.

In sepsis and septic shock, the goal of fluid resuscitation is to restore organ perfusion. Reassessment of both indices of organ perfusion as well as markers of fluid overload is critical to achieve the goals of fluid resuscitation without causing harm. Fluid resuscitation can be guided by improving lactate levels and mean arterial pressure (MAP) to >65 in adults. However, this requires experienced staff and the requisite equipment to measure blood pressure and perform blood chemistry analysis. When advanced haemodynamic monitoring is not available, adequate perfusion may be guided by physical examination findings including temperature of extremities, skin mottling, capillary refill time, urine output >0.5 mL/kg/hour, or response to fluid bolus as assessed by blood pressure and heart rate before and after. As in all aspects of critical care medicine, fluid resuscitation beyond the initial volume repletion is dependent on the frequent reassessment of volume status and indices of tissue perfusion and must be balanced with signs of volume overload including peripheral oedema, elevated jugular venous distention, increasing oxygen requirement, and/or evidence of pulmonary oedema. Separate recommendations for paediatric populations can be found in the 2020

Surviving Sepsis Campaign International Guidelines for the management of septic shock and organ failure (8).

Intravenous vasopressor medications are used in patients who have persistent hypotension despite adequate fluid resuscitation. Importantly, this requires the ability to precisely deliver vasopressor medications and closely monitor the patient. Due to the risk of tissue injury and necrosis if extravasation occurs, it is recommended that vasopressors be delivered through a CVC. The use of CVCs requires experienced personnel to insert the CVC and manage it to avoid infection, and the requisite equipment to safely place a CVC, including ultrasound for direct visualisation. Additionally, arterial lines are also recommended for continuous blood pressure monitoring to ensure the lowest amount of vasopressor necessary is used and to avoid drug-associated complications including arrhythmias and elevated blood pressure above the intended target.

In outbreaks of EBOD, patients often develop severe gastrointestinal symptoms, including voluminous diarrhoea and anorexia, quickly leading to hypovolaemia due to a combination of dehydration, sepsis, and septic shock. Early recognition and volume resuscitation are essential to maintain tissue perfusion and prevent organ dysfunction. Having the necessary equipment, trained personnel, systems for monitoring and responding, and a treatment unit that affords safe but continuous observation is essential to delivering life-saving critical care.

LABORATORY TESTING

Critically ill patients often have evidence of electrolyte and acid-base disturbances that can be life-threatening and require immediate management and close monitoring. Routine laboratory tests including clinical chemistry (e.g., sodium, potassium, chloride, blood urea nitrogen, creatinine, glucose, calcium, magnesium, phosphate, albumin, bilirubin, liver function tests, lactate, creatine kinase), haematology (e.g., white blood cell count, haemoglobin, haematocrit, platelet count), and arterial blood gas analysis (e.g., pH, pCO_2, arterial oxygen level, bicarbonate) are essential in the management of critically ill patients. The frequency of laboratory testing depends on the patient and available laboratory and clinical capacity.

In EBOD, profound diarrhoea, vomiting, and anorexia, coupled with end-organ dysfunction, contribute to perturbations of electrolytes and acid-base balance. Early identification and treatment prevent downstream complications including arrhythmias (9–11), altered mental status, and other organ failure. Additionally, life-threatening hypoglycaemia has been increasingly recognised in paediatric and adult populations infected with EBOD and requires close monitoring and treatment, especially in patients with altered mental status and seizures (12). Close monitoring of these laboratory values requires a laboratory infrastructure and systems in place to safely collect blood, transfer samples to the lab, report the results, and interpret the findings, and the resources to treat and monitor the response to treatments. In outbreaks of highly transmissible infectious diseases, these need to be conducted with rigorous infection prevention and control (IPC) procedures. Point-of-care devices can help facilitate daily or more frequent monitoring of clinical chemistry and haematology but often lack the full complement of laboratory tests needed and/or have a restricted dynamic range of analytes that can be tested.

ORGAN SUPPORTIVE CARE

End-organ dysfunction is an important modifiable risk factor for mortality in critical illness. Creatinine, a marker of acute renal failure, is associated with increased mortality in critically ill patients including those with sepsis and EBOD. Acute renal injury is potentially preventable if organ perfusion pressure can be restored and the underlying cause treated early. Diagnostic laboratory support can help identify the aetiology of renal failure and complications as well as monitor the response to treatment. In patients who develop renal failure, haemodialysis is sometimes required to treat complications such as acidosis, hyperkalaemia, volume overload, and uraemia. Similarly, acute hypoxic or hypercarbic respiratory failure and/or ventilatory insufficiency in the setting of metabolic acidosis are complications that require organ-specific supportive care including supplemental oxygenation, non-invasive ventilation (continuous positive airway pressure [CPAP] and bilevel positive airway pressure [BIPAP]), high-flow oxygen, invasive mechanical ventilation, and/or ECMO. Each of these tools of organ supportive critical care medicine is a resource-intensive therapy that requires an infrastructure of experienced personnel, equipment, and consumables, strategies for initiation, monitoring, and discontinuation, and specially designed treatment centres to safely deliver these therapies. Importantly, using any of these devices outside of the required infrastructure can lead to patient injury and/or death and increase the risk of infection in HCWs.

Acute respiratory distress syndrome (ARDS) is a severe inflammatory complication of the lungs that results from a variety of aetiologies, most commonly sepsis. Despite many clinical trials, only two interventions have been shown to consistently reduce mortality in patients with ARDS—low tidal volume ventilation and prone positioning. Low tidal volume ventilation refers to the use of tidal volumes of around 6 cc/kg of body weight. This reduces ventilator-induced lung injury. In the ARMADA trial, compared with patients who received tidal volumes of 12 cc/kg predicted body weight, patients randomised to a tidal volume of 6 cc/kg of body weight had a lower mortality rate (31 per cent versus 40 per cent) and a greater number of ventilator-free days (12 versus 10 days) (13). This is an important example of how advanced critical care requires experienced centres and the right infrastructure to avoid patient harm due to organ supportive interventions.

Prone ventilation reduces mortality in patients with moderate-to-severe ARDS. In the PROSEVA study (14), 466 patients receiving low tidal volume ventilation and requiring FiO_2 of >0.6 and PEEP >5 cm H_2O were randomised within 33 hours of intubation to prone ventilation for at least 16 hours or usual care. Compared with the supine ventilation group, patients who received prone ventilation had reduced 28-day (16 per cent versus 33 per cent) and 90-day mortality (24 per cent versus 41 per cent). With appropriately trained staff and when done in a setting that affords comprehensive care and continuous observation, proning is a low-tech intervention that can be operationalised in resource-limited settings.

ECMO is a form of prolonged mechanical cardiopulmonary support that is often used for patients with profound hypoxic and/or hypercapnic respiratory failure that is not responding to conventional mechanical ventilation. Two forms of ECMO exist including venovenous ECMO and venoarterial ECMO, with both providing respiratory support and only venoarterial ECMO also providing cardiac support. While clinical trials comparing the use of ECMO with conventional mechanical ventilation in patients with acute respiratory failure have produced mixed results, a consistent finding has been that patients who are transferred to experienced centres have improved outcomes, highlighting the role of experienced providers and established systems or strategies of care in addition to advanced technology in the safe and effective delivery of advanced critical care interventions.

> **Advanced critical care in Ebola virus outbreaks**
>
> In Ebola virus outbreaks, advanced critical care, including the use of RRT, non-invasive ventilation, and invasive mechanical ventilation, has largely been provided to patients who were treated outside of Africa. Of 27 patients with EVD treated in the U.S. or Europe, five (19 per cent) received RRT, four (15 per cent) received non-invasive ventilation, and seven (26 per cent) received invasive mechanical ventilation (15). Both intubation for mechanical ventilation and central line placement required careful consideration of the infection risks to HCWs. Intubation was conducted with rapid sequence induction and neuromuscular blockade followed by direct airway visualisation using video laryngoscopy to minimise the potential for aerosolisation. However, confirmation of endotracheal tube placement was challenging in some centres due to IPC practices. Continuous RRT was selected over intermittent haemodialysis to minimise HCW exposure to blood (12).
>
> Mechanical ventilation and RRT were operationalised for less than 1 per cent of patients in Guinea, Liberia, and Sierra Leone during the same 2014–2016 Ebola virus epidemic due to the lack of supplies and equipment, treatment units that enable the provision of advanced critical care, experienced providers, and strategies for implementing advanced critical care.
>
> Similarly, the recent COVID-19 pandemic revealed marked inequity in access to advanced critical care as the use of mechanical ventilation, ECMO, and even prone positioning, not to mention diagnostics, vaccinations, and therapeutics, was largely restricted to countries with well-resourced and experienced centres.

Central nervous system complications, including altered mental status, delirium, seizures, and encephalopathy, are important complications of critical illness and require prevention strategies, urgent treatment, and close monitoring. Using the Confusion Assessment Method for ICU patients (CAM-ICU) screening tool, delirium was reported in over 80 per cent of patients during their ICU stay (16). Multiple potential aetiologies of altered mental status, encephalopathy, and delirium should be considered, most commonly metabolic encephalopathy from fluid and electrolyte abnormalities (e.g., dehydration, hypoglycaemia, hypo/hypernatremia, hypo/hypercalcaemia), infection (e.g., sepsis, meningitis, and encephalitis), organ dysfunction (e.g., uraemia, hepatic encephalopathy), pain, and drug toxicity (e.g., sedation medications). Management includes treatment of the underlying condition, removal of an offending agent if present, provision of supportive care, and treatment of agitation. Importantly, multidisciplinary approaches can be taken to reduce the chance of developing delirium including the facilitation of physiologic sleep, early mobilisation (17), and avoidance of deliriogenic medications (18).

CO-INFECTIONS

Co-infections or secondary infections should be considered in all critically ill patients, particularly in outbreak settings given the non-specific nature of presenting signs/symptoms for many outbreak-prone pathogens. During Ebola virus outbreaks, co-infections with malaria have been reported in up to 24 per cent of patients (19). Bacterial co-infections have also been reported in case reports of patients with EBOD treated outside of West Africa. Additionally, prolonged hospitalisation for critically ill patients, coupled with invasive catheters needed for vasopressors and dialysis, the use of urinary catheters, and mechanical ventilation, increases the risk for nosocomial infections including central line-associated bloodstream infections, urinary tract infections, and ventilator-associated pneumonia. As a result, readily available testing, or consideration of empiric treatment, for common co-infections including malaria, respiratory viruses, and bacterial pathogens is an essential component of critical care. Similarly, systematic evaluation of antibiotic or antimalarial courses is of equal value to determine when antibiotics can be stopped or de-escalated to prevent the development of antibiotic-associated complications including the development of *Clostridium difficile* infections and/or drug resistance. In other words, knowing when to stop is as important as knowing when to start.

PSYCHOSOCIAL AND PALLIATIVE CARE

Psychosocial support and palliative care are essential aspects of critical care designed to reduce the psychological suffering of patients facing life-threatening illnesses. Patients' families are also important targets of this care. This includes the early identification of psychological suffering or distress and treatment focused on preventing and relieving suffering including managing physical and psychological symptoms, addressing social and economic needs, and providing religious and spiritual support. Treatment units that allow the safe visitation of family and community members can also play an important role in the relief of suffering of patients and their families, while also reducing rumours and misinformation about care during an outbreak.

TIME TO PATHOGEN-SPECIFIC TREATMENT AND INITIATION OF CRITICAL CARE

In critically ill patients, the early identification of the pathogen causing the illness and control of the source of infection is intimately linked with survival. This is particularly true in patients with sepsis or septic shock, where delays in the initiation of appropriate antibiotics are associated with worse outcomes. A retrospective study of almost 18,000 patients with sepsis and septic shock showed a linear increase in mortality for every hour delay in antibiotic administration (20), highlighting the importance of timely diagnosis and initiation of empiric pathogen-specific treatment.

The same is true in outbreaks. The PALM randomised controlled trial of four therapeutics for EVD found an 11 per cent increase in the odds of death for each day of symptoms before enrolment, again highlighting the link between early initiation of pathogen-specific treatment with survival. Similarly, the early initiation of influenza and anti-SARS-CoV-2 therapeutics was associated with lower rates of progression to severe disease including hospitalisation and mortality (21–25).

The same is also true for critical care. Data from observational and registry studies consistently demonstrate an increase in severity associated with delays in the admission of critically ill patients to an ICU. A retrospective observational cohort study including more than 14,000 patients who were admitted to an ICU in the Netherlands found that prolonged emergency department to ICU time (>2.4 hours) was associated with increased mortality (26). Studies in the U.S. found an increased mortality rate among those who remained in the emergency department for longer than six hours before transfer to an ICU (17 per cent vs 12.9 per cent; p<0.001) (27). The SPOTlight study, a prospective cohort study of consecutive hospitalised patients assessed for admission to an ICU, found that admission within four hours of assessment was associated with lower 90-day mortality (28). Importantly, this study also demonstrated that ICU admissions within four hours were less frequent as bed occupancy increased, highlighting that a surge of patients, as occurs during an outbreak, can quickly overwhelm the capacity of a healthcare system. The disparity in access to ICUs globally poses a significant challenge particularly during outbreaks in both well- and under-resourced settings. During outbreaks in settings without ICUs, consideration must be directed to installing treatment units that allow regular assessments and delivery of supportive care and advanced critical care. Experienced staff need to be at ratios that enable personalised care and have the necessary equipment and systems or strategies required to ensure equal access to care.

PROVIDING CRITICAL CARE IN OUTBREAKS: STAFF, STUFF, SYSTEMS, SPACE (4S'S)

The delivery of patient-centric critical care is logistically challenging in that it requires a complement of clinical expertise (staff), medical equipment and supplies, and supply chain (stuff), triage, treatment protocols and trainings, outbreak response plans (systems), and healthcare infrastructure that protects HCWs but also increases access between providers and patients (space) (1). Given the resource-intensive nature of critical care and the link between clinical outcomes and time from illness onset to ICU admission, considerable planning must be conducted to be able to provide critical care in an outbreak setting. Settings with no critical care capacities prior to an outbreak will struggle to introduce capacities in an infectious disease emergency. They need to be established as part of normal healthcare activities before an emergency and include national- and facility-level preparedness plans on how to surge in a public health emergency.

Staff

Critical care cannot be provided without sufficient numbers of experienced providers (staff). In studies evaluating outcomes in sepsis and ARDS, patients who receive care at more experienced centres consistently do better. Importantly, experienced providers are not limited to just critical care physicians and nurses but are complemented by those who enable critical care providers to do their jobs. This list includes respiratory therapists, subspecialty consultants including nephrologists, paediatricians, obstetrics and gynaecology providers, and laboratory technicians, as well as waste management staff and logistics coordinators who purchase equipment and consumables. Even with the right expertise, the care of critically ill patients requires sufficient staffing (provider-to-patient ratios) to assess, re-assess, and adapt the care needed to each patient. This is especially true in responding to outbreaks where surges of patients can quickly overwhelm healthcare system capacity, threatening not only patients who are infected with the outbreak pathogen but also patients with every other disease. As outbreaks are often extremely stressful for providers and their families, psychosocial support before, during, and following an outbreak can serve to improve the resilience of the workforce.

Stuff

The care of critically ill patients is a resource-intensive effort requiring equipment including oxygen, CPAP/BIPAP machines, high-flow nasal cannulas, mechanical ventilators, dialysis machines, ECMO machines, and laboratory machines, along with all the consumables that are required for their use, and the supply chain to ensure continued access to the necessary equipment and supplies. "Stuff" also includes essential infrastructure including reliable and consistent electricity supply, running water, and equipment for handling waste. The procurement of equipment and supplies and the maintenance of equipment is a time-intensive activity that requires considerable planning in advance of an outbreak as delivery takes time, especially when the destination is a resource-limited setting.

Systems

"Systems" refers to how the staff, stuff, and space function together. The implementation of IPC systems enables providers and patients to flow through a treatment unit in a specific and consistent manner to mitigate nosocomial transmission. The systematic evaluation and re-assessment of patients, the use of low tidal volume ventilation in patients with ARDS, and the WHO-optimised supportive care guidelines for patients with Ebola virus disease are examples of clinical care protocols that enable systems of care to ensure equal and effective care is afforded to all patients. The implementation of these systems requires training, practice, re-evaluation, and improvement to ensure systems are resilient and staff are prepared.

Space

The delivery of critical care is dependent on the ability to assess and re-assess patients to identify those who require emergent treatment and to adjust that treatment to maximise the benefit and minimise the side effects as the clinical course evolves. However, during outbreaks of highly transmissible infectious pathogens, infection control makes access to patients challenging. For example, during the 2014–2016 EVD epidemic, patients were isolated in opaque tents that limited the ability to directly and continuously monitor them, provide direct treatment, and enable visitation by families. This physical set up also limited the ability to mentor HCWs in patient care. Innovative treatment units such as the CUBE (**Figure 24.1**) (29) and other closed monitoring treatment spaces allow the continuous safe monitoring and treatment of patients without the use of personal protective equipment (PPE). It also allows less experienced providers, family members, and community members to be bedside to assist with care and build trust (29).

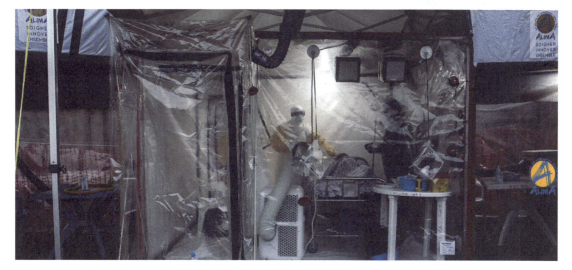

Figure 24.1: The Alliance for Medical Action (ALIMA) CUBE
ALIMA's game-changing innovation: the CUBE [Internet]. https://alima.ngo/en/alima-cube/; 2022.

The COVID-19 pandemic resulted in an unprecedented number of patients who required critical care. In some instances, this demand outstripped the local capacity, which led to increased mortality (30). Scaling up critical care capacity requires consideration of the 4S's. Critical care-trained providers without the necessary equipment, staffing ratios, care strategies, or in a healthcare setting that does not allow for continuous close monitoring and intervention will be limited in their ability to provide basic or advanced critical care. Similarly, increased numbers of mechanical ventilators without experienced healthcare providers or a continuous supply of oxygen will not only fail to help patients in respiratory failure but could lead to harm if this care is delivered incorrectly. Hospitals in the U.S. and Canada employed several interventions to rapidly increase critical care capacity including cancelling elective surgery, redeploying HCWs to critical care settings, and using general floor beds for non-ventilated critically ill patients and ICU telemedicine. As a result, surge capacity planning is an essential aspect of healthcare planning.

Case study – part 3

Back to our patient with EVD. He was initially treated with antipyretics, analgesics, a proton-pump inhibitor, intravenous antibiotics, and oral hydration. He started to deteriorate five days following admission with marked rises in aspartate aminotransferase (AST) out of proportion to alanine aminotransferase (ALT) and creatinine levels. Clinically, his urine output decreased to <0.5 mL/kg/hour and he developed altered mental status. Fever was noted and viraemia on polymerase chain reaction (PCR) was detected.

The patient's hospital course was complicated by hypotension (88/40 mmHg and 76/38 mmHg on two successive measurements) and hypoglycaemia. The patient was started on artesunate to treat a possible malaria infection. The bladder catheter and venous access catheters were also all changed but no soft tissue infection was observed clinically. Unfortunately, the provision of vasopressors was not possible due to the use of a tent for an ETU.

Because he was in the critical care section of the ETU, his low blood pressure was detected early and responded to volume resuscitation. Given the presence of a new fever and hypotension with evidence of end-organ failure with altered mental status and decreasing urine output, this patient's condition was identified immediately as septic shock, prompting appropriate fluid management and empirical antibiotics which resulted in the stabilisation of his condition.

OTHER IMPORTANT FACTORS IN CRITICAL CARE
Communication

Communication between staff, patients, and families is a key factor in all care, and especially in the ICU. Face-to-face communication is not always possible or can be compromised by masks, visors, and hoods that might obscure hearing and vision. One lesson of the COVID-19 pandemic was the importance of clear and timely communication from leadership (of all levels) that can help ease anxieties and provide support to HCWs, patients, and the affected communities (31–32). In EBOD outbreaks, continuous effort has been made to engage communities and families. The CUBE as a treatment space allows family members to see and speak to patients even while they are isolated and undergoing treatment, which builds trust and facilitates communication (29).

Special population groups

Special population groups may also require special provisions during outbreaks. Children differ from adults both physiologically and psychologically. Children with EBOD can die within the first 24 hours of admission to hospital (33) so timely triage and identification of a sick child is even more important. Normal values of vitals need to be adjusted for age, and any medications, including fluids, should be adjusted for age and weight.

Pregnant women are also physiologically different from other adults and will need specific treatments to protect them and their foetuses. As a result, clinicians should always check if patients of childbearing potential might be pregnant (6). Pregnant patients often require closer observation and monitoring and might require the use of different medications or dosages. Preparations for obstetric emergencies and neonatal care are essential (29).

Older populations are also vulnerable to infectious diseases and often suffer higher mortality and morbidity due to poorer physiological reserve and pre-existing conditions. Discussions about escalation plans should be made early with these patients while they are able to have conversations. Not all interventions in advanced supportive critical care may be suitable for them and some might lead to poor outcomes (34–35).

> **Case study – part 4**
>
> The learning points from the critical care Michel was fortunate enough to access are as follows:
> - early triage identified this patient as high risk for developing life-threatening illness given tachycardia, tachypnea, and borderline blood pressure necessitating admission to a critical care setting for supportive care and close monitoring
> - early diagnosis, continual assessment, and regular clinical and laboratory monitoring (haematology, biochemistry, biology, coagulation test, and antibiotic culture, among others) are essential aspects of good critical care
> - the delivery of critical care requires the 4S's: a treatment space that enables close monitoring and the ability to clinically intervene as needed, systems including triage and optimised supportive care protocol, critically-trained staff, and critical care supplies (stuff) including vasopressors

Learning in real time

The nature of outbreaks can be unpredictable, and many infectious pathogens (such as SARS-CoV-2) are able to evolve through outbreaks. In the face of profound uncertainty, acquiring knowledge about the disease and identifying interventions that are safe, effective, and accessible are paramount goals. Standardised data collection and reporting will remain important, and this needs to be linked to larger bodies of information (e.g., national information systems) so that data can continue to be collected and managed for further surveillance and response. Even in low-resource settings, research and innovation play a big part and there are lessons learnt throughout the management of outbreaks that can further inform best practices. Clinical research platforms with expedited ethical approvals, either fast-tracked or pre-approved for outbreak-prone pathogens in the region, present an important opportunity. Such platforms facilitate the collection of essential data on transmission patterns, host-, pathogen-, and disease-related factors associated with severe illness or death, and viral replication kinetics. This information can determine therapeutic windows which ultimately provide an evidence base for prevention and treatment strategies (**See Chapter 18, Research to inform practice; See Chapter 27, Research for therapeutics**).

CONCLUSION

The one certainty about outbreaks is that they will happen again. Transitioning from crisis response to "integrated systems of preparedness, response, and recovery" will not only improve the response to outbreaks but increase the resiliency of the healthcare infrastructure of affected communities. This will benefit the care of patients with every other disease. Enhanced outbreak preparedness will require consideration of the 4S's of clinical care. Critical care is an essential component particularly during times of uncertainty that come with outbreaks of new, highly pathogenic, or highly transmissible infectious diseases in which surges can overwhelm healthcare settings. In the past, outbreak response strategies to protect communities have focused on prevention through isolation. While isolation is effective at curtailing transmission, it offers little in the way of survival for patients who are isolated. Optimised clinical care, including critical care, is essential and effective at reducing mortality during outbreaks. During the 2014–2016 Ebola epidemic, the reduced case fatality ratio of patients with EVD who were treated outside of Africa (18.5 per cent) compared to the case fatality ratio reported in West Africa (estimated 82.9 per cent) is likely attributable to the availability and provision of advanced critical care (15,36). This is particularly true in the absence of effective therapeutics, where critical care provides life-sustaining treatment until an effective immune response can be mounted. While critical care is resource intensive, it cannot be acceptable to have two standards of care – one for those in well-resourced parts of the world and a lesser standard in countries with under-resourced healthcare infrastructure.

*In WHO terminology, EBOD refers to Ebola virus diseases where the exact type of filovirus causing the infection is still not known. EVD refers to Ebola virus disease where the Ebola virus is known to be the infective agent.

REFERENCES:

1. Anesi GL, Lynch Y, Evans L. A conceptual and adaptable approach to hospital preparedness for acute surge events due to emerging infectious diseases. Crit Care Explor. 2020 Apr;2(4):e0110. https://doi.org/10.1097/CCE.0000000000000110 PMID:32426752.
2. World Health Organization. Emergency Triage Assessment and Treatment (ETAT) course [Internet]. [cited 2023 Jun 12]. https://www.who.int/publications-detail-redirect/9241546875.
3. Iacorossi L, Fauci AJ, Napoletano A, D'Angelo D, Salomone K, Latina R, et al. Triage protocol for allocation of critical health resources during Covid-19 pandemic and public health emergencies. A narrative review. Acta Biomed. 2020 Nov;91(4):e2020162. https://doi.org/10.23750/abm.v91i4.10393 PMID:33525236.
4. World Health Organization. Case definition recommendations for Ebola or Marburg Virus diseases [Internet]. 2014. https://www.euro.who.int/__data/assets/pdf_file/0007/268747/Case-definition-recommendations-for-Ebola-or-Marburg-Virus-Diseases-Eng.pdf.

5. Hsu CH, Champaloux SW, Keïta S, Martel L, Bilivogui P, Knust B, et al. Sensitivity and specificity of suspected case definition used during West Africa Ebola epidemic. Emerg Infect Dis. 2018 Jan;24(1):9–14. https://doi.org/10.3201/eid2401.161678 PMID:29260687.

6. World Health Organization. Optimized supportive care for Ebola virus disease. 2019. https://www.who.int/publications/i/item/9789241515894.

7. Singer M, Deutschman CS, Seymour CW, Shankar-Hari M, Annane D, Bauer M, et al. The third international consensus definitions for sepsis and septic shock (Sepsis-3). JAMA. 2016 Feb;315(8):801–10. https://doi.org/10.1001/jama.2016.0287 PMID:26903338.

8. SCCM | Pediatric Patients [Internet]. Society of Critical Care Medicine (SCCM). [cited 2023 Jun 14]. https://sccm.org/SurvivingSepsisCampaign/Guidelines/Pediatric-Patients.

9. Schieffelin JS, Shaffer JG, Goba A, Gbakie M, Gire SK, Colubri A, et al.; KGH Lassa Fever Program; Viral Hemorrhagic Fever Consortium; WHO Clinical Response Team. Clinical illness and outcomes in patients with Ebola in Sierra Leone. N Engl J Med. 2014 Nov;371(22):2092–100. https://doi.org/10.1056/NEJMoa1411680 PMID:25353969.

10. Lyon GM, Mehta AK, Varkey JB, Brantly K, Plyler L, McElroy AK, et al.; Emory Serious Communicable Diseases Unit. Clinical care of two patients with Ebola virus disease in the United States. N Engl J Med. 2014 Dec;371(25):2402–9. https://doi.org/10.1056/NEJMoa1409838 PMID:25390460.

11. Hunt L, Gupta-Wright A, Simms V, Tamba F, Knott V, Tamba K, et al. Clinical presentation, biochemical, and haematological parameters and their association with outcome in patients with Ebola virus disease: an observational cohort study. Lancet Infect Dis. 2015 Nov;15(11):1292–9. https://doi.org/10.1016/S1473-3099(15)00144-9 PMID:26271406.

12. Jacob ST, Crozier I, Fischer WA 2nd, Hewlett A, Kraft CS, Vega MA, et al. Ebola virus disease. Nat Rev Dis Primers. 2020 Feb;6(1):13. https://doi.org/10.1038/s41572-020-0147-3 PMID:32080199.

13. Acute Respiratory Distress Syndrome Network; Brower RG, Matthay MA, Morris A, Schoenfeld D, Thompson BT, Wheeler A. Ventilation with lower tidal volumes as compared with traditional tidal volumes for acute lung injury and the acute respiratory distress syndrome. N Engl J Med. 2000 May;342(18):1301–8. https://doi.org/10.1056/NEJM200005043421801 PMID:10793162.

14. Guérin C, Reignier J, Richard JC, Beuret P, Gacouin A, Boulain T, et al.; PROSEVA Study Group. Prone positioning in severe acute respiratory distress syndrome. N Engl J Med. 2013 Jun;368(23):2159–68. https://doi.org/10.1056/NEJMoa1214103 PMID:23688302.

15. Uyeki TM, Mehta AK, Davey RT Jr, Liddell AM, Wolf T, Vetter P, et al.; Working Group of the U.S.–European Clinical Network on Clinical Management of Ebola Virus Disease Patients in the U.S. and Europe. Clinical management of Ebola virus disease in the United States and Europe. N Engl J Med. 2016 Feb;374(7):636–46. https://doi.org/10.1056/NEJMoa1504874 PMID:26886522.

16. Ely EW, Inouye SK, Bernard GR, Gordon S, Francis J, May L, et al. Delirium in mechanically ventilated patients: validity and reliability of the confusion assessment method for the intensive care unit (CAM-ICU). JAMA. 2001 Dec;286(21):2703–10. https://doi.org/10.1001/jama.286.21.2703 PMID:11730446.

17. Schweickert WD, Pohlman MC, Pohlman AS, Nigos C, Pawlik AJ, Esbrook CL, et al. Early physical and occupational therapy in mechanically ventilated, critically ill patients: a randomised controlled trial. Lancet. 2009 May;373(9678):1874–82. https://doi.org/10.1016/S0140-6736(09)60658-9 PMID:19446324.

18. Clegg A, Young JB. Which medications to avoid in people at risk of delirium: a systematic review. Age Ageing. 2011 Jan;40(1):23–9. https://doi.org/10.1093/ageing/afq140 PMID:21068014.

19. Kerber R, Krumkamp R, Diallo B, Jaeger A, Rudolf M, Lanini S, et al. Analysis of diagnostic findings from the European mobile laboratory in Guéckédou, Guinea, March 2014 through March 2015. J Infect Dis. 2016 Oct;214 suppl 3:S250–7. https://doi.org/10.1093/infdis/jiw269 PMID:27638946.

20. Ferrer R, Martin-Loeches I, Phillips G, Osborn TM, Townsend S, Dellinger RP, et al. Empiric antibiotic treatment reduces mortality in severe sepsis and septic shock from the first hour: results from a guideline-based performance improvement program. Crit Care Med. 2014 Aug;42(8):1749–55. https://doi.org/10.1097/CCM.0000000000000330 PMID:24717459.

21. Mehta RM, Bansal S, Bysani S, Kalpakam H. A shorter symptom onset to remdesivir treatment (SORT) interval is associated with a lower mortality in moderate-to-severe COVID-19: a real-world analysis. Int J Infect Dis. 2021 May;106:71–7. https://doi.org/10.1016/j.ijid.2021.02.092 PMID:33647517.

22. Gottlieb RL, Nirula A, Chen P, Boscia J, Heller B, Morris J, et al. Effect of bamlanivimab as monotherapy or in combination with etesevimab on viral load in patients with mild to moderate COVID-19: a randomized clinical trial. JAMA. 2021 Feb;325(7):632–44. https://doi.org/10.1001/jama.2021.0202 PMID:33475701.

23. Gupta A, Gonzalez-Rojas Y, Juarez E, Crespo Casal M, Moya J, Falci DR, et al.; COMET-ICE Investigators. Early treatment for Covid-19 with SARS-CoV-2 neutralizing antibody sotrovimab. N Engl J Med. 2021 Nov;385(21):1941–50. https://doi.org/10.1056/NEJMoa2107934 PMID:34706189.

24. Gottlieb RL, Vaca CE, Paredes R, Mera J, Webb BJ, Perez G, et al.; GS-US-540-9012 (PINETREE) Investigators. Early remdesivir to prevent progression to severe Covid-19 in outpatients. N Engl J Med. 2022 Jan;386(4):305–15. https://doi.org/10.1056/NEJMoa2116846 PMID:34937145.

25. Hammond J, Leister-Tebbe H, Gardner A, Abreu P, Bao W, Wisemandle W, et al.; EPIC-HR Investigators. Oral nirmatrelvir for high-risk, nonhospitalized adults with Covid-19. N Engl J Med. 2022 Apr;386(15):1397–408. https://doi.org/10.1056/NEJMoa2118542 PMID:35172054.

26. Groenland CN, Termorshuizen F, Rietdijk WJ, van den Brule J, Dongelmans DA, de Jonge E, et al. Emergency department to ICU time is associated with hospital mortality: a registry analysis of 14,788 patients from six university hospitals in The Netherlands. Crit Care Med. 2019 Nov;47(11):1564–71. https://doi.org/10.1097/CCM.0000000000003957 PMID:31393321.

27. Chalfin DB, Trzeciak S, Likourezos A, Baumann BM, Dellinger RP; DELAY-ED study group. Impact of delayed transfer of critically ill patients from the emergency department to the intensive care unit. Crit Care Med. 2007 Jun;35(6):1477–83. https://doi.org/10.1097/01.CCM.0000266585.74905.5A PMID:17440421.

28. Harris S, Singer M, Sanderson C, Grieve R, Harrison D, Rowan K. Impact on mortality of prompt admission to critical care for deteriorating ward patients: an instrumental variable analysis using critical care bed strain. Intensive Care Med. 2018 May;44(5):606–15. https://doi.org/10.1007/s00134-018-5148-2 PMID:29736785.

29. ALIMA. A comprehensive approach to essential critical care of Ebola patients: experience from outbreaks in Africa. 2021.

30. Bravata DM, Perkins AJ, Myers LJ, Arling G, Zhang Y, Zillich AJ, et al. Association of intensive care unit patient load and demand with mortality rates in US Department of Veterans Affairs hospitals during the COVID-19 pandemic. JAMA Netw Open. 2021 Jan;4(1):e2034266. https://doi.org/10.1001/jamanetworkopen.2020.34266 PMID:33464319.

31. Lasater KB, Aiken LH, Sloane DM, French R, Martin B, Reneau K, et al. Chronic hospital nurse understaffing meets COVID-19: an observational study. BMJ Qual Saf. 2021 Aug;30(8):639–47. https://doi.org/10.1136/bmjqs-2020-011512 PMID:32817399.

32. Ferrara F, Galmarini V, Tosco P, Molinari G, Capelli RM. Redeployment of specialist surgeons in the COVID-19 pandemic in a general hospital: critical issues and suggestions. Acta Biomed. 2021 May;92(2):e2021172. PMID:33988153.

33. World Health Organization. Updated guideline: paediatric emergency triage, assessment and treatment: care of critically-ill children [Internet]. Geneva; 2016 [cited 2022 Dec 26]. 74 p. https://apps.who.int/iris/handle/10665/204463.

34. Mehraeen E, Karimi A, Barzegary A, Vahedi F, Afsahi AM, Dadras O, et al. Predictors of mortality in patients with COVID-19-a systematic review. Eur J Integr Med. 2020 Dec;40:101226. https://doi.org/10.1016/j.eujim.2020.101226 PMID:33101547.

35. Kang SJ, Jung SI. Age-related morbidity and mortality among patients with COVID-19. Infect Chemother. 2020 Jun;52(2):154–64. https://doi.org/10.3947/ic.2020.52.2.154 PMID:32537961.

36. Forna A, Nouvellet P, Dorigatti I, Donnelly CA. Case fatality ratio estimates for the 2013-2016 West African Ebola epidemic: application of boosted regression trees for imputation. Clin Infect Dis. 2020 Jun;70(12):2476–83. https://doi.org/10.1093/cid/ciz678 PMID:31328221.

CHAPTER 25

HEALTHCARE FACILITIES AND INFRASTRUCTURE

by Shreya Dwarakacherla, Moi Lin Ling, and Craig Kenzie

Facility infrastructure design needs to take into account requirements in anticipation of a health emergency, including major outbreaks of infectious diseases. This includes planning for capacity to manage a surge in infectious disease patients. Essential health services must be enabled to safely continue during a crisis and capacities need to be able to be ramped up to deal with an increasing number of infectious patients. Expandability, convertibility, and adaptability are key concepts that would have been factored into a well-designed facility.

However, despite strategic design efforts afforded in the preceding infrastructure, new facilities may be required during a crisis. These can be specifically designed to move case management for an outbreak away from the usual facilities or may be considered only at the time to support (potentially) overwhelmed services. Location and local community buy-in are essential for any structure dealing with infectious patients and the design must factor in important nuances including security and enhanced infection control.

INTRODUCTION

Facility infrastructure design for infectious disease emergencies features in several distinct contexts. Hospitals, laboratories, outpatient healthcare facilities, and other physical structures are part of the usual health system. When designed and constructed, these should ideally have considerations for how they could adapt in an infectious disease emergency to meet infection control and surge capacity needs (1). When this cannot be done in a crisis, hospitals, indeed entire health systems, are at risk of being overwhelmed. When this happens, the case fatality rate for the outbreak-associated pathogen increases, as does overall mortality from other conditions. Public health authorities need to invest in significant planning and expertise as part of outbreak preparedness to ensure their facility infrastructure is sufficiently flexible to maintain both outbreak response and regular operations in an emergency.

When a component of a health system is at risk of being overwhelmed, the leadership of said system must respond urgently to provide alternative facilities beyond the pre-existing structures. These may be new hastily-built structures or repurposed existing buildings quickly fitted out to support the response (and therefore protect the health system). Additionally, these non-traditional health facilities may be established because a new role has emerged, such as an isolation or quarantine facility, or because the infectious agent cannot be managed safely in the usual hospital. Many international humanitarian organisations that specialise in emergency response have predesigned health facility templates for a variety of outbreak sizes and pathogens (2–3). These pre-validated plans can then be quickly adapted to the specific site/structure that has been identified, sometimes within days.

Despite the differing origins of facilities used in an outbreak response, there are general concepts that should be adhered to. In this chapter, we will highlight the strategic considerations and design principles pertaining to facility infrastructure and how they can enable an effective outbreak response. We will explore the considerations of placement and dispersal of facilities as well as the design of specific facilities. Whether the context is a high- or low-resource country, strategic considerations and design principles remain consistent, though the implementation challenges are greater when resources are constrained, and more compromises may have to be made.

When planning new infrastructure or reviewing existing infrastructure, the assessed state of the outbreak has implications on infrastructure design, especially as it relates to the expansion of bed capacity. The dynamics are not always easy to predict. Expansion plans should be integrated into the initial design to minimise future disruptive, messy, loud, and time-consuming work that can impact primary functions.

GENERAL DESIGN FEATURES

This section describes the general principles relevant to infrastructure requirements in an infectious disease emergency that apply to pre-existing, new, or repurposed structures. Whether a modification of an existing structure or creation of a new infrastructure, there are design elements that should be considered in the context of the facility's purpose (4–5).

Pre-existing healthcare facilities should have been designed factoring in the needs in infectious disease emergencies. These include the ability to expand, convert, and adapt. Likewise, even urgently designed new or repurposed structures should consider potential emerging needs.

Concept	Space strategy
Expandability	• Designate vacant, flat, accessible outdoor space in proximity to key facilities (e.g., emergency rooms) for temporary surge/overflow/mass casualty expansion or medium- to long-term semi-permanent/permanent construction • Create standardised modular infrastructure that allows flexibility in conversion and re-adaptation of spaces and quick turnaround response to changing operational space needs
Convertibility	• Unfurnished spaces (shell space) • Furnished spaces such as offices, ancillary spaces, and waiting areas can be repurposed with minimal construction to accommodate other functions (soft space) as administration spaces are less disruptive to relocate/decentralise
Adaptability	• Rooms of standard size with utilities to accommodate several possible uses (generic design) • Rooms are furnished and can be reconfigured and repurposed during an emergency

Table 25.1: Designing flexibilities in healthcare infrastructure (4,6)

Points of entry to the facility

The transmissibility of the pathogen and severity of the disease will determine the degree to which access to the facility may need to be controlled and restricted. Pathogens with high infectivity or that cause severe disease will require strict attention to staff, patient, and visitor movements (7–8). Effective designs enable enhanced screening and pre-emptive isolation, as well as safe entry to the facility or a particular service/department within a facility for the full spectrum of potential patients and staff (**Table 25.2**). The entry of symptomatic patients via a standard emergency department is a particular risk with highly infectious pathogens. Improperly adapted entry points can cause additional transmission and even superspreading events if screening and isolation are not undertaken (**See MERS-CoV outbreak from an emergency room**). Options for the design and management of the points of entry, their internal flow, and connectedness to other departments/services should be carefully considered during the preparedness and readiness phases.

Features	Explanation
Sufficient number of entrances to allow convenient access while allowing control in times of crises	• Patients need to have specific entrances where triage and screening can take place
Cater for patients with diverse medical needs	• Points of entry to a healthcare facility should cater to patients entering with low, highly suspect, or confirmed disease, patients with severe disease related to the outbreak pathogen, patients with other medical conditions, and patients who have died • Infrastructure should physically separate infected patients from those who are presenting for other reasons (**See Chapter 23, Essential services; See Chapter 26, IPC**) • Points of exit for discharging patients should be kept separate from points of entry. This applies whether they are discharged because they have tested negative, recovered, or are transferring to another facility. • A holding bay/isolation rooms at these sites can separate presenting patients with suspected disease, but the risk of transmission within these cohorts needs to be addressed. Appropriately ventilated isolation rooms at the emergency department should be well equipped to manage severe disease presentation, in cases where there is potential airborne transmission.
Facilitate contact between visitors and family members and the patient	• Space for registration and screening of visitors is crucial and visitors should be physically separated when they visit the patient • Fences outside the facility can work to support visitor control when it is not possible to control hospital lobby entrances and doors • These fences will require the deployment of appropriate staff to them, such as health promoters or security staff, or a mix of both, depending on circumstances. Automated turnstile visitor control systems are also available in some countries.
If space permits, facilitate scaled proactive screening and testing with rapid tests	

Table 25.2: Features of points of entry for outbreak readiness

The number of entrances should allow convenient access but be able to be controlled during an infectious disease emergency to enable more oversight of staff, patient, and visitor movement. Means of access may have to adapt to the potentially evolving facility layout and corresponding patient/material/staff flow. Patients presenting for assessment may need specific entrances, different to those for visitors and staff. At patient entry points, there should be capacity to physically separate those with confirmed from suspect infections, as well as those presenting with other conditions or who have died (**See Chapter 23, Essential services; See Chapter 26, IPC**). Clearly delineated isolation rooms/areas should be at these points of entry with appropriate infection prevention and control (IPC) measures (e.g., ventilation, spacing, barriers, personal protective equipment [PPE], etc.) to prevent transmission between occupants. These measures are essential to deal with the surges of potential cases that present, as there will be people in these areas who have not been infected. Confirmed cases can likely be cohorted (depending on the nature of the pathogen) but during outbreaks with highly infectious pathogens, those pending a test result should be separated. Specialised entry points and existing healthcare entry points (e.g., emergency departments) should be well equipped to manage severe case presentation with appropriate treatments, case management, and IPC measures.

Whenever possible, points of exit for discharging patients should be kept separate from points of entry. This applies regardless of whether they are discharged because they have tested negative, recovered, or are transferring to another facility.

The numbers of visitors will generally be limited during large-scale or highly infectious outbreaks. Still, space for registration and screening of visitors is needed as well as the capacity to communicate with patients who have been admitted. Tiers of fences or other physical barriers outside the facility can work to support visitor control when it is not possible to control areas within the health facility and entries. This would work if there is appropriate staff deployed to them. These could be health promoters or security staff, or a mix of both. Automated turnstile visitor control systems are also available in some countries. During the COVID-19 pandemic and after the introduction of rapid tests, scaled proactive screening and testing of visitors were implemented where resources allowed.

MERS-CoV outbreak from an emergency room in South Korea

At the Samsung Medical Center in South Korea, a 35-year-old man (patient 14) had been infected with MERS-CoV upon exposure to patient 1 at another hospital while being treated for community-acquired pneumonia (9). He arrived at the emergency room at Samsung Medical Center with deteriorating respiratory symptoms but was not initially identified as a suspect case. Therefore, he had not been isolated in a separate negative-pressure room; this had placed 675 patients, an estimated 683 visitors, and 218 healthcare workers (HCWs) at the risk of exposure. Of these, 33 patients, 41 visitors, and eight HCWs were ultimately confirmed to have MERS-CoV infection, sparking the largest Middle East respiratory syndrome (MERS) outbreak outside of the Middle East, eventually causing 186 laboratory-confirmed cases between May and July 2015, including 38 deaths.

> In an emergency department setting, there is an increased potential for the transmission of pathogens, especially highly infectious airborne pathogens. Overcrowding in hospital emergency rooms is almost inevitable in large-scale outbreaks and facilitates transmission. The best use of infrastructure in emergency rooms requires screening for patients to reveal a risk for unusual infections that can cause outbreaks, followed by their isolation.

Isolation capacity

Whether for a small isolation capacity in a conventional health facility or a dedicated outbreak screening/testing/management facility, designing how people are isolated and how those isolation systems interact with all associated non-isolation systems are essential. Likewise, a tiered and compartmentalised isolation system is essential for any highly infectious pathogen. The design of screening and triage zones can be particularly challenging due to the high volume of patient turnover and the significant risk of pathogen transmission. Undiagnosed individuals who are positive for an infectious disease may unknowingly spread the infection to others who are present for screening or other medical services. Therefore, meticulous attention to isolation systems within these spaces is essential to safeguard all individuals accessing the facility.

An organised patient, staff, and material flow in isolation areas can be enabled by well-considered infrastructure. The risk is greatest at emergency presentation (**See MERS-CoV outbreak from an emergency room**). In most outbreaks, once patients are confirmed to be positive with the outbreak pathogen, the need for isolation from each other is significantly reduced and cohorting (10) can be a more effective means of preventing transmission (11). Isolation capacity needs advanced consideration and planning and is possible in some form in any setting. It is required wherever an infected patient could have been (e.g., screening, emergency department, inpatient wards, operating theatre, labour ward, dialysis centre, radiology department). These areas where patients are in isolation (or cohort) ideally need designated areas for showering and toilets, separate entrances and exits for staff, patients, and visitors, separate flow paths for the incoming clean supply of materials and outgoing soiled waste and used materials, separate gown-up and gown-down rooms at the unit's entrance, and two-way lockers between the gown-up and gown-down rooms to separate the deposit and collection of belongings (4).

Inpatient care

As with all patient areas of health facilities, the design and flow of the ward are very important for the safe and effective treatment of patients. Good infrastructure is a great enabler. Staff, materials/medications, waste, and patients should all have a linear flow with as little backtracking and path-crossing as possible (12), especially in outbreaks with highly infectious pathogens.

As in conventional health facilities and systems, patient privacy should be prioritised as much as possible, but in large-scale and severe outbreak settings, this principle can conflict with other priorities which will need to be navigated with the management team. Private patient rooms maximise personal privacy and dignity but can mean a reduction in medical

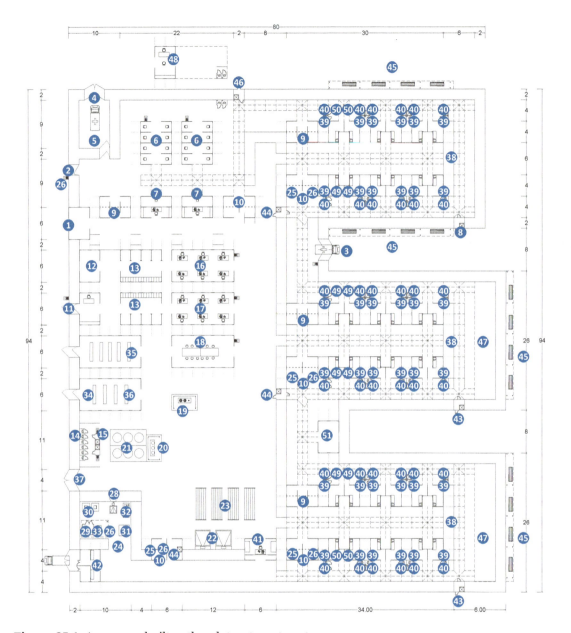

Figure 25.1: A purpose-built outbreak treatment centre

This purpose-built Ebola outbreak facility illustrates some of the key general principles of infrastructure design. Points of entry are very carefully considered, with different entries for confirmed and unconfirmed cases. The use of a geometrical design helps with the implementation of one-way patient flows. Staff-only spaces are generously designed. Access to visitors is given so that the facility is as visible to outsiders as possible, but in a carefully designed manner. Flows of inputs and outputs, including laundry and different forms of waste, are important to the overall design.

This is a model Ebola treatment facility layout drawn up by Techné, a World Health Organization (WHO) network of architects, engineers, designers, and public health practitioners from several institutions globally, which aims to make health settings and structures safer for health workers and patients and reduce the risk of hospital-acquired infections.

*Image is not publicly available but used with permission.

1. Screening	19. Kitchen	37. Vehicles entrance
2. Patients' entrance	20. Chlorination banks	38. Patients' treatment area
3. Confirmed patients' entrance	21. Water tanks	39. Patients' latrine
4. Ambulance entrance	22. Laundry	40. Patients' shower
5. Ambulance disinfection	23. Drying stand	41. Laboratory
6. Waiting room	24. Waste zone	42. Morgue
7. Triage	25. Chlorination taps	43. Discharge survivors
8. Discharge negative	26. Water tap stand	44. Caregivers' shower
9. Donning	27. Grease trap	45. Visitors' area
10. Doffing	28. Soakaway pit	46. Discharge non-case
11. Staff entrance	29. Waste storage	47. Patients' resting area
12. Scrubs distribution area	30. Ash pit	48. Psychosocial centre
13. Staff changing rooms	31. Sharp pit	49. Paediatric room
14. Staff latrine	32. Organic pit	50. Adolescent room
15. Staff shower	33. Incinerator	51. Family-friendly space for confirmed children and their caretakers
16. Medical office	34. Logistic warehouse	
17. Tech office	35. Pharmacy	
18. Staff canteen	36. Electrical equipment area	

oversight of the patient, especially when PPE is required. Large, open wards are the most efficient for cleaning and medical oversight and they require less space per patient.

The average length of inpatient stay is also a defining consideration on how to ensure adequate bed capacity in the facility, irrespective of whether it is built electively or as part of response (13). When calculating this, the length of stay must be considered, which may evolve over time as the relationship between patient and pathogen evolves, and with increasing immunity due to exposure, vaccines, or emerging treatments.

Flexibility and adaptability are integral to the design. Inpatient wards that are designated as potential cohort wards should be designed and future-proofed for conversion with the appropriate ventilation, whether that be open air or with sophisticated negative-pressure systems (14) for airborne pathogens.

Visibility of operations

Points of interaction between isolated patients and family members or visitors can be accomplished via multiple mechanisms such as by transparent barriers, spaced distances, some utilisation of PPE (requiring some level of training, donning/doffing areas, etc.), or via phone/ or digital media. In addition to being an important human element for patients and their loved ones, this promotes community acceptance by allowing external insight into the workings of the facility.

Outbreaks, especially those requiring high levels of public health measures, can lead to conspiracy theories about clinical practices. In times of significant public health measures to limit people's movement or interactions, there have been conspiracy theories of "empty" isolation units built to justify the restrictions on people for some other nefarious reason (15). Diseases with high mortality rates can lead to suspicion and mistrust of HCWs, for example, through rumours of blood or body part harvesting or medical experiments (16–17). To avoid or counter such scenarios, visitors and community leaders who view facilities can become important advocates for the health system. The media can also play a huge role in the acceptance or rejection of outbreak control measures by the community. Safely and ethically

Infectious Disease Emergencies: Preparedness & Response

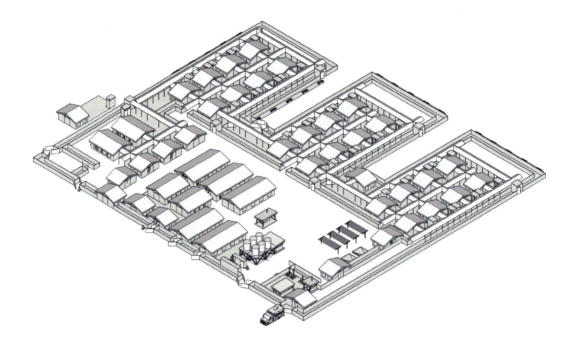

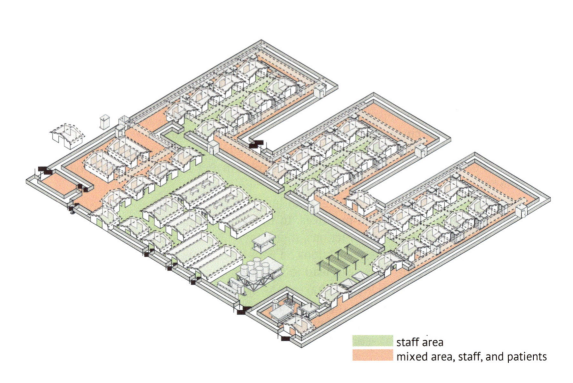

■ staff area
■ mixed area, staff, and patients

Healthcare Facilities and Infrastructure

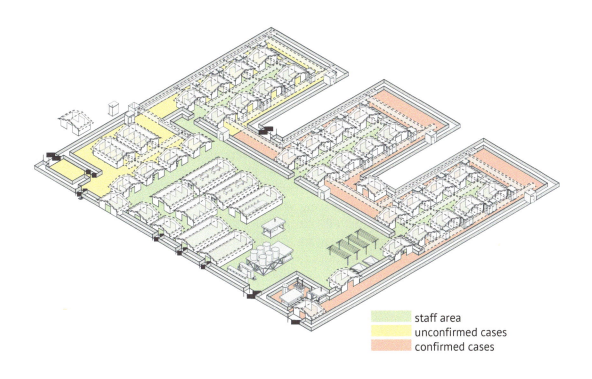

Figures 25.2, 25.3, and 25.4: Planning for isolation
Designing how people are isolated, and how those isolation systems interact with all associated non-isolation systems, is essential. Likewise, a tiered and compartmentalised isolation system is essential for any highly infectious pathogen. The design of screening and triage zones can be particularly challenging due to the high volume of patient turnover and the significant risk of pathogen transmission. Undiagnosed individuals who are positive for an infectious disease may unknowingly spread the infection to others who are present for screening or other medical services. Therefore, meticulous attention to isolation systems within these spaces is essential to safeguard all individuals accessing the facility. This plan for an Ebola Treatment Centre highlights the areas for staff and patient circulation, and furthermore, the different spaces for suspected and confirmed cases.

(Source: Ebola High Performance Tents layout, WHO Techné Report)
*Images are not publicly available but used with permission.

facilitating visits from the media and other actors/entities seen as credible by the community can be critical in any successful outbreak response. Effective IPC measures and patient confidentiality/consent need to be carefully weighed and considered in these cases, with the design of the facility potentially being able to support this.

Risk zones for staff

In the case of outbreaks involving highly transmissible pathogens, implementing a tiered risk system within the healthcare facility is generally an effective approach to manage staff safety without burdening lower risk areas with excessive PPE/IPC protocols. High-risk zones necessitate the use of transmission-based PPE packages and feature controlled donning and doffing areas to ensure staff safety when transitioning between zones. Medium-/low-risk areas, which serve different purposes, have distinct PPE requirements. A well-designed infrastructure can facilitate the safe movement between these zones, minimising any potential confusion among the staff. Additionally, patients and visitors can be strategically separated to enhance safety measures (**See Chapter 26, IPC**).

Laundry, sterilisation/equipment disinfection areas, supply network

Consideration is needed on the flow for clean and soiled linen and equipment including storage and disinfection. The infectiousness of the pathogen and nature of disinfection will influence whether the materials used during an outbreak response require a separate flow if used in a shared facility (18).

Storage and/or disinfection capacity may be required within isolation areas or individual departments/zones, or the flow may include passage from low- to high-risk areas. Considering the granular detail of how all activities will function within the constraints of a tightly controlled isolation system will enable smooth running and minimise additional transmission. Strategic decisions on what materials/equipment are realistically able to be disinfected (compared to single-use materials) should be considered ahead of time whenever possible as effective disinfection infrastructure and flow of materials can have a large impact on facility design.

Waste management/waste zone

Outbreaks create an increase in healthcare waste, and a safe and sustainable waste management system must also be scalable and adaptable. Medical and biological waste should be segregated from municipal solid waste. A separate waste collection, management, and disposal system is needed for medical and biological waste. Depending on the pathogen, infectious medical waste can include pharmaceutical supplies, soiled linen, meals/used wares, used sterile supplies, soiled items, patient specimens, and equipment. Infrastructure for the treatment and storage of infectious medical waste generated should be planned in accordance with operational needs.

There could be centralised and decentralised waste disposal areas and disposal routes which are discreet where possible. Infrastructure to store surges in waste, as well as potentially treat waste on-site, should be considered and weighed against the benefits of larger, centralised waste management systems across facilities. Adequate space for extra bins and biohazard containers should be planned should there be a surge in cases or disruption to external services (4).

Utilities planning

Whether designing a facility for baseline healthcare needs or during an outbreak response, the future roles and facility expansion with regard to the need for good access to utilities such as water, electricity, sewage, internet, and phone lines need to be considered. For instance, if a haemodialysis unit is likely to be moved in a major outbreak, then appropriate installation in an alternative site must be ensured (19). Equipment and infrastructure in areas within isolation zones of highly infectious outbreaks are likely to suffer gaps in maintenance, and repairs or upgrades may be delayed due to the additional complications of working in the area. Delays and complications may also be multiplied if they necessitate an external technical person.

Management of dead bodies

Morgue sizing is a sombre yet necessary task, especially in health facilities dealing with an outbreak causing a high mortality (20). Undersized morgues pose a safety risk to staff and compromise patient dignity which can have serious consequences with community acceptance. This can be exacerbated in settings where significant amounts of bulky and awkward PPE interfere with workflows and visibility and mobility are compromised. While it can be tempting to economise on space by establishing more elaborate tiered shelves in the morgue to store more bodies, the realistic mobility of the PPE-dressed HCWs needs to be pragmatically considered, as well as the potential psychological trauma for families and mortuary staff. Also, as a related function in contexts with highly transmissible and severe outbreaks, there may be a need to disinfect bodies/body bags before their handover to either burial teams or family members which may require important infrastructure considerations.

Expanding a morgue in Sierra Leone

There wasn't any way around it, and we couldn't wait any longer—we were going to have to make it bigger.

In a temperature of >40°C, we gathered our tools and materials, took a collective deep breath, and started the sequence of donning the layers of PPE to go into the high-risk area of the Ebola Management Centre in Kailahun, Sierra Leone.

The task was simple enough, at least in theory: remove the cumbersome door to the morgue and make the doorway bigger to bring in the shelves that were built in the workshop area to increase the number of dead bodies we could safely store in a dignified manner. The job would have been a couple of hours under normal circumstances, but these were anything but normal circumstances. Just a 15-minute walk from one end of the 100+ bed facility to the other would leave you covered in your own sweat due to the full-body suit, mask, boots, gloves, and goggles you had to wear in the High-Risk Zone; staying in the maximum of 45 minutes ensured that every bit of you would be soaked and you would be well into the start of heatstroke. In these conditions, even the most basic manual labour needed for the project was exhausting, sawing the doorframe became a Herculean task that fogged your goggles and pooled sweat in your gloves, hammering nails into the new boards seemed to require superhuman coordination, and manoeuvring the shelves into place resembled a rigged carnival game.

After several exhausting round trips into the High-Risk Zone, the job was done, and as we reflected while rehydrating and cooling down in the Low-Risk Zone, we hoped that we wouldn't need to expand the morgue again—both selfishly and for the sake of the people in the affected region.

Surrounding physical environment

Beyond the perimeter of the outbreak-related health facility, whether it be a dense urban environment or a remote patch of jungle, there are factors that need to be considered in the design, construction, and implementation of activities. General accessibility (for staff, patients, and ambulances), traffic, environmental impact including drainage, access to utilities, security considerations, and community sensitivities all need to be considered when deciding the appropriateness of an area.

Community acceptance factors can come into play, for example, when a site is seen to be too near a school or religious building, even if there are no tangible public health risks. Ambulance sirens, smoke from open burning pits or body cremation, and a perception of drawing infected people to the community could result in significant tensions, potentially leading to the facility being protested or blockaded by the community.

Reviewing the general location and consulting the host community will help foster relationships and integrate the facility into the community in a more constructive way. Such integration is an important contribution to ensure a more accepted and effective infrastructure (14).

Community acceptance of new health infrastructure

A biosafety level 4 (BSL-4) National Emerging Infectious Diseases Laboratory (NEIDL) was completed in downtown Boston in 2008 at a cost of US$ 192 million and two years after regulatory approval was granted by the federal government for its funding. There was strong community opposition to having dangerous pathogens in the vicinity and court injunctions meant that it was 2012 before even BSL level 2 research could be undertaken.

In 2014, a Boston City Councillor attempted to file a proposed ordinance to prohibit BSL-4 research in the city of Boston. The National Institutes of Health (NIH) sponsored an independent risk assessment which estimated that a community member could become infected once every 500 to 10,000 years. There were ten BSL-4 laboratories in North America with 100 years cumulative activity and there had never been a laboratory worker or community member infection (21). The superior court rejected a challenge to the risk assessment.

A prolonged programme of community engagement paralleled the legal defence and in December 2017, approval was finally given for BSL-4 work to begin with a focus on Ebola and Marburg viruses. In early 2020, this research was paused to enable research on SARS-CoV-2.

Laboratories and laboratory departments

Adapting or expanding existing infrastructure in laboratories and radiology departments during an outbreak is often poorly considered in advance. The pathology unit or laboratory must deliver continuous, prompt, and accurate results to handle an increase in test load, assist swift patient triage, and offer the necessary isolation precautions and patient care. To handle routine processes and simultaneously manage suspect infectious specimens in an outbreak or pandemic, laboratories should be built with spaces for specimen receiving, processing, storage, and disposal. When making plans for the laboratory, operational shifts and the physical separation between staff necessary during a pandemic should be taken into account (4). When an outbreak causes a surge in requests, several questions arise including:
- should we replicate these systems and tools in the facility?
- should a section be designated for isolation?
- should we forgo them or outsource if expansion isn't possible?

Infrastructure design can enable future activity if a plan is made in advance. Isolation capacity with suitable IPC measures such as ventilation should be considered in the design of radiology departments. Patient flow, room disinfection, and waste management should be intrinsic capacities in design and planning. In the laboratory, the same should be the case for specimens. Beyond the laboratory, designated areas should be established for site access, screening, triaging, testing (unknown status area), and treatment (confirmed area), as well as other specialised case areas (e.g., for pregnant women or unaccompanied minors) (4,18).

ENSURING CAPACITY FOR PERMANENT FACILITIES DEVELOPED AS PART OF THE HEALTH SYSTEM

Scalability is the ability of the structure to maintain functionality when confronted by a caseload surge. An outbreak-resilient healthcare facility requires a design that allows adaptation from regular caseloads to safely manage the surge in infectious patients while maintaining the required standard of care for conventional medical conditions in a safe way. Environmental and engineering controls should enable adapted workflows for patients, waste, materials, HCWs, and visitors, while optimising IPC standards and remaining patient centred. In addition to the design features listed above, which aim to facilitate safe adapted pandemic response of an established facility, we discuss adaptations to settings not likely to be part of new or repurposed structures.

Emergency department

The emergency department should be designed to handle rapid surges in patient volumes with plans for conversion in response to various outbreak stages. Key features for consideration include (4):
- separate drop-off points for arrival and flows of patients identified or suspected to have infectious diseases
- designated screening areas at both ambulance and walk-in entries to support diversion decisions
- pre-triage rapid screening and triage assessment areas

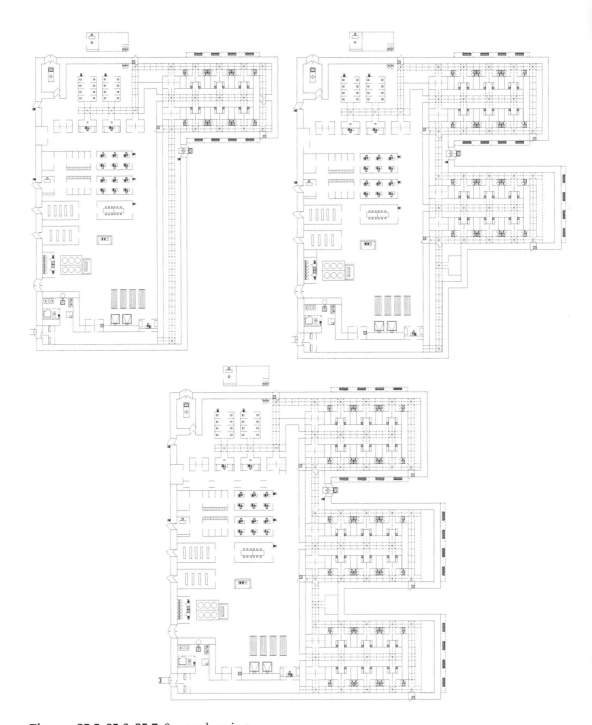

Figures 25.5, 25.6, 25.7: Surge planning
Even temporary purpose-built facilities should be planned with surge capacity in mind. This Techné design for an Ebola treatment facility using high performance tents can be expanded from a small to large size without undue disruption to ongoing operations.

(Source: Ebola High Performance Tents layout, WHO Techné Report)
*Images are not publicly available but used with permission.

- a fever/isolation area adjacent to screening facilities
  - consultation rooms, treatment rooms, imaging rooms (where required), support areas, and staff facilities (shower, toilets, lockers, and rest areas should be provided within the fever/isolation area to minimise staff movement in/out of the area)
- closely located near an operating theatre if there is to be one
- designated route to transfer high-risk patients to isolation operating theatres (ISO OT), intensive care units/high dependency units (ICUs/HDUs), and isolation wards, with a designated elevator if possible
- modular zones with each self-contained with critical resources, necessary equipment, and ventilation control to support ad hoc isolation in zones without affecting the operations of other areas of the department
- an area adjacent to the emergency department designed to support surge (22)
  - open and levelled area for mass casualty triage/treatment that can accommodate the rapid construction of temporary facilities such as tents and mobile units. It may be designed to be self-contained for patient treatment and observation, with a dedicated entrance and exit.
  - empty space allowing urgent construction of temporary or permanent facility expansion
- utilities supplies (e.g., power, oxygen, plumbing, and sanitary connections) are best designed and installed to be ready to support temporary and/or expansion facilities
- appropriate medical services and capacities within the area so as to not have to compromise between patient care and isolation
- space and infrastructure for ambulances and private cars that require disinfection are to be ideally placed well away from triage and patient areas
- a decontamination room which can be used to decontaminate patients prior to entering the emergency department, including those who have potentially been exposed to, or contaminated with, toxins, chemicals, radioactive materials, and other hazardous substances

Complex treatment units

These units include ICUs, HDUs, and OTs. Ideally, ICU and HDU patient rooms should be planned in modular zones, where each is self-contained, with critical resources and necessary equipment to support the containment capabilities of zones when needed without affecting the operations of other areas within the unit.

There should be designated and direct access between ICUs, HDUs, and the emergency department, and other key areas to support the transfers of patients and staff movement. The room area and layout of all ICU and HDU rooms should be similar and equipped with the capabilities to flex between ICU and HDU functions. Where resources allow, airflow control should be provided at designated ICU and HDU isolation rooms to accommodate patients with airborne transmission diseases (4).

NEW OR REPURPOSED BUILDINGS REQUIRED DURING A RESPONSE

The effective design of new or repurposed existing structures is more likely once the pathogen is understood, the outbreak strategy defined, and strategy for placement of sites decided. Irrespective of the setting and the type of infrastructure, there are overarching principles governing the design of outbreak-resilient healthcare facilities (**Figure 25.1**). In addition to the general design features listed above, new and repurposed buildings have specific nuances not applicable to permanent pre-existing healthcare structures.

Site selection

Strategically, planners should consider to what degree emergency healthcare infrastructure should be centralised or decentralised across a given geography (23). The geography of the outbreak is the first factor to consider, along with the availability of financial and human resources, ease of movement, the level of community acceptance of public health interventions, and the nature of the pathogen and outbreak progression (24).

In cases of very localised "hotspot" outbreak dynamics, it is generally better to have a localised infrastructure strategy to be more agile and responsive. This better enables infrastructure to be quickly established, suspended, decommissioned, and potentially re-activated. In such instances, these very decentralised/localised facilities can support community acceptance and outreach initiatives as well as counter community stigma regarding the outbreak and/or distrust of authorities—if needed. For a wider outbreak, centralised hubs may offer a more effective use of resources. A centralised response can evolve into a decentralised system especially if combined with robust community outreach and engagement, decentralised surveillance and screening mechanisms, and efficient referral capacities.

Like many aspects of healthcare infrastructure, it is generally helpful to think of these dynamics as along a spectrum rather than as binary options. Each end of the spectrum has their own positive and negative attributes, with most interventions operating somewhere in between the two extremes. As outbreaks themselves are highly dynamic, responses need to be adaptive, and may shift along that spectrum, sometimes dramatically, as the response evolves.

All relevant population and environmental elements should be considered when planning infrastructure strategies to ensure they are community centric. Dense urban environments may be best served by centralised hubs, while smaller and more spread-out communities tend to benefit from decentralised community facilities. Mobile facilities may be needed to support very sparse or nomadic populations.

An individual's ability to access facilities will influence where key infrastructure is positioned. The mode of pathogen transmission interacts with these concerns. Ideally, dedicated ambulances can be used to collect patients, especially when dealing with respiratory pathogens where travel to seek treatment may itself become an important nexus of transmission. Planners must understand whether people can access personal vehicles or rely on walking, bicycles, or livestock to travel. Public transportation should be discouraged in outbreaks with highly infectious pathogens (especially respiratory ones), while blood-borne and faecal-oral transmissible pathogens present a much lower risk of transmission in public transport. As population mobility increases, so can the centralisation of infrastructure hubs. Systems will need to support people with low personal mobility due to physical disabilities or income/resource challenges.

Road infrastructure and accessibility will also help determine the infrastructure model needed for an outbreak. Poor roads in the outbreak area threaten the continuity of supply and staff as well as the referrals of patients. This can be mitigated by a centralised model but reduces patient accessibility. Conversely, in areas where there is only intermittent road access, such as areas where rain or snow may make roads impassable for days or weeks at a time, a more decentralised and self-sufficient model may be more appropriate to reduce barriers for individuals and communities to access support. If this is only an issue for part of the year, a hybrid model that involves seasonal overstocking and/or short-term supplies of next-level care in outposts may be the most effective strategy.

During outbreaks, especially novel outbreaks, there can be significant distrust of government and health authorities. In some cases, necessary community-based infection control interventions may amplify pre-existing disconnection and mistrust (**See Chapter 33, RCCE**). This possibility needs to be anticipated in infrastructure planning (25). In general, central treatment and quarantine options are easier when there are good community relations. Equally, the decision to take a centralised strategy might require additional investment in community relations to head off and deal with concerns that might arise. In general, when trust is low, more decentralised and in-community models are more approachable and may be a better option in the spirit of transparency and relationship building (26–27).

Nature of the pathogen

For any given outbreak, the transmissibility, mode of transmission, attack rate (of infection from person to person), and severity of the disease caused by the pathogen will guide the level of biosecurity that needs to be implemented. This should be done in collaboration with relevant biosecurity/IPC referents. To ensure that facilities are fit for purpose and complementary to the activities that will be undertaken, individuals who should be consulted include experienced case management specialists, anthropologists, and logistics experts (28). The manner in which infectious patients are diagnosed during an outbreak influences the design of the treatment centre. For instance, in a cholera outbreak, confirmation is often based on clinical manifestations; thus, the treatment centre is designed according to disease severity. Conversely, Ebola diagnoses are conducted via polymerase chain reaction (PCR), and the treatment centre includes areas for both suspected and confirmed cases. All these types of variables can have significant impacts on facility design and overall intervention strategies—especially to what degree a response should/can be decentralised.

Managing Ebola outbreaks with standardised Ebola Treatment Units

Médecins Sans Frontières (MSF) has played a significant role in responding to Ebola outbreaks, often deploying Ebola Treatment Units (ETUs) to provide medical care and isolation for suspect and confirmed cases. An ETU was built in the Firestone District, Margibi County, Liberia, upon reporting of the first confirmed case of Ebola virus disease (EBOD) on 31 March 2014. Firestone implemented modifications to convert an outpatient health clinic separated from the main hospital to meet the infection control standards of an ETU following standard guidance developed by MSF (29). This facility housed up to 23 patients, including those classified as having confirmed, probable, or suspected EBOD. The construction of this ETU was completed by 9 April 2014 (30).

A site considered for an ETU should be large enough, and have access to clean water, electricity, and sanitation. In most cases, ETUs should be established as close as possible to the epicentre(s) of the outbreak to minimise travel time and improve ease of access for patients, visitors, and others. Any host community concerns or fears, along with security concerns and risks of civil unrest, should be assessed, with planners working as closely as possible with local community leaders to help build trust, ensure cultural sensitivity, and therefore, increase the chances of successful treatment and containment.

Once a suitable site has been identified and a design approved, the construction process can begin, setting up patient wards, triage areas, laboratory facilities, and areas for staff accommodation and support services. The time needed to set up an ETU depends on the urgency of the situation, local conditions, and available resources. However, MSF's standard design protocol allows for a very efficient deployment process, in the order of a few days in many cases.

In treatment centres, different facility design and infrastructure elements are needed depending on whether the pathogen is transmitted through physical contact, droplets, or the air. For pathogens with low infectivity in typical settings, such as those only transmitted through blood, conventional medical facilities and IPC measures are likely to suffice. However, when dealing with pathogens that can be transmitted through droplets or via the air, more stringent protocols and potentially intricate design elements become more important. Among these, airborne transmission presents the greatest challenge, generally requiring the most complex design considerations.

Beyond mode of transmission, a pathogen that causes more severe disease, such as the Ebola virus, may demand a high level of facility design despite it being only a moderately infectious pathogen (31). Such cases require additional infrastructure such as more space for patient screening and treatment, more complex flow and zoning considerations, additional staff, areas for storage and donning and doffing of PPE, and waste and dead body management.

ADAPTING NON-MEDICAL INFRASTRUCTURE

Taking existing infrastructure and adapting it to be able to cope with an outbreak surge can be a very effective strategy, especially in dynamic and rapidly expanding outbreaks (32). A key consideration before deciding to convert a structure is the importance of the facility for core societal functions. The use of facilities where their removal from regular function will have a detrimental effect on the social, economic, or cultural well-being of the community (e.g., schools, religious facilities [except with the agreement of the religious community], or critical markets) should be avoided. Furthermore, medical equipment, infrastructure, and IPC measures may require significant infrastructure modification, and community acceptance consequences need to be considered.

While not all scenarios can be anticipated, public health planners should periodically conduct reviews of potential sites from both public and private sectors, considering them for different outbreak scenarios. This review should account for the amount of materials needed for conversion, including beds and cots, wall dividers, portable toilets, mobile laboratory equipment, and improvement to ventilation.

After an outbreak peaks, infrastructure can be repurposed, and sites can be reduced in size or number. As outbreak forecasting is, by its nature, imperfect, having the flexibility to scale capacity up and down via the rapid commission, decommission, and potential re-commission of sites enables a more effective response.

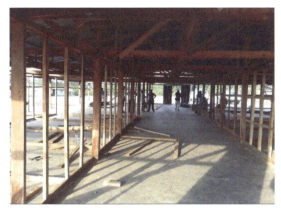

Figure 25.8: An ETU being built in Foya, Liberia, 2014
(Credit: Dale Fisher)

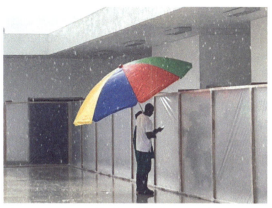

Figure 25.9: Medical staff talking with patients within the Marburg treatment centre in Bata, Equatorial Guinea, 2023
(Credit: Janet Diaz)

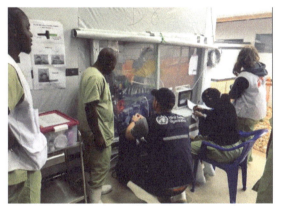

Figure 25.10: Medical staff monitoring a patient at the Ebola Treatment Centre in Katwa, Butembo, Democratic Republic of the Congo, 2019
(Credit: Ian Crozier)

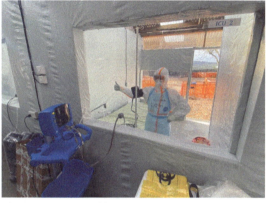

Figure 25.11: Staff testing materials at the Ebola Treatment Centre set up by Médecins Sans Frontières in Mubende, Uganda, 2021
(Credit: Luca Fontana)

Security situations and potential constraints

Militarised conflicts, terrorism, and criminal activity can significantly shape the strategy for infrastructure in response to an outbreak (33). The security situation not only impacts the design of specific facilities (e.g., physical security infrastructure), but also influences the overall location and placement of outbreak response infrastructure. In regions prone to instability, a decentralised infrastructure approach can help mitigate the risk of the main outbreak treatment capacity getting cut off from the broader outbreak area. Conversely, having decentralised facilities in areas with a higher likelihood of instability may increase the risk of at least some facilities being directly affected by the insecurity (34). Implementing a screening and referral model in insecure areas can minimise the infrastructure requirements, staffing needs, and equipment deployed in those regions. Alternatively, in locations where the movement of teams and vehicles poses a greater risk due to criminality, terrorism, or localised low-level conflicts, it might be preferable to establish one or more highly secure central hubs within or adjacent to the higher risk area to minimise the volume of potentially exposed movements and staff.

CONCLUSION

Infrastructure design for pandemic or outbreak management can occur in the preparedness, readiness, or response phases **(See Chapter 1, Introduction)**. Ideally, consideration of potential needs would happen at the time of healthcare facility design which would enable pre-planned and efficient adaptation to the circumstances. This applies particularly to hospitals and more specialised healthcare facilities. Where such planning has not occurred, the healthcare leadership will struggle to adapt infrastructure to cope with a surge in infected patients; this will be reflected in both patient outcomes and outbreak progression.

Well-prepared hospitals can effectively manage patients during infectious disease emergencies, minimising mortality from both the outbreak disease and other conditions. This preparation can also minimise the number of hospital-acquired infections among patients, staff, and visitors.

Outside of hospitals, there is the option to repurpose existing non-health facilities, modify smaller health facilities, or rapidly build temporary facilities in key areas for the outbreak. This chapter has outlined the principles that should be used to make and implement such decisions, but all actual decisions need to be very context, resource, pathogen, and outbreak specific. Healthcare infrastructure design enables the continuity of clinical care, IPC, and the maintenance of essential services, so it is highly important in any successful response and is intimately linked with both planned needs and workflows.

Health infrastructure design needs input from many stakeholders including architects, construction engineers, IPC practitioners, nurses and other clinicians, sanitation experts, and community leaders. Collaborative and multidisciplinary consultation is required, as is the consideration of what is needed to support safe and effective management of surging patient numbers during an outbreak. All these combined will help ensure a facility is effectively prepared for an outbreak.

REFERENCES:

1. Luxon L. Infrastructure - the key to healthcare improvement. Future Hosp J. 2015 Feb;2(1):4–7. https://doi.org/10.7861/futurehosp.2-1-4 PMID:31098066.
2. World Health Organization Regional Office for the Western Pacific. District health facilities: guidelines for development and operations. 1998. https://apps.who.int/iris/handle/10665/207020.
3. U.S. Department of Health and Human Services Centers for Disease Control and Prevention (CDC) Atlanta. Guidelines for Environmental Infection Control in Health-Care Facilities. Updated: July 2019. https://www.osha.gov/sites/default/files/CDC's_Guidelines_for_Environmental_Infection_Control.pdf.
4. Infrastructure_preparedness_and_response_for_disease_outbreaks__/20220621_PPHI_DRAFT3_main or? https://www.who.int/publications/i/item/9789240011311.
5. Anesi GL, Lynch Y, Evans L. A conceptual and adaptable approach to hospital preparedness for acute surge events due to emerging infectious diseases. Crit Care Explor. 2020 Apr;2(4):e0110. https://doi.org/10.1097/CCE.0000000000000110 PMID:32426752.
6. Łukasik M, Porębska A. Responsiveness and adaptability of healthcare facilities in emergency scenarios: COVID-19 experience. Int J Environ Res Public Health. 2022 Jan;19(2):675. https://doi.org/10.3390/ijerph19020675 PMID:35055493.

7. Centers for Disease Control and Prevention. Standard operating procedure (SOP) for triage of suspected COVID-19 patients in non-US healthcare settings: early identification and prevention of transmission during triage. https://www.cdc.gov/coronavirus/2019-ncov/hcp/non-us-settings/sop-triage-prevent-transmission.html.

8. Becky A Smith MD. COVID-19: general approach to infection prevention in the healthcare setting. https://www.uptodate.com/contents/covid-19-general-approach-to-infection-prevention-in-the-health-care-setting.

9. Cho SY, Kang JM, Ha YE, Park GE, Lee JY, Ko JH, Lee JY, Kim JM, Kang CI, Jo IJ, Ryu JG, Choi JR, Kim S, Huh HJ, Ki CS, Kang ES, Peck KR, Dhong HJ, Song JH, Chung DR, Kim YJ. MERS-CoV outbreak following a single patient exposure in an emergency room in South Korea: an epidemiological outbreak study. Lancet. 2016 Sep 3;388(10048):994-1001. https://doi.org/10.1016/S0140-6736(16)30623-7 PMID:27402381.

10. Whiteside T, Kane E, Aljohani B, Alsamman M, Pourmand A. Redesigning emergency department operations amidst a viral pandemic. Am J Emerg Med. 2020 Jul;38(7):1448–53. https://doi.org/10.1016/j.ajem.2020.04.032 PMID:32336583.

11. Rosenberger LH, Hranjec T, Politano AD, Swenson BR, Metzger R, Bonatti H, Sawyer RG. Effective cohorting and "superisolation" in a single intensive care unit in response to an outbreak of diverse multi-drug-resistant organisms. Surg Infect (Larchmt). 2011 Oct;12(5):345-50. https://doi.org/10.1089/sur.2010.076 PMID:21936667.

12. Ali S. Al-Shareef, Azzah Al Jabarti, Kholoud A. Babkair, Maan Jamajom, Abduallah Bakhsh, Syed Sameer Aga. Strategies to improve patient flow in the emergency department during the COVID-19 pandemic: a narrative review of our experience. Emergency Medicine International, vol. 2022, Article ID 2715647, 7 pages, 2022. https://doi.org/10.1155/2022/2715647.

13. Vekaria B, Overton C, Wiśniowski A, Ahmad S, Aparicio-Castro A, Curran-Sebastian J, et al. Hospital length of stay for COVID-19 patients: data-driven methods for forward planning. BMC Infect Dis. 2021 Jul;21(1):700. https://doi.org/10.1186/s12879-021-06371-6 PMID:34294037.

14. Najafi M, Khah DE, Asadi-Yeganeh MR. The factors affecting the location of medical centers in Tehran City Case Study: District 1 of Teherán Municipality. Tehran, Iran. Innovaciencia. 2019;7(2):1–15. https://doi.org/10.15649/2346075X.767.

15. Ahmed W, López Seguí F, Vidal-Alaball J, Katz MS. COVID-19 and the "Film Your Hospital" conspiracy theory: social network analysis of Twitter data. J Med Internet Res. 2020 Oct;22(10):e22374. https://doi.org/10.2196/22374 PMID:32936771.

16. Muzembo BA, Ntontolo NP, Ngatu NR, Khatiwada J, Ngombe KL, Numbi OL, et al. Local perspectives on Ebola during its tenth outbreak in DR Congo: a nationwide qualitative study. PLoS One. 2020 Oct;15(10):e0241120. https://doi.org/10.1371/journal.pone.0241120 PMID:33091054.

17. Peter Mwai and Rachel Schraer. Ebola in Uganda: the people spreading misinformation online. BBC Reality Check. 29 November 2022. https://www.bbc.com/news/63741125.

18. National Infection Prevention and Control Committee (Nipc). The National Infection Prevention and Control Guidelines for Acute Healthcare Facilities. 2017. https://www.moh.gov.sg/docs/librariesprovider4/default-document-library/the-national-infection-prevention-and-control-guidelines-for-acute-healthcare-facilities---2017.pdf.

19. Badru M, Morrison E, Woodside JC. Flexible and adaptable hospital MEP systems: smart planning helps to ensure hospital infrastructure systems can handle any contingency safely, effectively and efficiently. April 30, 2023. Health Facilities Management. https://www.hfmmagazine.com/articles/4710-flexible-and-adaptable-hospital-mep-systems.

20. COVID-19: authorities must urgently plan ahead to ensure the dead are properly handled. Geneva, International Committee of the Red Cross. 22 April 2020. https://www.icrc.org/en/document/covid-19-authorities-must-urgently-plan-ahead-ensure-dead-bodies-are-properly-handled.

21. BU questions claims behind ordinance to Ban BSL-4 research: city council hearing on April 16. https://www.bu.edu/neidl/2014/03/bu-questions-claims-behind-proposed-ordinance/.

22. Bagdasarian N, Mathews I, Ng AJ, Liu EH, Sin C, Mahadevan M, et al. A safe and efficient, naturally ventilated structure for COVID-19 surge capacity in Singapore. Infect Control Hosp Epidemiol. 2021 May;42(5):630–2. https://doi.org/10.1017/ice.2020.309 PMID:32578525.

23. Sreeramareddy CT, Sathyanarayana T. Decentralised versus centralised governance of health services. Cochrane Libr. 2019;2019(9):CD010830. https://doi.org/10.1002/14651858.CD010830.pub2.

24. Carter P, Megnin-Viggars O, Rubin GJ. What factors influence symptom reporting and access to healthcare during an emerging infectious disease outbreak? A rapid review of the evidence. Health Secur. 2021;19(4):353–63. https://doi.org/10.1089/hs.2020.0126 PMID:33416425.

25. Commission on a Global Health Risk Framework for the Future; National Academy of Medicine, Secretariat. The Neglected Dimension of Global Security: A Framework to Counter Infectious Disease Crises. Washington (DC): National Academies Press (US); 2016 May 16. 3, Strengthening Public Health as the Foundation of the Health System and First Line of Defense. https://www.ncbi.nlm.nih.gov/books/NBK368392/.

26. Tavakkoli M, Karim A, Fischer FB, Monzon Llamas L, Raoofi A, Zafar S, et al. From public health policy to impact for COVID-19: a multi-country case study in Switzerland, Spain, Iran and Pakistan. Int J Public Health. 2022 Aug;67:1604969. https://doi.org/10.3389/ijph.2022.1604969 PMID:36119450.

27. Dhillon RS, Kelly JD. Community trust and the Ebola endgame. N Engl J Med. 2015 Aug 27;373(9):787-9. https://doi.org/10.1056/NEJMp1508413 PMID:26222382.

28. Infection Prevention and Control of Epidemic- and Pandemic-Prone Acute Respiratory Infections in Health Care. Geneva: World Health Organization; 2014. Annex B, Isolation precautions. https://www.ncbi.nlm.nih.gov/books/NBK214342/; Guidelines for Environmental Infection Control in Health-Care Facilities. U.S. Department of Health and Human Services Centers for Disease Control and Prevention (CDC) Atlanta. Updated: July 2019. https://www.osha.gov/sites/default/files/CDC's_Guidelines_for_Environmental_Infection_Control.pdf.

29. Sterk, E. Filovirus haemorrhagic fever guidelines. Médecins Sans Frontières; 2008. https://www.nursingworld.org/globalassets/practiceandpolicy/work-environment/health--safety/medicins.pdf.

30. Reaves EJ, Mabande LG, Thoroughman DA, Arwady MA, Montgomery JM. Control of Ebola virus disease - Firestone District, Liberia, 2014. MMWR Morb Mortal Wkly Rep. 2014 Oct;63(42):959–65. https://www.ncbi.nlm.nih.gov/pmc/articles/PMC5779472/ PMID:25340914.

31. Hewlett, A., Vasa, A. M., Cieslak, T. J., Lowe, J. J., & Schwedhelm, S. (2017). Viral hemorrhagic fever preparedness. Infection Prevention: New Perspectives and Controversies, 197–211. https://doi.org/10.1007/978-3-319-60980-5_21.

32. Fang D, Pan S, Li Z, Yuan T, Jiang B, Gan D, et al. Large-scale public venues as medical emergency sites in disasters: lessons from COVID-19 and the use of Fangcang shelter hospitals in Wuhan, China. BMJ Glob Health. 2020 Jun;5(6):e002815. https://doi.org/10.1136/bmjgh-2020-002815 PMID:32546589.

33. Khisa, M., & Rwengabo, S. (2023). Militarism and the politics of Covid-19 response in Uganda. Armed Forces and Society, 0095327X231162848. https://doi.org/10.1177/0095327X231162848.

34. Blackburn CC, Lenze PE Jr, Casey RP. Paul E. Lenze Jr., and Rachel Paige Casey. Conflict and cholera: Yemen's man-made public health crisis and the global implications of weaponizing health. Health Secur. 2020;18(2):125–31. https://doi.org/10.1089/hs.2019.0113 PMID:32324073.

CHAPTER 26

STRENGTHENING INFECTION PREVENTION AND CONTROL SYSTEMS

by Amy R. Kolwaite, S. Kushlani Jayatilleke, Folasade T. Ogunsola, and Benjamin Park

Infection prevention and control (IPC) is a central function of healthcare facilities and health systems as they respond to rapidly emerging infectious diseases. Recent events, such as the West Africa Ebola outbreak and the COVID-19 pandemic, have put these capabilities to the test in many different settings. This chapter will present an overview of IPC in managing these infectious disease outbreaks or pandemics and look at the most recent ideas for how to implement emergency IPC programmes, based on adapted and feasible IPC policies.

INTRODUCTION: THE ROLE OF HEALTHCARE SETTINGS IN OUTBREAKS

Sick people seek healthcare. While obvious, recognising this statement is crucial to understanding why healthcare settings are essential for epidemic detection, response, and ultimately, prevention. Because potentially infectious persons visit healthcare facilities during their most infectious periods, healthcare facilities are often where emerging infections are first identified. This was the case during South Korea's Middle East respiratory syndrome (MERS) outbreak in 2015 (1). As such, facilities play a key and central part in any effort to prevent, detect, and respond to emerging threats. However, as outbreaks take root, healthcare transmission can then become a major driver of the overall epidemiology, with infections occurring among healthcare workers (HCWs) and patients. Infections may become amplified in healthcare environments, and then spill over to communities (2). Third, as outbreaks evolve into epidemics or pandemics, weak IPC and the healthcare transmission that results can lead to public perceptions that healthcare facilities are unsafe. Patient avoidance of healthcare settings, and subsequent major declines in essential health services such as routine immunisations, maternal health, and treatment for HIV and tuberculosis, may come back to stress and even contribute to the collapse of a healthcare system. Although the term "health system resiliency" can mean many things, one key component of a resilient system is undoubtedly the ability to protect its staff (3). Fourth, some outbreaks of dangerous pathogens *start* in healthcare settings and spread to the community, as is sometimes the case with infections caused by antimicrobial resistant organisms.

IPC is much more than the provision of personal protective equipment (PPE) health workers use to care for infectious patients. IPC is a clinical and public health specialty based on a practical, evidence-based approach that protects patients, HCWs, and visitors to healthcare facilities by preventing avoidable infections (4–5). Providing PPE without the supportive infrastructure needed to properly use it is akin to providing specialty medical equipment or treatments without the guidance, training, or staff to use and oversee them properly. Improperly used PPE has little protective value and can be harmful. The examples below show how IPC preparation can be challenged in outbreaks.

The 2014–2016 West Africa Ebola outbreak resulted in more than 28,000 reported cases of Ebola virus disease (EBOD) and more than 11,000 reported deaths (6). Of these, 881 HCWs were reported to have contracted EBOD and 513 (58.2 per cent) died. The Ebola outbreak overwhelmed the affected countries' healthcare systems which were precariously under-resourced before the outbreak. A meta-study covering research from Liberia, Guinea, and Sierra Leone reported an 18 per cent reduction in essential health services delivery due to the EBOD epidemic, including services such as outpatient visits, deliveries, other inpatient care, malaria, HIV and tuberculosis services, and immunisation (6).

More recently, a key feature of the COVID-19 pandemic was healthcare-associated SARS-CoV-2 acquisition among HCWs and patients admitted for non-COVID-19-related reasons (7). Reports from Asia and the U.S. suggest that 19–29 per cent of COVID-19 cases involved HCWs (8). This aligns with data from the 2002–2003 severe acute respiratory syndrome (SARS) epidemic, in which globally, HCWs accounted for 21 per cent of all cases, most of which were believed to be healthcare associated (8). Major challenges faced during the COVID-19 pandemic included shortages of PPE, infections among HCWs, and insufficient preparations for a surge of patients with severe disease (9). Despite the challenges, there are examples of healthcare facilities which experienced very low rates of HCW infections. The National University Hospital in Singapore took a whole-of-hospital approach in their response to the COVID-19 pandemic, resulting in no healthcare-associated SARS-CoV-2 infections through the first 18 months (10). They implemented many of the strategies which will be discussed in this chapter including planning for surge capacity, prioritising HCW well-being and safety, transparent communication, and ensuring solid IPC systems (10).

The West Africa Ebola outbreak and the COVID-19 pandemic illustrate the ways in which many healthcare facilities and health systems may give way in the crisis conditions caused by rapidly emerging infectious diseases (9). A mature and functional IPC programme can effectively prepare for and respond to emerging threats through the development, adaptation, and implementation of policies and protocols to respond to situations as they develop and support decision-making across all levels to ensure the continual operation of the health system (11). During the West Africa EBOD outbreak, HCWs accounted for 97 (12 per cent) of the 810 cases reported in Liberia by mid-August 2014 (12). In early 2015, a single transmission chain led to 166 non-Ebola Treatment Unit (ETU) HCWs being exposed to the virus at ten facilities; however, only one HCW became infected. This low transmission may be due to the intensive response from Liberia's newly developed IPC programme (12).

OVERVIEW OF TECHNICAL IPC CONCEPTS

A functional IPC programme provides oversight, monitoring, and supportive supervision to implement policies and improve practices to prevent hospital-acquired infections (HAI) and combat antimicrobial resistance (AMR). Supported by many colleagues in the field of IPC, the World Health Organization (WHO) released comprehensive recommendations in the WHO Guidelines on Core Components of Infection Prevention and Control Programmes (13). At both national and healthcare facility levels, the core components of an IPC programme are:
- IPC programme (dedicated team to support best practices)

- evidence-based guidelines
- education and training
- surveillance (guiding IPC practice and the detection of outbreaks)
- multimodal strategies (several elements implemented in an integrated way)
- monitoring, audit, and feedback
- workload, staffing, and bed occupancy (specific to healthcare facility)
- built environment, materials, and equipment for IPC (specific to healthcare facility)

Implementing all the core components is necessary for a functional, comprehensive IPC programme. However, implementing such a complex programme also takes sustained and resourced commitment. The WHO and its partners have developed a set of minimum requirements that represents the starting points for countries and facilities as they build towards full implementation of all the IPC core components (14).

Hierarchy of controls

The hierarchy of controls is a framework which may be used to determine the relative effectiveness of IPC interventions (**Figure 26.1**) (9). According to this particular framework, the most effective prevention measure is elimination of the risk factor, followed by substitution, engineering, administrative controls, and PPE. Controls become less effective as you move down the hierarchy of controls pyramid due to human behavioural factors.

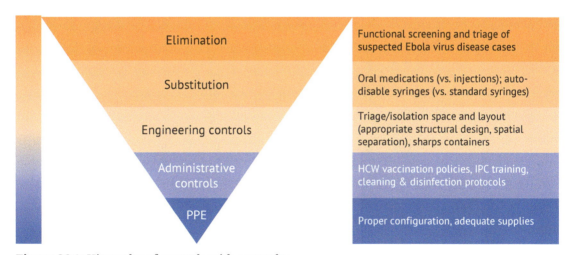

Figure 26.1: Hierarchy of controls with examples
(Figure developed by the International Infection Control Program, Division of Healthcare Quality Promotion, Centers for Disease Control and Prevention)

Elimination and substitution

The most effective measure for reducing the risk of healthcare transmission is to physically eliminate the risk from the environment. Examples of successful elimination measures in IPC include screening and triaging and/or testing patients, visitors, and HCWs for early detection of potentially infectious persons before they enter the healthcare setting. In these interventions, the early identification of such persons, followed by their isolation (where they are physically separated from susceptible persons to prevent transmission) or exclusion (where they are asked not to enter the facility at all) eliminates the risk to the rest of the healthcare environment. When patients are isolated, telehealth tools can often be used to provide routine care or care for mild or moderate infections, thereby reducing the need to visit emergency departments and urgent care facilities (9). Common telehealth modalities include live video teleconferencing, remote patient monitoring, mobile health applications, text, and email (15). Substitution involves replacing the hazard with another less risky hazard, such as treating a disease with an oral instead of an injectable medication.

Engineering controls

Engineering controls are used to reduce or control the risk of exposure at the source through physical means. Examples of engineering controls include facility design measures such as ventilation, barriers, screens, or holding bays for suspect cases at points of entry to a healthcare facility. Other examples of engineering controls are auto-disable syringes which help to prevent re-use, and germicidal technology, such as ultraviolet B lights, to reduce tuberculosis burden.

Administrative controls

Administrative controls establish work practices that reduce the duration, frequency, or intensity of exposure to hazards, and are meant to reduce risk by changing the way people work through policies such as visitor restrictions, employee training, appropriate supervision, and written policies and procedures (9). Because administrative controls are dependent on human behaviour, they are often less effective than engineering controls and often require multiple modalities to ensure behaviour change. For example, adhering to complex IPC protocols typically necessitates clear guidance, effective competency-based training, supportive supervision/mentorship, and quality assurance/quality improvement. Other examples of administrative controls include reducing the burden of organisms through hand hygiene, regular disinfection of the environment, safe waste disposal, and cohorting of patients.

Although often overlooked, environmental cleaning is an administrative control and a service critical for a well-functioning IPC programme. Environmental cleaners are often poorly educated and receive little training or supportive supervision, yet their task of decontaminating the healthcare environment is crucial to reduce infectious disease transmission (16–17). Their work could also be supported with engineering controls, for example, changing an environment to make it easier to clean.

PPE

PPE is worn by individuals as a barrier to protect against exposure to an infectious agent, but it does not eliminate the risk of infection (4). PPE only provides protection when used properly and should only be worn when exposure to an infectious agent is possible or likely. This risk might include visible blood or body fluids (e.g., vomit, urine, faeces), or it might be invisible agents, as with airborne pathogens. The correct PPE must be used to mitigate the risk; for example, using a particulate respirator for an airborne virus. Staff must know which type of infectious agent might be present and which type of PPE is indicated. PPE used incorrectly could result in ineffective risk reduction and potentially promote a false sense of security. An example of this is improperly donning (putting on) or doffing (taking off) of PPE when caring for a patient with Ebola. PPE must also be removed immediately following the exposure; failure to do so could unintentionally spread the pathogen to others.

Ensuring that HCWs have sufficient PPE during an outbreak or epidemic is critical. Shortages have led to worker strikes (18). In these situations, a resilient and flexible supply chain is needed to surge supplies of PPE to affected locations. These considerations will be discussed below.

IMPLEMENTING IPC PROGRAMMES FOR OUTBREAK PREPAREDNESS, READINESS, AND RESPONSE AT NATIONAL AND FACILITY LEVELS

IPC is a specialty that involves complex technical programming to have a robust system and it requires well-trained and well-resourced IPC practitioners to implement these programmes. The WHO has developed national-level and healthcare facility-level frameworks and toolkits to provide guidance and tools for decision-makers responsible for the prevention and control of infectious diseases with outbreak potential in the healthcare setting (19).

This WHO guidance is based on three phases: preparedness, readiness, and response. The preparedness section of the framework covers planning for *potential* infectious disease threats. The readiness and response sections cover planning for *existing* threats. Preparedness activities ensure that baseline IPC activities are adequate in the event of future communicable disease threats (19). Readiness activities link preparedness efforts to a specific identified threat or communicable disease with the potential to cause an outbreak within the next six months, for example, a measles outbreak in a neighbouring region. If an outbreak with the potential to be amplified in the healthcare setting is declared, then the response phase should be activated.

National IPC stakeholders and healthcare facilities should use the framework and toolkit at the appropriate outbreak management phase, reflecting the reality on the ground. Throughout all three phases, emphasis should be given to the following key areas:
- evaluation of IPC capacity
- preparedness, readiness, and response plans
- outbreak response teams
- IPC outbreak guidance
- IPC outbreak training
- surveillance and reporting programmes
- IPC communications strategy
- IPC surge capacity
- IPC partners mapping and networks
- system assessment/audit

Evaluation of IPC capacity

Evaluation of IPC function and capacity at both the national and healthcare facility levels identifies IPC areas that need to be strengthened. It can translate into an action plan to meet WHO minimum requirements (19).

Many settings may not have the resources to physically assess all healthcare facilities. Nigeria has 36 States, the Federal Capital Territory, and 774 Local Government Areas. Its healthcare system is composed of public and private providers (20). Given the vast number of facilities, a web-based survey was conducted to assess healthcare facility preparedness for safely identifying and managing suspect and confirmed cases of COVID-19. The survey found public health facilities were better prepared than private health facilities (20). The Nigeria

Centre for Disease Control (NCDC) used findings from the survey to develop interventions to improve IPC among private health facilities and to provide contact details of state Ministry of Health and NCDC officials for better coordination (20).

> **Baseline IPC assessments for Ebola in Uganda**
>
> During the readiness or response phase, it may be necessary to conduct disease-specific assessments to ensure that the necessary, appropriate IPC practices are in place. In August 2018, an EBOD outbreak was declared in the Democratic Republic of the Congo (DRC) (19). Cross-border movement between the DRC and Uganda provided a risk for the importation of Ebola into Uganda. As part of the readiness phase, baseline IPC assessments specific to EBOD were performed at healthcare facilities in Uganda. These assessments focused on the facilities' readiness to prevent Ebola transmission, including the ability to safely and systematically screen for and isolate patients with signs and symptoms of Ebola, and to report those patients to the required public health authorities (19). Data indicated that IPC readiness was lacking in several important areas within each of these three domains. In response, a training curriculum was implemented, and mentorship was provided to priority healthcare facilities within high-risk districts.

Preparedness, readiness, and response plans

IPC preparedness, readiness, and response plans at the national and healthcare facility levels are crucial in order to plan IPC measures for local implementation. Different plans may be required for different disaster types (21). If an epidemic or pandemic preparedness plan already exists, it is important to ensure that IPC components are added or strengthened. At a minimum, an overview of IPC goals and objectives in outbreaks, surge capacity, and ways to monitor IPC supplies may be considered (19).

During a response, plans may be updated as new information and scientific evidence become available. When developing or modifying plans, it is important to consider issues from a hierarchy of controls perspective, including transmission-based precautions, environmental cleaning and disinfection, waste management, PPE requirements, and controls to limit the number of visitors (19).

Outbreak response teams

During the readiness or response phases, as emergency operations teams are established at both the national and healthcare facility levels, it is crucial to ensure that IPC is established as a key pillar. The national-level IPC response team should ensure that roles are well defined to minimise the duplication of efforts and focus on rapidly identifying and adapting national or subnational materials specific to the outbreak. Similarly, for preparedness phases, IPC must be represented in these teams to ensure that planning is coordinated across partners and that IPC is a part of overall preparedness programming.

> **Outbreak response taskforce for Ebola in Liberia**
>
> In Liberia in September 2014, many months after the start of the Ebola outbreak, a national IPC response taskforce was established. Prior to the 2014–2015 Ebola outbreak, IPC activities in Liberian healthcare facilities were rudimentary. During the outbreak, over 30 organisations were contributing to the IPC response in Liberia, including international partners and local NGOs, but with no significant coordination and each teaching and providing guidance from their own protocols and processes (21). The IPC Task Force provided sustained authority and balance between international and local expertise and implemented several initiatives crucial to the response, including standardising protocols and messages, overseeing resource needs, establishing IPC standards, and providing tools to assess compliance. Numerous guidelines, posters, and training materials were rapidly developed for non-ETUs in Liberia, all carrying the "Keep Safe - Keep Serving" logo.
>
> The most significant issue reported by HCWs was the need for consistent and clear guidance for PPE. In response, a simple two-tier, risk-based PPE protocol was issued, with enhanced PPE recommended for all high-risk activities. The national IPC Task Force created a system that would ensure a safe working environment for all HCWs and would also restore pre-existing health services. By December 2014, over 4,000 HCWs were trained on EBOD IPC precautions.

IPC outbreak guidance

The need for harmonised evidence-based IPC guidance is one of the most critical components for preparedness, readiness, or response efforts. Often, this guidance may be based on international guidance but adapted to a national context, particularly to ensure that the guidance is appropriate for local settings. With a new or emerging infectious disease, it is also advisable to continually monitor new data to rapidly adapt guidance. Ensuring that this guidance can be efficiently disseminated to health workers is similarly necessary (19). When developing and disseminating guidance, best practices include (22–23):

- developing a clear document that demonstrates alignment among local and national guidance but is adapted to local contexts
- adapting to evolving scientific information, but balancing the incorporation of new data with consistent messaging
- support from visible leaders, including public health and national IPC experts or professional organisations
- planning for operationalising guidance, including scalable and sustainable training and monitoring
- including all health workers, which includes support staff

IPC outbreak training

All HCWs should receive training and education in IPC strategies based on national guidance. During readiness and response phases, external outbreak training programmes can be used or adapted for use. It is essential to remember to train key personnel in outbreak preparedness, including a dedicated IPC response team (19). Training should focus on how the infection is caused and transmitted and how the different elements of an IPC strategy are meant to contain it (22). Before an outbreak (preparedness phase), attention should be given to developing pre-service and in-service training, ensuring that all HCWs meet basic competencies in IPC practices, including hand hygiene and donning and doffing of PPE (19).

> **IPC outbreak training for Ebola in Guinea**
>
> During the 2014–2016 Ebola epidemic, large-scale IPC training efforts were implemented to prevent Ebola transmission in healthcare settings. In October–December 2014, at the height of the Ebola epidemic, Guinea implemented a comprehensive IPC strategy that included training, supervision, provision of PPE and other IPC supplies, and monitoring and evaluation (24). Two IPC courses were developed and conducted for non-ETU settings. The first course targeted trainers of the curriculum (training of trainers approach) and IPC supervisors and included conducting rapid IPC needs assessments for non-ETU facilities using a standard quality control checklist. The second IPC course targeted frontline HCWs from non-ETU healthcare facilities. To assess changes in knowledge associated with the training, a 30-question, multiple-choice test was developed and administered to all participants at the beginning and end of each IPC training. Among the IPC supervisors and IPC trainers, post-course knowledge of Ebola symptoms and transmission was high; the median post-training score was 28 out of 30 (93 per cent). For frontline HCWs, the median number of correct answers increased from 17 to 25 on the pre- and post-training tests (25). Most participants experienced donning and doffing of PPE for the first time during the IPC training.
>
> Although the IPC trainings were a success, logistical challenges were encountered, including finding clean training spaces, arranging a consistent power supply, obtaining and transporting training materials, and identifying all frontline HCWs in public, private, and informal healthcare facilities to include in the training sessions. Following the training, IPC supervisors provided IPC supervision and support to healthcare facilities and HCWs during the Ebola response. Providing IPC supervision and ongoing mentoring following initial training was key to success.

It is important to understand that training does not always alter behaviour, not without other supportive measures such as leadership buy-in, supportive supervision and mentorship, oversight and monitoring, an adequate supply chain (e.g., soap, water, supplies for cleaning and disinfection), and quality improvement initiatives. These multimodal strategies are evidence-based ways to improve IPC and HCW behaviour and are recommended by the WHO (13).

Surveillance and reporting programmes

Having a timely system for identifying and reporting cases is critical in outbreak preparedness, readiness, and response. Surveillance data should guide activities by directing resources to high-risk outbreak areas. It also allows for monitoring the impact of interventions, as effective interventions should lead to a decrease in new cases. Parties should coordinate with existing surveillance networks, adapt surveillance definitions as needed, strengthen microbiology and laboratory capacity at the healthcare facility level, generate regular reports, analyse available reports at the local, national, and international levels, and disseminate key information to facility leadership (19). Healthcare facilities may also consider implementing HCW surveillance and ongoing patient surveillance to quickly identify and mitigate spread within the healthcare facility, such as the HCW surveillance system established in one Singapore hospital.

> **COVID-19 HCW surveillance system at a hospital in Singapore**
>
> One institution in Singapore successfully detected and contained a cluster of SARS-CoV-2 infections among HCWs early in the pandemic through an integrated strategy focused on the surveillance of acute respiratory illness (ARI) symptoms for early case detection, outbreak management, and compliance at the individual level. HCWs with ARI symptoms were asked to report to the staff clinic or emergency department, were given five days of medical leave, and instructed to rest at home. Investigations were initiated when ground-level supervisors reported above-average numbers of staff in their work areas reporting sick for ARI, or heat maps suggested an unusual aggregation of HCWs with fever or ARI symptoms in a specific location. This strategy minimised disruption to service and prevented the closure of the medical social services department during the initial acute phase of the outbreak.

IPC communications strategy

Policies and guidelines may be updated frequently during a pandemic as the scientific community learns more about the infectious organism and methods for preventing and controlling transmission. Therefore, it is critical that healthcare facilities have effective internal and external communication methods during an outbreak. Many options exist for communicating with HCWs during an outbreak, including daily emails, a living document or webpage, a text group or online chat board, and a mobile phone app or podcast. Best practices for communication recommend that it be bidirectional, easy to access, and frequent. It may be important to adapt existing communications strategies to the outbreak/pandemic threat at hand and ensure it is integrated with the broader outbreak communications strategy at the national or subnational level. It may also be crucial to disseminate IPC information to various groups and ensure hospital leadership and administration are supportive and involved in decision-making and their communications (19).

IPC surge capacity

Surge capacity refers to the ability to increase key resources in affected areas during an emergency. Such resources include commodities such as PPE or disinfectants, equipment, and human and financial resources. During the readiness phase, it is recommended that plans be adapted to address surge capacity and IPC resources specific to the outbreak at hand, in collaboration and partnership with subnational (regional/district/local) and national level agencies and networks. It is important to map any existing inventory of IPC capacity pertaining to the threat at hand, including the consideration of human resources and financial and logistical issues (19). Examples include PPE stocks, isolation ward capacities, HCWs to provide surge capacity, trainers and training venues, waste management facilities, and cleaning supplies.

Once an outbreak has occurred, existing plans for surge capacity and IPC resources will need to be activated, specific to the outbreak at hand, including staff, hand hygiene, PPE, and disinfection supplies. It is important to ensure that supplies are being distributed equitably across healthcare facilities while also considering high-risk areas where resources may be of most need. A recent Global Fund report found that during the COVID-19 pandemic, inadequate availability of respirators was reported in three out of four public and private primary care facilities in Nigeria and about half of specialised care facilities. In Malawi, stockouts of respirators were twice as high in rural compared to urban facilities (24).

In outbreak situations, the availability of commodities like PPE might become a major concern, especially in low-resource settings where availability may already be limited. In these situations, the safe adaptation of IPC measures may need to be considered, but only if there are IPC experts available who can evaluate and approve these adaptations. Early in the West Africa EBOD outbreak, a lack of beds in the ETU resulted in EBOD patients being cared for at home or in community care centres (25). Response efforts to acknowledge and support community care were slow due to concerns of amplifying an already critical situation, but without healthcare facility capacity, there was no alternative. In September 2014, a community IPC strategy was created by a group formed of relevant non-governmental organisations and Ministry of Health and Social Welfare staff, resulting in community workers trained and equipped to provide safe household care (25).

During outbreaks, some interventions may have been implemented that were not recommended and are potentially harmful. Guidelines issued by personnel who are not IPC experts frequently do not take into consideration effectiveness, unintended consequences, equity, or feasibility. Other examples of adaptations intended to extend the availability of IPC resources but not grounded in evidence include modifying surgical masks to improve fit to provide respiratory protection and reusing non-reusable gloves following disinfection. While some adaptations are clearly necessary, it is important to consult with IPC technical experts to avoid adaptations that might be harmful.

IPC partners mapping and networks

During an emergency response, there is the potential to have multiple national and international partners supporting the local government. This can often lead to confusion if partners do not follow the same response plan or use standardised technical documents. Prior to a response, stakeholders that can be engaged during an emergency should be identified to ensure a coordinated approach to IPC activities. This is essential since it allows government officials to quickly mobilise partners, facilitates information sharing, unifies messages and actions, and minimises the duplication of efforts.

System assessment/audit

Assessment or monitoring of the IPC system is a cyclical and ongoing process for continual improvement that may occur during all phases. During the preparedness phase, it is important to define core indicators of preparedness, considering all the above key components and using a strategy to evaluate and assess these indicators to identify gaps (19). Ongoing analysis and use of the data to inform programme improvement are critical. Ideally, resources and programming should focus on the crucial areas identified through the assessments. Countries may consider using national health systems, such as DHIS2, to collect and analyse these data. Once a threat has been identified, it may be important to rapidly re-evaluate the current status of the IPC system and adapt or modify the IPC programme (19).

CONCLUSION

As the world moves forward from COVID-19, one of the pressing questions will certainly be how to minimise the impact of the next pandemic. Many people saw, and now understand, how health systems can be impacted by a fast-moving outbreak, and how essential health services can suffer as a result. We live in an increasingly globalised world, and outbreaks are rarely contained to one geographic area. It is essential that partners across communities, healthcare specialties (e.g., health administrators, clinicians, pharmacists, nurses, environmental services), governments, and partner organisations work together to ensure that we are prepared and ready to respond to the next threat. As countries focus on preparedness, readiness, and response, having sound, well-resourced IPC systems will always be a core pillar for focus.

REFERENCES:

1. Ki M. 2015 MERS outbreak in Korea: hospital-to-hospital transmission. Epidemiol Health. 2015 Jul;37:e2015033. https://doi.org/10.4178/epih/e2015033 PMID:26212508.
2. Shears P, O'Dempsey TJ. Ebola virus disease in Africa: epidemiology and nosocomial transmission. J Hosp Infect. 2015 May;90(1):1–9. https://doi.org/10.1016/j.jhin.2015.01.002 PMID:25655197.
3. Baller A, Padoveze MC, Mirindi P, Hazim CE, Lotemo J, Pfaffmann J, et al. Ebola virus disease nosocomial infections in the Democratic Republic of the Congo: a descriptive study of cases during the 2018-2020 outbreak. Int J Infect Dis. 2022 Feb;115:126–33. https://doi.org/10.1016/j.ijid.2021.11.039 PMID:34883237.
4. WHO's Infection Prevention & Control Department [Internet]. [cited 2022 Sep 1]. https://www.who.int/teams/integrated-health-services/infection-prevention-control.
5. Global report on infection prevention and control [Internet]. [cited 2022 Sep 23]. https://www.who.int/publications-detail-redirect/9789240051164.
6. Mæstad O, Shumbullo EL. Ebola outbreak 2014-2016: effects on other health services. CMI Brief [Internet]. 2020 [cited 2022 Aug 29];2020:03. https://www.cmi.no/publications/7212-ebola-outbreak-2014-2016-effects-on-other-health-services.
7. Abbas M, Robalo Nunes T, Martischang R, Zingg W, Iten A, Pittet D, et al. Nosocomial transmission and outbreaks of coronavirus disease 2019: the need to protect both patients and healthcare workers. Antimicrob Resist Infect Control. 2021 Jan;10(1):7. https://doi.org/10.1186/s13756-020-00875-7 PMID:33407833.
8. Lentz RJ, Colt H, Chen H, Cordovilla R, Popevic S, Tahura S, et al. Assessing coronavirus disease 2019 (COVID-19) transmission to healthcare personnel: the global ACT-HCP case-control study. Infect Control Hosp Epidemiol. 2021 Apr;42(4):381–7. https://doi.org/10.1017/ice.2020.455 PMID:32900402.
9. Godshall CE, Banach DB. Pandemic preparedness. Infect Dis Clin North Am. 2021 Dec;35(4):1077–89. https://doi.org/10.1016/j.idc.2021.07.008 PMID:34752221.
10. Lum BX, Liu EH, Archuleta S, Somani J, Bagdasarian N, Koh CS, et al. Establishing a new normal for hospital care: a whole of hospital approach to COVID-19. Clin Infect Dis. 2021 Nov 2;73(9):e3136-e3143. https://doi.org/10.1093/cid/ciaa1722 PMID:33179039.
11. Loveday H, Wilson J. Pandemic preparedness and the role of infection prevention and control - how do we learn? J Infect Prev. 2021 Mar;22(2):55–7. https://doi.org/10.1177/17571774211001040 PMID:33859721.
12. Nyenswah TG, Kateh F, Bawo L, Massaquoi M, Gbanyan M, Fallah M, et al. Ebola and its control in Liberia, 2014-2015. Emerg Infect Dis. 2016 Feb;22(2):169–77. https://doi.org/10.3201/eid2202.151456 PMID:26811980.
13. World Health Organization. Guidelines on core components of infection prevention and control programmes at the national and acute health care facility level [Internet]. World Health Organization; 2016 [cited 2022 Sep 23]. 90 p. https://apps.who.int/iris/handle/10665/251730.

14. World Health Organization. Minimum requirements for infection prevention and control programmes [Internet]. World Health Organization; 2019 [cited 2022 Sep 23]. x, 55 p. https://apps.who.int/iris/handle/10665/330080.
15. Lurie N, Carr BG. The role of telehealth in the medical response to disasters. JAMA Intern Med. 2018 Jun;178(6):745–6. https://doi.org/10.1001/jamainternmed.2018.1314 PMID:29710200.
16. Tyan K, Cohen PA. Investing in our first line of defense: environmental services workers. Ann Intern Med. 2020 Aug;173(4):306–7. https://doi.org/10.7326/M20-2237 PMID:32357202.
17. Doll M, Stevens M, Bearman G. Environmental cleaning and disinfection of patient areas. Int J Infect Dis. 2018 Feb;67:52–7. https://doi.org/10.1016/j.ijid.2017.10.014 PMID:29102556.
18. US Centers for Disease Control and Prevention. Standard Precautions for All Patient Care | Basics | Infection Control | 2019 [cited 2022 Sep 3]. https://www.cdc.gov/infectioncontrol/basics/standard-precautions.html.
19. Geneva: World Health Organization. Framework and toolkit for infection prevention and control outbreak preparedness, readiness and response at the health care facility level. 2021.
20. Joy Okwor T, Gatua J, Umeokonkwo CD, Abah S, Ike IF, Ogunniyi A, et al. An assessment of infection prevention and control preparedness of healthcare facilities in Nigeria in the early phase of the COVID-19 pandemic (February-May 2020). J Infect Prev. 2022 May;23(3):101–7. https://doi.org/10.1177/17571774211060418 PMID:35502165.
21. Best S, Williams SJ. What have we learnt about the sourcing of personal protective equipment during pandemics? Leadership and management in healthcare supply chain management: a scoping review. Front Public Health. 2021 Dec;9:765501. https://doi.org/10.3389/fpubh.2021.765501 PMID:34957018.
22. Houghton C, Meskell P, Delaney H, Smalle M, Glenton C, Booth A, et al. Barriers and facilitators to healthcare workers' adherence with infection prevention and control (IPC) guidelines for respiratory infectious diseases: a rapid qualitative evidence synthesis. Cochrane Database of Systematic Reviews [Internet]. 2020 [cited 2022 Sep 11];(4). https://www.cochranelibrary.com/cdsr/doi/10.1002/14651858.CD013582/full.
23. Tomczyk S, Storr J, Kilpatrick C, Allegranzi B. Infection prevention and control (IPC) implementation in low-resource settings: a qualitative analysis. Antimicrob Resist Infect Control. 2021 Jul;10(1):113. https://doi.org/10.1186/s13756-021-00962-3 PMID:34332622.
24. Transforming the medical PPE ecosystem: joint action can protect healthcare workers with effective and high-quality personal protective equipment - World | ReliefWeb [Internet]. [cited 2022 Sep 26]. https://reliefweb.int/report/world/transforming-medical-ppe-ecosystem-joint-action-can-protect-healthcare-workers.
25. Salmon S, McLaws ML, Fisher D. Community-based care of Ebola virus disease in West Africa. Lancet Infect Dis. 2015 Feb;15(2):151–2. https://doi.org/10.1016/S1473-3099(14)71080-1 PMID:25749064.

CHAPTER 27

ENABLING RESEARCH FOR THERAPEUTICS

by Xin Hui Sam, Marissa Alejandria, John Amuasi, and Barnaby Young

Research is a vital part of the effective response to a disease outbreak. Given the wide spectrum of potential outbreaks and the varying therapeutic research questions, it is challenging to develop a generic, broadly applicable clinical trial protocol as part of outbreak research preparedness. However, when considering approaches, there are common threads which can be pulled together and examples of best practice which have facilitated an effective outbreak response via research in the past. These can be replicated or adapted. This chapter will consider these common themes and discuss relevant examples that can facilitate timely, relevant, and clinically meaningful research on therapeutics during an outbreak.

INTRODUCTION

As early as 1960, research was understood to represent an important component of the pandemic preparedness framework (1). However, it was not until 1978 that the first U.S. pandemic plan was drafted by the Federal Interagency Working Group on Influenza, and only in 2006 that the Biomedical Advanced Research and Development Authority (BARDA) was established with the aim of coordinating the research and development of vaccines, therapeutics, and diagnostics against infectious disease threats. A respiratory virus pandemic has long been considered one of the top ten threats to global health, and in the wake of COVID-19, globally coordinated efforts to mitigate the *next* pandemic have become a priority. Sustaining this commitment to pandemic research preparedness is a critical challenge for the coming years if recent progress is not to be lost (2).

Clinical trials are the fundamental research method for establishing whether therapeutics and treatment protocols are safe, efficacious, and can improve patient outcomes. Despite the challenge of conducting clinical trials during a health emergency when resources may already be stretched, this research must be prioritised as an essential part of an effective outbreak response (3). The COVID-19 pandemic has clearly shown that even during an outbreak, well-designed trials can provide timely answers to critical clinical questions, reduce morbidity and mortality, and combat misinformation.

Enabling clinical research during an outbreak relies on preparation and planning (4). This includes the following:
- surveillance efforts to predict likely zoonotic pathogens
- basic research to identify promising therapeutic agents
- the development and maintenance of clinical trial research networks and expertise
- the establishment of file drawer protocols of appropriate trial designs

Designing trials in anticipation of need will ensure that time and effort are not wasted by studies which are not able to lead to valid and clinically useful conclusions (**Figure 27.1**) (5). To achieve these goals, active trial collaborations outside of an outbreak must be fostered and then switched with agility to address urgent outbreak questions. Ethics guidelines and expertise, research agreements, regulatory approval, and funding mechanisms need to be developed ahead of time to streamline rapid implementation. These all rely on the foundation of a strong healthcare system and robust clinical research infrastructure across geographical borders (6).

Detailed planning for therapeutic research must consider the wide diversity of potential pathogens, therapeutics, and clinical settings, with the flexibility to adapt to the contextual demands of each outbreak.

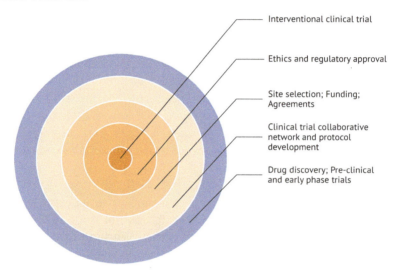

Figure 27.1: A summary of the key factors that are required such that the target—a clinical trial on a therapeutic during an outbreak—can proceed

Pathogens and populations

Novel pathogens may emerge with no available therapy, such as the severe acute respiratory syndrome coronavirus 1 (SARS-CoV-1) outbreak in 2002–2003 and the COVID-19 pandemic. In other cases, treatments may be available but the effectiveness of the medications may be uncertain, as is the case currently with tecovirimat for mpox and neuraminidase inhibitors for severe influenza (7). Even when treatments exist, it is often necessary to confirm the effectiveness of therapeutics against new variants or strains, remain vigilant for the emergence of resistance-associated mutations, and provide further information regarding any observed uncommon adverse effects. Further study may also be necessary to understand the impacts of treatments in important populations at increased risk of severe illness, such as children, pregnant women, and the immunocompromised, where efficacy and safety data is limited.

Treatments

The research questions to be investigated in a therapeutic trial can vary from investigating the safety and efficacy of pathogen- or host-directed therapies to understanding optimal treatment strategies or the timing of interventions.

Experimental agents may have very limited human safety data or may require first-in-man evaluation. There are many examples of novel products which entered clinical development during the COVID-19 pandemic, from small molecule antivirals to monoclonal antibodies. Alternatively, drugs may have been developed for other conditions and are being repurposed. Robust safety, tolerability, and pharmacological data may already be available, speeding progression to efficacy trials. For example, remdesivir had been tested in the West Africa and Democratic Republic of the Congo (DRC) Ebola virus disease (EBOD) epidemic and so could be rapidly brought into phase III efficacy trials for COVID-19 (8). A large range of other repurposed drugs were tested during the COVID-19 pandemic, largely on the basis of *in vitro* susceptibility data, but with little success (9). When the experimental data is robust, conducting rapid efficacy trials of these drugs is important, both for the early identification of effective treatments and to prevent misinformation filling a treatment vacuum (10–11). However, the manner by which it is decided which repurposed drugs enter into clinical trials is often opaque; international coordination, a clear framework, and inclusion of different stakeholder opinions can help address this.

The pathogenesis of an infection is typically a consequence of both the pathogen and the host immune response. Host-directed treatments which modulate damaging inflammatory responses have become part of the standard of care for COVID-19. While clinical trial evidence is currently limited, they are likely to have a similar importance in other respiratory virus infections, and potentially other viral infections from mpox to EBOD.

Research on therapeutics must also consider the appropriate timing of treatments in relation to illness onset and severity. For example, it has become clear that small molecule antivirals and monoclonal antibodies in COVID-19 are most effective when administered as early as possible during the illness. This may then be followed by host-directed therapy if there is evidence of a developing dysfunctional inflammatory response. Administration either too late or too early mitigates benefit and may potentially cause harm. Strategy trials that consider the appropriate sequence of interventions, combination therapy, or the role of biomarkers can be challenging to conduct and struggle to attract industry funding, but are highly instructive for clinical practice, as has been evident from the Randomized Embedded Multifactorial Adaptive Platform for Community-acquired Pneumonia (REMAP-CAP) studies (12). It is also important to consider the role of therapeutics across the full natural history of an infection, from post-exposure to early infection, hospitalisation to critical illness, and post-recovery.

Settings

Outbreaks may be global with the general population susceptible, such as with the 2009 H1N1 influenza A and COVID-19 pandemics. Alternatively, infections may be geographically disseminated but concentrated among individuals with specific risk factors, as has been observed to date with mpox. There may also be ongoing sporadic zoonotic outbreaks of varying size, but with limited human-to-human transmission, such as avian influenza and Middle East respiratory syndrome coronavirus (MERS-CoV). Outbreaks may be regional or limited to single countries and may occur across varying political, socioeconomic, and geographical contexts. Finally, outbreaks may be by emerging pathogens about which little is known, a result of changing disease epidemiology (e.g., vector-borne diseases such as dengue or Zika) or a consequence of natural disasters such as flooding, drought, and earthquakes (e.g., leptospirosis and plague) (13).

Summary

Given this wide spectrum of potential outbreaks, and the varying therapeutic research questions in each, it is challenging to develop a generic research protocol which can cover all eventualities. However, there are common themes which emerge when considering the obstacles to successful drug discovery and development. This chapter will consider these common themes and discuss relevant examples that can enable effective research on therapeutics during an outbreak. The method by which clinical trial results will be implemented into clinical practice needs to be considered throughout this process.

Drug development

Conducting pre-clinical and phase I testing *before* an outbreak can substantially reduce the time to availability of treatments, as was evident during the COVID-19 pandemic. Due to extensive clinical testing during earlier EBOD outbreaks, remdesivir was issued with an emergency use authorisation (EUA) for the treatment of severe COVID-19 by the U.S. Food and Drug Administration (U.S. FDA) on 1 May 2020. This was less than three months after the first person was enrolled in the pivotal Adaptive COVID-19 Treatment Trial (ACTT-1) (14).

Granting of the next EUA for a small molecule antiviral would not occur until June 2021. Both drugs authorised then—a nirmatrelvir precursor and molnupiravir—were discovered prior to the COVID-19 pandemic and were at various stages of pre-clinical development, including in animal studies of coronavirus infection models. However, progress was slow and first-in-man studies for both agents only occurred in 2021 (15–16). Despite the rapidity of subsequent clinical development and approval, the course of the COVID-19 pandemic may have been substantially altered if oral antivirals had been available earlier. Funding mechanisms are needed to incentivise this work by industry and/or academia outside of an outbreak when the clinical and commercial impact are unpredictable.

OUTBREAK PREPAREDNESS RESEARCH & DEVELOPMENT PLATFORMS

Outbreak preparedness

A key pillar of outbreak preparedness is investment in research and development (R&D) with the aim of shortening the time between the emergence of a pathogen and the approval of candidate therapeutics. There are three critical areas:
- surveillance to identify the most likely emerging and re-emerging pathogens, particularly those at the animal-human interface (**See Chapter 13, One Health**)
- establishing a library of therapeutic candidates that can be rapidly investigated in the event of an outbreak by a specific pathogen
- building international capacity and networks for clinical trials (this will be discussed in more detail later in this chapter)

For purpose and repurposed drugs

Under normal circumstances, the process from drug discovery to marketing of a registered therapeutic product takes up to 15 years (17). Without compromising on safety or efficacy evaluations, this traditional drug development timeline clearly needs to be expedited for an outbreak (**Figure 27.2**). Drug development is also expensive. After accounting for the costs of failed trials, it was estimated in 2020 that the median capitalised R&D investment to bring a new systemic anti-infective drug to market was US$ 1.3 billion (18).

Manufacturing capacity and logistics are a crucial step from authorisation/approval of a therapeutic agent to it entering clinical care. Assurance that supplies will be sufficient for both performing the necessary studies and subsequent clinical use should be obtained before planning a clinical trial during a crisis. Shortages of remdesivir limited its use in many countries, particularly when demand surged as waves of new variants emerged. Costs were also prohibitive for many low- and middle-income countries.

Repurposing generic drugs can also have an enormous positive impact, for example, the use of the corticosteroid dexamethasone. This medication has long been in clinical use and is widely available and inexpensive. The large-scale, U.K.-based Randomised Evaluation of COVID-19 Therapy (RECOVERY) trial publicly released the results that established dexamethasone as the standard of care for severe COVID-19 on 16 June 2020, and the U.S. National Institutes of Health COVID-19 treatment guidelines were updated to recommend its use for severe COVID-19 within 10 days (14). Attention should also be paid to ensuring that the new use of a repurposed drug does not threaten its supply for other essential clinical indications. To support this, one of the key recommendations from the Independent Panel for Pandemic Preparedness and Response was to establish regional capacity for the manufacturing, regulation, and procurement of "equitable access to vaccines, therapeutics, diagnostics ... and for clinical trials" (15).

A small molecule antiviral toolbox

In its 2022–2026 strategy document, the Coalition for Epidemic Preparedness Innovations (CEPI) set out a list of initiatives with the aim of delivering a vaccine for use within 100 days from the moment that a new pathogen is sequenced (16). A similar aspiration has been put forward for diagnostics and therapeutics, as articulated in the 100 Days Mission report by the G7 (19). The Rapidly Emerging Antiviral Drug Development Initiative (READDI), in collaboration with the Intrepid Alliance, among others, is working to develop 25 high-quality therapeutic candidates that have completed phase I studies in humans, and so are ready for entry into confirmatory phase II/III trials in the event of the identification of a new pandemic. As the 100 Days Mission report notes, success of this initiative will also rely on improving clinical trial capability and regulation processes.

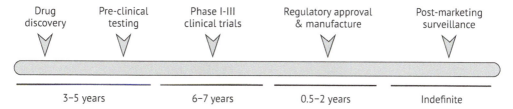

Figure 27.2: Traditional drug discovery and development timeline

Impacts for outbreak research will require shortening the overall timeline for drug development, reducing the failure rate at each step, and increasing the involvement of participants and investigators/sites in clinical research (17).

ADMINISTRATIVE FRAMEWORK
Research ethical preparedness
Whether or not associated with an outbreak, health research must always uphold fundamental ethical principles (respect for persons, beneficence, and justice) and protect the rights, safety, and well-being of participants and staff involved in the research (20). A rapidly changing situation, the need for decisions to be made quickly amidst scientific uncertainty, and limited knowledge about the clinical outcomes from a novel pathogen can challenge ethical study conduct if relevant issues have not been considered ahead of time. Ethical preparedness involves establishing appropriate ethics review committees, frameworks, and regulations before an outbreak. It also means ensuring that the underpinning moral principles and values are clearly understood by decision-makers and generally accepted by the public.

Establishing in advance a process for an expedited independent ethics review of outbreak-focused clinical trials is an important practical measure. Additional training of review board members on adaptive and innovative trial designs, biosafety requirements, isolation protocols, and current management guidelines may be necessary. Mechanisms should also be in place to prioritise the review of potentially practice-changing research such as international platform study designs versus conventional small-scale clinical trials of more limited scope. The capacity of regulatory and ethical oversight review committees should continue to be developed and enhanced to better support and understand the benefits of innovative trial designs in emerging disease conditions where speed and rigour needs to be carefully balanced, and the exploitation of disadvantaged populations remains a concern (21).

The process of ethics committee review of research can also be streamlined by establishing central institutional review boards (IRBs) or accepting cross-recognition of ethics approvals. The use of a central IRB facilitated the rapid implementation of ACTT-1 by Special Pathogens Research Network (SPRN) partner sites in the U.S. (22). Another notable example would be the African Vaccine Regulatory Forum (AVAREF) which has a mission to help national regulatory authorities, ethics committees, and sponsors achieve consensus on ethical and regulatory questions surrounding the R&D of medical products in Africa. Its primary aim is to improve access to medical products across the continent by reducing the review and approval times for clinical trial applications, while also optimising the quality of regulatory processes (23). However, while such mechanisms can help minimise duplicative work, there is a continued requirement for individual sites to conduct local reviews, particularly in international studies where regulatory approaches and ethical guidelines may differ.

Regulatory framework
The U.S. FDA's Accelerated Approval pathway was established in 1992 as part of the response to the HIV/AIDS crisis (24). This provided a mechanism for the regulatory approval of drugs shown to have a beneficial effect via a surrogate or intermediate clinical endpoint—such as viral loads. This system was modified in 2012 and expanded to include various other approval mechanisms including Fast Track Designation and Priority Review. Even with these,

the timeline for regulatory approvals by the U.S. FDA remained too long for an emergency setting. In 2004, the U.S. FDA was given the power to grant EUA of unapproved products against a threat to public health and safety after formal declaration of an emergency by the U.S. Department of Health and Human Services (HHS) (25). EUAs were given to several antivirals during the 2009 H1N1 pandemic, including the neuraminidase inhibitors oseltamivir and zanamivir (both previously approved for seasonal influenza). Similar systems are in place with other regulators, such as the Conditional Marketing Authorisation (CMA) by the European Medicines Agency (EMA). The African Medicines Regulatory Harmonization (AMRH) programme was started in 2009 by the African Union (AU). AMRH helps address the challenges faced by regulatory authorities in Africa by aiming to facilitate the harmonisation of medicine regulation and improve access to quality, safe, efficacious, and affordable medicines in the region (26).

To the frustration of researchers, contract negotiation is often a time-consuming process. While not always feasible, an agreement template outlining key matters such as data sharing, storage, transfer, and analysis of samples, governance structure, post-trial access to interventions, supply chain, intellectual property ownership, and so on should be developed between outbreaks (27).

Funding/investment

The COVID-19 pandemic highlighted the importance of nurturing and sustaining research capacity at the local level, especially in low- and middle-income countries. Equipping local healthcare workers with the research skills and knowledge when there is no outbreak is a key enabler to therapeutic research by facilitating a rapid shift to conducting clinical trials when the need arises during an emergency. Necessary research infrastructure such as electronic data capture (EDC) platforms, safe and secure storage facilities, and cold chains for the transportation of samples is also important for the conduct of research activities (28).

While funding for therapeutic discovery is important, there should also be funding to ensure downstream accessibility such as product registration and affordability (including via national and private insurance coverage) in these countries or regions where resources are limited. For research projects taking place at remote locations where resources may be constrained, funding needs to consider the costs to host organisations of using their tangible and intangible assets. Examples of tangible assets are power, water, and food, while examples of intangible assets include staff time and diversion from other essential health system and healthcare delivery functions (29).

Public–private partnerships (PPP) can provide essential incentives for collaboration and coordination between governmental agencies and industry (30). Examples include Operation Warp Speed (OWS) initiated by the U.S. government, and the pre-existing PPP between the U.S. National Institute of Allergy and Infectious Diseases (NIAID) and Moderna Therapeutics (31). With these PPPs in place, pharmaceutical companies were supported by the authorities in terms of R&D work, regulatory review of clinical trials, approval for clinical use for potential agents, and scaling up of manufacturing capacity.

Another financing mechanism designed to offer equitable access during an outbreak is the Pandemic Emergency Financing Facility (PEF) created by the World Bank Group in 2016 to offer rapid mobilisation of funding from capital-rich markets to contain a large-scale outbreak in regions without funding. Although activation criteria were carefully set, the PEF was widely criticised for approving funds too late, having set too high a bar for its activation criteria, and offering over-generous returns to investors (32). The PEF was officially closed on 30 April 2021. The new World Bank Financial Intermediary Fund (FIF) for Pandemic Prevention, Preparedness and Response (PPR) was officially established in September 2022. The FIF aims to address critical gaps identified before and during the COVID-19 pandemic through investments and technical support to strengthen PPR capabilities in regions with no funding (33). This includes a focus on building capacity in low- and middle-income countries, promoting the international sharing of epidemiological data, and strengthening the coordination of responses. Strengthening and financing international health agencies such as the World Health Organization (WHO) is also a key requirement (34).

Local engagement

To integrate research as part of the emergency response, stakeholders should be engaged at the initial stage of research protocol development and planning (35). Engaging with local communities is an essential component to build trust between researchers and individuals in the community and to avoid suspicion, resistance, and resentment. For example, in 2015, the Partnership for Research on the Ebola Virus in Liberia (PREVAIL 1) trial opened after rapid work by the Liberian and U.S. teams but was halted after launch because local communities were opposed to the study (36). A series of meetings involving local stakeholders was subsequently held to address the various issues that were of concern.

Improving general public health and clinical care infrastructure is critical to form the foundation for sustainable conduct of research activities especially in underdeveloped settings (37). There is an urgent need to invest to improve the health workforce and infrastructure in lesser developed countries as some of these countries are at the greatest risk of emerging infectious disease outbreaks. However, resources and capacity are not the only requirements. Capacity to act is not helpful without transparency. High levels of trust and cooperation between countries are essential so that responses can be mobilised quickly. Establishing frameworks for data sharing and collaboration before an outbreak is important and can be a vital scientific resource. This was shown, for example, with GISAID, a PPP for the rapid sharing of genetic, clinical, and epidemiological data from priority pathogens including influenza, SARS-CoV-2, and monkeypox.

STUDY DESIGN AND IMPLEMENTATION
Study designs

Core trial protocols that can flexibly accommodate the changing and unpredictable features of an outbreak are needed. The randomised controlled trial (RCT) is undoubtedly the ideal design to evaluate the therapeutic effectiveness of an agent. However, rather than the traditional fixed-sample trial, the use of adaptive trial designs can be more efficient and informative without compromising methodologic rigour and ethics (38). Adaptive trial platforms facilitate simultaneous or sequential evaluation of multiple candidate products using a common control arm, with potentially fewer trial participants, as ineffective agents can be dropped from evaluation more quickly, and the generation of useful data is accelerated. This design can also accommodate the merging of traditionally discrete trial phases, for example, the Therapeutics for Inpatients with COVID-19 (TICO) platform (39). The SOLIDARITY trial, conducted by the WHO in collaboration with national ministries of health, is another example that uses the adaptive trial design to allow the continuation of a study with promising investigational drug(s) while stopping futile treatment arms based on the ongoing review of evidence generated in a global pandemic condition (40).

Large-scale, pragmatic clinical trial designs are a useful approach to expand subject recruitment while minimising the burden on clinical teams and supporting the involvement of a broader variety of trial sites. Understanding and selecting relevant endpoints are critical to assess the effectiveness of an intervention for new emerging diseases. The use of surrogate endpoints at the initial phase of exploring a new therapy drives the research effort and can help accelerate approvals (41). As the situation progresses, the evidence should be re-evaluated to identify an appropriate primary outcome and meaningful effect sizes for robust scientific evidence to confirm therapy usefulness.

Equity in study recruitment and therapeutic distribution in vulnerable populations

Conventionally, pregnant or lactating women, children, prisoners, and in some cases, immunocompromised individuals are excluded from trials. In some instances, this has been true even when these special populations are particularly vulnerable to adverse outcomes following infection. The exclusion of these vulnerable individuals eventually hampers their access to experimental therapeutics due to the absence of directly relevant safety and efficacy data. The rationale of this practice remains debatable. Some may argue that when dealing with a highly contagious deadly disease, the probable risk to these individuals from the investigational therapeutic is not greater than the probable risk from the disease itself. Ensuring diversity, equity, and inclusivity during the experimental phase helps generalise therapeutics with proven clinical benefits among all groups of patients. Establishing stoppage rules for the participation of these vulnerable individuals is one of the many ways to minimise potential harm from the investigational interventions (42).

Embracing technological innovation

The COVID-19 pandemic accelerated the adoption of digital work processes in many sectors, including the conduct of clinical trials (43). On the ground, the deployment of ethically acceptable technological tools should be allowed to overcome the limitations imposed by trial personnel's inability to meet participants physically and perform visits or investigations. Electronic consent taking is an alternative to traditional paper consent-seeking, and with planning, can adhere to legislative and ethical requirements without compromising participant rights (44). Virtual consultations and follow-up are useful for the continuity of study conduct and essential data collection. These can be less of a burden than physical visits for study participants and teams even outside of outbreak settings, hence reducing study withdrawals and missing data. Remote monitoring by project managers ensures vigilant trial oversight and timely communication for any safety concern and reporting.

Shifting to online data collection may involve considerable effort to build the functionality into the trial database. The standardisation of data collection translates to a harmonised dataset that can simplify subsequent analysis and promote rapid visualisation of data for sharing with relevant stakeholders (45). Data preparedness testing needs to be conducted to ensure the integrity, security, and privacy of data collection systems before an outbreak emerges. Despite the promise of information systems and technology to enable research, digital disparity in some countries poses a significant challenge. Enhancing IT infrastructure universally is a key area to focus on for better collaboration and coordination of future global health crises. The objective should be to use all the available tools as flexibly and innovatively as necessary, while working to enhance data quality and adhering to fundamental ethical and research standards and duty of care.

Clinical trial networks

Well-developed clinical trial networks are a vital resource for the rapid implementation of therapeutic research in an emergency. Active participation by investigators and sites in such networks outside of an outbreak requires substantial investment but builds capacity that can be redeployed as needed. These networks also function as a resource and avenue for experienced investigators and trained research staff to offer training, education, and consultation to strengthen the research capability of other network members. Having a core team of staff that can shift to lead a trial, armed with planning documents delineating staffing needs according to the size of enrolment and scale of study, would expedite trial activation (22).

Inclusion and diversity are important within all parts of a clinical trial network—from trial leadership to study sites, study teams, and research participants. This includes promoting geographic and economic diversity among sites, and demographic and cultural diversity among study teams (46). Such diversity can help ensure clinical trial results are generalisable to historically under-represented populations, while also promoting the understanding of issues such as cost or sociocultural factors that may limit global equitable access. In countries/regions lacking clinical trial resources or expertise, support is available from international initiatives such as the Global Outbreak Alert and Response Network (GOARN), which has the capacity to contribute resources to international disease outbreak response, and the Council on Health Research for Development (COHRED) that helps optimise research and innovation in lower income countries, while the Special Programme for Research and Training in Tropical Diseases (TDR) is co-sponsored by international organisations including the WHO and the World Bank to reduce the burden of infectious diseases that contributes to poverty.

The ISARIC clinical research networks

The International Severe Acute Respiratory and emerging Infection Consortium (ISARIC) is a global federation of clinical research networks with more than 50 ratified networks from different global regions including developed and less developed countries. It has a vision to provide proficient, coordinated, and agile research response to outbreak-prone infectious diseases.

Since its inception in 2011, ISARIC has responded to emerging infectious diseases such as MERS, Ebola, Zika, COVID-19, and many others by gathering clinical evidence from patients, both between and during outbreaks, to improve patient care and inform public health strategies. The ISARIC-WHO clinical record form was quickly adopted at the onset of the COVID-19 pandemic and is accessible for analyses. Researchers, clinicians, industry, national and international public health bodies, and non-governmental organisations (NGOs) can exchange knowledge and ideas through the network to form partnerships or collaborate for synergistic output from participating members.

> Other than operational, administrative, technical, and project management support, essential tools were also created for investigators to collect and store data in a standardised way for accessibility by its members. The existence of standardised platforms and datasets eases effective data collection from multiple institutes for rapid analysis, as with the example of the ISARIC-COVID-19 dataset in response to a new outbreak (47).

Data sharing and dissemination of findings

Research data sharing from multicentre international trials provides the aggregation of data to support key regulatory agencies in accelerating the review and approval of therapeutics for emergency use (48). Information could be kept on a secured platform under the custody of a reputable entity to govern the accessibility within ethical guidelines. The global community needs a coordinated effort to put together all the available knowledge and resources in a central repository, on the principles of open science and raw data sharing. In the case of COVID-19, the WHO created a collection of articles about COVID-19 compiled in a publicly accessible database (15). However, the articles did not cover all the work done and the veracity and originality of some data could not be easily ascertained.

Ensuring research data is made available to the scientific community—particularly when that research is publicly funded—promotes ongoing evaluation and reflection as the situation evolves and can accelerate scientific discovery. The Wellcome Open Research platform, developed by the Wellcome Trust, allows rapid and transparent publication of researchers' work so that source data, details of data processing, and findings are openly shared (taking into account ethical and security considerations). Open Research Europe (ORE) is another open access publishing platform launched by the European Commission where the publishing cost is fully covered. The platform is open access for full text and data and can be mined by researchers as well as the public. Due to the many unknowns in any emerging infection, sharing via platforms like these can help prevent an outbreak from becoming a public health emergency.

CONCLUSION

The phases of an outbreak (preparedness, readiness, and response) discussed in the Introduction apply equally to research. Effective therapeutic research for an outbreak requires extensive preparation *before* an outbreak emerges. It is critical that the sense of urgency, collaboration, and commitment that emerges in the aftermath of a global pandemic is sustained, and that attention is not diverted to other issues which may appear more pressing in the short term.

Preparedness requires work in many areas. Research infrastructure and research networks should allow for the design and implementation of adaptive platform trials which can be activated once a public health emergency is detected. The ethical framework in the context of public health emergencies needs to be established to allow for cross-recognition of ethics approvals and the incorporation of local context. The harmonisation of processes among ethical review boards and regulatory agencies is necessary to streamline the governance process and avoid redundant and bureaucratic regulations. Sustained funding is also required to develop and enhance clinical research infrastructure and capacity.

REFERENCES:

1. Iskander J, Strikas RA, Gensheimer KF, Cox NJ, Redd SC. Pandemic influenza planning, United States, 1978-2008. Emerg Infect Dis. 2013 Jun;19(6):879–85. https://doi.org/10.3201/eid1906.121478 PMID:23731839.
2. Micah AE, Bhangdia K, Cogswell IE, Lasher D, Lidral-Porter B, Maddison ER, et al.; Global Burden of Disease 2021 Health Financing Collaborator Network. Global investments in pandemic preparedness and COVID-19: development assistance and domestic spending on health between 1990 and 2026. Lancet Glob Health. 2023 Mar;11(3):e385–413. https://doi.org/10.1016/S2214-109X(23)00007-4 PMID:36706770.
3. Saxena A, Bouvier PA, Shamsi-Gooshki E, Köhler J, Schwartz LJ. WHO guidance on ethics in outbreaks and the COVID-19 pandemic: a critical appraisal. *J Med Ethics* 2021; medethics-2020-106959. https://doi.org/10.1136/medethics-2020-106959.
4. Carlson CJ. From PREDICT to prevention, one pandemic later. Lancet Microbe. 2020 May;1(1):e6–7. https://doi.org/10.1016/S2666-5247(20)30002-1 PMID:32835320.
5. Goossens H, Derde L, Horby P, Bonten M. The European clinical research response to optimise treatment of patients with COVID-19: lessons learned, future perspective, and recommendations. Lancet Infect Dis. 2022 May;22(5):e153–8. https://doi.org/10.1016/S1473-3099(21)00705-2 PMID:34951954.
6. Gostin LO, Friedman EA. A retrospective and prospective analysis of the west African Ebola virus disease epidemic: robust national health systems at the foundation and an empowered WHO at the apex. Lancet. 2015 May;385(9980):1902–9. https://doi.org/10.1016/S0140-6736(15)60644-4 PMID:25987158.
7. Jefferson T, Jones M, Doshi P, Spencer EA, Onakpoya I, Heneghan CJ. Oseltamivir for influenza in adults and children: systematic review of clinical study reports and summary of regulatory comments. BMJ. 2014 Apr;348 apr09 2:g2545. https://doi.org/10.1136/bmj.g2545 PMID:24811411.
8. Mulangu S, Dodd LE, Davey RT Jr, Tshiani Mbaya O, Proschan M, Mukadi D, et al.; PALM Writing Group; PALM Consortium Study Team. A randomized, controlled trial of Ebola virus disease therapeutics. N Engl J Med. 2019 Dec;381(24):2293–303. https://doi.org/10.1056/NEJMoa1910993 PMID:31774950.
9. Horby PW, Mafham M, Bell JL, Linsell L, Staplin N, Emberson J, et al.; RECOVERY Collaborative Group. Lopinavir-ritonavir in patients admitted to hospital with COVID-19 (RECOVERY): a randomised, controlled, open-label, platform trial. Lancet. 2020 Oct;396(10259):1345–52. https://doi.org/10.1016/S0140-6736(20)32013-4 PMID:33031764.
10. Bramante CT, Huling JD, Tignanelli CJ, Buse JB, Liebovitz DM, Nicklas JM, et al; COVID-OUT Trial Team. Randomized trial of metformin, ivermectin, and fluvoxamine for Covid-19. N Engl J Med. 2022 Aug 18;387(7):599-610. https://doi.org/10.1056/NEJMoa2201662 PMID:36070710.
11. Maziarz M, Stencel A. The failure of drug repurposing for COVID-19 as an effect of excessive hypothesis testing and weak mechanistic evidence. Hist Philos Life Sci. 2022 Oct;44(4):47. https://doi.org/10.1007/s40656-022-00532-9 PMID:36258007.
12. Angus DC, Berry S, Lewis RJ, Al-Beidh F, Arabi Y, van Bentum-Puijk W, et al. The REMAP-CAP (Randomized Embedded Multifactorial Adaptive Platform for Community-acquired Pneumonia) study. rationale and design. Ann Am Thorac Soc. 2020 Jul;17(7):879–91. https://doi.org/10.1513/AnnalsATS.202003-192SD PMID:32267771.
13. Mora C, McKenzie T, Gaw IM, Dean JM, von Hammerstein H, Knudson TA, et al. Over half of known human pathogenic diseases can be aggravated by climate change. Nat Clim Chang. 2022;12(9):869–75. https://doi.org/10.1038/s41558-022-01426-1 PMID:35968032.
14. Horby P, Lim WS, Emberson JR, Mafham M, Bell JL, Linsell L, et al.; RECOVERY Collaborative Group. Dexamethasone in hospitalized patients with Covid-19. N Engl J Med. 2021 Feb;384(8):693–704. https://doi.org/10.1056/NEJMoa2021436 PMID:32678530.
15. Main Report & Documents. Indep. Panel Pandemic Prep. Response. https://theindependentpanel.org/documents/ (accessed Nov 5, 2022).
16. CEPI's 100 Days Mission. CEPI. https://100days.cepi.net/ (accessed Nov 5, 2022).
17. Hughes JP, Rees S, Kalindjian SB, Philpott KL. Principles of early drug discovery. Br J Pharmacol. 2011 Mar;162(6):1239–49. https://doi.org/10.1111/j.1476-5381.2010.01127.x PMID:21091654.
18. Wouters OJ, McKee M, Luyten J. Estimated research and development investment needed to bring a new medicine to market, 2009-2018. JAMA. 2020 Mar;323(9):844–53. https://doi.org/10.1001/jama.2020.1166 PMID:32125404.
19. 100 Days Mission: First Implementation Report - HTML. https://www.gov.uk/government/publications/100-days-mission-first-implementation-report/100-days-mission-first-implementation-report-html.

20. Ethical preparedness. Nuffield Counc. Bioeth. https://www.nuffieldbioethics.org/blog/ethical-preparedness (accessed Dec 12, 2022).
21. Weigmann K. The ethics of global clinical trials: in developing countries, participation in clinical trials is sometimes the only way to access medical treatment. What should be done to avoid exploitation of disadvantaged populations? EMBO Rep. 2015 May;16(5):566–70. https://doi.org/10.15252/embr.201540398 PMID:25851646.
22. Levine CB, Vasistha S, Persson CC, Larson LR, Kratochvil CJ, Mehta AK, et al. Prepared to act: lessons learned by the Special Pathogens Research Network, based on collaborations with the NIAID-led Adaptive COVID-19 Treatment Trial. Health Secur. 2022 Jun;20 S1:S20–30. https://doi.org/10.1089/hs.2021.0178 PMID:35483093.
23. African Vaccine Regulatory Forum (AVAREF). WHO Reg. Off. Afr. 2023; published online April 17. https://www.afro.who.int/health-topics/immunization/avaref (accessed April 18, 2023).
24. Kepplinger EE. FDA's Expedited approval mechanisms for new drug products. Biotechnol Law Rep. 2015 Feb;34(1):15–37. https://doi.org/10.1089/blr.2015.9999 PMID:25713472.
25. Tran A, Witek TJ Jr. The emergency use authorization of pharmaceuticals: history and utility during the COVID-19 pandemic. Pharmaceut Med. 2021 Jul;35(4):203–13. https://doi.org/10.1007/s40290-021-00397-6 PMID:34453703.
26. Sillo H, Ambali A, Azatyan S, Chamdimba C, Kaale E, Kabatende J, et al. Coming together to improve access to medicines: the genesis of the East African Community's Medicines Regulatory Harmonization initiative. PLoS Med. 2020 Aug;17(8):e1003133. https://doi.org/10.1371/journal.pmed.1003133 PMID:32785273.
27. Rojek AM, Horby PW. Offering patients more: how the West Africa Ebola outbreak can shape innovation in therapeutic research for emerging and epidemic infections. Philos Trans R Soc Lond B Biol Sci. 2017 May;372(1721):20160294. https://doi.org/10.1098/rstb.2016.0294 PMID:28396467.
28. Evans NG, Hills K, Levine AC. How should the WHO Guide access and benefit sharing during infectious disease outbreaks? AMA J Ethics. 2020 Jan;22(1):E28–35. https://doi.org/10.1001/amajethics.2020.28 PMID:31958388.
29. National Academies of Sciences, Engineering, and Medicine, Health and Medicine Division, Board on Health Sciences Policy, Board on Global Health, Committee on Clinical Trials During the 2014-2015 Ebola Outbreak. Integrating Clinical Research into Epidemic Response: The Ebola Experience. Washington (DC): National Academies Press (US), 2017 http://www.ncbi.nlm.nih.gov/books/NBK441679/ (accessed Nov 5, 2022).
30. Olliaro P, Torreele E. Global challenges in preparedness and response to epidemic infectious diseases. Mol Ther. 2022 May;30(5):1801–9. https://doi.org/10.1016/j.ymthe.2022.02.022 PMID:35218930.
31. Lurie N, Keusch GT, Dzau VJ. Urgent lessons from COVID 19: why the world needs a standing, coordinated system and sustainable financing for global research and development. Lancet. 2021 Mar;397(10280):1229–36. https://doi.org/10.1016/S0140-6736(21)00503-1 PMID:33711296.
32. Brim B, Wenham C. Pandemic Emergency Financing Facility: struggling to deliver on its innovative promise. BMJ. 2019 Oct;367:l5719. https://doi.org/10.1136/bmj.l5719 PMID:31597630.
33. Financial Intermediary Fund for Pandemic Prevention, Preparedness and Response – PPR FIF. World Bank. https://www.worldbank.org/en/programs/financial-intermediary-fund-for-pandemic-prevention-preparedness-and-response-ppr-fif (accessed April 18, 2023).
34. A Package of Reforms for Financing Pandemic Preparedness and Response for the G7. Cent. Glob. Dev. Ideas Action. https://www.cgdev.org/publication/package-reforms-financing-pandemic-preparedness-and-response-g7 (accessed Dec 12, 2022).
35. Dean NE, Gsell PS, Brookmeyer R, Crawford FW, Donnelly CA, Ellenberg SS, et al. Creating a framework for conducting randomized clinical trials during disease outbreaks. N Engl J Med. 2020 Apr;382(14):1366–9. https://doi.org/10.1056/NEJMsb1905390 PMID:32242365.
36. Larson GS, Baseler BR, Hoover ML, Pierson JF, Tegli JK, Johnson MP, et al. Conventional wisdom versus actual outcomes: challenges in the conduct of an Ebola vaccine trial in Liberia during the International Public Health Emergency. Am J Trop Med Hyg. 2017 Jul;97(1):10–5. https://doi.org/10.4269/ajtmh.16-1015 PMID:28719299.
37. Singh S, Cadigan RJ, Moodley K. Challenges to biobanking in LMICs during COVID-19: time to reconceptualise research ethics guidance for pandemics and public health emergencies? J Med Ethics. 2022 Jul;48(7):466–71. https://doi.org/10.1136/medethics-2020-106858 PMID:33980656.

38. Pallmann P, Bedding AW, Choodari-Oskooei B, Dimairo M, Flight L, Hampson LV, et al. Adaptive designs in clinical trials: why use them, and how to run and report them. BMC Med. 2018 Feb;16(1):29. https://doi.org/10.1186/s12916-018-1017-7 PMID:29490655.

39. Murray DD, Babiker AG, Baker JV, Barkauskas CE, Brown SM, Chang CC, et al. Design and implementation of an international, multi-arm, multi-stage platform master protocol for trials of novel SARS-CoV-2 antiviral agents: Therapeutics for Inpatients with COVID-19 (TICO/ACTIV-3). Clin Trials. 2022 Feb;19(1):52–61. https://doi.org/10.1177/17407745211049829 PMID:34632800.

40. Pan H, Peto R, Henao Restrepo AM, Preziosi MP, Sathiyamoorthy V, Karim QA, et al.; WHO Solidarity Trial Consortium. Remdesivir and three other drugs for hospitalised patients with COVID-19: final results of the WHO Solidarity randomised trial and updated meta-analyses. Lancet. 2022 May;399(10339):1941–53. https://doi.org/10.1016/S0140-6736(22)00519-0 PMID:35512728.

41. Schilling WH, Jittamala P, Watson JA, et al. Pharmacometrics of high-dose ivermectin in early COVID-19 from an open label, randomized, controlled adaptive platform trial (PLATCOV). Elife. 2023 Feb 21;12:e83201. https://doi.org/10.7554/eLife.83201. PMID:36803992.

42. Nichol AA, Antierens A. Ethics of emerging infectious disease outbreak responses: using Ebola virus disease as a case study of limited resource allocation. PLoS One. 2021 Feb;16(2):e0246320. https://doi.org/10.1371/journal.pone.0246320 PMID:33529237.

43. Mitchell EJ, Ahmed K, Breeman S, Cotton S, Constable L, Ferry G, et al. It is unprecedented: trial management during the COVID-19 pandemic and beyond. Trials. 2020 Sep;21(1):784. https://doi.org/10.1186/s13063-020-04711-6 PMID:32917258.

44. Skelton E, Drey N, Rutherford M, Ayers S, Malamateniou C. Electronic consenting for conducting research remotely: a review of current practice and key recommendations for using e-consenting. Int J Med Inform. 2020 Nov;143:104271. https://doi.org/10.1016/j.ijmedinf.2020.104271 PMID:32979650.

45. Kraft CS, Kortepeter MG, Gordon B, Sauer LM, Shenoy ES, Eiras DP, et al. The Special Pathogens Research Network: enabling research readiness. Health Secur. 2019 Feb;17(1):35–45. https://doi.org/10.1089/hs.2018.0106 PMID:30779607.

46. Sharma A, Palaniappan L. Improving diversity in medical research. Nat Rev Dis Primers. 2021 Oct;7(1):74. https://doi.org/10.1038/s41572-021-00316-8 PMID:34650078.

47. Knight SR, Ho A, Pius R, Buchan I, Carson G, Drake TM, et al.; ISARIC4C investigators. Risk stratification of patients admitted to hospital with covid-19 using the ISARIC WHO Clinical Characterisation Protocol: development and validation of the 4C Mortality Score. BMJ. 2020 Sep;370:m3339. https://doi.org/10.1136/bmj.m3339 PMID:32907855.

48. Bhimraj A, Morgan RL, Shumaker AH, Baden L, Cheng VC, Edwards KM, et al. Lessons learned from coronavirus disease 2019 (COVID-19) therapies: critical perspectives from the Infectious Diseases Society of America (IDSA) COVID-19 Treatment Guideline Panel. Clin Infect Dis. 2022 May;74(9):1691–5. https://doi.org/10.1093/cid/ciab882 PMID:34668008.

CHAPTER 28

PANDEMIC VACCINE DEVELOPMENT

by Qi Rou Yap, Wei Chuen Tan-Koi, John C.W. Lim, and Eng Eong Ooi

The COVID-19 pandemic has emphatically underscored the value of vaccines in the control of viral outbreaks. The rapid development of vaccines with potent immunogenicity, production, and global distribution, along with efficiently executed mass vaccination or ring vaccination programmes, are all likely key components of future response to viral outbreaks. Each of these components is a rapidly developing field in its own right; positive developments would not only be relevant for pandemic preparedness but would also benefit the prevention of endemic and childhood diseases. The Coalition for Epidemic Preparedness Innovations (CEPI) has set the target of vaccine discovery and development to be completed within a hundred days to tackle future pandemics. The authors will discuss the regulatory process behind vaccine development, the intellectual property (IP) rights involved, the transfer of liability, and access to vaccines. Issues around vaccine hesitancy will be explored in the next chapter.

INTRODUCTION

According to the World Health Organization (WHO), 105 million infants worldwide were vaccinated with all three doses of the diphtheria-tetanus-pertussis (DTP3) vaccine in 2021 (1). This high vaccination rate explains the low prevalence of these diseases which afflict children with potentially life-threatening consequences. For instance, in the U.S., only 1,609 cases of pertussis were reported in 2021, a far cry from the 200,000 or more cases (2) reported annually in the 1930s before DTP vaccines were developed. Similar trends have also been seen with regard to the incidence of poliomyelitis, measles, and rubella, where these debilitating and sometimes fatal childhood diseases have been effectively controlled and even eliminated wherever vaccination rates are high. Besides preventing childhood infections, the use of vaccines through emergency mass vaccination or ring fencing of cases has also led to early outbreak control (3) and even smallpox eradication (4). With the world now increasingly facing emerging novel viruses, as experienced with the emergence of amongst others, SARS-CoV, avian influenza H5N1, and SARS-CoV-2 in this century alone, the development of and access to new vaccines will feature prominently in any pandemic preparedness programme. This chapter explores the regulatory aspects of vaccine development, related IP rights, vaccine access and allocation, and the transfer of liability.

Modern-day vaccines are developed on the foundation laid by Edward Jenner and Louis Pasteur. Jenner, considered the trailblazer of vaccinology, pioneered the concept in 1796, when he successfully immunised a young boy against smallpox by inoculating him with the genetically-related cowpox that caused localised skin lesions but conferred lifelong immunity against smallpox. In the 1800s, Pasteur built on this discovery, injecting inactivated rabies virus from the dried spinal cord of an afflicted rabbit into experimental dogs which became immune to the virus thereafter (5). Since then, advancements in the understanding of molecular genetics, immunology, and virology have enabled vaccinology to make leaps and bounds in innovative new vaccines against a number of different infections and even cancers caused by infections such as hepatitis B and the human papillomavirus (HPV).

Vaccines can be administered in several different ways. While the goal of vaccines against HPV, influenza, tetanus, pertussis, and diphtheria is for control of these diseases, other childhood vaccination programmes against diseases such as polio, measles, and rubella aim to obtain coverage high enough to achieve herd immunity. Herd immunity refers to the protection of unimmunised subjects from either infection or disease by the high proportion of immunised subjects in the population; infection of the immunised subjects would effectively be dead ends for the virus (6). Consequently, pathogen transmission is halted or reduced by vaccination.

During an outbreak, achieving herd immunity is challenging, although not impossible, as mass vaccination across all age groups would be needed. An alternative approach to mass vaccination is ring vaccination. Ring vaccination is the vaccination of confirmed contacts of a patient as well as contacts of those contacts (7). It is a viable option when the infection has a sufficiently long incubation period for vaccine-induced adaptive immunity to develop before disease onset (8). Ring vaccination can reduce disease incidence and continued spread of the pathogen and may be the right choice when vaccines are limited.

These approaches represent the ends of a spectrum that also involve the vaccination of special populations (e.g., the elderly and the immunocompromised), as well as pre-travel vaccination. However, while there exist multiple strategies to immunise susceptible populations, the approaches will depend on the existence of licensed vaccines.

VACCINE DEVELOPMENT PROCESS

While Jenner and Pasteur were able to experiment independently on their own subjects, the development of vaccines today is governed by strict rules and regulations. There are three main stages (9) in developing and delivering a vaccine:
- research and development, and regulatory review
- manufacturing and procurement
- delivery and access

Research and development, and regulatory review

The first stage (4) involves investment in research on specific viruses and the identification of immune responses that protect against infection. These findings would also be predicated on the availability of suitable animal models and tractable clinical trials of vaccine candidates to ascertain their safety and efficacy profiles. After completion of all phases of clinical trials with satisfactory results, an application for approval will be filed to regulatory authorities such as the U.S. Food and Drug Administration (U.S. FDA) and European Medicines Agency (EMA) for the review of relevant scientific data before marketing authorisation is granted.

During research and development (R&D), scientists identify the immune responses that would protect against infection or illness and then decide on the type of vaccine that would elicit those immune responses. Vaccines work by stimulating protective responses against microbial organisms and the diseases they cause. The protective response can either be in the form of neutralising antibodies or a combination of humoral and cellular immunity against the pathogen. Many vaccines have been developed based on the assumption that antibodies, especially neutralising antibodies alone, would protect against infection. For instance, while the most widely considered assessment of COVID-19 vaccine immunogenicity was neutralising antibody titres against SARS-CoV-2, the clinical development of vaccine candidates did not weigh the merits of cellular immunity (although it was measured for completeness during the trials). T cell responses have since appeared to be particularly useful in protecting against SARS-CoV-2 variants of concern (VOCs), thereby and fortuitously contributing to the low rates of severe COVID-19 cases despite the VOCs.

In a typical R&D phase, several different teams would take on the challenge of examining if their favoured vaccine platform would be suitable to develop vaccine candidates against specific diseases. These platforms range from live-attenuated viruses to specific viral antigen subunits that can induce protective antibodies (10). Once proof-of-concept has been demonstrated and selected for development, the vaccine candidate is formulated and tested in animals to evaluate for immunogenicity, as well as local reaction, systemic toxicity, and toxicity reversibility (11). If these pre-clinical studies are promising, the vaccine candidate can progress to clinical trials.

Vaccine development and platforms

As noted above, most vaccines are developed on the assumption that the stimulation of neutralising antibodies will be enough to protect against the pathogen. In the initial stages of vaccine development, researchers must first target specific antigens within the disease-causing pathogen. These antigens, foreign substances that trigger antibody production when introduced into the human body, can then be integrated into vaccines in various formats (**Table 28.1**). Following this, vaccine developers conduct research to ascertain which vaccine type can most effectively induce an immune response in a host.

Type of vaccine	Information	Examples
Live-attenuated vaccines	Contain live pathogens that immunise by causing a mild or asymptomatic infection	Measles, mumps, and rubella Rotavirus Smallpox Chickenpox
Inactivated vaccines	Contain inactivated pathogens	Hepatitis A Polio Rabies Ebola virus
Subunit vaccines	Contain part of the pathogen which stimulates an immune response in the host	Hepatitis B HPV Pneumococcal Shingles
Toxoid vaccines	Contain inactivated toxins from the pathogen	Diphtheria Tetanus

Type of vaccine	Information	Examples
Viral vector vaccines	Utilise a harmless virus to deliver the genetic code of a protein antigen into vaccinees' cells	COVID-19
mRNA vaccines	Contain the genetic code of a protein antigen. The host body produces a specific protein unique to the virus which triggers an immune response in the host without causing disease.	COVID-19

Table 28.1: Types of vaccines and examples

A phase I trial is a blinded, dose-ranging, placebo-controlled study involving around 20–80 people. It studies the safety profile of the vaccine candidate in healthy human volunteers (12) and the immune response after administration. If the phase I trial demonstrates safety of the vaccine, the studies progress.

A phase II trial is a randomised, double-blind, placebo-controlled study involving a larger cohort of 100–300 participants. It yields more details on the safety and immunogenicity profile and dose schedule of the vaccine candidate to be utilised in the next phase. It determines the ideal dose of the vaccine—the lowest dose required to elicit an adequate immune response with acceptable side effects (11).

A phase III trial typically involves thousands to tens of thousands of people and is a randomised, double-blind, placebo-controlled trial to primarily determine vaccine efficacy. Phase III trial data also add to the body of evidence on the safety of the vaccine candidate.

Following the success of a phase III trial, data from the pre-clinical studies and all the different clinical trials will be rigorously reviewed by national regulatory authorities (NRAs) before marketing authorisation is granted (4). The role of the NRAs is to ensure that the products being released for public distribution have been evaluated properly and meet national standards of quality, safety, and efficacy. The WHO prequalification programme then ensures the availability of quality vaccines to countries in need. It does this by ensuring that the vaccines are safe, enforcing Good Manufacturing Practices (GMP), Good Laboratory Practices (GLP), and strict post-qualification requirements for continued good vaccine quality, as well as investigating all vaccine quality complaints. It also works with NRAs which help regulate the quality of vaccines in their own countries.

Despite the cumulative tens of thousands of participants in phase I to III clinical trials, there is a low probability that rare but severe adverse events following vaccination are detected, a finding that shapes the overall safety profile of any vaccine. Events that occur in one out of 100,000 vaccinations, for instance, would be unlikely to be detected throughout these stages of clinical development. Similarly, trials may miss outcomes that have delayed onset or occur in subpopulations excluded from or who are under-represented in clinical trials. Thus, following licensing, the WHO may recommend, and NRAs may require, phase IV clinical trials or equivalent post-marketing studies. Such studies not only add to the safety profile of vaccines, but also provide vaccine effectiveness data that collectively inform vaccination policies. Thus, studies on vaccines do not end with phase III clinical trials. Other surveillance measures may be advisable after vaccines are introduced.

Rigour and transparency: WHO vaccine prequalification and WHO Listed Authority

The WHO vaccine prequalification programme plays a pivotal role in ensuring a safe and effective vaccine supply to global procurement agencies such as Gavi, UNICEF, and the International Federation of Red Cross and Red Crescent Societies (IFRC) (13).

Manufacturers who want to participate in the WHO vaccine prequalification programme require marketing authorisation of the vaccine from the NRA of the country of manufacture, provided that the NRA is considered to be functional for a vaccine-exporting country or assessed and determined to meet the requirements of an NRA operating at a minimum Maturity Level (ML) 3.

The new WHO Listed Authority (WLA) framework replaces the previous procurement-oriented concept of stringent regulatory authorities. A WLA is an NRA which has been certified through WHO as a well-functioning regulatory system of ML 3 or an advanced regulatory system of ML 4, and has undergone a performance evaluation process (14).

Post-marketing surveillance and rotavirus vaccine-associated intussusception

Based on the Global Burden of Disease 2019 Study (GBD 2019), rotavirus infection is one of the leading causes of diarrhoeal death among children aged below 5 years, particularly affecting low-resourced countries with challenges in sanitation and timely medical access (15). A national childhood immunisation programme to protect against rotavirus is needed.

Rotashield® was the first rotavirus vaccine licensed in 1998. However, shortly after its licensure, the U.S. Vaccine Adverse Event Reporting System (VAERS) detected an increased risk of intussusception among infants administered with Rotashield®.

Intussusception can occur in one out of 2,000 to 3,000 infants. Five cases were reported among 10,054 vaccine recipients compared to one case among 4,633 who received placebo in the pre-licensing trials of Rotashield®. This was assessed as statistically insignificant, and no association was established. Nonetheless, as a precautionary measure, intussusception was listed as a possible side effect on the package insert. Upon approval and use in the real world, more infants were given Rotashield® and more cases were reported to the VAERS. Upon investigation, the U.S. Centers for Disease Control and Prevention (U.S. CDC) estimated that with every 10,000 infants vaccinated with Rotashield®, there will be one or two additional cases of intussusception with the highest risk window being two weeks after the administration of the first dose. In 1999, the U.S. Advisory Committee on Immunization Practices (ACIP) voted to no longer recommend the use of Rotashield® vaccines for infants, weighing the serious nature of intussusception against the ready availability of oral rehydration to treat rotavirus in the U.S. In 1999, the manufacturer voluntarily withdrew from the market (16).

Since the withdrawal of Rotashield®, other rotavirus vaccines have been developed and licensed, with the appropriate risk management plans and communications put in place. Positive cost-effectiveness studies have been reported in over 100 countries and there is a continual body of evidence to support the inclusion of the rotavirus vaccine into national immunisation programmes (17). In this case, post-marketing surveillance serves to detect and characterise safety signals in the real world and facilitate evidence-based benefit-risk assessment and decision-

> making. However, this case also reiterates many key points flagged out in this chapter and discussed in detail in the other chapters, namely the liability of manufacturers, the importance of risk communication, and the need for no-fault compensation.

Manufacturing and procurement

After a vaccine is approved, manufacturing can commence and, depending on the type of vaccine, takes weeks to months from production to fill and finish. Vaccine manufacturing was once done domestically through licensing from the discoverer or original developer. With the development of more sophisticated vaccine technologies and adjuvants, however, centralisation of manufacturing has become common practice. Hence, while many countries manufactured polio vaccines for their own use, COVID-19 vaccines were manufactured mostly in Europe, North America, China, and India, and shipped to other parts of the world. Regardless of the site of manufacture, raw materials that constitute the ingredients of any vaccine will need to be obtained and processed into active ingredients to generate the antigen used in the vaccine, with appropriate stabilisers, preservatives, and adjuvants to create the final product (18). The completed formulation is filled aseptically into a vial or syringe and is ready for shipping and use (19). Quality control checks are applied throughout the manufacturing process and take up to 70 per cent of manufacturing time (19).

The manufacturing process, materials used, and distribution process must comply with widely accepted guidelines such as GMP and GLP. GMP ensures that the starting materials, premises, equipment, training, and hygiene of the staff are maintained according to quality standards (20), while GLP guarantees the quality and integrity of non-clinical laboratory studies used to support the marketing permits for the vaccines (21). These guidelines are legal requirements of many, if not all, NRAs to ensure that the vaccines are safe, uncontaminated, and effective. Failure to adhere to these guidelines can result in legal consequences including fines, seizure, and jail time (22).

There are many other challenges to be overcome during the manufacturing and distribution process, including working out the total number of vaccine doses required for a population and in which countries, finding adequate manufacturing facilities, establishing supply chains, and dealing with IP and regulatory requirements in each country, as well as deciding on a price that will keep the vaccine affordable but allow the developer to cover R&D costs (9).

These issues are usually tackled by governments as well as Gavi, a vaccine alliance formed by a public–private partnership, whose goal is to increase the equitable and sustainable use of vaccines (23). Gavi and its core partners—the WHO, UNICEF, the World Bank, and the Bill & Melinda Gates Foundation—negotiate directly with the manufacturers to purchase vaccines at more affordable prices for low- and middle-income countries (9). Gavi also invests in vaccine stockpiles and works with UNICEF to secure contracts for the long-term procurement of vaccines. This helps ensure a consistent and reliable vaccine supply which in turn, strengthens preparedness against future outbreaks as well as access to vaccines for poorer countries. This is to ensure that access to live-saving vaccines during an outbreak is not limited to the richest countries (23).

Delivery and access

After the vaccines have been successfully manufactured and procured, they can then be moved, whilst maintaining necessary storage conditions such as a cold chain (24), to the countries of intended usage. To ensure that the vaccines are given safely, staff and volunteers will have to be trained to administer the vaccinations properly as well as manage the cold chain.

Vaccines will have their greatest impact when there is high coverage in the target population. Public health education, timely and transparent information dissemination, and the engagement of focus groups for those unwilling to be vaccinated may be required to achieve this. Information and engagement are critical elements of any successful vaccination programme, as are vaccine education, hesitancy, misinformation, and risk communication and community engagement (RCCE) (**See Chapter 29, Vaccine implementation; See Chapter 33, RCCE; See Chapter 34, Infodemics**). These important functions are undertaken by both government and non-governmental organisations, as seen in the calls for COVID-19 vaccination globally (25). Influential individuals and community leaders also play important roles in managing misinformation.

Beyond the role of national health agencies, transnational organisations and multilateral development banks play an important role in helping to ensure equitable vaccine access. Equitable access is critical for meeting a fundamental tenet of human rights, but varying levels of herd immunity should also be considered. For example, as part of the global pandemic response in 2020, the COVID-19 Vaccines Global Access Facility (COVAX) was created as a collaboration among CEPI (**See CEPI**), Gavi, and the WHO to promote global access to COVID-19 vaccines (26). It provided countries with gross national income per capita of less than US$ 4,000 with COVAX-subsidised vaccines to vaccinate up to 20 per cent of their population (26). It also follows the WHO guidelines for fair and equitable access to COVID-19 vaccines, which recommend the vaccination of high-risk and vulnerable people before rolling out the vaccination programme to the rest of the population.

Finally, while structures are in place for equitable access, the reality remains far from ideal. With the distribution of COVID-19 vaccines largely based on financial competition, high-income countries were able to obtain prioritised access to the vaccines through deals with pharmaceutical companies, depleting the global supply. COVAX had no choice but to either wait or rely on voluntary donations, many of which were unusable after being donated only close to expiry (27). Models for equitable access must remain a policy research priority of the global pandemic preparedness agenda.

THE ECONOMICS OF VACCINE DEVELOPMENT, PROCUREMENT, AND DISTRIBUTION

The development of any vaccine is a costly undertaking. Capital investment ranging from US$ 500 million to US$ 1 billion or more may be needed, depending on the complexity of the vaccines. This includes all phases from R&D to the building of manufacturing facilities and infrastructure (28). Besides capital investment, funding can also come from a variety of sources such as public funding, public–private partnerships, and philanthropic foundations. The cost of vaccine development must also be weighed against the development of other products in the pipeline of any company. Thus, although there was no shortage of interest in the development of COVID-19 vaccines during the early months of the pandemic, the economics of developing vaccines for viral diseases that threaten but have yet to emerge at anticipated scale, remain uncertain.

In 2017, CEPI, a collaboration among public, private, philanthropic, and civil society organisations, was launched. It is an international fund supporting the R&D of vaccine candidates, subsequent trials, and the production of a stockpile when the commercial market is insufficient to justify private investment in the development of the vaccine (29). It has three clearly defined goals (30):
- to advance the development of vaccines against known priority pathogens and create a stockpile before an epidemic starts
- to finance novel and innovative platform technologies that accelerate the development and manufacture of vaccines against previously unknown pathogens
- to support and coordinate global response to epidemics as well as advance the regulatory science behind product development

CEPI

CEPI is an international not-for-profit organisation whose mission is to accelerate vaccine development against emerging infectious diseases. The 2014–2016 Ebola outbreak in West Africa emphatically underscored the need for a well-coordinated global response to developing vaccines for future epidemics and pandemics. At the 2016 World Economic Forum in Davos, Switzerland, discussions were held on the formation of a global coalition to address the economic challenges that hamper epidemic preparedness. This discussion led to the formation of CEPI shortly after, with the governments of Norway and India, the Bill & Melinda Gates Foundation, the Wellcome Trust, and the World Economic Forum as founding members. The membership has since grown to include partner countries from all continents, except Antarctica. Amongst the vaccines prioritised for development by CEPI are those against Middle East respiratory syndrome (MERS), Lassa fever, Nipah encephalitis, Rift Valley fever, Chikungunya, and Ebola fever, as well as Disease X (a term adopted by the WHO in 2018 to describe a hypothetical unknown pathogen that could cause a future epidemic).

Before the creation of CEPI, the development and funding of vaccines was poorly coordinated (31), with no international body specifically managing and coordinating the efforts of individual countries to tackle global threats together (32). Such fragmented vaccine development efforts were unable to address global epidemics efficiently, resulting in many missed opportunities to bring a successful vaccine to the market before an epidemic struck (32). A prime example would be the 2014–2016 Ebola outbreak in West Africa, where vaccine development was hindered by insufficient investment due to the business model at that time which prioritised the development of vaccines with a larger market potential. The outbreak and its impact on vaccine development will be further discussed later in this chapter.

The COVID-19 pandemic has highlighted the crucial links across health, development, and economic growth. Multilateral development banks, which originated in the aftermath of World War II to rebuild war-ravaged nations and stabilise the global financial system, played critical roles by providing financing for the procurement and distribution of vaccines, especially in low-resourced settings. Clearly, sustainable financing for vaccines should be an important discussion in the "lab-to-jab" journey (33).

IP AND PATENTS

Patents are a type of IP, referring to creations of the mind, encompassing inventions, literary and artistic works, designs, and symbols, as well as names and images used in commerce (34). In the development of vaccines, patents grant the inventors the right to prevent others from creating, utilising, or selling the invention without a license from the inventor. This in turn helps inventors and developers protect their investment and reap due rewards (35).

With the high costs that research companies spend on creating vaccines, patenting their invention allows them to protect their investment and be duly accountable to their shareholders (36). It allows the companies to sell their vaccines at a price which would allow them to earn back their investment without worrying about their invention being copied by another company and launched into the market at a lower price made possible by not investing in its development (36).

As IP and technology transfer are part and parcel of vaccine development, production, and distribution, case studies on COVID-19 suggested that improving licensing conditions may facilitate more equitable distribution (37).

THE 2014–2016 WEST AFRICA EBOLA OUTBREAK AND PARADIGM SHIFT IN VACCINE DEVELOPMENT

The Ebola virus was first identified almost five decades ago and research into a vaccine commenced shortly after its discovery (38). Despite the knowledge and experience of devastating outbreaks of Ebola haemorrhagic fever (mortality rates can be as high as 90 per cent), the development and funding of vaccines was not prioritised (31). The clinical development of candidate vaccines was delayed as data on safety, immunogenicity, and dosing in humans for licensing decisions of Ebola vaccines were then not clearly defined, making the investment in vaccine trials risky (31).

As cases began to mount in July 2014, international attention to the outbreak, if not panic, grew greatly (39). The World Bank pledged US$ 200 million to help contain the infections and develop the public healthcare system of the affected countries, while global communities including the African Union, China, Cuba, the European Union, the U.K., the U.S., the International Monetary Fund, and United Nation (UN) agencies mobilised to assist in the response (39). The WHO convened an international meeting to review all available data on Ebola vaccines at that point in time to hasten vaccine development. Together with the African Vaccine Regulatory Forum, the WHO also organised key meetings between international regulators and experts to accelerate the authorisation of clinical trials. As a result, by the end of 2015, there were various phase I to III trials in place for the vaccines (40).

Despite these remarkable efforts during the outbreak, the lack of pre-planned coordination of vaccine development with outbreak response efforts led to missed opportunities. Specifically, during the 2014–2016 Ebola outbreak in West Africa, many clinical trials only started when the epidemic was already waning, and many trials were halted due to an insufficient number of cases for statistically meaningful analysis. Not only does such an outcome serve as a deterrent for investment in pandemic preparedness, but the victims of the outbreak have also arguably been deprived of live-saving vaccines.

Nonetheless, in December 2019, the Ebola vaccine ERVEBO® was approved by the U.S. FDA, just five years after clinical trials began (41). This was much quicker than the 10–15 years usually required to create a vaccine. This was achieved through trials like STRIVE (Sierra

Leone Trial to Introduce a Vaccine against Ebola), with the safety and immunogenicity of ERVEBO® evaluated through immediate (within seven days of enrolment) and deferred (18 to 14 days post-enrolment) vaccination (42).

> **Ebola ça Suffit vaccination trial**
>
> The Ebola ça Suffit ring vaccination trial was conducted in 2015 and compared the outcomes of immediate vaccination with the rVSV-ZEBOV Ebola vaccine versus delayed vaccination 21 days after exposure to the virus (43). Once a definitive case of Ebola was identified, a ring of the individual's contacts as well as the contacts' contacts was picked out and randomised to receive either immediate vaccination or be vaccinated 21 days post-randomisation. The pre-specified primary outcome was laboratory-proven Ebola infection with onset 10 days or more after the randomisation (43). The result was that there were zero cases in the group with immediate vaccination versus 11 confirmed cases in the group with delayed vaccination.
>
> This was unlike a traditional randomised placebo-controlled trial as it would not fully withhold a potentially effective intervention from the control group. It was also different from traditional ring vaccination trials as it used an unproven vaccine instead of one that had already been proven effective (44). It was developed due to the urgent need to evaluate trial vaccines against the Ebola virus. Subsequent trials such as the STRIVE trial were developed based on the Ebola ça Suffit trials.

Although many had advocated for changes to vaccine development for outbreak preparedness prior to 2014, the Ebola outbreak in West Africa initiated a paradigm shift. Firstly, the WHO developed an R&D Blueprint priority list of diseases with the potential to cause a public health emergency and which required urgent research and countermeasure development. This effort raised awareness on the urgent and unmet needs from highly infectious diseases for which few to no pharmaceutical countermeasures exist (45). It was to ensure that we would not face another situation where the world was grossly unprepared due to the uncertainty of economic returns from any investment in pandemic countermeasures.

> **WHO R&D Blueprint and COVID-19**
>
> The WHO R&D Blueprint is a global strategy and preparedness plan which allows R&D efforts to be quickly activated during epidemics (46). The Blueprint covers severe emerging diseases for which there are inadequate or no existing medical countermeasures or ways to produce them. It aims to decrease the time between the outbreak of a public health emergency and when effective diagnostic tests, vaccines, and treatments become available (47). In order to achieve this, it develops a Target Product Profile (TPP) which describes the minimally acceptable and preferred criteria for products created in response to an epidemic.

As part of the WHO's response to COVID-19, the R&D Blueprint was activated to improve the coordination between international scientists and healthcare personnel to accelerate the creation of effective countermeasures toward COVID-19. It developed the COVID-19 TPP which helped outline the desired attributes of the tests, vaccines, and therapeutics developed in response to COVID-19 (46). It was an important step to help developers define the appropriate criteria for their products, aiding them through the development process in order to meet consumer demands all while ensuring the clinical utility, safety, and effectiveness of the products (48).

The WHO Emergency Use Listing Procedure (EUL) is used to assess and list unlicensed vaccines, therapeutics, and tests, with the goal of expediting the availability of these products in an epidemic (49). During COVID-19, the TPP created was used as a tool to evaluate the adequacy of the novel products created against the pandemic, with vaccines like Comirnaty from Pfizer and Spikevax from Moderna being approved for global usage (50).

STREAMLINING VACCINE DEVELOPMENT FOR FUTURE PANDEMICS
Regulatory agility

Besides investing in vaccine research as well as providing the economic impetus for the development of vaccines to safeguard against impending pandemics, smoothening the pathway from vaccine discovery to licensing would also accelerate vaccine access.

In 2020, with COVID-19 quickly spreading across the world and causing an unprecedented global pandemic, there was a need to apply lessons of regulatory agility from the 2014 Ebola outbreak and recent trends among regulators to expedite innovative therapeutic approvals to ensure the rapid development and adequate access to a vaccine (51). Regulatory agility is the domain of NRAs and refers to the use of risk-based, context-driven approaches and regulatory cooperation based on sound scientific evidence and information (52). The adoption of regulatory agility in a pandemic ensures that a vaccine can be developed and made available in a quicker time without substantively compromising on its quality, safety, and efficacy. This is facilitated by providing emergency use authorisation (EUA) or expedited pathways that allow conditional authorisation of newly developed vaccines with less information than is traditionally expected for regulatory review, allowing rolling submission of new data as trials progress, and concurrently stepping up pharmacovigilance monitoring of adverse events (51). The enhancement of post-market monitoring to balance faster pre-market review of data is important for enabling regulatory agility while maintaining appropriate robustness of public health protection. An example is the authorisation of the Pfizer/BioNTech vaccine for emergency use in December 2020 after the U.S. FDA reviewed data from an ongoing phase I/II/III trial in approximately 44,000 participants and found it adequately safe and effective for use (53).

What is described above can be achieved by open access to information, transparency among regulatory agencies, and expedition of the vaccine development process based on informed, risk-based decisions. For example, the International Coalition of Medicines Regulatory Authorities (ICMRA), established following discussions among NRAs in 2012 to support strategic and international coordination, initiated regular virtual seminars early in the pandemic to discuss regulatory considerations for COVID-19 clinical trials with the goal of streamlining the development, approval, and availability of COVID-19 treatments internationally (33).

Regulatory agencies can also speed up the development of a vaccine by expediting regulatory approaches based on context-relevant data for approving diagnostic tests, treatments, and vaccines (51). This means that the regulatory bodies take new pandemic standards and measures into context when making decisions. The U.S. FDA's Coronavirus Treatment Acceleration Program (CTAP) provides guidance to developers as well as information on quality assessments and relevant pathways to materialise the treatments as quickly as possible without compromising on safety and efficacy. The EMA has also allowed the rolling submission of data from vaccine clinical trials so that regulators can assess the available information on vaccines and treatments in real time and approve them for emergency use if the data are adequate. They have also reduced review times from 210 to 150 days or less, as long as promising clinical data are provided while accommodating the need for inputs from member states.

> **Regulatory reliance: mechanism to facilitate faster vaccine access**
>
> Regulatory reliance is a principle which promotes leveraging the regulatory outputs of other NRAs for expedited or conditional regulatory approvals. This facilitates faster patient access, reduces the duplication of efforts, helps streamline efforts to focus on national level regulatory activities, and enhances regulatory capacity building. Early adopters include Singapore's Health Sciences Authority (HSA) with its abridged verification routes introduced in the first decade of the 21st century for faster patient access if products had been approved by its trusted reference agencies. During the COVID-19 pandemic, regulatory reliance to promote faster patient access to the new vaccines was greatly in evidence globally. The ICMRA was first established in 2012 following discussions among NRAs for a need to support strategic and international coordination. During the pandemic, the value of this network as originally envisaged was significantly realised. It spearheaded regular virtual seminars early in the pandemic to discuss regulatory considerations for COVID-19 clinical trials with the goal of streamlining the development, approval, and availability of COVID-19 treatments internationally (33).

Another way of speeding up the development process is to authorise a new product into the market earlier under a provisional market authorisation, relying on data from a smaller phase III trial. The phase III trials continue alongside the provisional market authorisation until 1,000 to 3,000 people have been in contact with the virus. However, this means that there is a higher chance of adverse effects in people during the provisional market authorisation as the product has not yet been tested in a large number of subjects in regular phase III trials. This also means that liability claims against the manufacturer may arise when the vaccine is released into the market under a provisional authorisation (54). Protection against liability will be explored further in this chapter.

The rapid sharing of gene sequences

Advancements in genomic sequencing (**See Chapter 21, Genomics**) and the creation of digital vaccines have also helped with the sharing of information between countries (55). While traditional vaccines required cultivation of the pathogen to produce an analogue vaccine, the genetic code of the virus can now be digitally uploaded to the internet where multiple laboratories and manufacturers can download it and begin developing a vaccine. This allowed the sequence of the SARS-CoV-2 spike protein to be shared publicly online on 10 January 2020, after which hundreds of laboratories across the world were able to download it and start developing vaccines without the need to ship the virus. The Moderna vaccine was able to commence clinical testing in just 66 days and the Pfizer vaccine was approved by the U.S. FDA just one year after the first confirmed COVID-19 case (55).

> **The development of the COVID-19 vaccine**
>
> COVID-19 vaccine development began soon after the SARS-CoV-2 genomic sequence was published online in January 2020. Multiple vaccine companies and academic and research institutions embarked on this quest using different approaches and technologies. In the lead were partnerships such as Moderna-NIH, Pfizer-BioNTech, and Oxford-AstraZeneca, using platforms such as mRNA and chimpanzee adenoviral vector vaccines. Johnson and Johnson, Sinovac, and Sinopharm used more conventional technologies such as human adenoviral vector and whole virus inactivation technologies. Novavax used recombinant protein technology to produce a protein subunit vaccine and combined it with their proprietary adjuvant.
>
> The first clinical trial was initiated as early as March 2020 by the Moderna-NIH partnership. Other trials started soon after in April 2020. By December 2020, EUA was given to the mRNA vaccines developed by Pfizer-BioNTech and Moderna-NIH by the U.S. FDA, while the U.K. authorised the Oxford-AstraZeneca vaccine for emergency use.
>
> That vaccines could be developed and tested in pre-clinical studies and phase I–III clinical trials within a year from the discovery of the SARS-CoV-2 genomic sequence is remarkable but should not be considered surprising. These efforts were built on the foundational research conducted on mRNA technologies, severe acute respiratory syndrome (SARS), and MERS vaccine development, as well as the experience in accelerating the development of the Ebola vaccines in response to the West Africa Ebola outbreak of 2014. The unprecedented speed in COVID-19 vaccine development now serves as a benchmark and springboard for the even more ambitious challenge by CEPI to develop and produce vaccines in less than 100 days as a response to future pandemics.

Protection against liability

The potential liability and fear of lawsuits is something pharmaceutical companies must manage as they release their products into the market. This has previously hindered the release of certain vaccines, such as the 2009 H1N1 influenza vaccine. To tackle this, governments can offer manufacturers either full or partial protection against civil liabilities with no-fault compensation systems (54). A no-fault compensation scheme allows for a person to seek compensation without having to prove fault against the opposite party (56). They are eligible to seek compensation as long as they can prove that a medical intervention caused their injury, irrespective of the exact party at fault (57). Meanwhile, exemption from civil liability would absolve the manufacturers of the responsibility to make payments to those affected by their vaccines.

With a guarantee that manufacturers are immune from lawsuits regarding the usage and administration of their products for a certain period of time, the risk-benefit relationship of rapid vaccine development is further enhanced. During the COVID-19 pandemic, despite clinical trials being conducted in countries with a high infection rate, any requirement for the vaccine to be tested in specific diverse groups of individuals would have seen marketing delayed by perhaps six months (54).

Different countries have been tackling this approach in their own way, with the U.S. developing no-fault compensation schemes for vaccinations since the 1980s. In 2005, the U.S. Congress enacted the Public Readiness Emergency Preparedness (PREP) Act. When a threat is assessed to have the potential to cause a public health emergency, the PREP Act can be issued, providing the relevant parties immunity from liability for claims of loss resulting or relating to the use of their products. In 2020, the U.S. Secretary for Health and Human Services issued a PREP Act of Declaration encompassing COVID-19 tests, drugs, and vaccines to protect the manufacturers, distributors, healthcare professionals, and other qualified people identified by the Secretary. This meant that they were protected from liability and lawsuits with respect to their products or their administration as long as there was no wilful misconduct.

During the COVID-19 pandemic, the COVAX No-Fault Compensation Programme was created. It is the world's first and only international vaccine injury scheme which provides a lump sum compensation to individuals affected by certain serious adverse events after receiving a COVID-19 vaccine distributed by COVAX. This allowed them to provide COVID-19 vaccines to many low- and middle-income countries by easing the potential financial burdens caused by the adverse effects of the vaccine on these countries. It is funded by a small levy charged on each dose of the vaccine distributed by COVAX to these countries (58).

With immunity against liability for their products, pharmaceutical companies are more willing to release their vaccines into the market earlier without waiting for full completion of their phase III trials, greatly speeding up the development process and vaccination rates.

CONCLUSION

The vaccine development process is traditionally long and arduous but recent developments in technology, adaptability in legal frameworks, and agility in regulatory processes have enabled remarkable reductions in the time taken for communities to be able to access vaccines during an outbreak. The establishment of global collaborations like CEPI and Gavi has made it easier to coordinate international efforts during infectious disease emergencies. There is potential for further streamlining of processes to shorten the wait time even more but there are arguably bigger threats to vaccine uptake than manufacture. Some of the most pressing challenges relate to issues of vaccine access and equity, community engagement and education, and combating aggressive misinformation.

With health authorities and the scientific community shaken into action by the overt lack of vaccine readiness exposed in 2014 during the Ebola epidemic, it is a tribute to all involved that during the COVID-19 pandemic, so many lives were saved globally as a result of deliberate steps enabling the rapid development and distribution of safe and effective vaccines.

REFERENCES:

1. World Health Organization. Immunization coverage [Internet]; 2021. https://www.who.int/news-room/fact-sheets/detail/immunization-coverage.
2. Centers for Disease Control and Prevention. Pertussis [Internet]; 2019. https://www.cdc.gov/pertussis/surv-reporting.html.

3. Watson OJ, Barnsley G, Toor J, Hogan AB, Winskill P, Ghani AC. Global impact of the first year of COVID-19 vaccination: a mathematical modelling study. Lancet Infect Dis. 2022 Sep;22(9):1293–302. https://doi.org/10.1016/S1473-3099(22)00320-6 PMID:35753318.
4. History of Vaccines. Vaccine development, testing, and regulation [Internet]; 2022. https://historyofvaccines.org/vaccines-101/how-are-vaccines-made/vaccine-development-testing-and-regulation.
5. DPMA | Pasteur, Jenner and history vaccines [Internet]. Deutsches Patent- und Markenamt. https://www.dpma.de/english/our_office/publications/milestones/greatinventors/pasteur/index.html.
6. John TJ, Samuel R. Herd immunity and herd effect: new insights and definitions. Eur J Epidemiol. 2000;16(7):601–6. https://doi.org/10.1023/A:1007626510002 PMID:11078115.
7. Centers for Disease Control and Prevention. Ring vaccination [Internet]; 2019. https://www.cdc.gov/smallpox/bioterrorism-response-planning/public-health/ring-vaccination.html.
8. Wells C, Yamin D, Ndeffo-Mbah ML, Wenzel N, Gaffney SG, Townsend JP, et al. Harnessing case isolation and ring vaccination to control Ebola. PLoS Negl Trop Dis. 2015 May;9(5):e0003794. https://doi.org/10.1371/journal.pntd.0003794 PMID:26024528.
9. Wellcome. The vaccine journey: from idea to immunisation | News [Internet]. https://wellcome.org/news/vaccine-journey-idea-immunisation-covid-19-coronavirus.
10. Chakravarti DN, Fiske MJ, Fletcher LD, Zagursky RJ. Application of genomics and proteomics for identification of bacterial gene products as potential vaccine candidates. Vaccine. 2000 Nov;19(6):601–12. https://doi.org/10.1016/S0264-410X(00)00256-5 PMID:11090710.
11. Artaud C, Kara L, Launay O. Vaccine development: from preclinical studies to phase 1/2 clinical trials. Methods Mol Biol. 2019;2013:165–76. https://doi.org/10.1007/978-1-4939-9550-9_12 PMID:31267501.
12. Vax Report - Understanding vaccine trials [Internet]; 2015. https://www.vaxreport.org/vax-1-1-august-2003/869-understanding-vaccine-trials.
13. Vaccines | WHO - Prequalification of Medical Products (IVDs, Medicines, Vaccines and Immunization Devices, Vector Control) [Internet]. [cited 2023 Oct 30]. https://extranet.who.int/prequal/vaccines.
14. World Health Organization. Evaluating and publicly designating regulatory authorities as WHO listed authorities: policy document. https://www.who.int/publications/i/item/9789240023444.
15. Du Y, Chen C, Zhang X, Yan D, Jiang D, Liu X, et al. Global burden and trends of rotavirus infection-associated deaths from 1990 to 2019: an observational trend study. Virol J. 2022 Oct;19(1):166. https://doi.org/10.1186/s12985-022-01898-9 PMID:36266651.
16. Centers for Disease Control and Prevention. Rotavirus vaccine (rotashield) and intussusception. Retrieved January 1999;3:2013.
17. Janko MM, Joffe J, Michael D, Earl L, Rosettie KL, Sparks GW, et al. Cost-effectiveness of rotavirus vaccination in children under five years of age in 195 countries: a meta-regression analysis. Vaccine. 2022 Jun;40(28):3903–17. https://doi.org/10.1016/j.vaccine.2022.05.042 PMID:35643565.
18. World Health Organization. How are vaccines developed? [Internet]; 2020. https://www.who.int/news-room/feature-stories/detail/how-are-vaccines-developed.
19. Vaccines Europe. How are vaccines produced? [Internet]. https://www.vaccineseurope.eu/about-vaccines/how-are-vaccines-produced.
20. International Society for Pharmaceutical Engineering. Good Manufacturing Practice (GMP) Resources [Internet]. https://ispe.org/initiatives/regulatory-resources/gmp#:~:text=Good%20Manufacturing%20Practice%20(GMP)%20is.
21. Teuscher N. What is GLP (Good Laboratory Practice)? [Internet]. Certara. 2013. https://www.certara.com/knowledge-base/what-is-glp-good-laboratory-practice/.
22. International Society for Pharmaceutical Engineering. What is GMP? [Internet]. https://ispe.org/initiatives/regulatory-resources/gmp/what-is-gmp#:~:text=GMP%20regulations%20address%20issues%20including.
23. Gavi. About our Alliance [Internet]; 2016. https://www.gavi.org/our-alliance/about.
24. Lloyd J, Cheyne J. The origins of the vaccine cold chain and a glimpse of the future. Vaccine. 2017 Apr;35(17):2115–20. https://doi.org/10.1016/j.vaccine.2016.11.097 PMID:28364918.
25. NetHope. Global Covid-19 vaccination efforts: the world's leading NGOs unite [Internet]. https://nethope.org/articles/global-covid-19-vaccination-efforts-the-worlds-leading-ngos-unite/.

26. Yoo KJ, Mehta A, Mak J, Bishai D, Chansa C, Patenaude B. COVAX and equitable access to COVID-19 vaccines. Bull World Health Organ. 2022 May;100(5):315–28. https://doi.org/10.2471/BLT.21.287516 PMID:35521037.

27. Pilkington V, Keestra SM, Hill A. Global COVID-19 vaccine inequity: failures in the first year of distribution and potential solutions for the future. Front Public Health. 2022 Mar;10:821117. https://doi.org/10.3389/fpubh.2022.821117 PMID:35321196.

28. Plotkin SA, Mahmoud AA, Farrar J. Establishing a global vaccine-development fund. N Engl J Med. 2015 Jul;373(4):297–300. https://doi.org/10.1056/NEJMp1506820 PMID:26200974.

29. Plotkin SA. Vaccines for epidemic infections and the role of CEPI. Hum Vaccin Immunother. 2017 Dec;13(12):2755–62. https://doi.org/10.1080/21645515.2017.1306615 PMID:28375764.

30. CEPI | New Vaccines For A Safer World [Internet]; 2018. https://cepi.net/.

31. Nath S, Mahajan A, Tandon V. New vaccines against epidemic infectious diseases. JK Science. 2018 Apr;20(2):55.

32. Wong G, Qiu X. Funding vaccines for emerging infectious diseases. Hum Vaccin Immunother. 2018 Jul;14(7):1760–2. https://doi.org/10.1080/21645515.2017.1412024 PMID:29194012.

33. International Coalition of Medicines Regulatory Authorities (ICMRA). COVID-19 | [Internet]. https://icmra.info/drupal/covid-19.

34. WIPO. What is Intellectual Property? [Internet]; 2016. https://www.wipo.int/about-ip/en/.

35. Johnston J, Wasunna AA; Hastings Center. Patents, biomedical research, and treatments: examining concerns, canvassing solutions. Hastings Cent Rep. 2007;37(1):S1–36. https://doi.org/10.1353/hcr.2007.0006 PMID:17348259.

36. Mahoney RT, Pablos-Mendez A, Ramachandran S. The introduction of new vaccines into developing countries. III. The role of intellectual property. Vaccine. 2004 Jan;22(5-6):786–92. https://doi.org/10.1016/j.vaccine.2003.04.001 PMID:14741174.

37. Sridhar S. Clinical development of Ebola vaccines. Ther Adv Vaccines. 2015 Sep;3(5-6):125–38. https://doi.org/10.1177/2051013615611017 PMID:26668751.

38. Abbott FM. Intellectual property and technology transfer for COVID-19 vaccines: assessment of the record. Geneva, Switzerland. World Intellectual Property Organization; 2023. https://www.wipo.int/publications/en/details.jsp?id=4684&plang=EN.

39. Moon S, Sridhar D, Pate MA, Jha AK, Clinton C, Delaunay S, et al. Will Ebola change the game? Ten essential reforms before the next pandemic. The report of the Harvard-LSHTM Independent Panel on the Global Response to Ebola. Lancet. 2015 Nov;386(10009):2204–21. https://doi.org/10.1016/S0140-6736(15)00946-0 PMID:26615326.

40. Henao-Restrepo AM, Preziosi MP, Wood D, Moorthy V, Kieny MP; WHO Ebola Research, Development Team. On a path to accelerate access to Ebola vaccines: the WHO's research and development efforts during the 2014-2016 Ebola epidemic in West Africa. Curr Opin Virol. 2016 Apr;17:138–44. https://doi.org/10.1016/j.coviro.2016.03.008 PMID:27180074.

41. US Food and Drug Administration. First FDA-approved vaccine for the prevention of Ebola virus disease, marking a critical milestone in public health preparedness and response. Silver Spring (MD). FDA; 2019. https://www.fda.gov/news-events/press-announcements/first-fda-approved-vaccine-prevention-ebola-virus-disease-marking-critical-milestone-public-health.

42. Annex I summary of product characteristics. https://www.ema.europa.eu/en/documents/product-information/ervebo-epar-product-information_en.pdf

43. Henao-Restrepo AM, Camacho A, Longini IM, Watson CH, Edmunds WJ, Egger M, et al. Efficacy and effectiveness of an rVSV-vectored vaccine in preventing Ebola virus disease: final results from the Guinea ring vaccination, open-label, cluster-randomised trial (Ebola Ça Suffit!). Lancet. 2017 Feb;389(10068):505–18. https://doi.org/10.1016/S0140-6736(16)32621-6 PMID:28017403.

44. Rid A, Miller FG. Ethical rationale for the Ebola "ring vaccination" trial design. Am J Public Health. 2016 Mar;106(3):432–5. https://doi.org/10.2105/AJPH.2015.302996 PMID:26794172.

45. Mehand MS, Millett P, Al-Shorbaji F, Roth C, Kieny MP, Murgue B. World Health Organization methodology to prioritize emerging infectious diseases in need of research and development. Emerg Infect Dis. 2018 Sep;24(9):e171427. https://doi.org/10.3201/eid2409.171427 PMID:30124424.

46. World Health Organization. Background to the WHO R&D Blueprint pathogens [Internet]. [cited 2024 Jan 29]. https://www.who.int/observatories/global-observatory-on-health-research-and-development/analyses-and-syntheses/who-r-d-blueprint/background.

47. Mehand MS, Al-Shorbaji F, Millett P, Murgue B. The WHO R&D Blueprint: 2018 review of emerging infectious diseases requiring urgent research and development efforts. Antiviral Res. 2018 Nov;159:63–7. https://doi.org/10.1016/j.antiviral.2018.09.009 PMID:30261226.

48. Soong R, Bradford E, Yeh KB, Olinger G Jr. Using a target product profile (TPP) to guide innovation for future in vitro diagnostic (IVD) developments in the United States. Glob Secur Health Sci Policy. 2023 Aug;8(1):2244561. https://doi.org/10.1080/23779497.2023.2244561.

49. Krause PR, Arora N, Dowling W, Muñoz-Fontela C, Funnell S, Gaspar R, et al. Making more COVID-19 vaccines available to address global needs: considerations and a framework for their evaluation. Vaccine. 2022 Sep;40(40):5749–51. https://doi.org/10.1016/j.vaccine.2022.07.028 PMID:35941036.

50. Pfizer/BioNTech. Comirnaty [Internet]. [cited 2024 Jan 29]. https://covid19.trackvaccines.org/vaccines/6/.

51. Soumyanarayanan U, Choong M, Leong J, Lumpkin MM, Rasi G, Skerritt JH, et al. The COVID-19 crisis as an opportunity to strengthen global regulatory coordination for sustained enhanced access to diagnostics and therapeutics. Clin Transl Sci. 2021 May;14(3):777–80. https://doi.org/10.1111/cts.12954 PMID:33314667.

52. Lim JC. Wither ASEAN regulatory agility and convergence in the ongoing COVID-19 pandemic. Singapore: SingHealth Duke-NUS Global Health Institute. https://www.duke-nus.edu.sg/core/think-tank/core-regulatory-perspective/whither-asean-regulatory-agility-and-convergence-in-the-ongoing-covid-19-pandemic.

53. RADM Denise M. H. EUA [Internet]. US Food and Drug Administration. FDA; 2020. https://fm.cnbc.com/applications/cnbc.com/resources/editorialfiles/2020/12/11/Pfizer-BioNTech%20COVID-19%20Vaccine%20LOA_0_0.pdf.

54. A vaccine for COVID-19: risks and liabilities from an international perspective [Internet]. [cited 2023 Oct 30]. https://www.twobirds.com/en/insights/2020/netherlands/a-vaccine-for-covid-19-risks-and-liabilities-in-international-perspective.

55. FDA. FDA approves first COVID-19 vaccine [Internet]; 2021. https://www.fda.gov/news-events/press-announcements/fda-approves-first-covid-19-vaccine.

56. USLegal, Inc. No-Fault Compensation Law and Legal Definition [Internet]. [cited 2023 Oct 30]. https://definitions.uslegal.com/n/no-fault-compensation/.

57. Gaine WJ. No-fault compensation systems. BMJ. 2003 May;326(7397):997–8. https://doi.org/10.1136/bmj.326.7397.997 PMID:12742898.

58. World Health Organization. COVAX no fault compensation [Internet]. [cited 2024 Jan 29]. https://www.who.int/initiatives/act-accelerator/covax/no-fault-compensation.

CHAPTER 29

VACCINE IMPLEMENTATION STRATEGIES: EQUITY AND HESITANCY

by Jolyn Koh, Leesa Lin, and Heidi J. Larson

Vaccines are crucial in protecting against infectious diseases. Their equitable distribution is important in tackling infectious disease health crises and intricately related to questions of social justice. However, vaccination rates are highly uneven between and within countries. In a digital age with highly unequal geographies, even if vaccines are easily accessible, vaccine hesitancy has also emerged as a significant barrier. This chapter seeks to explore the issue of vaccine equity and identify barriers to attaining it. The particular theme of vaccine hesitancy will be highlighted and analysed. A critical perspective will be presented, focusing on structural and systematic barriers to vaccine uptake, and how they intersect with one another across various levels.

INTRODUCTION

Vaccination is a crucial means of preventing infectious diseases and outbreaks (1). However, vaccine uptake rates for these diseases vary across countries, communities, and individuals. This serves as a barrier toward achieving vaccine equity (2). It is important that we address vaccine inequity as it translates to the widening of health inequalities and more broadly, deeply implicates the ethical and moral question of social justice (3–4). This chapter seeks to:
- provide a brief thematic overview of barriers to vaccine uptake
- identify barriers to achieving vaccine uptake across various levels within global and national contexts
- highlight vaccine hesitancy as a pertinent obstacle in the contemporary context

This chapter presents the argument that a multilevel and place-specific approach should be taken to address vaccine equity issues in all its complexities. In particular, more attention should be paid to tackling vaccine hesitancy and the spread of misinformation in a digital age. This chapter makes a key contribution by resituating vaccine equity in its historical context of disease prevention and immunisation. As made evident during the COVID-19 pandemic, vaccine inequity exacerbates existing social inequalities, and rampant vaccine misinformation contributes to hesitancy and reduced uptake. It is thus important to pursue the goal of vaccine equity, given the significant ethical and practical implications if we fail to do so.

VACCINE EQUITY
Context and development of the concept

Medical advancements have led to the advent of vaccines as a key preventative measure to protect against certain diseases, reducing related morbidity and mortality rates. Vaccinations are projected to prevent about 5.1 million deaths each year globally, at least if current World Health Organization (WHO) coverage targets are met (5), and the impact will be greater in low- and middle-income countries that are more susceptible to the spread of infectious diseases (6).

There has been significant progress in rolling out new vaccinations over the last two decades, in part due to the establishment of global initiatives and programmes. Gavi, the Vaccine Alliance, is an international organisation established in 2000 seeking to promote equitable access to vaccinations worldwide. Gavi engages with both public and private sector actors to fund vaccine initiatives in countries with an average per capita income of less than US$ 1,730 (7). Gavi has played a crucial role in funding vaccination for almost half of the world's children. The organisation supports vaccination against 17 infectious diseases and has funded about 1.8 billion vaccine doses between 2000 and 2022. Through its support of routine immunisation programmes, the organisation has helped vaccinate more than one billion children in 77 countries within this period. This translates to the prevention of more than 17.3 million deaths (8–9).

The Coalition for Epidemic Preparedness Innovations (CEPI), established in 2017, is another important organisation that operates more specifically in the realm of infectious diseases. Similar to Gavi, CEPI is a global coalition of public, private, philanthropic, and non-governmental organisations, but focuses on financing the development of vaccines and other biologic countermeasures against emerging infectious diseases and helps ensure their equitable distribution in an outbreak context (10). For instance, CEPI, together with Gavi and the WHO, formed the COVID-19 Vaccines Global Access (COVAX) alliance in 2020 to accelerate the development of the COVID-19 vaccine and procure adequate doses to distribute to the poorest countries (11).

For multilateral agreements, the Global Vaccine Action Plan (GVAP) is a global immunisation framework endorsed by the World Health Assembly in 2012 for the period of 2011–2020. The primary goal of GVAP was to ensure equitable access to vaccinations across all communities, such that vaccine-preventable diseases could be eradicated or significantly reduced. The goals included meeting vaccination coverage targets within every locality, developing vaccines and relevant technologies, embedding immunisation as a key priority on national agendas, and ensuring public health education on the importance of being vaccinated (12).

Although the GVAP introduced a valuable monitoring framework, it has challenges, and the Immunization Agenda 2030 (IA2030) will focus more on national ownership and locally tailored strategies to address differences across countries and settings. Conflicts, climate change, migration, and urbanisation have prompted the Immunization Agenda to include the importance of more flexibility to emerging issues (13). IA2030 sets new goals in the face of changing contexts, including tackling misinformation and sustaining public trust in vaccinations, renewing a focus on inequality, especially at the subnational level, and disease monitoring in the face of climate change-specific contexts (13).

Nonetheless, inequities in vaccination coverage across countries still exist. Out of some 20 million children who have not received the recommended three doses of diphtheria-tetanus-pertussis (DTP3) immunisation coverage, more than half of them reside in ten countries (12). Within countries, studies have shown that vaccination coverage is stratified along lines of intersecting social inequalities—across socioeconomic, ethnic, race, gender, age, and nationality divides (6,9,12,14–16).

The COVID-19 pandemic, with its uneven vaccination coverage, has mirrored these long-standing trends. Furthermore, existing inequalities are further magnified through the health crisis itself, including the disruption of routine immunisation (RI) (17). Globally, this is estimated to have resulted in at least a 5 per cent increase in the number of people who are not fully vaccinated against vaccine-preventable diseases, and 5.22 per cent more deaths (6) (**See Chapter 23, Essential services**).

Vaccine equity broadly entails equity in the **accessibility, affordability, and acceptability** of vaccines (4). At the global level, this is highly intertwined with global production chains, and inequities are prevalent from the upstream stages of research to distribution and procurement. Research funding, international governance of intellectual property rights and patents, geographical differences in manufacturing stratified across international divisions of labour, and geopolitical considerations, amongst others, are other prominent issues (4). At the national level, even after countries procure vaccine doses, vaccination uptake may remain low or highly uneven due to issues of access and acceptance within populations (18).

The next section will elaborate more on the barriers to vaccine equity. At the global level, **vaccine nationalism** is a prominent issue. At the national level, **social inequalities** are determinants of **vaccine inequities**. Lastly, at both national and global levels, vaccine hesitancy is an increasing problem, lowering vaccine uptake and confidence in immunisation efforts. Nonetheless, it is important to note these factors are not mutually exclusive and influence overall vaccine equity in mutually constitutive ways, through controls on vaccine access, affordability, and acceptance.

Obstacles to attaining vaccine equity: vaccine nationalism and global supply chains

Vaccine nationalism refers to the phenomenon whereby vaccine supplies are concentrated in certain countries while excluding others (19). As vaccine production is a highly complex and expensive process involving patented technologies, research and manufacturing capacities are highly segmented geographically, concentrated in regions with relevant expertise and resources. Pre-COVID-19 data showed that vaccine production was dominated by the European Union (EU), U.S., and India. This composition has changed slightly since COVID-19, with China playing a more prominent role in vaccine production and export (20–21). Nonetheless, vaccine production and distribution remain highly uneven processes, concentrated within specific localities.

Arguably, vaccine nationalism is made more prominent in an epidemic/pandemic context, characterised by high infection rates across a wide geographical area. The fast spread of diseases and rapid rise in cases may be attributed to the emergence of a new or modified pathogen which requires the development of novel vaccines (20). Due to the lack of readily available supplies of these new vaccines in the context of a pressing health crisis, countries often put health interests of their own populations first, and as such, securing vaccine supplies becomes a national priority. Briefly, the result is differential access to procuring vaccines, stratified across wealth and production capacities.

First, high-income countries can more easily secure access to the development of new vaccines through financing agreements. This was observed during COVID-19, when developed countries such as the U.S. and U.K. secured a bulk of the vaccines during the initial development stage through advance market commitments (AMCs) or advance purchase agreements (APAs) (22). These agreements are presented as "innovative funding mechanisms" operating on free market principles. Governments sign legally binding commitments with vaccine manufacturers to provide initial funding for vaccine development and production, on the condition that these companies will also commit to sell these vaccines to developing countries at an "affordable" price (23). Funding is provided through richer countries committing to pre-ordering a percentage of doses of a potential vaccine (22). As only high-income countries have the financial means to bulk order and purchase a large amount of vaccine doses, participation in these agreements is limited. A study has shown that more than half of the AMCs attributed to COVID-19 vaccine orders were placed by rich countries (24). Theoretically, this free market mechanism could have incentivised and facilitated vaccine innovation and production, and as manufacturing capacities scale up, vaccine supply will increase and the doses will be made available to less developed countries at more affordable prices. This presents itself as a win-win solution whereby every country will eventually be able to obtain sufficient vaccinations for their populations. However, in reality, countries with first-hand access to vaccine doses engaged in hoarding practices as manufacturing capacities were unable to scale up quickly enough to meet global demand. This phenomenon is made most evident in an outbreak context when there is a need to rapidly scale up supply. During the COVID-19 pandemic, national interests were put first, and more than 70 countries imposed export regulations on medicines, vaccines, medical equipment, and personal protective supplies (19). Such practices were also observed during the H1N1 pandemic in 2009 when high-income countries purchased almost all the vaccine supply following its development (25).

Second, the disparity between high- and low-income countries in their capacities to secure vaccine supplies goes beyond their fiscal positions and is further attributed to longstanding geographical unevenness in vaccine supply chains. Dominant pharmaceutical players are mostly based within developed contexts, where scientific research is supported through generous public funding, an educated labour force, and established expertise in scientific research (26). Vaccine developments emergent from these contexts are also protected under a regime of intellectual property rights, preventing the export of vaccine production capacities (21). Due to existing agglomeration dynamics and protection laws, low-income countries are unable to expand domestic vaccine production to meet local demand and remain in a position of structural disadvantage as net vaccine importers (21). Notably, technology transfer programmes have been launched by the WHO during COVID-19 (COVID-19 Technology Access Pool [C-TAP]) and the 2011 influenza pandemic (Pandemic Influenza Preparedness [PIP] Framework) (26). While such initiatives are positive steps towards vaccine equity, their success remains highly limited as major pharmaceutical players do not proactively engage in voluntary one-way technology transfers (26). Hence, low-income countries will continue to face prominent challenges in achieving security in vaccine supplies unless scientific and manufacturing capacities can be shored up locally (21).

Beyond restricting access, vaccine inequity and hoarding further drives up demand while supplies remain limited. This inflates prices with the greatest impacts falling upon low- and middle-income countries. Such acts also undermine global cooperation, especially important in the event of future outbreaks. Countries that are unable to secure initial stocks of vaccines may use leverage with critical production ingredients or different sorts of medical equipment to gain access to vaccine supplies (19). In the long term, the erosion of global cooperation and amplified global inequalities will worsen the issue of vaccine inequity, with every disease outbreak exacerbating these fault lines.

Geopolitical tensions and global supply chains during COVID-19

At the start of the pandemic, the Trump administration invoked the Defense Production Act against the mask-producing company 3M. The Act mandates a company to prioritise orders from the U.S. government over others. The administration demanded 3M stop mask exports and send masks made in overseas factories to the U.S. This, however, presents the risk of other countries doing the same and stopping exports of medical supplies to the U.S. (27). This similarly applies to the procurement of raw materials and equipment needed for vaccine development and production (e.g., adjuvants which may only be available within certain countries with the available resources and/or technology) (28). The multistep and complicated process of vaccine production itself makes it susceptible to bottlenecks within the supply chain that can be used as geopolitical leverage.

Furthermore, with limited supplies, countries with production capacities may reduce vaccine exports to ensure local supplies. India dramatically reduced the volume of COVID-19 vaccine exports in the face of its own surge of disease. This had major implications for low-income countries that historically depended on India for their vaccine supplies (20). On the other hand, China increased its export volume dramatically compared to the pre-COVID period. Multiple scholars (29–31) have argued that China's commitment to supplying its vaccines to the global market can be interpreted as a diplomatic strategy. It is noted that many of the recipient countries of Chinese vaccines were developing countries in Southeast Asia and Africa and are involved in China's Belt and Road Initiative (BRI) (31). Hence, in the face of scarcity, vaccine production and distribution become more strategic and contentious, intrinsically linked to geopolitics and geographical dependencies in global supply chains.

There are global and multilateral initiatives seeking to redistribute vaccine supplies and ensure vaccine equity. However, their non-legally binding nature means that countries are not responsible for ensuring that their poorer counterparts receive sufficient doses. For example, COVAX was launched in 2020 to increase the accessibility to and affordability of COVID-19 vaccines, especially for low-income countries, through its various financing and procurement strategies (21). However, as of October 2022, vaccine doses distributed through this programme only accounted for 12 per cent out of 15 billion vaccine doses administered (21). Looking at how vaccine distribution in the current and previous pandemics played out, the lack of legally binding or legislative frameworks that facilitate a more diverse and inclusive geography of vaccine production and access will continue to realise inequitable distribution globally, particularly in an outbreak context. Hence, while global initiatives play a crucial role, they must also be made more robust to better plan for scenarios that serve as obstacles to vaccine equity.

The issue of vaccine nationalism goes beyond the pitting of rich and poor countries against one another, but also involves consideration of the geopolitics and spatial-temporal aspects in the geography of vaccine production (e.g., where production capacities are located, historical patterns of export and import, and historical dependencies). Given the highly stratified geographies, robust transnational and global forms of cooperation and governance will be crucial in addressing this.

Obstacles to attaining vaccine equity: intersectional social inequalities

Nationally, vaccination rates differ between individuals and communities due to factors that reduce the access, affordability, and acceptability of vaccines. Overall, marginalised populations are disproportionately affected with lower vaccination rates. These populations live in regions with little or no access to healthcare services, are more susceptible to misinformation that deters them from getting vaccinated, are unaware of the benefits of vaccination, are unable to afford the costs of getting vaccinations, or experience structural discrimination that undermines their confidence in governments and vaccination programmes. These groups include the elderly, females, ethnic and racial minorities, and low-income individuals.

A recent global study (3) that sought to investigate longstanding inequalities in vaccine coverage found that overall, the poorest individuals—defined as within the lowest wealth quintile band—were 27 per cent less likely to be fully vaccinated than those within the richest band. Females were also 3 per cent less likely to be fully vaccinated compared to males. Education levels also significantly determined vaccination rates, particularly for children. Children born to mothers with no formal education were 27 per cent less likely to be fully vaccinated than those who were born to mothers with at least a primary education level.

A systematic review (15) of 24 peer-reviewed studies revealed that ethnic minority communities (e.g., Hispanic, African, Asian, etc.) in the U.K. were more hesitant to receive a COVID-19 vaccination. This was attributed to factors of misinformation, distrust in governance systems due to experience of structural discrimination, barriers to information pertaining to the risk and use of vaccines to make informed decisions, and lack of access to healthcare services.

Similarly, another scoping review (14) investigated vaccination uptake by minority ethnic communities. An identified barrier was the cost of vaccines and travelling to vaccination sites. For example, in a survey conducted amongst an uninsured population in Suffolk County in New York, of which 80 per cent were Hispanic/Latino, the high costs of influenza vaccines were a significant barrier. About 76 per cent of the participants were willing to seek vaccination if offered for free (compared to 17 per cent previously) (32). Another barrier was higher levels of distrust in vaccines due to bad experiences with local healthcare systems, which was particularly accentuated for historically marginalised minority populations (33–35).

A separate survey conducted in November 2020 by the National Association for the Advancement of Coloured People (NAACP) in the U.S. found that only 14 per cent of Black survey respondents trusted the safety of COVID-19 vaccines and only 18 per cent planned to get vaccinated (36). The higher rates of vaccine hesitancy are associated with mistrust in local healthcare due to the everyday racism they experience with these systems (37). Microencounters such as being given lower quality treatment or services and being treated with negligence or suspicion contribute to and reinforce mistrust, heightening the anxieties that can increase susceptibility to misinformation (38). During the COVID-19 pandemic, narratives circulated online of how Black communities were receiving inferior vaccine doses (e.g., with lower efficacy rates) due to their race and socioeconomic status. Despite authorities justifying the choice of vaccine based on logistical constraints, the belief that vaccine distribution was discriminatory and racist was still widespread (39). Therefore, the structural and systemic racism experienced within Black communities in the U.S. contributed to heightened COVID-19 vaccine hesitancy, putting these populations at further risk of infection and associated vulnerabilities (39).

Crucially, the intersectional, context-dependent, and complex nature of vaccine inequity needs to be highlighted. Due to different historical, social, cultural, economic, and political contexts of different countries (noting their potential overlaps), the determinants of vaccine inequity also vary across localities. Hence, it is important to recognise the context dependency of vaccine equity, and conduct local analyses to sift out the specific factors that systematically influence access, affordability, and acceptance of vaccines across different social groups.

The context-specific determinants of vaccine acceptance influencing vaccine equity

In Sierra Leone, children are often vaccinated through routine immunisation programmes. Locals are well acquainted with the idea of vaccinations, so much so that it has its own term—'*maklat*'—within the national language.

These programmes were carried out by the local health ministry, acting through its network of rural health services. However, trust in the public health system eroded following the Ebola health crisis, due to the perceived unethical measures taken by the local authorities (e.g., excessively spraying patients with chlorine). Hence, in this post-Ebola context, there was low confidence in the COVID-19 vaccines distributed by the government, despite individuals being well aware of the benefits of vaccination itself.

Additionally, villagers also felt that there was no need for vaccination due to the apparent low transmission rates that are likely to have been an artefact of lack of testing. COVID-19 was perceived as less severe compared to Ebola, which had visibly worse symptoms and higher mortality rates.

Vaccine hesitancy was further fuelled by the spread of misinformation through social media that built upon the denial of the severity of COVID-19. Information about the life-threatening side effects of taking the vaccine circulated within communities. For example, one rumour on social media suggested that the Sinopharm vaccine, developed by the Chinese, was an invention to wipe out African people.

A confluence of historical and socio-political factors in Sierra Leone resulted in low uptake of the vaccine despite available supplies. Hence, in this context, overcoming vaccine hesitancy required instilling confidence in public health systems and tackling misinformation (40).

Seniors in Singapore, Hong Kong, and later, mainland China, demonstrated a specific cultural hesitancy in vaccination against COVID-19 largely over worries of side effects and the lack of recommendations from healthcare professionals. This hesitancy was correlated with solitary living and being diagnosed with a higher number of health impairments. The greater anxiety of this group was not targeted with advocacy, including social media usage, that could emphasise the importance of vaccination to seniors (41).

> In contrast to the Sierra Leone example, the use of social media in Singapore and Hong Kong was encouraged to dispel anxieties around receiving vaccinations. This vaccine hesitancy was associated with lacking exposure to sufficient information that could reinforce the importance of vaccination, dispel myths, and provide information on where to access vaccinations.

VACCINE HESITANCY IN A DIGITAL AGE

Vaccine hesitancy is the "state of indecision and uncertainty that precedes a decision whether to become vaccinated" (42). It was highlighted as one of the top ten threats to global health by the WHO in 2019 (43). Vaccine hesitancy is not a new issue and has been observed for multiple vaccines, especially the whole-cell pertussis, human papillomavirus (HPV), dengue, and measles-mumps-rubella (MMR) vaccines. It was amplified during the COVID-19 pandemic.

The spread of misinformation and conspiracy theories driving vaccine hesitancy was cited as one of the factors preventing adequate COVID-19 vaccine uptake (44). Some of the misinformation that circulated included messages that COVID-19 was a virus developed by the Chinese government as a type of bioweapon (45), that vaccines cause autism (a myth that has been consistently debunked by multiple scientific studies) (42,44,46–47), and the circulation of dystopian tales such as Bill Gates microchipping individuals through vaccines to create a global surveillance network (48).

The increasing prevalence of social and online media in disseminating information plays a particular role in the amplification of hesitancy and risk perception through their hyper-connective modalities (42). Marginalised communities will be more susceptible to misinformation, building upon previous mistrust in local authorities (49). The differences in vaccine acceptance between social groups will then further amplify vaccination and health inequalities (**See Chapter 34, Infodemics**).

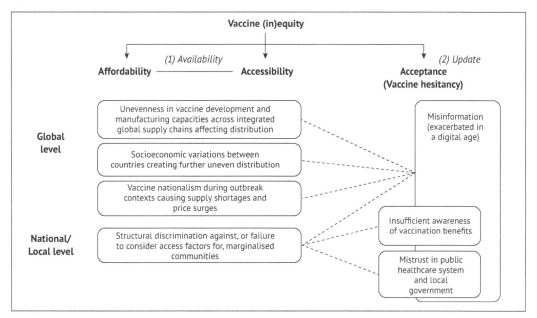

Figure 29.1: An overview of vaccine (in)equity and hesitancy

> **Increased risk of vaccine hesitancy influenced by structural factors**
>
> In 2015, two planned Ebola vaccine trials to be conducted in Ghana were suspended before they started, largely due to rumours and public distrust. A discourse analysis study (38) highlighted that misinformation on media platforms played a crucial role in invoking negative public sentiments toward the trials. The Coalition for Ghana's Independence Now (CGIN), a political party, openly criticised these trials as inhumane. The Ebola vaccine trials were seen as an experiment that was threatening to participants, associated with the common misconception that individuals would have to be "infected" first before the vaccines were developed. This was influenced by misinformation and "half-truths" spreading across media outlets and by user comments (e.g., the use of language such as "infected" versus "developing immunity"). Such fears were propagated effectively in the context of Ghanaian society, whereby there has been longstanding mistrust in the local authorities due to a historical association of scientists with corruption and working for personal gains.

Given that disease outbreaks are likely to become even more commonplace in a globalised world (50) and may require the constant development of novel vaccines (1), the amplified levels of vaccine hesitancy create a "landscape of uncertainty" (18) for future preparedness.

Vaccine mandates have been proposed (particularly in the COVID-19 pandemic) to address the challenge of vaccine hesitancy, but more sustainable solutions are needed. In these instances, non-vaccinated individuals are subjected to a suite of disincentives hoping to encourage them to get vaccinated (e.g., potential denial of entry into certain venues or particular modes of travel for non-vaccinated individuals). While mandatory vaccinations can help increase vaccination rates in the short term, such approaches are not sustainable as this approach does not address the root causes of vaccine hesitancy and refusal, particularly aggravated by compulsory measures and perceptions of being controlled. In some cases, the mandates have actually increased resentment, and one study in France reported that even though some people were vaccinated to be able to attend public places and travel, their negative sentiments around vaccines persisted (51).

CONCLUSION

It is ironic that the status of vaccine development, production, innovation, and programme implementation has reached new levels of advancement but is being matched by seemingly increasing levels of inequity and hesitancy.

COVID-19 has exacerbated health inequalities, and also exposed existing vaccine inequities—from development to distribution and acceptance. During the crisis, intensified inequities, as well as their contributing factors (e.g., vaccine nationalism, social inequalities, vaccine hesitancy), were brought to the fore. This presents as a learning opportunity for politicians, health authorities, and healthcare professionals to identify gaps in vaccination policies, public attitudes, and institutional capacities, concomitantly adapting current and future approaches to ensure vaccine equity. In an increasingly globalised world where infectious diseases are becoming more commonplace and severe, while faced with other global challenges such as climate change, conflict, and migration, attaining vaccine equity is more crucial than ever.

REFERENCES:

1. Dubé E, Gagnon D, MacDonald N. Between persuasion and compulsion: the case of COVID-19 vaccination in Canada. Vaccine. 2022 Jun;40(29):3923–6. https://doi.org/10.1016/j.vaccine.2022.05.053 PMID:35637068.
2. Global Dashboard for Vaccine Equity. UNDP Data Futures Platform. Accessed April 11, 2023. https://data.undp.org/vaccine-equity/.
3. Rydland H, Friedman J, Stringhini S, Link B, Eikemo T. The radically unequal distribution of Covid-19 vaccinations: a predictable yet avoidable symptom of the fundamental causes of inequality. Humanit Soc Sci Commun. 2022;9(1):61. https://doi.org/10.1057/s41599-022-01073-z.
4. van der Graaf R, Browne JL, Baidjoe AY. Vaccine equity: past, present, and future. Cell Rep Med. 2022 Feb;3(3):100551. https://doi.org/10.1016/j.xcrm.2022.100551 PMID:35474741.
5. Carter A, Msemburi W, Sim S, Gaythorpe K, Lindstrand A, Hutubessy R. Modeling the impact of vaccination for The Immunization Agenda 2030: deaths averted due to vaccination against 14 pathogens in 194 countries from 2021–2030. *SSRN* Electronic Journal. Published online January 1, 2021. https://doi.org/10.2139/ssrn.3830781.
6. Ali HA, Hartner AM, Echeverria-Londono S, Roth J, Li X, Abbas K, et al. Vaccine equity in low and middle income countries: a systematic review and meta-analysis. Int J Equity Health. 2022 Jun;21(1):82. https://doi.org/10.1186/s12939-022-01678-5 PMID:35701823.
7. Gavi. Eligibility. Accessed April 11, 2023. https://www.gavi.org/types-support/sustainability/eligibility.
8. Gavi@20. Accessed April 11, 2023. https://www.gavi.org/gavi-at-20.
9. Gavi. Facts and figures. Accessed January 26, 2024. https://www.gavi.org/sites/default/files/programmes-impact/our-impact/Gavi-Facts-and-figures-October-2023.pdf.
10. CEPI. Why we exist. Accessed April 11, 2023. https://cepi.net/about/whyweexist/.
11. Bown CP, Bollyky TJ. How COVID-19 vaccine supply chains emerged in the midst of a pandemic. World Econ. 2022 Feb;45(2):468–522. https://doi.org/10.1111/twec.13183 PMID:34548749.
12. WHO. Global vaccine action plan 2011-2020. Accessed April 11, 2023. https://www.who.int/publications-detail-redirect/global-vaccine-action-plan-2011-2020.
13. WHO. Immunization Agenda 2030: a global strategy to leave no one behind. Accessed April 11, 2023. https://www.who.int/publications/m/item/immunization-agenda-2030-a-global-strategy-to-leave-no-one-behind.
14. Bhanu C, Gopal DP, Walters K, Chaudhry UA. Vaccination uptake amongst older adults from minority ethnic backgrounds: a systematic review. PLoS Med. 2021 Nov;18(11):e1003826. https://doi.org/10.1371/journal.pmed.1003826 PMID:34735440.
15. Hussain B, Latif A, Timmons S, Nkhoma K, Nellums LB. Overcoming COVID-19 vaccine hesitancy among ethnic minorities: a systematic review of UK studies. Vaccine. 2022 May;40(25):3413–32. https://doi.org/10.1016/j.vaccine.2022.04.030 PMID:35534309.
16. Pietraszek A, Sobieszczańska M, Makuch S, Dróżdż M, Mazur G, Agrawal S. Identification of barriers limiting the use of preventive vaccinations against influenza among the elderly population: a cross-sectional analysis. Vaccines (Basel). 2022 Apr;10(5):651. https://doi.org/10.3390/vaccines10050651 PMID:35632407.
17. UNICEF 2023 State of the World's Children Report. SOWC-2023-full-report-English.pdf (unicefusa.org).
18. de Figueiredo A, Simas C, Karafillakis E, Paterson P, Larson HJ. Mapping global trends in vaccine confidence and investigating barriers to vaccine uptake: a large-scale retrospective temporal modelling study. Lancet. 2020 Sep;396(10255):898–908. https://doi.org/10.1016/S0140-6736(20)31558-0 PMID:32919524.
19. Bollyky TJ, Bown CP. The tragedy of vaccine nationalism. Foreign Aff. 2020 Sep/Oct. Accessed April 11, 2023. https://www.foreignaffairs.com/articles/united-states/2020-07-27/vaccine-nationalism-pandemic.
20. A world divided: global vaccine trade and production. Bruegel | The Brussels-based economic think tank. Published March 9, 2023. Accessed April 11, 2023. https://www.bruegel.org/blog-post/world-divided-global-vaccine-trade-and-production.
21. WHO. Global Vaccine Market Report. 2023: A shared understanding for equitable access to vaccines. Accessed February 11, 2024. https://iris.who.int/bitstream/handle/10665/367213/9789240062726-eng.pdf?sequence=1.
22. Chimpango B. Vaccine nationalism and equitable access to COVID-19 pharmaceuticals: TRIPS Agreement under trial (again). J Int Trade Law Policy. 2021 Oct;20(3):166–83. [cited 2023 Apr 11] https://doi.org/10.1108/JITLP-03-2021-0012.

23. World Bank. Advance Market Commitment. Accessed April 11, 2023. https://fiftrustee.worldbank.org/en/about/unit/dfi/fiftrustee/fund-detail/amc.
24. Duke Global Health Institute. Will low-income countries be left behind when COVID-19 vaccines arrive? Accessed April 11, 2023. https://globalhealth.duke.edu/news/will-low-income-countries-be-left-behind-when-covid-19-vaccines-arrive.
25. Riaz MM, Ahmad U, Mohan A, Dos Santos Costa AC, Khan H, Babar MS, et al. Global impact of vaccine nationalism during COVID-19 pandemic. Trop Med Health. 2021 Dec;49(1):101. https://doi.org/10.1186/s41182-021-00394-0 PMID:34963494.
26. Thambisetty S, McMahon A, McDonagh L, Kang HY, Dutfield G. Addressing vaccine inequity during the COVID-19 pandemic: the TRIPS intellectual property waiver proposal and beyond. Camb Law J. 2022 Jul;81(2):384–416. https://doi.org/10.1017/S0008197322000241.
27. Swanson A, Kanno-Youngs Z, Haberman M. Trump seeks to block 3M mask exports and grab masks from its overseas customers. The New York Times. https://www.nytimes.com/2020/04/03/us/politics/coronavirus-trump-3m-masks.html. Published April 3, 2020. Accessed April 11, 2023.
28. Fisher M, Kharenko K, Ucel C, Yadav P. Building the supply chain for COVID-19 vaccines. Harvard Business Publishing. 2021.
29. Liu L, Huang Y, Jin J. China's vaccine diplomacy and its implications for Global Health Governance. Healthcare. 2022; 10(7):1276. MDPI. https://doi.org/10.3390/healthcare10071276.
30. Kobierecka A. Post-covid China: 'vaccine diplomacy' and the new developments of Chinese foreign policy. Place Branding Public Dipl. 2023 Sep;19(3):280–93. https://doi.org/10.1057/s41254-022-00266-2.
31. van Dijk RJ, Lo CY. The effect of Chinese vaccine diplomacy during COVID-19 in the Philippines and Vietnam: a multiple case study from a soft power perspective. Humanit Soc Sci Commun. 2023;10(1):1–12. https://doi.org/10.1057/s41599-023-02073-3.
32. Chen G, Kazmi M, Chen D, Phillips J. Identifying associations between influenza vaccination status and access, beliefs, and sociodemographic factors among the uninsured population in Suffolk County, NY. J Community Health. 2020 Dec;45(6):1236–41. https://doi.org/10.1007/s10900-020-00873-1 PMID:32607750.
33. Cameron KA, Rintamaki LS, Kamanda-Kosseh M, Noskin GA, Baker DW, Makoul G. Using theoretical constructs to identify key issues for targeted message design: African American seniors' perceptions about influenza and influenza vaccination. Health Commun. 2009 Jun;24(4):316–26. https://doi.org/10.1080/10410230902889258 PMID:19499425.
34. Harris LM, Chin NP, Fiscella K, Humiston S. Barrier to pneumococcal and influenza vaccinations in Black elderly communities: mistrust. J Natl Med Assoc. 2006 Oct;98(10):1678–84. PMID:17052061.
35. Sengupta S, Corbie-Smith G, Thrasher A, Strauss RP. African American elders' perceptions of the influenza vaccine in Durham, North Carolina. N C Med J. 2004;65(4):194–9. https://doi.org/10.18043/ncm.65.4.194 PMID:15481486.
36. Bajaj SS, Stanford FC. Beyond Tuskegee - vaccine distrust and everyday racism. N Engl J Med. 2021 Feb;384(5):e12. https://doi.org/10.1056/NEJMpv2035827 PMID:33471971.
37. Powell W, Richmond J, Mohottige D, Yen I, Joslyn A, Corbie-Smith G. Medical mistrust, racism, and delays in preventive health screening among African-American men. Behav Med. 2019;45(2):102–17. https://doi.org/10.1080/08964289.2019.1585327 PMID:31343960.
38. Thompson EE. Botched Ebola vaccine trials in Ghana: an analysis of discourses in the media. Vaccines (Basel). 2021 Feb;9(2):177. https://doi.org/10.3390/vaccines9020177 PMID:33669759.
39. First Draft. Covid-19 vaccine misinformation and narratives surrounding Black communities on social media. Accessed April 11, 2023. https://firstdraftnews.org/long-form-article/covid-19-vaccine-misinformation-black-communities/.
40. Leach M, MacGregor H, Akello G, Babawo L, Baluku M, Desclaux A, et al. Vaccine anxieties, vaccine preparedness: perspectives from Africa in a Covid-19 era. Soc Sci Med. 2022 Apr;298:114826. https://doi.org/10.1016/j.socscimed.2022.114826 PMID:35228096.
41. Zhang D, Zhou W, Poon PK, Kwok KO, Chui TW, Hung PH, et al. Vaccine resistance and hesitancy among older adults who live alone or only with an older partner in community in the early stage of the fifth wave of COVID-19 in Hong Kong. Vaccines (Basel). 2022 Jul;10(7):1118. https://doi.org/10.3390/vaccines10071118 PMID:35891283.
42. Larson HJ, Gakidou E, Murray CJ. The vaccine-hesitant moment. N Engl J Med. 2022 Jul;387(1):58–65. https://doi.org/10.1056/NEJMra2106441 PMID:35767527.

43. WHO. Ten health issues WHO will tackle this year. Accessed April 11, 2023. https://www.who.int/news-room/spotlight/ten-threats-to-global-health-in-2019.

44. Lee SK, Sun J, Jang S, Connelly S. Misinformation of COVID-19 vaccines and vaccine hesitancy. Sci Rep. 2022 Aug;12(1):13681. https://doi.org/10.1038/s41598-022-17430-6 PMID:35953500.

45. Romer D, Jamieson KH. Conspiracy theories as barriers to controlling the spread of COVID-19 in the U.S. Soc Sci Med. 2020 Oct;263:113356. https://doi.org/10.1016/j.socscimed.2020.113356 PMID:32967786.

46. Hotez PJ. COVID19 meets the antivaccine movement. Microbes Infect. 2020;22(4-5):162–4. https://doi.org/10.1016/j.micinf.2020.05.010 PMID:32442682.

47. Larson HJ, Lin L, Goble R. Vaccines and the social amplification of risk. Risk Anal. 2022 Jul;42(7):1409–22. https://doi.org/10.1111/risa.13942 PMID:35568963.

48. Reuters. False claim: Bill Gates planning to use microchip implants to fight coronavirus. https://www.reuters.com/article/uk-factcheck-coronavirus-bill-gates-micr-idUSKBN21I3EC. Published January 6, 2022. Accessed April 11, 2023.

49. Jaiswal J, LoSchiavo C, Perlman DC. Disinformation, misinformation and inequality-driven mistrust in the time of COVID-19: lessons unlearned from AIDS denialism. AIDS Behav. 2020 Oct;24(10):2776–80. https://doi.org/10.1007/s10461-020-02925-y PMID:32440972.

50. Pang T, Guindon GE. Globalization and risks to health. EMBO Rep. 2004 Oct;5(S1 Suppl 1):S11–6. https://doi.org/10.1038/sj.embor.7400226 PMID:15459728.

51. Ward JK, Gauna F, Gagneux-Brunon A, Botelho-Nevers E, Cracowski JL, Khouri C, et al. The French health pass holds lessons for mandatory COVID-19 vaccination. Nat Med. 2022 Feb;28(2):232–5. https://doi.org/10.1038/s41591-021-01661-7 PMID:35022575.

CHAPTER 30

MANAGING RISK IN MASS GATHERINGS

by Jacob Lewis, Ziad Memish, and Brian McCloskey

Mass gatherings present specific challenges to public health systems and need effective and comprehensive public health planning. The COVID-19 pandemic demonstrated both perceived and actual risks of mass gatherings, in the context of novel infectious diseases, leading to many gatherings being cancelled or postponed. Learning, experience, and evidence from mass gatherings over recent decades have shown that risks can be managed but only if they are recognised, with appropriate mitigation measures put in place and with those measures tested and monitored. Effective planning for mass gatherings can allow important events to proceed safely with reassurance to organisers, participants, and communities that they will not be put at undue risk.

INTRODUCTION

Mass gatherings are held for a variety of social, religious, and cultural reasons. Humans are inherently social animals and gatherings are necessary and important in a developed and high-functioning community. However, alongside the benefits are risks associated with large gatherings, including potential sources for a disease outbreak. There are many reasons why an outbreak might be easily spread among a large, dense population.

The field of mass gathering healthcare has been developing for a decade (1–3) and key considerations in mass gathering planning from a global healthcare perspective are well documented, particularly in the 2015 World Health Organization (WHO) manual (4).

The WHO defines mass gatherings as "a planned or spontaneous event where the number of people attending could strain the planning and response resources of the community or country hosting the event. The Olympic Games, The Hajj, and other major sporting, religious, and cultural events are all examples of a mass gathering."

Much of the evidence base and guidance for mass gatherings pre-dated the COVID-19 pandemic but has been updated to reflect the newly recognised realities and impacts of COVID-19 on the organisation of large groups of people. Advice for preventing the spread of this respiratory disease was based around public health and social measures (PHSMs), including principles of limiting human contact, national and more focused lockdowns in various forms, and the use of personal protective equipment (PPE) at an individual as well as institutional level, alongside the deployment of vaccination and treatment options as these were developed. This application of guidance in most settings of society required a large shift in behaviour and an extension of protocols from the clinical environment to workplaces, home, schools, and social environments. Mass gatherings were viewed as likely superspreader events and were often banned by national authorities. This was met with mixed opinions from experts and the public (5–7).

This chapter focuses on the assessment and running of mass gatherings and how guidance can optimise safety while allowing the event to proceed during an infectious disease emergency.

More recent mass gatherings can provide examples of both well-implemented guidance and strategies that required improvement. Considering the recent pandemic and several high-profile outbreak cases, it is clear that, as with all potential public health hazards, a risk assessment and response system is a vital part in the organisation of mass gatherings.

CANCELLATION OF MASS GATHERINGS DURING A MAJOR INFECTIOUS DISEASE OUTBREAK

Prior to the emergence of COVID-19 in 2020, the focus of mass gathering advice was primarily on assessing the risks and developing mitigation strategies to ensure risks were appropriately managed when the event took place. COVID-19 highlighted the need for a more radical approach addressing the question of whether mass gatherings should be cancelled entirely in the context of a pandemic. Prior to the development of testing, treatment, and vaccination options for COVID-19, cancellation seemed to be the only effective means of mitigating the risk of mass gatherings escalating the global spread of COVID-19.

Through late 2020 and 2021, a wide range of mass gatherings including festivals, sporting events, and religious gatherings was cancelled. Cancelling planned mass gatherings has significant consequences both in economic and social terms and these affect the organisers of the events, the participants, and the communities in which the events were scheduled to happen. In most cases, the costs of staging the event will already have been committed before cancellation, and if the event is cancelled, the opportunity to recover costs through income from participants is lost. For individuals, the costs of tickets and travelling to the event may not be fully reimbursed, for communities, the associated benefits for travel, hospitality, and retail businesses will not materialise, while for sponsors, the opportunities to generate new business will be lost. There are also non-financial costs such as the psychological impact of cancelling a much anticipated event and the negative impact on well-being of reinforcing the feeling that COVID-19 was permanently disrupting society.

As understanding of the impact of public health measures on the risk of spread of COVID-19 evolved in 2021 and 2022, and as options to mitigate the risk including testing, treatment, and vaccinations expanded, the focus of mass gathering planning shifted again to a robust risk assessment of each event to decide whether the risk could be sufficiently mitigated to allow the event to go ahead without creating an unacceptable public health risk. Thus, the Tokyo 2020 Olympic and Paralympic Games were not cancelled but postponed until the summer of 2021 to allow the organisers and governments to review the progress with potential mitigation measures and develop protocols that would allow the Games to be held safely in 2021.

In Formula 1 motor racing, the 2020 season was almost entirely cancelled due to a combination of risk assessments and travel and quarantine restrictions in host cities. However, in 2021, a limited series went ahead with races rescheduled and substituted, or held in "bio bubbles", including several held without spectators. By 2022, a refined COVID-19 protocol allowed an almost normal season to run.

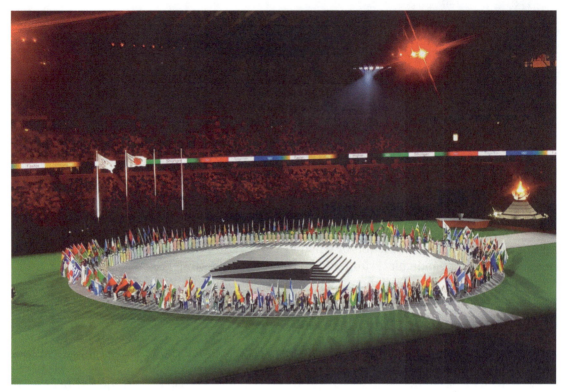

Figure 30.1: Closing of the Tokyo Olympics, 2021
(Courtesy Brian McCloskey)

Similarly, the Hajj pilgrimage in the Kingdom of Saudi Arabia was scaled back in 2020 so that only a limited number of Saudi residents could attend. In 2021, foreign attendees were still banned but a larger number of residents was permitted. In 2022, international visitors were allowed again and the numbers were scaled up to one million attendees.

In 2023, in line with learning from mass gatherings during the pandemic and a generalised easing of COVID-19 restrictions globally, the default assumption was again that mass gatherings could now be held safely if appropriate mitigation and risk reduction measures are taken. However, the decision to continue or cancel should remain as an important consideration for all mass gatherings in the local and global contexts.

PLANNING MASS GATHERINGS

Planning for a mass gathering can be considered in key stages, each of which need to be carefully actioned.

Risk assessment and mitigation

A formal risk assessment should inform the thinking on whether a mass gathering can be held safely, assessing all risks and factoring in feasible mitigation measures. A decision can then be made based on the risk assessment and the importance of the event. Organisers and local public health organisations must appreciate the key issues and understand where the major risks are and what mitigation measures will be required to manage the risks. This allows an informed decision on the appropriateness, or otherwise, of proceeding with the mass gathering. It can also set the basis for risk communication that is an integral part of the planning and execution of mass gatherings. Initial insights into the specific challenges and risks associated with any mass gathering can be developed using the WHO Mass Gathering Risk Assessment Tool (8).

Strategic risk assessment is paramount to event preparation and must reflect context. For example, a music festival taking place outdoors in the summer will need an assessment of heat conditions and the ability to respond to related health emergencies. Organisers need to be confident that the local health system can cope with the additional demand on services caused by the mass gathering, due to environmental and context-dependent factors, as well as any further demand due to an outbreak, should it occur.

Testing and exercising

Risk mitigation measures should be tested via exercises to see whether they are adequate, fit for purpose, and capable of being effectively implemented. Adaptations and improvements are designed in response to the exercise findings. Pre-event testing and exercises also assess whether the mass gathering has the capability and capacity to carry out protocols for mass gathering emergencies and is prepared for low- to high-level healthcare provision if needed. Testing and exercising are used to train staff, identify potential shortcomings, and validate plans. Exercises can be in the form of rehearsals, drills, or discussions, and can range widely in the number and type of personnel needed. Both daily operations and emergency responses need to be tested to get an understanding of how outcomes can be optimised.

Testing can also examine whether appropriate standards, for example for food and water, are in place and can be monitored as detailed in ongoing guidance (9).

Monitoring and surveillance

A fundamental requirement for successfully managing a mass gathering is for the health sector to know what is happening during the mass gathering. This is especially relevant in the case of infectious disease issues. This requires disease surveillance systems that are timely and sensitive. An early priority for organisers and local authorities is to review whether the existing systems are sufficient for the task or whether enhancements will be necessary.

"Knowing what is happening makes life more comfortable"

A general strategy to review the disease surveillance systems is as follows:
- Assess existing systems and identify strengths and weaknesses in the context of the planned mass gathering
- Use the mass gathering risk assessment to identify particular challenges that might arise and prioritise conditions to survey
- Determine resources required and plan to ensure that these resources will be in place
- Develop plans for disease surveillance. These include:
    - Objectives
    - Data to be collected
    - Where to collect data?
    - Who will collect data, how will data collection be done, how will data be transmitted?

- How will data be reviewed and what constitutes signals requiring further investigation?
- How will data be reported?
- How long will the systems operate?

• Identify and train stakeholders
• Test and evaluate any systems

Mass gatherings can produce unique demands on disease surveillance systems that may not be easily met by the routine systems in place.

"Expect the unexpected"

One such demand arises from the speed with which issues can escalate in the context of a mass gathering, driven both by the nature of the mass gathering event itself and by the political interest in the success (or failure) of the event organisation. Such rapid escalation requires surveillance systems that can also react as fast as the situation requires and that can function well in the face of uncertainty.

Another unique facet of mass gatherings is that the basic paradigm for disease surveillance can shift. In normal practice, disease surveillance systems are designed to alert public health authorities when something unusual happens so that they can respond quickly. In a mass gathering, what is often needed is a surveillance system that can reassure organisers and politicians that *nothing* is happening—and that is a very different challenge. Proving a negative in science is difficult, and in a mass gathering, the best, perhaps only, way to enable this is by using multiple parallel surveillance systems. Multiple systems all showing no signals of unusual issues make it easier to reassure organisers and politicians. Multiple systems are often in place in national public health surveillance (laboratory notifications and clinician notifications, syndromic surveillance, event-based surveillance, etc.), but an important part of the risk assessment is to review how well this can be delivered.

COMMAND, CONTROL, AND COMMUNICATION

As noted above, mass gatherings can move and escalate at great speed and produce multiple demands on public health systems. This means that management of the mass gathering needs a clear process of command, control, and communication alongside contingency plans for adverse events. Surveillance systems tell organisers what is happening at the mass gathering, whereas Command, Control, and Communication (C3) systems are what enable an effective response to a signal.

The C3 system at a mass gathering will determine how the different agencies involved will coordinate with each other and how responsibilities will be agreed across different agencies. The C3 plans and protocols will also set out how information about a potential issue will be analysed, how information will be shared (and with whom), who will be responsible for initiating action, who will be responsible for implementing each action, and who will monitor the outcomes. Very importantly, the C3 plan will set out how information will be shared with the public and how public health advice will be formulated, agreed to, and issued.

It is obvious that in an outbreak, the primary aim should be to control the spread of infection and reduce the impact as much as possible, but this can only happen with clear and

agreed upon responsibilities and leadership delivered through an effective C3 system. The C3 system is there to avoid (4):
- unclear lines of authority
- too many people reporting to one supervisor
- inadequate and incompatible communication between agencies
- terminology differences between agencies
- unclear or unspecified incident objectives
- different emergency response organisational structures
- multijurisdictional issues
- high public and media visibility
- excessive risks to property, life, and health
- excessive cost of the response and poor results

All these problems can lead to confused and inefficient decision-making and unclear advice being given to the organisers, local authorities, and ultimately, to the public.

Health sector coordination bodies must be established as part of any C3 protocol. This will generally require a physical Emergency Operating Centre (EOC) to act as a contact point for all agencies and as a source of consolidated health advice. The setup, staffing, and management of the EOC must be part of the testing and exercising programme prior to the mass gathering to ensure that it functions well and to establish its role as the main point of contact for public health issues during the mass gathering.

RESPONSE AND COMMUNICATION

Following the identification of a public health issue at a mass gathering, a rapid and decisive response is necessary. This should be based on the normal public health systems and practices in the host city or country, but these may need to be strengthened or enhanced to work at a pace that may become necessary in a mass gathering situation and to reflect the complexity of the organisation of the mass gathering.

> **The Hajj**
>
> The annual pilgrimage to Mecca, Saudi Arabia, the Hajj attracts around two million people from 185 countries. It is a setting for acute respiratory illness caused by influenza, rhinovirus, coronaviruses, pneumococcus, and haemophilus. Studies have shown infection rates as high as 50 and 93 per cent, depending on the year and methodology of screening. In addition, diarrhoeal illness can affect up to 23 per cent and is mostly caused by bacteria (10).

In response, authorities and planning groups have developed several strategies and policies to counter outbreaks, such as:
- health education and awareness campaigns
- water and food supply alongside safe sanitation
- pre- and post-travel advice and vaccination opportunities
- control at ports of entry
- clinic and hospital care integration

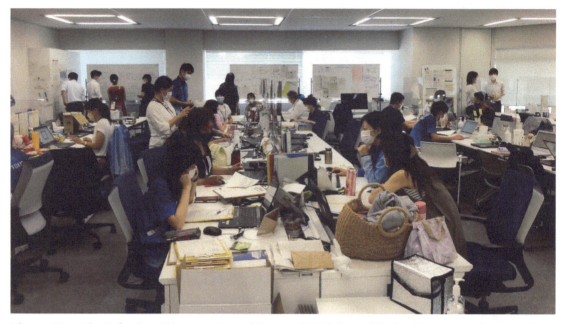

Figure 30.2: The Infectious Diseases Control Centre (IDCC) for public health preparedness and response during the Tokyo 2020 Games

The IDCC acted as the hub between the Tokyo government, local governments, and the polyclinic in the Olympic/Paralympic village. The IDCC worked on public health preparedness and response, including daily screening and confirmatory testing, surveillance, transport, isolation, and epidemiological response for all athletes and stakeholders during the Tokyo 2020 Games.
(Courtesy Brian McCloskey)

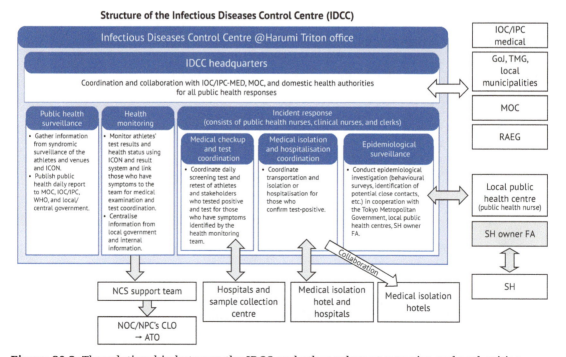

Figure 30.3: The relationship between the IDCC and other relevant agencies and authorities

The C3 system described above should set out in advance who is responsible for what and how they will coordinate with each other. For example, in a food-borne outbreak, the different responsibilities of public health staff, food safety agencies, environmental or sanitary inspectors, food retailers and distributors, the hosting organisation, and local or national governments should all be agreed on and tested in exercises before the mass gathering so that if something happens during the mass gathering, there is clarity on who is responsible for each element of the response.

"In a mass gathering, even the 'ordinary' can become extraordinary"

Equally, event medical services (EMS) must be coordinated as part of the organisers' efforts and fall under key decision-making processes in planning. They must be able to provide a comprehensive and effective general medical service, as well as deal with more serious situations. This includes primary care provision, treatment of minor injuries or illnesses, and symptomatic relief. Even in a worst-case outbreak scenario, EMS should be capable of preventing a large surge in local hospital admissions and stop the hospitals from being overloaded.

Adequate risk assessment should consider local medical services and capacity in the area. Context is also important when planning EMS provision. Respiratory illness, minor injury, heat-related injury, and headaches make up 80 to 90 per cent of injuries at mass gatherings (4). Nevertheless, the type of event matters. For example, drug overdoses may be more likely at concerts. Logistically, the location and number of medical stations is crucial as there is a possibility of an extremely delayed response due to the crowd at a mass gathering.

The actions necessary in an outbreak situation will be based on standard public health responses to address key issues such as identifying the source of infection, routes of transmission, and at-risk populations, and implementing appropriate interventions to block or limit further harm including infection prevention and control measures. Such measures should be pre-planned based on the mass gathering risk assessment.

As has been seen during the COVID-19 pandemic and at previous mass gatherings, good communication and information sharing with the population is essential to facilitate community engagement and support for the actions recommended.

Crisis communication is therefore essential for acute problem management and must be built on a foundation of risk communication which is integrated into the host public health system (**See Chapter 33, RCCE**). In a crisis, communication flows in two main directions: to the mass gathering host organisation and local and national politicians who will be instrumental in formulating the messages, and to the public who will be asked to implement the advice.

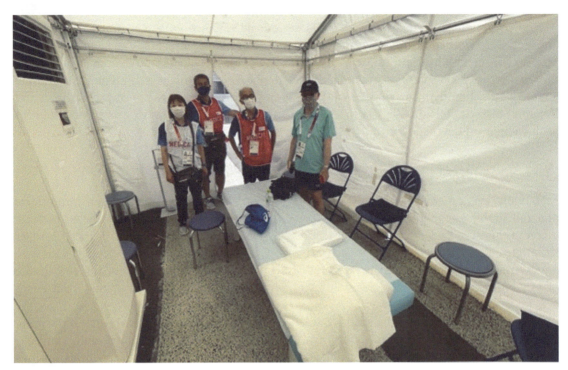

Figure 30.4: COVID-19 isolation facility at the Tokyo 2020 Games
(Courtesy Brian McCloskey)

Communication with local and national authorities must be quick, easily understood, scientifically credible, and implementable. Much of the advice that might be needed can be pre-planned based on the risk assessment and shared with authorities before the mass gathering event so that they are familiar with the issues before anything happens and before they are asked to make decisions rapidly in a world of uncertainty.

"Politics can drive decision-making faster than science drives answers"

Communicating with the public rapidly and with clarity is crucial, so targeted use of social and conventional media platforms as well as internal systems is needed. Control and limitation of misinformation is important (**See Chapter 34, Infodemics**). Social media enables the spread of pseudoscientific, political, and misinformed views, and this can potentially disrupt organised responses. The best management of public health emergencies comes from utilising modern public communication methods based on a variety of channels to meet the needs of every participant. For example, with younger attendees, the use of social networks such as Instagram and TikTok is high, whereas older participants might rely on traditional outlets such as radio and TV broadcasts and the Facebook platform. Understanding how to harness the power of these networks for good enables organisers to tackle the issues of misinformation with an informed plan. Strategies to engage with the public and stakeholders must be started early (before the mass gathering), be based on building relationships and trust, and be transparent and dynamic.

EVALUATION AND LEGACY PLANNING

The event needs to be evaluated to inform future event planning. Infectious disease outbreaks at a mass gathering are rare occurrences but if they happen, a superspreading event can ensue with consequent mass morbidity and possible mortality on individuals and impact on the health system. Increasing the effectiveness of outbreak prevention at mass gatherings over time is possible through shared learning from one mass gathering to the next and sharing with the mass gathering planning and hosting communities. The reintroduction of mass gatherings in 2022 and 2023 as the COVID-19 pandemic continued shows that the use of modern technologies, higher speeds of surveillance and information sharing, and better engagement with the public and authorities can mitigate risks and allow the safe hosting of mass gatherings. However, such measures depend on sharing and learning.

Further research into this area is vital and ongoing due to the myriad potential contexts that need exploring (e.g., the ability of strategies from higher resourced communities to be transferred to lower resource settings). The evaluation of public health interventions in mass gatherings should also be an ongoing endeavour, as should inquiries into medium and smaller mass gatherings (11).

The legacy of mass gathering-related research and implementation of new guidance is as important as current management, and the WHO documentation previously cited identified several areas of 'legacy and improvement':

- surveillance systems and situational awareness
- regulations, legislation, and policies
- emergency preparedness and response
- environmental health (e.g., food and water safety and quality, air quality)
- health promotion, awareness, enhanced knowledge, and understanding
- strengthening communication networks and collaborations within and between organisations
- internal organisational capacity and capability building and C3

The role of post-mass gathering debriefs has been highlighted as important in maintaining standards in subsequent mass gatherings as well as identifying areas for improvement after an event. In short, legacy work following mass gatherings is important for many reasons, not least of which is ultimately the viability of mass gatherings and the safety of future event attendees (12).

Mass gatherings, especially very large sporting events and religious pilgrimages, have worldwide and potentially substantial financial significance. Information and travel accessibility has enabled people to reach mass gatherings more easily—this creates opportunities and threats that are proportionate to the increase in visitor potential. These all increase the range and diversity of potential stakeholders in the mass gathering planning process.

Planning and management of mass gatherings should therefore be based on a mixture of regulation, advice, and guidance that is broadly applicable regardless of country, but which can be tailored to the specific context of the mass gathering and the legal framework of the host community.

Mass gatherings that are cross-national or international in nature should be planned and executed within the public health framework of the host country but also within the framework of the International Health Regulations (e.g., in relation to travel advice and information sharing) (13). This is key to ensuring the safety of the participants, as well as maintaining a consistent standard approach across nations regarding risk communication and information sharing. Host nations can learn from the principles of the International Health Regulations and sharing of information can be encouraged and reciprocated (1).

There is a largely untapped potential for health promotion and public information campaigns at mass gatherings. Context-dependent advertisements are already in use at some venues and events (14), but there is considerable scope for improvement in this area. However, the evidence base for their efficacy is not yet robust enough and needs greater emphasis.

The Ottawa Charter in 1986 provides a useful framework for the development of health promotion interventions at mass gatherings (15). Key points include the integration of public policy, a supportive environment, community action, and personal skills of staff and associated key figures.

CONCLUSION

Mass gatherings are, at their best, a representation of humanity coming together and celebrating the social force of a shared experience. They are opportunities for public good and promoting well-being in communities and individuals. They are also opportunities to review, test, and improve public health systems and enhance public safety. However, they can also create public health risks and cause, or amplify, severe outbreaks of disease.

Experience from mass gatherings during the COVID-19 pandemic shows that the risks are real, but can be managed. As new tests, treatments, and vaccines are developed, and evidence and experience are accumulated, the balance of risk versus benefit can be shifted toward the safe and successful hosting of mass gatherings and the realisation of the potential societal benefits.

As Dr Tedros Adhanom Ghebreyesus, the Director-General of the WHO, declared at the beginning of the rescheduled Tokyo Olympic Games in 2021 (16):

"The Games bring the nations of the world together in celebration: a celebration of sport; of health; of excellence, friendship, and respect. But ultimately, they are a celebration of something even more important – of something that our world needs now, more than ever: a celebration of hope. I repeat: the world needs now more than ever a celebration of hope. The celebrations may be more muted this year, but the message of hope is all the more important ... May the message of hope resound from Tokyo around the world in every nation, every village, and every heart."

Although not all mass gatherings are on the scale of the Hajj or the Olympic Games, they are all opportunities to engage with communities, bring people together, and improve lives. They do come with risks and may have to be revised to meet specific challenges but a robust, honest, and transparent approach to recognising and managing risks can help deliver safe and healthy events.

REFERENCES:

1. Memish ZA, Zumla A, McCloskey B, Heymann D, Al Rabeeah AA, Barbeschi M, et al. Mass gatherings medicine: international cooperation and progress. Lancet. 2014 Jun;383(9934):2030–2. https://doi.org/10.1016/S0140-6736(14)60225-7 PMID:24857704.

2. Arbon P. Mass-gathering medicine: a review of the evidence and future directions for research. Prehosp Disaster Med. 2007;22(2):131–5. https://doi.org/10.1017/S1049023X00004507 PMID:17591185.
3. Memish ZA, Steffen R, White P, Dar O, Azhar EI, Sharma A, et al. Mass gatherings medicine: public health issues arising from mass gathering religious and sporting events. Lancet. 2019 May;393(10185):2073–84. https://doi.org/10.1016/S0140-6736(19)30501-X PMID:31106753.
4. McCloskey B, et al. WHO Collaborating Centre for Mass Gatherings Medicine. Public Health for Mass Gatherings: Key Considerations. WHO Library Cataloguing-in-Publication Data. WHO Press, World Health Organization; 2015. https://www.who.int/publications/i/item/public-health-for-mass-gatherings-key-considerations.
5. Sparrow AK, Brosseau LM, Harrison RJ, Osterholm MT. Protecting Olympic participants from Covid-19 - the urgent need for a risk-management approach. N Engl J Med. 2021 Jul;385(1):e2. https://doi.org/10.1056/NEJMp2108567 PMID:34033274.
6. Kato T. Opposition in Japan to the Olympics during the COVID-19 pandemic. Humanit Soc Sci Commun. 2021;8(1):327. https://doi.org/10.1057/s41599-021-01011-5.
7. Hoang VT, Al-Tawfiq JA, Gautret P. The Tokyo Olympic Games and the risk of COVID-19. Curr Trop Med Rep. 2020;7(4):126–32. https://doi.org/10.1007/s40475-020-00217-y PMID:33145147.
8. WHO. WHO Mass Gathering Risk Assessment Tool. ISO; 2023. https://www.who.int/publications/i/item/WHO-2023-Generic-Mass-gatherings-All-Hazards-RAtool-2023-1.
9. Carter RJ, Rose DA, Sabo RT, Clayton J, Steinberg J, Anderson M, et al.; CDC COVID-19 Response Team. Widespread severe acute respiratory syndrome coronavirus 2 transmission among attendees at a large motorcycle rally and their contacts, 30 US jurisdictions, August-September, 2020. Clin Infect Dis. 2021 Jul;73 Suppl 1:S106–9. https://doi.org/10.1093/cid/ciab321 PMID:33912907.
10. Hoang VT, Gautret P. Infectious diseases and mass gatherings. Curr Infect Dis Rep. 2018 Aug;20(11):44. https://doi.org/10.1007/s11908-018-0650-9 PMID:30155747.
11. Mountjoy M, McCloskey B, Bahr R, Hull JH, Kemp J, Thornton JS, et al. Hosting international sporting events during the COVID-19 pandemic: lessons learnt and looking forward. Br J Sports Med. 2023 Jan;57(1):3–4. https://doi.org/10.1136/bjsports-2022-106096 PMID:35985809.
12. Smallwood CA, Arbuthnott KG, Banczak-Mysiak B, Borodina M, Coutinho AP, Payne-Hallström L, et al. Euro 2012 European Football Championship Finals: planning for a health legacy. Lancet. 2014 Jun;383(9934):2090–7. https://doi.org/10.1016/S0140-6736(13)62384-3 PMID:24857705.
13. World Health Organization. International Health Regulations. 2005. https://www.who.int/publications/i/item/9789241580496.
14. Memish ZA, Zumla A, Alhakeem RF, Assiri A, Turkestani A, Al Harby KD, et al. Hajj: infectious disease surveillance and control. Lancet. 2014 Jun;383(9934):2073–82. https://doi.org/10.1016/S0140-6736(14)60381-0 PMID:24857703.
15. World Health Organization. Ottawa Charter for Health Promotion. https://www.who.int/teams/health-promotion/enhanced-wellbeing/first-global-conference.
16. WHO Director General: "May these games be the moment that unites the world, and ignites the solidarity and determination we need to end the pandemic together" - Olympic news [Internet]. International Olympic Committee; 2021. https://olympics.com/ioc/news/who-director-general-may-these-games-be-the-moment-that-unites-the-world-and-ignites-the-solidarity-and-determination-we-need-to-end-the-pandemic-together.

CHAPTER 31

MENTAL HEALTH AND PSYCHOSOCIAL SUPPORT

by Heather Boagey, Maha Barakat, and Cristina Carreño Glaría

While efforts to contain the spread of an infectious agent can be highly effective, containing the impact of those efforts on the mental health of the population can be considerably more complex. A pandemic introduces new stressors, including anxiety surrounding the contagion itself. Restriction of freedom can heighten existing sources of stress, such as relationships and finances. Many of the coping mechanisms we rely on become less accessible as socialising and entertainment options are limited. The mental health of different groups is affected in a variety of ways, depending on the extent of disruption to daily life, levels of exposure to infection, and the specific consequences of infection for individuals. Existing users of psychiatric services may find these disrupted, triggering an acute deterioration in their mental state. By implementing an organised programme of mental health and psychosocial support, the potential for both acute and chronic damage can be mitigated. This approach integrates care with existing services in a sustainable fashion, with preventative and curative arms reaching both those who present to services and those requiring identification in the population.

INTRODUCTION

An outbreak brings about an overwhelming variety of emotions in the affected population, from indifference to confusion, panic, helplessness, and fear. The upheaval in daily life gives rise to new stressors and impacts our existing coping mechanisms. Some groups, such as those with high levels of exposure or risk, are particularly vulnerable. Consequences are far reaching, with widespread increases in mental health concerns including anxiety and depressive disorders. Rates of suicidal ideation, suicide attempts, and self-harm were shown in a meta-analysis to be increased compared to levels before the COVID-19 pandemic (1). The psychological support during and following such a response must therefore be comprehensive to limit suffering, improve quality of life, and mitigate the potential for maladaptive coping which can later give rise to intergenerational trauma. Psychological support is also important given the relationship between mental health and infection control. During the 2014–2015 West Africa Ebola virus disease (EBOD) outbreak, depression and post-traumatic stress disorder (PTSD) were associated with subsequent disease-spreading behaviours and lower levels of prevention behaviours, while anxiety was associated with greater adherence to preventative measures (2). In this chapter, we will explore the impact of outbreaks and pandemics on mental health, and how damage can be minimised by targeting at-risk groups and protecting mental health services.

REASONS FOR MENTAL ILLNESS IN AN OUTBREAK
Stressors

The threat of infection is itself a significant new source of stress during an outbreak. Anxiety is induced by the prospect of contracting the disease and its consequences for an individual's health, especially in high-risk or high-exposure populations. Anxiety is also associated with the risk of spreading disease, along with feelings of shame and guilt arising from the prospect or the reality of infecting individuals who are vulnerable, or those for whom self-isolation would be financially or psychosocially impactful. Societal stigma, often cultured to deter risky behaviours, and the spread of misinformation, may heighten these emotions. This can lead to groups with a higher risk of pathogen exposure becoming ostracised from society and isolated from essential support. Individuals with existing anxiety disorders may find these exacerbated. A positive correlation exists between those with health anxiety and the development of new generalised anxiety or depressive symptoms during the COVID-19 pandemic (3), and symptoms were reported to worsen in individuals with obsessive-compulsive disorder (OCD), especially among those with preoccupations of contamination (4).

When a disease spreads, such that restrictions are imposed by individuals or the government, significant disruption to daily lives is unavoidable. For example, movement within a certain area may be restricted, limited to a specific time of day as part of a curfew, or apply to specific individuals during quarantine. The overall restriction of freedom and autonomy by authorities can exacerbate the stress response. As daily routines are lost, often without clear timescales for resumption, feelings of uncertainty prevail. Some individuals have difficulty tolerating uncertainty and this has been associated with increased psychological distress (5). This is worse for those also struggling to provide for themselves and their families, with psychological distress shown to be greatest for individuals who do not have sufficient supplies and those who are least affluent (6). The closure of sectors that are deemed non-essential or that cannot continue in accordance with social distancing, as well as requirements for self-isolation, both affect an individual's ability to work. This loss of role and financial instability are additional sources of stress. Notably, loss of employment and subsequent socioeconomic deprivation are both risk factors for suicidality (7), rates of which have been shown to increase during a pandemic (1).

Loss of protective coping mechanisms

During an outbreak, many of the coping mechanisms we rely on to maintain good mental well-being become inaccessible. Distraction through entertainment is more difficult, as arts and leisure industries limit their services. There may be restrictions on exercising outdoors, reducing our physical activity and interaction with nature, with negative implications for mental health.

During a lockdown, the number of daily interpersonal interactions falls due to social isolation and enforced distancing. While this may temporarily alleviate stress for those with social anxiety, for most individuals, the loss of this coping mechanism is detrimental. Although electronic communication between contacts may be ongoing, it may not be possible to develop new relationships unless in a covert way. Feelings of loneliness become widespread, increasing in all groups including those already living alone (8). Conversely, the length of time spent with those in your household increases, with mixed results. Mental health outcomes during the COVID-19 pandemic were better among those in a high-satisfaction relationship compared to those who were single, but worse among those in a relationship with low levels of satisfaction. The responsibility of dependents may exacerbate this, as the rates of anxiety and suicidal ideation and the risk of intimate partner violence were highest for individuals in a low-commitment relationship with children in the household (9).

Loss of time socialising with peers particularly affects the mental health of children and adolescents who rely on these interactions for social development. Lockdown itself is associated with an increased prevalence of self-harm behaviours, with presentations amongst children increased in proportion to the stringency of lockdown and degree of social isolation (10). Although technology has been beneficial in facilitating socialising online amongst young people, this remains harder to access for older people and is dependent on financial and geographical circumstances.

Socialising provides more than entertainment and distraction. When contact is limited, collective coping mechanisms, such as religious gatherings and rituals celebrating important life events, are affected. There is also a lack of practical support for individuals with physical or psychosocial disabilities, the elderly, and new parents, as well as a lack of respite for carers, whose workload may have increased to limit the number of individuals their dependent is exposed to.

In times of crisis, many turn to substance use as a maladaptive coping mechanism, leading to an increased demand for addiction services. The impact of this is culturally specific. For example, the impact on alcohol consumption is dependent on governmental attitude, ranging from sales being prohibited or designated as essential. During the COVID-19 pandemic, there was an increase globally in the number of presentations of alcohol withdrawal, alcohol-related suicide attempts, and methanol toxicity, as well as a rise in binge drinking (11). Risk factors included living alone, being older or male, being a parent, being unemployed, or having poor mental or physical health (12).

THE SPECTRUM OF DISORDERS AND OUTCOMES

Due to variable disease risk, exposure, and access to services, different groups can have vastly different experiences during a pandemic. Poorer mental health outcomes are found in those with a high risk of infection, high exposure to infection, or those with reduced access to services. When these factors are controlled, there remain differences between individuals' risk of developing mental illness in response to the same stressor, as a result of their pre-morbid personality and mental health status. For example, during the COVID-19 pandemic, generalised anxiety and depressive symptoms were more likely in individuals with higher neuroticism and less likely in those with high extraversion, independent of the risk of the infectious disease (3). Risk assessment in mental health should involve consideration of various features as it pertains to an individual or a subpopulation. Intervention can then be tailored to meet specific needs and be delivered most effectively.

Factors associated with poorer mental health outcomes following an infectious disease outbreak

High risk of severe disease
- Physical illness

- Elderly
- Children
- Pregnant people

High risk of disease exposure
- Healthcare workers (HCWs)
- Other essential workers (e.g., emergency services, education, food industry)
- Carers
- Disease survivors
- Contacts of cases

Limited access to healthcare
- Prisoners, refugees, and asylum seekers
- Victims of intimate partner violence
- Individuals of low socioeconomic status
- Rural and indigenous communities

PRE-EXISTING VULNERABILITIES OF INDIVIDUALS AND COMMUNITIES: PHYSIOLOGICAL VULNERABILITIES

Individuals who are at greater risk of harm from contracting the infectious agent are at an increased risk of mental illness due to high levels of anxiety and the social isolation instigated to shield them from the population. This includes carers, those at the extremes of age, or those with physical health conditions that increase risk (either directly or indirectly via the use of immune-compromising medications).

Pregnant people are also particularly vulnerable, at a time when there is often little evidence base for the impact of the emerging pathogen, vaccination, and management on their pregnancy. The prevalence of anxiety and depression in this group is raised, but social support and physical exercise appear to be protective (13). In cases where offspring were affected by a viral infection, such as microencephaly following Zika virus infection, the anxiety levels of mothers were greater and adversely affected by a lack of understanding (14). Psycho-education of new mothers is therefore essential to help reduce and process negative emotions. Psycho-education teaches individuals and their communities about emotions, behaviours, and how both relate to mental health and illness, which empowers recipients to cope and support each other.

PREVENTING MENTAL ILLNESS IN AN OUTBREAK

The psychological impact of movement restrictions, including lockdowns, can be minimised by ensuring that lockdown duration is as short as possible and that regulations are consistent. Providing as much information and communication as possible, as well as access to essential resources, also reduces stress. Where possible, there should be a voluntary component to restrictions to help engender a sense of control and empowerment, and an emphasis on altruism to foster feelings of community at a time when social isolation can become the norm (15). The creation of support bubbles to allow contact within fixed groups can also mitigate the emotional burden on groups such as new parents. Although this may create resentment among individuals not meeting the criteria for this opportunity, the individuals involved can evaluate whether this increased level of exposure is acceptable to them, restoring a degree of autonomy.

THE ORGANISATION OF MENTAL HEALTH RESPONSE IN OUTBREAKS

Practitioners from international organisations, non-governmental organisations (NGOs), and the research community have, over the last 20 years, developed a structured methodology and framework to help in the delivery of mental health and psychosocial support (referred to as MHPSS) in times of emergency (16). This programme should be included in the emergency preparedness programmes of countries, districts, and individual hospitals. MHPSS is an evidence-based approach (17) based on core principles used to cope with other forms of humanitarian crises. It aids both those who seek help from services and those whose needs require detection in the community. For example, individuals with reduced access to or engagement with healthcare due to homelessness or refugee status may require more active surveillance.

MHPSS programmes seek to protect psychological well-being and identify, prevent, and manage mental illness as it arises. Often delivered by aid organisations, MHPSS involves the integration of mental health support into other services, such as hospitals, schools, or businesses. Continuity and sustainable impact are achieved by recruiting locally and providing on-the-job training, which must be tailored to social and cultural contexts. Where traditional and indigenous medicine plays a prominent role in society and is not harmful, a collaborative approach is beneficial.

PREVENTATIVE EFFORTS OF MHPSS

One strategy of MHPSS is to target those most at risk with timely interventions. For example, key workers should be prioritised for supplies and vaccination and supported to take breaks away from the working environment. The involvement of environmental teams is also important to ensure practices around death and burial are supported as much as possible.

For those in the wider community in contact with survivors, psycho-education is recommended to promote coping by sharing information about common mental health reactions associated with the disease. The environment of the treatment facility where intervention for physical health is received should be optimised to humanise care. Peer support is encouraged, but health promotion teams also need to engage with communities directly to support the reintegration of survivors and should be equipped to cope with the strong reactions they may face.

Specific attention should be paid to those at the extremes of age. Support groups providing age-appropriate, structured activities are recommended for affected children and can help families form supportive networks. Social activities, psycho-education of staff, and prioritising family contact are recommended for care homes.

MANAGEMENT OF MENTAL ILLNESS

The Inter-Agency Standing Committee on MHPSS in emergency settings (IASC) was established in 2007, linking United Nations (UN) organisations, NGOs, and researchers in an international collective of groups providing humanitarian assistance. The committee visualises MHPSS response as a pyramid of services (**Figure 31.1**), with tiers catering for the needs of progressively smaller proportions of the population. All individuals require that basic services are implemented with consideration to the promotion of mental well-being. Without active provision of support in the form of social measures, such as social network strengthening and assisted mourning, people with mental health conditions can have impaired daily functioning and strained relationships. A smaller number of individuals will need psychological first aid that can be provided by primary care (**Figure 31.2**). Yet smaller but still significant numbers will require support from specialist psychiatric services.

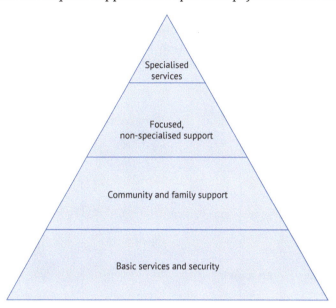

Figure 31.1: Pyramid of MHPSS services
(adapted from Interagency Standing Committee (IASC) (18))

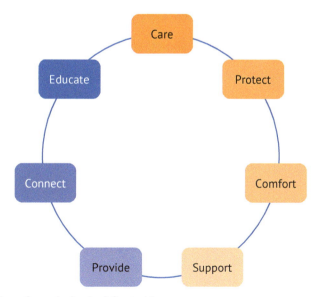

Figure 31.2: Principles of psychological first aid

For those who show signs of development of mental illness, treatment should be initiated according to local guidelines. For acute reactions, self-help for stress management and psychological first aid may be sufficient. For example, the World Health Organization (WHO) has developed the WHO Self-Help Plus (WHO SH+) stress management intervention based on acceptance and commitment therapy, cognitive behavioural therapy (CBT), and mindfulness to increase psychological resilience and flexibility. Using a pre-recorded course and a self-help book, WHO SH+ can be delivered in small groups to those affected by a humanitarian crisis. Those requiring specialist psychiatric input should be managed with a personalised formulation of psychological therapy or specific medications with appropriate follow-up depending on clinical need (**Table 31.1**).

Preventative measures	Curative measures
Flexibility of restrictions	Self-help
Psycho-education	Psycho-education
Support groups	Psychological therapy
Health promotion	Medication

Table 31.1: MHPSS intervention toolkit

There is an increasing role for telemedicine in MHPSS which removes the need for infection control measures. Most virtual interventions require only audio which may be more feasible in some contexts. However, access to networks and devices and the need for privacy remain important considerations (19).

Emergency services

As with other services, psychiatric services must continue in an emergency. Although the lockdown during the COVID-19 pandemic in the U.K. resulted in fewer psychiatric presentations, research showed that those who presented had more severe symptoms and were more likely to be detained and admitted under the mental health act (20). Altering existing pathways may be necessary.

Scotland, 2020

In response to the increased pressure on unscheduled psychiatric care in Scotland during the COVID-19 pandemic in 2020, services in Glasgow were consolidated to create specialist mental health assessment units (MHAUs) based at psychiatric hospitals. Instead of attending the emergency department, eligible patients were diverted to MHAUs by primary care clinicians, paramedics, or police, where they would be assessed by specialist mental health nurses with additional support from a psychiatric consultant on call if needed. From here, patients would either be admitted to the psychiatric hospital directly or discharged with appropriate follow-up from unscheduled care teams in the community. This allowed faster access to specialist care, limited transmission, and reduced the strain on general hospital receiving units. Condensing resources also compensated for staff shortages due to sickness or redeployment.

Community and inpatient services

Special attention must also be provided to individuals already under the care of services. Notably, the risk of disease transmission is higher among self-contained communities such as those in inpatient and supported living settings due to the continued requirement for external support staff. Vaccination of inpatient groups should be prioritised. It is essential that services, including the uninterrupted supply of medicines and delivery of therapy, continue despite logistical barriers. Furthermore, psychiatric medications are associated with increased physical health burden, and individuals on these medications may therefore continue to require routine physical health checks.

Outpatient mental health services should be encouraged to develop telemedicine services. Telemedicine is the use of electronic methods of communication to provide healthcare when face-to-face contact is not possible, such as due to distance or infection risk, and includes phone services and internet-based messaging and videocalls. However, services should be encouraged to maintain face-to-face appointments for individuals who require in-person assessment, such as those on long-acting antipsychotics or without access to technology.

El Salvador, April 2020

In order to continue providing psychotherapeutic care during COVID-19–related movement restrictions, Médecins Sans Frontières (MSF) abruptly transitioned part of its mental health activities to remote formats. Psychological consultations were done by phone. Only patients with severe symptomatology were referred to face-to-face services.

SPECIAL POPULATIONS

Disease survivors

Individuals who have contracted an emerging disease, faced the uncertainty of illness course and societal isolation, survived, and faced reintroduction to society have often been through unprecedented levels of stress. Unsurprisingly, rates of new mental health diagnoses are high amongst survivors. For example, among EBOD survivors, the prevalence of anxiety was found to be 14 per cent, depression 15 per cent, and insomnia 22 per cent (21). This is higher than the estimated prevalence of mood disorders (3–10 per cent) and anxiety disorders (6–16 per cent) in the African population (21), and an estimated prevalence of insomnia of 6–10 per cent according to the National Institute for Health and Care Excellence. This may be associated with disease severity or degree of functional impairment. Among survivors of COVID-19, the time spent bedridden was found to be associated with long-term mental morbidity (22). Intensive support from the multidisciplinary team, including physiotherapy and occupational therapy, is important to help patients re-establish mobility and independence as quickly as possible, to protect their mental health.

Bereaved

As death rates climb during a pandemic, so too does the number of recently bereaved, coming to terms with their loss in new and unstable circumstances. The manner of death impacts response. During the COVID-19 pandemic, bereavement secondary to infection was associated with greater severity of prolonged grief reaction than when death was attributed to other complications, such as cardiac disease or fever (23). Limitations on gatherings mean that traditions around end-of-life care and burial are disrupted, which can lead to resentment, anger, and fear of spiritual or religious consequences (24). To minimise the development of prolonged grief reactions, mourning practices should be encouraged to continue with feasible modifications for infection control compliance. Screening programmes enable individuals who are at higher risk of prolonged grief reaction to be identified for psycho-education (25). Participants are encouraged to consider how the development of negative patterns of thinking, emotions, and behaviour, collectively known as a maladaptive schema, affects how we perceive ourselves and the world, the potential for harmful consequences, and how this can be mitigated.

Key workers

While many people are prevented from carrying out their jobs as normal, essential services such as food provision, education, healthcare, power, and waste and emergency services must continue, and workers are needed. Workers in these high-exposure groups experience increased psychological burden as increased occupational demands bring additional shift work, loss of flexible working hours, and redeployment. Workers may feel underprepared for working in difficult and evolving situations and may face ethical challenges, with an increased risk of moral injury (26). Moral injury can itself lead to negative self-perception and feelings of guilt that increase the risk of depression.

> **Burdens on key workers**
>
> **Burnout:** Feelings of exhaustion, emotional distancing, or negativism related to one's job, and a sense of ineffectiveness resulting from chronic unmanaged workplace stress (27).
> **Vicarious trauma:** Trauma experienced by professionals as a result of listening to and supporting individuals who have experienced trauma.
> **Moral injury:** Feelings of guilt or shame following exposure to ethically challenging situations involving conflict with an individual's moral code.

Healthcare workers (HCWs)

HCWs are a subset of key workers. Help-seeking by this group may be affected by their marginalisation and that of their close contacts due to their high perceived levels of pathogen exposure. Caring for infected individuals can be traumatic itself, and carers may experience vicarious trauma, as well as symptoms of burnout. A systematic review showed that 34 per cent of nurses experienced burnout during the COVID-19 pandemic (28).

As well as being a negative experience for an individual, burnout has consequences for workplace dynamics. As work becomes unfulfilling, individuals become more cynical and levels of passive and passive-aggressive disrespect increase (26). Productivity is impaired, and the risk of medical error is twice as likely among those experiencing burnout (29).

Among healthcare staff, rates of psychological distress and PTSD are higher in staff caring for patients affected by the disease than those caring for other patients. Risk factors for psychological distress included being younger, being more junior, being the parents of dependent children, or having an infected family member, as well as quarantine, lack of practical support, and stigma. Clear communication, access to adequate personal protection, adequate rest, and both practical and psychological support were associated with reduced morbidity (30). Research has shown that the most successful interventions for this group make use of adaptation for local needs, effective communication, and positive safe learning environments (30).

Singapore, 2021

In 2021, as Singapore reimposed movement restrictions and home-schooling in response to an increase in Delta-variant cases of COVID-19, HCWs received a cash bonus of thousands of dollars. Hospitals had been providing free lunches since February 2020 and food treats were regularly personally delivered to offices and wards. One hospital had a weekly free ice cream stall and provided weekly updates from the management which offered information as well as inspirational messages of appreciation. Staff were better able to manage travel bans, redeployment, extra shifts, quarantine, and social stigma.

United Arab Emirates (UAE)

In the UAE, a dedicated federal office was set up to support frontline workers, and a registry for them was launched registering over 135,000 individuals from all sectors involved in frontline response, including the non-healthcare sectors and volunteers. Numerous initiatives were rolled out to help with education needs for frontline workers and their children. Health insurance top-ups, increased healthcare access, mental health support, discounts on groceries and essential services, and assistance from the Central Bank for loan repayments were all on offer. For the families of fallen heroes, the dedicated office looked after the needs of surviving spouses and children, including schooling, healthcare, and housing.

Although professionals working with patients infected with COVID-19 exhibited significantly higher levels of stress, burnout, secondary trauma, anxiety, and depression, this group was also twice as likely to ask for psychological support than those working with uninfected patients (31). This bodes well for the uptake of psychological support in the workplace, though it must be acknowledged that help-seeking can also be adversely affected by the public's idolisation of HCWs.

Support for HCWs

Interventions for healthcare staff should also be guided by specialist policy advice. Self-care and peer support groups are valuable, but it should be stressed that intervention is also the responsibility of employers who should facilitate these opportunities. Due consideration should be given to the tasks and shifts that are undertaken to share the workload equitably. Preparation is essential and need not be resource intensive. It has been shown that computer-assisted resilience training for HCWs under pandemic conditions is beneficial (32). For this, participants completed an online course comprising knowledge-based lectures, quizzes, relaxation techniques, and self-assessment using psychological questionnaires to characterise their own individual coping styles.

Policy advice in prioritising HCWs' mental health
- Evidence-based interventions
- Distribution of resources across healthcare networks
- National knowledge bases (information, tools, and resources)
- Ensure adequate staffing and fair pay
- Encourage help-seeking and ensure support is available
- Condemn and combat the stigmatisation of HCWs
- Facilitate dialogue about mental health in the workplace
- Engage frontline workers in the decision-making process
- Sufficient funding for research into optimising preparedness of frontline workers
- Consider the use of digital technology for training and support

(adapted from Front Public Heal [Internet]. 2021 May 7;9)

Support for those with pre-existing mental health conditions

Individuals with a pre-existing mental health condition are invariably affected during a pandemic, and there is often a shift in disease burden with some conditions requiring more support than others. For example, while social anxiety may improve, OCD symptoms may worsen. Rates of depression have been found to generally increase, irrespective of a country's economic status (33), and increased levels of distress irrespective of cause are a risk factor for relapse. By contrast, amongst individuals with a diagnosis of personality disorder, there is no increase in self-destructive actions (34). This has been linked to the increase in time spent at home in the company of others.

While patient demands may be variable, disruption across psychiatric services is frequent. As reported by the WHO, 93 per cent of countries reported disruptions to their provision of mental, neurological, and substance use services during June–August 2020 secondary to the COVID-19 pandemic (35). This risks the sudden discontinuation of therapy or medication due to a lack of supply, redeployment of personnel, or issues with patient concordance, with dangerous consequences for patient safety.

CONCLUSION

Outbreaks bring new challenges to the mental health of all individuals affected. Until recently, the risk and fallout have been under-recognised and undermanaged. The risk of infection as well as restrictions on leisure and social activities, with societal lockdown at the extreme, push many beyond their coping limits. Assessment of the pre-existing vulnerabilities of individuals and communities helps streamline preventative and curative efforts and can be organised under the MHPSS framework. Specific consideration of special populations including disease survivors, the bereaved, and key workers should be provided in the form of monitoring and implementing prevention measures, and in some cases, specialist support.

REFERENCES:

1. Dubé JP, Smith MM, Sherry SB, Hewitt PL, Stewart SH. Suicide behaviors during the COVID-19 pandemic: a meta-analysis of 54 studies. Psychiatry Res. 2021 Jul;301:113998. https://doi.org/10.1016/j.psychres.2021.113998 PMID:34022657.
2. Betancourt TS, Brennan RT, Vinck P, VanderWeele TJ, Spencer-Walters D, Jeong J, et al. Associations between mental health and ebola-related health behaviors: a regionally representative cross-sectional survey in post-conflict Sierra Leone. PLoS Med. 2016 Aug;13(8):e1002073. https://doi.org/10.1371/journal.pmed.1002073 PMID:27505186.
3. Nikčević AV, Marino C, Kolubinski DC, Leach D, Spada MM. Modelling the contribution of the Big Five personality traits, health anxiety, and COVID-19 psychological distress to generalised anxiety and depressive symptoms during the COVID-19 pandemic. J Affect Disord. 2021 Jan;279:578–84. https://doi.org/10.1016/j.jad.2020.10.053 PMID:33152562.
4. Guzick AG, Candelari A, Wiese AD, Schneider SC, Goodman WK, Storch EA. Obsessive–compulsive disorder during the COVID-19 pandemic: a systematic review [Internet]. Curr Psychiatry Rep. 2021 Oct;23(11):71. https://doi.org/10.1007/s11920-021-01284-2 PMID:34613498.
5. Rettie H, Daniels J. Coping and tolerance of uncertainty: predictors and mediators of mental health during the COVID-19 pandemic. Am Psychol. 2021 Apr;76(3):427–37. https://doi.org/10.1037/amp0000710 PMID:32744841.
6. Rehman U, Shahnawaz MG, Khan NH, Kharshiing KD, Khursheed M, Gupta K, et al. Depression, anxiety and stress among Indians in times of COVID-19 lockdown. Community Ment Health J. 2021 Jan;57(1):42–8. https://doi.org/10.1007/s10597-020-00664-x PMID:32577997.
7. Iob E, Steptoe A, Fancourt D. Abuse, self-harm and suicidal ideation in the UK during the COVID-19 pandemic. Br J Psychiatry. 2020 Oct;217(4):543–6. https://doi.org/10.1192/bjp.2020.130 PMID:32654678.
8. Wilson-Genderson M, Heid AR, Cartwright F, Collins AL, Pruchno R. Change in loneliness experienced by older men and women living alone and with others at the onset of the COVID-19 pandemic. Res Aging. 2022;44(5-6):369–81. https://doi.org/10.1177/01640275211026649 PMID:34344251.
9. Till B, Niederkrotenthaler T. Romantic relationships and mental health during the COVID-19 pandemic in Austria: a population-based cross-sectional survey [Internet]. Front Psychol. 2022 Apr;13:857329. https://doi.org/10.3389/fpsyg.2022.857329 PMID:35572322.
10. Wong BH, Vaezinejad M, Plener PL, Mehdi T, Romaniuk L, Barrett E, et al. Lockdown stringency and paediatric self-harm presentations during COVID-19 pandemic: retrospective cohort study [Internet]. BJPsych Open. 2022 Mar;8(2):e75. https://doi.org/10.1192/bjo.2022.41 PMID:35322782.
11. Murthy P, Narasimha VL. Effects of the COVID-19 pandemic and lockdown on alcohol use disorders and complications. Curr Opin Psychiatry. 2021 Jul;34(4):376–85. https://doi.org/10.1097/YCO.0000000000000720 PMID:34016817.
12. Roberts A, Rogers J, Mason R, Siriwardena AN, Hogue T, Whitley GA, et al. Alcohol and other substance use during the COVID-19 pandemic: a systematic review. Drug Alcohol Depend. 2021 Dec;229 Pt A:109150. https://doi.org/10.1016/j.drugalcdep.2021.109150 PMID:34749198.

13. Ahmad M, Vismara L. The psychological impact of COVID-19 pandemic on women's mental health during pregnancy: a rapid evidence review. Int J Environ Res Public Health. 2021 Jul;18(13):7112. https://doi.org/10.3390/ijerph18137112 PMID:34281049.
14. Romero-Acosta K, Marbán-Castro E, Arroyo K, Arrieta G, Mattar S. Perceptions and emotional state of mothers of children with and without microcephaly after the Zika virus epidemic in rural Caribbean Colombia. Behav Sci (Basel). 2020 Sep;10(10):147. https://doi.org/10.3390/bs10100147 PMID:32992703.
15. Brooks SK, Webster RK, Smith LE, Woodland L, Wessely S, Greenberg N, et al. The psychological impact of quarantine and how to reduce it: rapid review of the evidence. Lancet. 2020 Mar;395(10227):912–20. https://doi.org/10.1016/S0140-6736(20)30460-8 PMID:32112714.
16. Kola L, Kohrt BA, Hanlon C, Naslund JA, Sikander S, Balaji M, et al. COVID-19 mental health impact and responses in low-income and middle-income countries: reimagining global mental health. Lancet Psychiatry. 2021 Jun;8(6):535–50. https://doi.org/10.1016/S2215-0366(21)00025-0 PMID:33639109.
17. Cénat JM, Mukunzi JN, Noorishad PG, Rousseau C, Derivois D, Bukaka J. A systematic review of mental health programs among populations affected by the Ebola virus disease. J Psychosom Res. 2020 Feb;131:109966. https://doi.org/10.1016/j.jpsychores.2020.109966 PMID:32087433.
18. Interagency Standing Committee (IASC). IASC common monitoring and evaluation framework for mental health and psychosocial support in emergency settings: with means of verification (Version 2.0) [Internet]. Interagency Standing Committee (IASC); 2021 Sep. https://interagencystandingcommittee.org/iasc-reference-group-mental-health-and-psychosocial-support-emergency-settings/iasc-common-monitoring-and-evaluation-framework-mental-health-and-psychosocial-support-emergency.
19. Ibragimov K, Palma M, Keane G, Ousley J, Crowe M, Carreño C, et al.; M. S. F. Mental Health Working Group. Shifting to tele-mental health in humanitarian and crisis settings: an evaluation of Médecins Sans Frontières experience during the COVID-19 pandemic. Confl Health. 2022 Feb;16(1):6. https://doi.org/10.1186/s13031-022-00437-1 PMID:35164807.
20. Mukadam N, Sommerlad A, Wright J, Smith A, Szczap A, Solomou S, et al. Acute mental health presentations before and during the COVID-19 pandemic. BJPsych Open. 2021 Jul;7(4):e134. https://doi.org/10.1192/bjo.2021.970 PMID:34266510.
21. Acharibasam JW, Chireh B, Menegesha HG. Assessing anxiety, depression and insomnia symptoms among Ebola survivors in Africa: a meta-analysis [Internet]. PLoS One. 2021 Feb;16(2):e0246515. https://dx.plos.org/10.1371/journal.pone.024651510.1371/journal.pone.0246515 https://doi.org/10.1371/journal.pone.0246515 PMID:33544772.
22. Magnúsdóttir I, Lovik A, Unnarsdóttir AB, McCartney D, Ask H, Kõiv K, et al.; COVIDMENT Collaboration. Acute COVID-19 severity and mental health morbidity trajectories in patient populations of six nations: an observational study. Lancet Public Health. 2022 May;7(5):e406–16. https://doi.org/10.1016/S2468-2667(22)00042-1 PMID:35298894.
23. Tang S, Xiang Z. Who suffered most after deaths due to COVID-19? Prevalence and correlates of prolonged grief disorder in COVID-19 related bereaved adults [Internet]. Global Health. 2021 Feb;17(1):19. https://doi.org/10.1186/s12992-021-00669-5 PMID:33573673.
24. Van Bortel T, Basnayake A, Wurie F, Jambai M, Koroma AS, Muana AT, et al. Psychosocial effects of an Ebola outbreak at individual, community and international levels [Internet]. Bull World Health Organ. 2016 Mar;94(3):210–4. https://doi.org/10.2471/BLT.15.158543 PMID:26966332.
25. Diolaiuti F, Marazziti D, Beatino MF, Mucci F, Pozza A. Impact and consequences of COVID-19 pandemic on complicated grief and persistent complex bereavement disorder [Internet]. Psychiatry Res. 2021 Jun;300:113916. https://doi.org/10.1016/j.psychres.2021.113916 PMID:33836468.
26. Søvold LE, Naslund JA, Kousoulis AA, Saxena S, Qoronfleh MW, Grobler C, et al. Prioritizing the mental health and well-being of healthcare workers: an urgent global public health priority. Front Public Health. 2021 May;9:679397. https://doi.org/10.3389/fpubh.2021.679397 PMID:34026720.
27. ICD-11 for Mortality and Morbidity Statistics. https://icd.who.int/browse11/l-m/en#/http://id.who.int/icd/entity/129180281.
28. Galanis P, Vraka I, Fragkou D, Bilali A, Kaitelidou D. Nurses' burnout and associated risk factors during the COVID-19 pandemic: a systematic review and meta-analysis. J Adv Nurs. 2021 Aug;77(8):3286–302. https://doi.org/10.1111/jan.14839 PMID:33764561.
29. Balch CM, Oreskovich MR, Dyrbye LN, Colaiano JM, Satele DV, Sloan JA, et al. Personal consequences of malpractice lawsuits on American surgeons. J Am Coll Surg. 2011 Nov;213(5):657–67. https://doi.org/10.1016/j.jamcollsurg.2011.08.005 PMID:21890381.

30. Kisely S, Warren N, McMahon L, Dalais C, Henry I, Siskind D. Occurrence, prevention, and management of the psychological effects of emerging virus outbreaks on healthcare workers: rapid review and meta-analysis. BMJ. 2020 May;369:m1642. https://doi.org/10.1136/bmj.m1642 PMID:32371466.

31. Trumello C, Bramanti SM, Ballarotto G, Candelori C, Cerniglia L, Cimino S, et al. Psychological adjustment of healthcare workers in Italy during the COVID-19 pandemic: differences in stress, anxiety, depression, burnout, secondary trauma, and compassion satisfaction between frontline and non-frontline professionals. Int J Environ Res Public Health. 2020 Nov;17(22):8358. https://doi.org/10.3390/ijerph17228358 PMID:33198084.

32. Maunder RG, Lancee WJ, Mae R, Vincent L, Peladeau N, Beduz MA, et al. Computer-assisted resilience training to prepare healthcare workers for pandemic influenza: a randomized trial of the optimal dose of training. BMC Health Serv Res. 2010 Mar;10(1):72. https://doi.org/10.1186/1472-6963-10-72 PMID:20307302.

33. Kumar M, Kumar P. Impact of pandemic on mental health in lower- and middle-income countries (LMICs). Glob Ment Health (Camb). 2020 Dec;7:e35. https://doi.org/10.1017/gmh.2020.28 PMID:34191999.

34. Hartveit Kvarstein E, Zahl KE, Stänicke LI, Pettersen MS, Baltzersen ÅL, Johansen MS, et al. Vulnerability of personality disorder during COVID-19 crises: a multicenter survey of mental and social distress among patients referred to treatment. Nord J Psychiatry. 2021 Aug:1–12. https://doi.org/10.1080/08039488.2021.1942980 PMID:34369842.

35. The impact of COVID-19 on mental, neurological and substance use services. Results of a rapid assessment. https://www.who.int/publications/i/item/978924012455.

CHAPTER 32

PROTECTING THE VULNERABLE

by Elyssa Liu and Louisa Sun

A community's most vulnerable populations are often placed starkly in the spotlight in times of public health emergencies. Vulnerable groups can include, but are not limited to, women, children, the elderly, healthcare workers, indigenous peoples, people with disabilities or pre-existing conditions, migrants, refugees, and other individuals and communities marginalised by language, geography, and educational level. Vulnerability may be related to the groups' inability to fully care for themselves (e.g., the frail elderly) or those who are more able but are vulnerable by virtue of their poor living or working conditions or the stigma and prejudice they face in society.

Even before emergencies occur, these groups struggle with healthcare challenges, and during infectious disease outbreaks, their difficulties are compounded. They tend to suffer more from disease, encounter greater barriers to healthcare access, face exclusion from public health initiatives, and are at an increased risk of violence, exploitation, and harm. Vulnerable populations bring to light the existing cracks within healthcare systems, emergency response plans, national policies, and institutional frameworks that failed to adequately anticipate their needs, and which only become more pronounced under the pressure of crisis. The vulnerabilities of these specific groups are not isolated phenomena but indicative of broader societal weaknesses, making it clear that addressing their needs effectively strengthens the entire community's resilience against infectious disease emergencies.

INTRODUCTION

The nature and the degree of risk of vulnerable populations in an outbreak depend on many factors including disease, country context, and the severity of the health emergency, as well as pre-existing social, cultural, and financial disadvantages. Failure to consider vulnerable individuals, groups, and sub-communities will inevitably see poorer outcomes in their physical and mental health as well as social concerns. All populations have vulnerable groups who will suffer disproportionately during an infectious disease emergency.

The risk levels of these individuals are intensified if they fall under several vulnerable categories, as the convergence of socioeconomic, health, and structural factors only further exacerbates their challenges. For example, an elderly person with a disability may feel more isolated and anxious than most if a quarantine is mandated, and as a result, their mental health may suffer more (1), an undocumented migrant with HIV may delay seeking medical care due to concerns of being criminalised and deported, and a refugee displaced by an ongoing humanitarian crisis may face language barriers that render it impossible to communicate their symptoms (2). Recognising and addressing the vulnerabilities of these at-risk groups are essential to achieving a more equitable health emergency response. Additionally, it is sometimes very difficult to predict which vulnerabilities become salient in particular emergencies.

The vulnerable may be predisposed to worse health outcomes (e.g., risk of infection or severe infection, unidentified new health problems, and failure to receive satisfactory preventative care or care for new acute or chronic conditions). Furthermore, there is an increased risk across the spectrum of mental illness. Finally, and sadly, a vulnerability can be seen as a risk factor for violence, or sexual, financial, or physical abuse.

IDENTIFYING VULNERABLE POPULATIONS

The vulnerabilities of each at-risk population are unique and require solutions that are sensitive to their needs. To adequately determine a package of interventions in health emergencies for these populations, we first need to identify them.

Women and girls

There is documented evidence of a disproportionate impact on women and girls during past health outbreaks, such as during the 2014 Ebola crisis in West Africa (3), the 2016 cholera outbreak in Yemen, the 2015 Zika outbreak (4), and most recently, the COVID-19 pandemic (5). Across these outbreaks was a culmination of key factors rooted in pre-existing gender inequality that led to women and girls being at a greater risk of violence and harm, bearing a greater burden of disease, experiencing limitations to healthcare access, and having their needs inadequately met through preparedness, mitigation, and response measures.

In societies where gender inequality is deeply embedded in social and cultural norms, women and girls often have a lower status in the household. This can affect their ability to make independent decisions about seeking medical care (3). They may also have a lower financial standing and less control over household resources and spending. If women and girls have lower levels of education and literacy, they may have greater difficulty in understanding public health messaging about the outbreak or directions on medications or prevention (6). As primary caregivers in their families, women are at a greater risk of exposure to disease. This role can also have a severe mental and emotional toll.

There are typically also power dynamics at play related to consent, putting women and girls at an increased risk of gender-based violence (GBV) and sexual manipulation and abuse (7). According to data released by the World Health Organization and United Nations (UN) Women, an estimated 736 million women, or approximately one in three women worldwide, have experienced either physical or sexual intimate partner violence in their lifetimes (8).

GBV during health emergencies

The prevalence of GBV faced by women and girls escalates in emergency scenarios (9). The Democratic Republic of the Congo (DRC) has an extremely high prevalence of GBV, with 68 per cent of women in 2015 reporting exposure to physical, sexual, or emotional violence (9). This worsened during the 2018–2020 Ebola outbreak, where there was a notable rise in the reported incidence of physical violence, including increased sexual exploitation and abuse of women and girls. The ongoing conflict in North Kivu further amplified the risk, with sexual violence remaining widespread. Between 2021 and 2022 alone, there was a 91 per cent increase in reported GBV cases in the area. In Guinea, GBV data released by the government showed a 4.5 per cent increase in cases, including a doubling of rape cases during the 2014–2016 Ebola epidemic. Similarly, since the start of the COVID-19 pandemic, violence against women and girls has intensified, with 45 per cent of women globally reporting that they or a woman they know had become a victim of GBV.

It is important to note that diseases do not intrinsically increase the risk of GBV. However, disease outbreaks magnify the underlying flaws in systems and policies that are inadequate in protecting women and girls from harm and reveal the existing inequalities in societies rooted in patriarchal norms.

In volatile settings, women and girls are also at an increased risk of exploitation. In these instances of deep uncertainty, transactional sex and sexual exploitation, where sexual acts are coerced in exchange for food, can become more commonplace, just so women and girls can find a means of survival. Women and girls have reported sexual assaults while collecting water, food, or firewood during unusual hours or over long distances (10). On a particularly sinister level is the sexual exploitation and abuse of women and girls by health and aid workers, UN peacekeepers, and other individuals in positions of authority (11). It is the ultimate betrayal to have GBV perpetrated by a trusted person, especially one deployed to protect communities in emergencies.

Sexual exploitation in emergency response

With corroboration from aid agencies and local non-governmental organisation (NGO) workers, 51 women shared, in interviews, on the numerous instances of sexual exploitation and abuse they encountered by international workers from major UN and aid organisations during the DRC's 2018–2020 Ebola crisis. While pushing alcohol on these women, they were forced to exchange sexual favours for the promise of a job, or had their jobs terminated if they refused (12).

Incidences of sexual exploitation and abuse by interveners and emergency deployees severely—and sometimes, permanently—erodes their organisations' credibility. This hampers their capacity to respond efficiently to the ongoing emergency, and also acts as a substantial obstacle for these organisations to participate in future response efforts (13). Despite the establishment of policy and institutional frameworks aimed at preventing sexual exploitation and abuse and the introduction of accountability measures, peacekeeping and aid personnel persist in committing sexual exploitation and abuse (14). Given the perpetrators' positions of authority and the power dynamics that arise from it, victims may refrain from reporting these incidents due to concerns about potential retaliation or job loss.

Women also make up 70 per cent of the health workforce globally (15) yet hold only 25 per cent of leadership roles in health (16), which inherently exposes them to a greater risk of disease and limits their decision-making powers, particularly around policies that affect them. In health emergencies, they face gender-based occupational hazards, such as not having appropriate personal protective equipment (PPE). Most PPE is marked as unisex, but the designs are generally modelled after traditional male proportions (17) which may be ill-fitting on women health workers and compromise their protection from infection when treating patients and doing community visits, making them more vulnerable to infections as they perform their work. Women health workers also noted that menstruation posed an additional difficulty when wearing PPE, as PPE suits are not easily removable when visiting the restroom and need to be discarded (18).

Children

Children have unique physiological, developmental, and dependency needs that are often overlooked in times of crisis. During acute emergencies, essential services such as vaccination, nutrition, and education can be severely disrupted, placing children at an increased risk of disease (19). These disruptions can represent critical threats to their overall health and development. Missed vaccinations during emergencies can lead to outbreaks of vaccine-preventable diseases, on top of the existing emergency the country is responding to, which further endanger children's health (20).

Disruptions are not just constrained to health services. Education is pivotal to the development of children, and this is often halted in times of emergencies as a result of quarantine measures. During the COVID-19 pandemic, UNICEF warned that the scale of the loss of education for children was "nearly insurmountable", with around 616 million students affected worldwide (21). While some countries and schools have the resources to soften the disruption with distance or online learning, many low- and middle-income countries do not have the means to continue children's education until the end of the acute emergency. In these contexts, it is estimated that the impact of school closures has led to significant learning losses, with as many as 70 per cent of 10-year-olds now unable to read or comprehend a basic text, a substantial increase from 53 per cent before the pandemic (21). Additionally, the concerns are compounded among children from low-income backgrounds who rely on school meals for sustenance. UNICEF estimates that over 370 million children globally were deprived of school meals due to school closures during the COVID-19 pandemic (21).

Moreover, the psychological impact of health emergencies on children cannot be overstated. Experiencing or even witnessing the upheaval caused by pandemics, natural disasters, or conflict can lead to long-term emotional and psychological distress. This is particularly poignant for children who may lose family members, face displacement, or witness violence and instability (22). Such experiences can interrupt their developmental trajectory, leading to educational setbacks and emotional difficulties. During the 2014–2016 Ebola outbreak in West Africa, over 30,000 children lost one or both parents, and many children witnessed the deaths of their loved ones (23). A growing body of evidence shows that COVID-19 has caused high rates of anxiety and depression among children and young people, with some studies finding that girls, adolescents, and those living in rural areas most likely to experience these problems (24).

Refugees and internally displaced persons

Refugees and internally displaced persons (IDPs) face a different set of unique challenges during health emergencies that exacerbates their vulnerability. Often residing in overcrowded makeshift camps or shelters, these populations struggle with inadequate access to healthcare services, sanitation facilities, and clean water supplies (25–26). The dense living conditions not only make social distancing virtually impossible, but also facilitate the rapid spread of infectious diseases. The scarcity of clean water and sanitation infrastructure further compounds the risk, making basic hygiene practices difficult to maintain and increasing susceptibility to disease outbreaks (26).

The precarious legal status of many refugees and IDPs, coupled with the fear of deportation, also significantly hinders their ability to seek medical help or access emergency services (27). This fear is compounded by disrupted social networks, as the displacement process often separates individuals from their communities and traditional support systems. Without the ability to rely on established social ties for assistance or navigate the complex landscape of aid due to legal and logistical barriers, refugees and IDPs are left in a highly vulnerable position, facing heightened health risks with limited means to mitigate them (25,27).

Refugees and IDPs can also be excluded from national response plans for health emergencies, as they are often not counted in the official population, or their actual numbers are unknown. They also face linguistic obstacles in health communications and outreach efforts. This poses clear problems in outbreak response, particularly in the distribution of medical supplies or during nationwide vaccination drives, where refugees and IDPs are left behind. During the COVID-19 pandemic, refugees were left out of vaccination drives and other interventions, making disease containment much more challenging. Of course, such gaps then impact the wider population (28).

People with disabilities

People with physical and intellectual disabilities also encounter barriers during health emergencies that significantly amplify their vulnerability (29–30). Challenges in accessing emergency and health services are prevalent, often due to physical and infrastructure barriers, communication issues, and a general lack of accommodation that considers their unique needs. Important public health information may not be provided in accessible formats, such as sign language, braille, or audio formats, resulting in individuals with hearing or visual impairments being deprived of crucial knowledge needed to protect themselves in emergencies. This exclusion is common in general, but even more prevalent during health emergencies where communication materials are often urgently published without much time to consider audiences with disabilities (31).

The disruption of support networks and services during emergencies can have a profound impact on people with disabilities, particularly their mental health (29). Many depend on routine care and assistance for daily activities, which can be severely disrupted during disasters or pandemics. Assistive devices and personalised support systems, essential for their autonomy and well-being, may become unavailable or inaccessible, further exacerbating their isolation and making it difficult to receive support or social and medical services.

Indigenous populations

Indigenous populations also face heightened vulnerabilities during health emergencies (32–33). Addressing the vulnerabilities of these diverse populations requires an approach that respects cultural practices, involves community leaders in planning and response efforts, and ensures equitable access to healthcare and emergency services.

Many indigenous communities reside in remote areas that are far removed from healthcare facilities and the general population, making access to medical care and emergency response significantly challenging, as well as presenting obstacles for public health-related community outreach and engagement. This geographical isolation, coupled with the limited infrastructure in these regions, impedes the timely delivery of healthcare services and critical supplies during emergencies, leaving these communities disproportionately affected by health crises.

Cultural barriers and historical mistrust toward governmental and medical institutions can also deter indigenous populations from seeking help or accepting assistance during outbreaks and emergencies. Trust is a key challenge in successful health emergency outcomes, even in communities that are part of the larger population. Language barriers and a lack of culturally sensitive healthcare provisions further exacerbate this divide, preventing effective communication and engagement with these communities (34). "One-size-fits-all" messaging campaigns are unlikely to work effectively, and public health responses need to tailor campaigns by paying more attention to the specific socioeconomic, historical, and cultural contexts of indigenous populations (35).

A common solution for these challenges can be found in community health worker (CHW) programmes that aim to reach rural communities. However, in the case of utilising CHWs to reach indigenous populations, there are even greater difficulties in establishing relationships of trust unless the CHWs are part of the indigenous communities themselves or are very aware of their culture, customs, and practices. The importance of community engagement is illustrated by the example of the Community Health Representatives (CHRs), which are part of the wider CHW programme that serves the Navajo Nation (36). The resilience and dedication of the CHRs have been pivotal as they adapt to their community's evolving needs. During the COVID-19 pandemic, more than a hundred Diné men and women exceeded their conventional duties as health advocates and links between tribal members and healthcare professionals, taking on roles in crisis management. They have played key roles in enforcing tribal orders, such as regular curfews, and are involved in distributing medicines, food, and kitchen essentials to quarantined individuals and families. They also play an important role in translating COVID-19 health guidelines and related information, as well as linking people with resources to support them in maintaining social distance. This shift to a prolonged emergency response is undertaken amidst the backdrop of their own communities and families grappling with significantly high rates of infection and mortality (36).

The elderly

The elderly population is particularly susceptible to the impacts of health emergencies, largely due to a higher prevalence of pre-existing health conditions that can be exacerbated under such circumstances. Conditions such as heart disease, diabetes, and respiratory illnesses make them more vulnerable to severe complications from infectious diseases, including heightened mortality risks. Respiratory infections from outbreaks such as severe acute respiratory syndrome (SARS), Middle East respiratory syndrome (MERS), and COVID-19 can also worsen existing conditions (37). Additionally, many elderly individuals rely on regular healthcare services and medications to manage chronic conditions, which can be disrupted or less accessible during emergencies (38). The challenge of navigating healthcare systems during crises, coupled with potential shortages of essential medications, further jeopardises healthcare in the elderly.

Elderly individuals commonly face mobility issues, vision impairment, or cognitive decline, all of which require tailored interventions. As with people living with disabilities, their needs are often left behind in emergency response, particularly in terms of health messaging and communication campaigns (38).

Social isolation and mental health issues further compound their vulnerability; many elderly individuals live alone or are separated from their families, reducing their ability to receive help when needed (39). This isolation can also exacerbate feelings of loneliness and distress during times when social support is most needed. Addressing the needs of the elderly in health emergencies requires targeted interventions that ensure they have access to health care, support services, and clear communication tailored to their specific needs.

Impact of COVID-19 on the elderly in Italy

During the COVID-19 pandemic, Italy's nursing home residents, particularly the elderly, were severely impacted due to the high proportion of elderly citizens in the country and the rapid spread of the virus in such facilities. The situation was exacerbated by close living quarters, the slow adoption of infection control measures, and the residents' pre-existing health conditions, leading to a high mortality rate (40). The enforced isolation measures, aimed at virus containment, also isolated residents from their families and social networks, worsening their psychological stress.

The Lost in Lombardy project conducted a study on the psychological well-being of elderly individuals in Italy and revealed a significant rise in mental health issues during the pandemic (41). The findings showed that symptoms of depression surged by 112 per cent, anxiety symptoms by 136 per cent, instances of insufficient sleep by 12 per cent, and unsatisfactory sleep quality by 15 per cent. Additionally, feelings of hopelessness were observed to be more common in women than men and tended to increase with age.

Migrant workers

Migrant workers face unique challenges that stem from their often precarious living and working conditions (42). Many migrant workers live in overcrowded accommodation, work in environments with limited health and safety protection, and have restricted access to healthcare services, making them particularly vulnerable to the spread of infectious diseases, given that it is often impossible to keep a distance from others. Ironically, while they often live in crowded accommodation, they can also face exceptional degrees of social isolation due to being away from their usual support networks and families with limited resources to contact them. This social isolation, on top of the mental health challenges faced in outbreaks, exacerbates their vulnerabilities.

> **Migrant workers in Singapore**
>
> During the early stages of the COVID-19 pandemic, Singapore witnessed a significant outbreak among its migrant worker population, particularly those residing in densely packed dormitories. For some time and for this reason, migrant workers were at a higher risk of COVID-19 than the general population (42). Despite Singapore's initial success in controlling the spread of the virus among the general population, the cramped living conditions in these dormitories facilitated a rapid transmission of the virus among migrant workers (43).
>
> The outbreak among migrant workers shed light on the vulnerabilities faced by this group, including limited access to healthcare, language barriers, and the fear of job loss or deportation if they reported illness (44). In response, the Singapore government implemented measures such as mass testing and movement restrictions to reduce further spread from this group of more than 300,000 men. The government guaranteed maintenance of their pay and enabled improvements to living conditions. The situation brought to the forefront the need for policies that ensure equitable access to healthcare and safe living conditions for migrant workers, not just during pandemics but as a standard practice, to protect them from such disproportionate impacts in future emergencies.

Additionally, migrant workers frequently face language barriers and a lack of knowledge about the healthcare systems in their host countries. This can prevent them from understanding public health advisories or knowing how to navigate their host country's healthcare system, such as calling an emergency number for ambulance services for urgent care, obtaining COVID-19 tests, or contacting a designated COVID-19 healthcare facility (45). In addition to the language barriers, migrant workers might not have ready access to the internet and usual forms of media where information about outbreaks is circulated (46).

AMPLIFIERS OF VULNERABILITIES

Circumstances that change during an infectious disease emergency can amplify vulnerabilities contributing to a compounding effect. A population could already be vulnerable on the basis of gender, age, or disability status, and change can increase their risk. For instance, a child, already vulnerable, if orphaned during the emergency, may be placed into care facilities that can be crowded. On top of their existing vulnerabilities as children, they would then face the additional risk of disease transmission from being in a very populated space.

Vulnerable populations face mental health risks which are amplified during an infectious disease emergency due to the fear of infection, social isolation measures, and the like, leading to increased anxiety, depression, and loneliness. Additional stressors include the uncertainty of the situation, wage loss, discrimination, fear of deportation, and concern for distant family members.

The loss of jobs and payments to the vulnerable during illness or quarantine can push individuals into poverty (47), forcing them to compromise on health, nutrition, and education. Migrant workers support their families in their home country so a migrant worker's job loss can have far-reaching consequences. Children's education and support can be collateral damage after a job loss, amplifying their existing vulnerability and increasing their risk of malnutrition or being forced into labour to support the family, which in turn presents additional risks of exploitation and abuse.

Disruptions in supply chains affect the availability of necessities, including food and medical supplies, hitting hardest those who are economically disadvantaged or living in remote areas. This can lead to increased food insecurity and hinder access to essential medications, further endangering vulnerable populations. In outbreaks of zoonoses, emergency response may include the culling of livestock, as seen in previous avian flu outbreaks, which can completely devastate livelihoods and food security (48). The outbreak of avian flu in the U.S. in 2022 led to the loss of around 40 million animals, with the economic impact estimated between US$ 2.5 and US$ 3 billion (49).

Finally, fear and misinformation can drive stigma and discrimination directed at vulnerable groups. This can further restrict their access to healthcare and support services in outbreaks through fear of being targeted, increasing their marginalisation. This was observed in women who had been performing caretaking duties for their family members with Ebola virus disease and Asian migrant workers who faced racial discrimination during the COVID-19 pandemic.

STRATEGIES FOR PROTECTING VULNERABLE POPULATIONS DURING AN OUTBREAK

To adequately address the unique needs and challenges faced by vulnerable populations during outbreaks and public health emergencies, it is imperative to introduce appropriate channels that facilitate adequate representation from these groups in the discussion and decision-making processes during the early stages of preparedness planning. Allowing their voices and perspectives to be more directly heard is vital to developing more comprehensive and inclusive strategies that ensure their equitable access to resources and services during a crisis (50–51). Basic principles of effectively engaging vulnerable communities include clear, tailored, and sensitive communication, as well as implementing community-based outreach initiatives that promote ongoing trust-building. By adopting a collaborative and community-led model, outbreak preparedness and emergency plans can be better aligned with the specific needs and cultural contexts of diverse populations (52–55). These broad approaches are key to empowering vulnerable populations with the knowledge required to navigate complex healthcare systems, and ensuring they have the means to access necessary support during times of need.

Current emergency response planning often lacks adequate coverage to maintain health system capacity for essential services alongside surge responses. Importantly, planning for this should extend beyond the institutional health systems level, and involve the integration of essential health services and emergency responses into community-based frameworks which can better reach remote, marginalised, or underserved populations. A multifaceted approach with greater participation from stakeholders responsible for non-emergency health programmes should be considered to help bridge this gap and enhance health system resilience. Such an approach should include prioritisation of special populations and account for equitable distribution of resources and services during emergencies. Business continuity measures must also be implemented to facilitate continuity of care for individuals with chronic health conditions throughout the crisis period (52–53,56–57). To overcome the barrier of delivering vital medical services to remote or underserved areas, it is worthwhile to consider investing in mobile and community-based clinics, district and rural health posts, as well as community health worker programmes, to improve access to and utilisation of healthcare. Community-based workers (including local residents) who have gained trust and rapport in the communities they serve and have a natural understanding of the local context, are additional valuable assets in promoting sustainability (58–59). Additionally, customised telemedicine programmes and digital technology are important aides that can expand care delivery when it is not feasible to provide physical consultations (60–62). Lastly, in order to improve the acceptance and comprehension of health messaging, education materials and health literacy programmes must be carefully tailored and contextualised, taking into account the unique social, cultural, and linguistic characteristics of the priority audiences (53,63–65).

Aside from enhancing health system resilience, outbreak preparedness planning must also take on a more universal approach that addresses systemic causes of vulnerability and other disparities limiting access to healthcare and essential social services. These may include underlying structural issues, such as inadequate social safety nets, and socioeconomic inequalities like poverty, low education status, and discrimination and stigmatisation. Social support systems such as financial aid incentives, emergency food banks, temporary housing assistance schemes, and psychological counselling services are indispensable tools for providing overall more effective and practical aid to vulnerable populations during health emergencies. These programmes should be designed not only to provide immediate relief during crises, but also incorporate more holistic strategies to tackle and overcome fundamental systemic disparities (65–67). The important role of legislature and policy must not be overlooked in emergency planning to achieve more inclusive and effective responses. For example, implementing anti-discrimination policies in healthcare settings can promote fair and inclusive treatment for vulnerable individuals during public health emergencies (67–68).

Learning from past experiences

Mpox provides an excellent example of how acknowledging and learning from past mistakes are crucial for improving the effectiveness of outbreak responses and public health programmes. In the 2022 global outbreak, at-risk individuals notably expanded among homosexual, bisexual, and other men who have sex with men (GBMSM). The past HIV epidemic had clearly demonstrated how stigma can obstruct effective prevention, education, and research initiatives, culminating in a significant detrimental impact on most affected populations. To improve outcomes and response strategies for mpox, it is important to recognise that mpox transmission routes, including sexual contact, necessitate customised health communication and education strategies for different societies and communities. Messaging must balance inclusivity with sensitivity, and especially avoid stigmatisation of the largest at-risk populations. This enables individuals to better understand and take actions to reduce their personal risk, and encourages them to seek appropriate care when required. However, to effectively combat the mpox outbreak, this does not only involve tailored health messaging. It is all the more essential to review policies, legislature, and funding structures that collectively safeguard these vulnerable populations from discrimination (68).

Social and community resilience is equally important in helping vulnerable groups withstand and recover from public health emergencies. Studies have shown that vulnerable populations exhibit remarkable adaptability in the face of health emergencies. Recognising and enhancing their inherent resilience and community cohesiveness are essential in parallel to other response measures. To improve resilience through promoting and preserving a sense of identity, belonging, and shared purpose, it is important to understand and leverage important and deeply-rooted cultural, religious, or faith-based practices, traditions, and rituals which hold meaningful significance to specific communities. Immigrant and refugee communities have relied on cultural traditions to establish informal support systems during disease outbreaks. Religious institutions and faith-based community networks in particular, often play a significant role as key stakeholders, serving as vital hubs for disseminating information, mobilising resources, offering emotional support, and encouraging healthcare seeking behaviours. Faith and spiritual practices can also be an important catalyst for fostering emotional strength and community cohesion during crises (67,69–76). Furthermore, it has been well reported that indigenous communities have cultivated a deep understanding of their environments and often utilise natural health approaches and healing practices which can be synergistic with modern medical interventions (77–78).

Roles of faith-based and religious organisations and leaders in alleviating risk to the most vulnerable

Greyling et al (74) examined the Ebola outbreak in West Africa in 2013, highlighting the instrumental role of faith-based organisations in the response efforts. Populations most affected in this region inherently include those most vulnerable to significant health and social disparities. Through their trusted and respected status within local communities, and the establishment of platforms and networks for outreach, faith-based organisations proved an indispensable partner to the government and public health agencies, as well as international aid organisations and other healthcare responders, in managing this epidemic. Their contributions included:

- enhancing the delivery and acceptance of medical care and health interventions, and utilising existing community healthcare infrastructure and operational frameworks
- disseminating accurate and timely health messages and education about Ebola, including preventive measures, while dispelling myths and addressing misinformation
- providing spiritual and emotional support to affected populations, which was vital in moderating the psychological impact caused by the outbreak
- facilitating the mobilisation of valuable local resources and managing volunteers to support the efforts of international aid organisations and coordinate intervention strategies

Wijesinghe et al (75) report that religious leaders in Sri Lanka were key players during the COVID-19 pandemic, working together with international health and aid organisations to enhance the successful implementation of prevention and response strategies. It was recognised that establishing a successful community model of care relied heavily on the role of these leaders to act as a bridge between local residents and external organisations, broaden outreach to disseminate health messages effectively, and support the implementation of evidence-based healthcare interventions including vaccination. In particular, the authors report that these religious leaders performed a critical function in identifying and building trust and connecting with difficult-to-reach vulnerable groups, facilitating their access to health education and healthcare. They played an important role in reducing stigma and discrimination, and were a key pillar in the provision of spiritual, psychosocial, and welfare support to these groups.

In summary, recognising and comprehensively addressing the needs of vulnerable populations in outbreak preparedness and health emergencies planning is a practical necessity for achieving effective outbreak response and crisis management. The unique challenges faced by these groups demand tailored approaches that go beyond improving conventional institutional-based health system frameworks and protocols. Increasing focus should be placed on developing more flexible and community-based models that prioritise the needs of vulnerable populations and examining ways to effectively deliver holistic support to these target groups. Finally, by leveraging on the strengths of community representation, cultural practices, and local knowledge during the planning processes, more responsive and inclusive strategies can be developed to better protect vulnerable communities, as well as augment their inherent resilience and adaptability.

CONCLUSION

This chapter explores the multifaceted vulnerabilities faced by various populations during public health emergencies, emphasising how these crises exacerbate pre-existing disparities, and the challenges vulnerable populations already face. There is an urgent need for inclusive, culturally-sensitive, and equitable emergency response strategies that proactively address the unique needs of vulnerable groups including women, children, refugees, IDPs, people with disabilities, indigenous communities, the elderly, and migrant workers. However, even this list is not comprehensive. The experiences of these and other vulnerable populations during recent health emergencies highlight systemic flaws in healthcare systems, emergency preparedness, and response mechanisms that fail to adequately protect those most at risk.

To mitigate these vulnerabilities and ensure a more effective response to future health emergencies, targeted interventions and policies that prioritise the inclusion and protection of vulnerable populations are needed. This includes improving access to healthcare, ensuring the availability of critical supplies, enhancing communication and support services, and addressing the socioeconomic and structural barriers that contribute to vulnerability. It is not acceptable to redirect resources away from essential social services during an infectious disease emergency, essentially because the adverse impacts suffered by the vulnerable are less visible. By learning from past experiences and integrating these lessons into policy-making and planning, we can build more resilient communities and healthcare systems that are capable of withstanding the challenges of future public health emergencies, ensuring that no one is left behind.

REFERENCES:

1. Steptoe A, Di Gessa G. Mental health and social interactions of older people with physical disabilities in England during the COVID-19 pandemic: a longitudinal cohort study. Lancet Public Health. 2021 Jun;6(6):e365–73. https://doi.org/10.1016/S2468-2667(21)00069-4 PMID:33894138.
2. Deblonde J, Sasse A, Del Amo J, Burns F, Delpech V, Cowan S, et al. Restricted access to antiretroviral treatment for undocumented migrants: a bottle neck to control the HIV epidemic in the EU/EEA. BMC Public Health. 2015 Dec;15(1):1228. https://doi.org/10.1186/s12889-015-2571-y PMID:26654427.
3. African Development Bank Group. Women's resilience: integrating gender in the response to Ebola. 2016. https://www.afdb.org/fileadmin/uploads/afdb/Documents/Generic-Documents/AfDB_Women_s_Resilience_-_Integrating_Gender_in_the_Response_to_Ebola.pdf.
4. Meinhart M, Vahedi L, Carter SE, Poulton C, Mwanze Palaku P, Stark L. Gender-based violence and infectious disease in humanitarian settings: lessons learned from Ebola, Zika, and COVID-19 to inform syndemic policy making. Confl Health. 2021 Nov;15(1):84. https://doi.org/10.1186/s13031-021-00419-9 PMID:34801062.

5. Ahinkorah BO, Hagan JE Jr, Ameyaw EK, Seidu AA, Schack T. COVID-19 pandemic worsening gender inequalities for women and girls in Sub-Saharan Africa. Front Glob Womens Health. 2021 Jul;2(686984):686984. https://doi.org/10.3389/fgwh.2021.686984 PMID:34816232.

6. Nkangu MN, Olatunde OA, Yaya S. The perspective of gender on the Ebola virus using a risk management and population health framework: a scoping review. Infect Dis Poverty. 2017 Oct;6(1):135. https://doi.org/10.1186/s40249-017-0346-7 PMID:29017587.

7. Menéndez C, Lucas A, Munguambe K, Langer A. Ebola crisis: the unequal impact on women and children's health. Lancet Glob Health. 2015 Mar;3(3):e130. https://doi.org/10.1016/S2214-109X(15)70009-4 PMID:25618242.

8. World Health Organization. Violence against women. 2021. https://www.who.int/news-room/fact-sheets/detail/violence-against-women.

9. Tlapek SM. Women's status and intimate partner violence in the Democratic Republic of Congo. J Interpers Violence. 2015 Sep;30(14):2526–40. https://doi.org/10.1177/0886260514553118 PMID:25315479.

10. International Red Cross. République Démocratique du Congo : Rapport d'évaluation pour Planification Post Ebola, Mars 11-24, 2020 - Democratic Republic of the Congo | ReliefWeb. 2020 [cited 2024 Mar 5]. https://reliefweb.int/report/democratic-republic-congo/r-publique-d-mocratique-du-congo-rapport-d-valuation-pour.

11. Vahedi L, Bartels SA, Lee S. 'Even peacekeepers expect something in return': a qualitative analysis of sexual interactions between UN peacekeepers and female Haitians. Glob Public Health. 2021 May;16(5):692-705. https://doi.org/10.1080/17441692.2019.1706758 PMID:31887070.

12. Flummerfelt R, Peyton N. The aid sector's newest sex abuse scandal. The New Humanitarian. 2020. https://www.thenewhumanitarian.org/2020/09/29/exclusive-more-50-women-accuse-aid-workers-sex-abuse-congo-ebola-crisis.

13. Westendorf JK, Searle L. Sexual exploitation and abuse in peace operations: trends, policy responses and future directions. Int Aff. 2017 Mar;93(2):365–87. https://doi.org/10.1093/ia/iix001.

14. Datta D. The elephant in the room: addressing sexual exploitation and abuse at international NGOs. Humanit Soc Sci Commun. 2023 May;10(1):261. https://doi.org/10.1057/s41599-023-01776-x.

15. World Health Organization. Gender equity in the health workforce: analysis of 104 countries. 2019. https://www.who.int/publications/i/item/gender-equity-in-the-health-workforce-analysis-of-104-countries.

16. Women in Global Health. Gender-responsive pandemic preparedness, prevention, response and recovery. [cited 2024 Mar 5]. https://womeningh.org/gender-responsive-pandemicppreparedness/.

17. Janson DJ, Clift BC, Dhokia V. PPE fit of healthcare workers during the COVID-19 pandemic. Appl Ergon. 2022 Feb;99:103610. https://doi.org/10.1016/j.apergo.2021.103610 PMID:34740070.

18. Eco-Business. Medical PPE unfit for women on Covid-19 frontlines. 2021 [cited 2024 Mar 5]. https://eco-business.com/news/medical-ppe-unfit-for-women-on-covid-19-frontlines/.

19. Dziuban EJ, Peacock G, Frogel M. A child's health is the public's health: progress and gaps in addressing pediatric needs in public health emergencies. Am J Public Health. 2017 Sep;107 S2:S134–7. https://doi.org/10.2105/AJPH.2017.303950 PMID:28892439.

20. UNICEF. Childhood immunization begins recovery after COVID-19 backslide. 2023. https://www.unicef.org/press-releases/childhood-immunization-begins-recovery-after-covid-19-backslide#:~:text=According%20to%20data%20published%20today.

21. UNICEF. COVID-19 scale of education loss "nearly insurmountable", warns UNICEF. 2022. https://www.unicef.org/press-releases/covid19-scale-education-loss-nearly-insurmountable-warns-unicef.

22. Denis-Ramirez E, Sørensen KH, Skovdal M. In the midst of a "perfect storm": unpacking the causes and consequences of Ebola-related stigma for children orphaned by Ebola in Sierra Leone. Child Youth Serv Rev. 2017 Feb;73:445–53. https://doi.org/10.1016/j.childyouth.2016.11.025.

23. UNICEF. Children and the DRC Ebola outbreak: 4 things you need to know. 2018. https://www.unicef.org/stories/children-and-drc-ebola-outbreak-4-things-you-need-know.

24. Merrill KA, William TN, Joyce KM, Roos LE, Protudjer JL. Potential psychosocial impact of COVID-19 on children: a scoping review of pandemics and epidemics. J Glob Health Rep. 2021 Jan;4. https://doi.org/10.29392/001c.18229.

25. Ojeleke O, Groot W, Pavlova M. Care delivery among refugees and internally displaced persons affected by complex emergencies: a systematic review of the literature. J Public Health (Berl.). 2022;30:747–762. https://doi.org/10.1007/s10389-020-01343-7.

26. Cantor D, Swartz J, Roberts B, Abbara A, Ager A, Bhutta ZA, et al. Understanding the health needs of internally displaced persons: a scoping review. J Migr Health. 2021 Oct;4:100071. https://doi.org/10.1016/j.jmh.2021.100071 PMID:34820657.

27. El Arab RA, Somerville J, Abuadas FH, Rubinat-Arnaldo E, Sagbakken M. Health and well-being of refugees, asylum seekers, undocumented migrants, and internally displaced persons under COVID-19: a scoping review. Front Public Health. 2023 Apr 26;11:1145002. https://doi.org/10.3389/fpubh.2023.1145002 PMID: 37181725.

28. Ismail SA, Lam ST, Bell S, Fouad FM, Blanchet K, Borghi J. Strengthening vaccination delivery system resilience in the context of protracted humanitarian crisis: a realist-informed systematic review. BMC Health Serv Res. 2022 Oct;22(1):1277. https://doi.org/10.1186/s12913-022-08653-4 PMID:36274130.

29. Pearce E, Kamenov K, Barrett D, Cieza A. Promoting equity in health emergencies through health systems strengthening: lessons learned from disability inclusion in the COVID-19 pandemic. Int J Equity Health. 2022 Oct;21(S3 Suppl 3):149. https://doi.org/10.1186/s12939-022-01766-6 PMID:36284335.

30. Lunsky Y. The impact of stress and social support on the mental health of individuals with intellectual disabilities. Salud Publica Mex. 2008;50 Suppl 2:s151–3.] https://doi.org/10.1590/S0036-36342008000800007 PMID:18470342.

31. Bailey A, Harris MA, Bogle D, Jama A, Muir SA, Miller S, et al. Coping with COVID 19: health risk communication and vulnerable groups. Disaster Med Public Health Prep. 2021 Jul;17:e22. https://doi.org/10.1017/dmp.2021.225 PMID:34247692.

32. Power T, Wilson D, Best O, Brockie T, Bourque Bearskin L, Millender E, et al. COVID-19 and Indigenous Peoples: an imperative for action. J Clin Nurs. 2020 Aug;29(15-16):2737–41. https://doi.org/10.1111/jocn.15320 PMID:32412150.

33. Groom AV, Jim C, Laroque M, Mason C, McLaughlin J, Neel L, et al. Pandemic influenza preparedness and vulnerable populations in tribal communities. Am J Public Health. 2009 Oct;99(Suppl 2 Suppl 2):S271–8. https://doi.org/10.2105/AJPH.2008.157453 PMID:19461107.

34. Richards P, Mokuwa E, Welmers P, Maat H, Beisel U. Trust, and distrust, of Ebola Treatment Centers: a case-study from Sierra Leone. Schieffelin J, editor. PLoS ONE. 2019 Dec 2;14(12):e0224511. https://doi.org/10.1371/journal.pone.0224511.

35. Driedger SM, Cooper E, Jardine C, Furgal C, Bartlett J. Communicating risk to Aboriginal Peoples: First Nations and Metis responses to H1N1 risk messages. McVernon J, editor. PLoS One. 2013 Aug 7;8(8):e71106. https://doi.org/10.1371/journal.pone.0071106.

36. Rosenthal EL, Menking P, Begay MG. Lives on the line—Community Health Representatives' roles in the pandemic battle on the Navajo Nation. J Ambul Care Manage. 2020;43(4):301–5. https://doi.org/10.1097/JAC.0000000000000354 PMID:32858729.

37. Doraiswamy S, Mamtani R, Ameduri M, Abraham A, Cheema S. Respiratory epidemics and older people. Age Ageing. 2020 Oct;49(6):896–900. https://doi.org/10.1093/ageing/afaa151 PMID:32857159.

38. Alam MS, Sultana R, Haque MA. Vulnerabilities of older adults and mitigation measures to address COVID-19 outbreak in Bangladesh: a review. Soc Sci Humanit Open. 2022;6(1):100336. https://doi.org/10.1016/j.ssaho.2022.100336 PMID:36124099.

39. Guo Y, Wang A, Zheng R. Editorial: Reducing health disparities: promoting vulnerable older adults' psychological health. Front Psychol. 2023 Apr;14:1187403. https://doi.org/10.3389/fpsyg.2023.1187403 PMID:37151340.

40. Cuomo A, Amore M, Arezzo MF, De Filippis S, De Rose A, La Pia S, et al. Mental health in Italy after two years of COVID-19 from the perspective of 1281 Italian physicians: looking back to plan forward. Ann Gen Psychiatry. 2022 Aug;21(1):30. https://doi.org/10.1186/s12991-022-00410-5 PMID:35948983.

41. Amerio A, Stival C, Lugo A, Fanucchi T, d'Oro LC, Iacoviello L, et al.; "LOST in Lombardia" Study Investigators. COVID-19 pandemic impact on mental health in a large representative sample of older adults from the Lombardy region, Italy. J Affect Disord. 2023 Mar;325:282–8. https://doi.org/10.1016/j.jad.2023.01.006 PMID:36627059.

42. Liem A, Wang C, Wariyanti Y, Latkin CA, Hall BJ. The neglected health of international migrant workers in the COVID-19 epidemic. Lancet Psychiatry. 2020 Apr;7(4):e20. https://doi.org/10.1016/S2215-0366(20)30076-6 PMID:32085842. Koh D. Migrant workers and COVID-19. Occup Environ Med. 2020 Sep;77(9):634–636. https://doi.org/10.1136/oemed-2020-106626 PMID: 32513832.

43. Gorny AW, Bagdasarian N, Koh AH, Lim YC, Ong JS, Ng BS, et al. SARS-CoV-2 in migrant worker dormitories: geospatial epidemiology supporting outbreak management. Int J Infect Dis. 2021 Feb;103:389–94. https://doi.org/10.1016/j.ijid.2020.11.148 PMID:33212260.

44. Yee K, Peh HP, Tan YP, Teo I, Tan EU, Paul J, et al. Stressors and coping strategies of migrant workers diagnosed with COVID-19 in Singapore: a qualitative study. BMJ Open. 2021 Mar;11(3):e045949. https://doi.org/10.1136/bmjopen-2020-045949 PMID:33741672.

45. Nahari TH, Alkhidir MA, Ibrahim HM, Al Mamun M. Mohammad Al Mamun. Migrant workers with COVID-19: a major challenge for Gulf Cooperation Council (GCC) countries to curb the spread of infection. Glob Health Promot. 2024 Jan;17579759231216108. https://doi.org/10.1177/17579759231216108.

46. Tam WJ, Gobat N, Hemavathi D, Fisher D. Risk communication and community engagement during the migrant worker COVID-19 outbreak in Singapore. Sci Commun. 2022 Apr;44(2):240–51. https://doi.org/10.1177/10755470211061513 PMID:35440864.

47. Karpman M, Zuckerman S, Peterson G. Adults in families losing jobs during the pandemic also lost employer sponsored health insurance. 2020. https://www.urban.org/sites/default/files/publication/102533/adults-in-families-losing-jobs-in-the-pandemic-also-lost-employer-sponso_1.pdf.

48. Mcleod A, Morgan N, Prakash A, Hinrichs J. Economic and social impacts of avian influenza. https://www.fao.org/3/ag035e/ag035e.pdf.

49. FOUR PAWS International - Animal Welfare Organisation. Billion dollar cost of the global bird flu outbreak. https://www.four-paws.org/our-stories/press-releases/september-2023/billion-dollar-cost-of-the-global-bird-flu-outbreak.

50. World Health Organization. Framework on integrated, people-centred health services. Report by the Secretariat [Internet]. 2016. https://apps.who.int/gb/ebwha/pdf_files/WHA69/A69_39-en.pdf.

51. Hutchins SS, Truman BI, Merlin TL, Redd SC. Protecting vulnerable populations from pandemic influenza in the United States: a strategic imperative [Internet]. Am J Public Health. 2009 Oct;99(Suppl 2 Suppl 2):S243–8. https://doi.org/10.2105/AJPH.2009.164814 PMID:19797737.

52. Dehaven M, Gimpel N, Carmichael HK. Working with communities: meeting the health needs of those living in vulnerable communities when primary health care and universal health coverage are not available. 2020 Jul 16. https://doi.org/10.22541/au.159493336.63441482.

53. Bedson J, Jalloh MF, Pedi D, Bah S, Owen K, Oniba A, et al. Community engagement in outbreak response: lessons from the 2014-2016 Ebola outbreak in Sierra Leone [Internet]. BMJ Glob Health. 2020 Aug;5(8):e002145. https://doi.org/10.1136/bmjgh-2019-002145 PMID:32830128.

54. Toppenberg-Pejcic D, Noyes J, Allen T, Alexander N, Vanderford M, Gamhewage G. Emergency risk communication: lessons learned from a rapid review of recent gray literature on Ebola, Zika, and yellow fever [Internet]. Health Commun. 2019 Apr;34(4):437–55. https://doi.org/10.1080/10410236.2017.1405488 PMID:29558199.

55. Häfliger C, Diviani N, Rubinelli S. Communication inequalities and health disparities among vulnerable groups during the COVID-19 pandemic - a scoping review of qualitative and quantitative evidence [Internet]. BMC Public Health. 2023 Mar;23(1):428. https://doi.org/10.1186/s12889-023-15295-6 PMID:36879229.

56. Mustafa S, Zhang Y, Zibwowa Z, Seifeldin R, Ako-Egbe L, McDarby G, et al. COVID-19 Preparedness and Response Plans from 106 countries: a review from a health systems resilience perspective [Internet]. Health Policy Plan. 2022 Feb;37(2):255–68. https://doi.org/10.1093/heapol/czab089 PMID:34331439.

57. White DB, Villarroel L, Hick JL. Inequitable access to hospital care - protecting disadvantaged populations during public health emergencies [Internet]. N Engl J Med. 2021 Dec;385(24):2211–4. https://doi.org/10.1056/NEJMp2114767 PMID:34874647.

58. Yu SW, Hill C, Ricks ML, Bennet J, Oriol NE. The scope and impact of mobile health clinics in the United States: a literature review [Internet]. Int J Equity Health. 2017 Oct;16(1):178. https://doi.org/10.1186/s12939-017-0671-2 PMID:28982362.

59. Cone PH, Haley JM. Mobile clinics in Haiti, part 1: preparing for service-learning [Internet]. Nurse Educ Pract. 2016 Nov;21:1–8. https://doi.org/10.1016/j.nepr.2016.08.008 PMID:27665303.

60. Alnasser Y, Proaño A, Loock C, Chuo J, Gilman RH. Telemedicine and pediatric care in rural and remote areas of middle-and-low-income countries: narrative review. J Epidemiol Glob Health. 2024 Sep;14(3):779–86. https://doi.org/10.1007/s44197-024-00214-8 PMID:38478166.

61. Mohammadzadeh N, Rezayi S, Saeedi S. Telemedicine for patient management in remote areas and underserved populations. Disaster Med Public Health Prep. 2022 May;17:e167. https://doi.org/10.1017/dmp.2022.76 PMID:35586911.

62. Blocker A, Datay MI, Mwangama J, Malila B. Development of a telemedicine virtual clinic system for remote, rural, and underserved areas using user-centered design methods. Digit Health. 2024 May;10:20552076241256752. https://doi.org/10.1177/20552076241256752 PMID:38812852.

63. Feinberg IZ, Owen-Smith A, O'Connor MH, Ogrodnick MM, Rothenberg R, Eriksen MP. Strengthening culturally competent health communication. Health Secur. 2021 Jun;19 S1:S41–9. https://doi.org/10.1089/hs.2021.0048 PMID:33961489.

64. Barron GC, Laryea-Adjei G, Vike-Freiberga V, Abubakar I, Dakkak H, Devakumar D, et al.; Lancet Commission on COVID-19: Task Force on Humanitarian Relief, Social Protection and Vulnerable Groups. Safeguarding people living in vulnerable conditions in the COVID-19 era through universal health coverage and social protection. Lancet Public Health. 2022 Jan;7(1):e86–92. https://doi.org/10.1016/S2468-2667(21)00235-8 PMID:34906331.

65. Patel JA, Nielsen FB, Badiani AA, Assi S, Unadkat VA, Patel B, et al. Poverty, inequality and COVID-19: the forgotten vulnerable. Public Health. 2020 Jun;183:110–1. https://doi.org/10.1016/j.puhe.2020.05.006 PMID:32502699.

66. Zhai Y, Du X. Disparities and intersectionality in social support networks: addressing social inequalities during the COVID-19 pandemic and beyond. Humanit Soc Sci Commun. 2022;9(1):143. https://doi.org/10.1057/s41599-022-01163-y.

67. Öcek ZA, Geise M, Volkmann AM, Basili A, Klünder V, Coenen M. Strengthening the social resilience of people living at the intersection of precariousness and migration during pandemics: action recommendations developed in Munich, Germany. Front Public Health. 2023 Aug;11:1201215. https://doi.org/10.3389/fpubh.2023.1201215 PMID:37601211.

68. Titanji B. Protect the vulnerable from monkeypox. Science. 2022 Sep;377(6611):1129. https://doi.org/10.1126/science.ade7115 PMID:36074834.

69. Alonge O, Sonkarlay S, Gwaikolo W, Fahim C, Cooper JL, Peters DH. Understanding the role of community resilience in addressing the Ebola virus disease epidemic in Liberia: a qualitative study (community resilience in Liberia). Glob Health Action. 2019;12(1):1662682. https://doi.org/10.1080/16549716.2019.1662682 PMID:31507254.

70. Morton MJ, Lurie N. Community resilience and public health practice. Am J Public Health. 2013 Jul;103(7):1158–60. https://doi.org/10.2105/AJPH.2013.301354 PMID:23678934.

71. Kelly L, Hajistassi M, Ramasundram S. Migrant and refugee communities strengthening disaster resilience. Australian Journal of Emergency Management [Internet]. 2024 Jul;(No. 3):49–58. https://doi.org/10.47389/39.3.49.

72. Fadhlia TN, Sauter DA, Doosje B. Fear, anger, and hope: adversity, emotion, and resilience among Syrian refugees in the Netherlands. 2022 Jul 7. https://doi.org/10.21203/rs.3.rs-1823019/v1.

73. Jacinto E, Figueiredo Dalla Costa Ames MC, Serafim MC, Zappellini MB. Religion-spirituality influences in the governance of faith-based organizations during the Covid pandemic. Public Organ Rev. 2013;23(2):531–50. https://doi.org/10.1007/s11115-023-00704-6.

74. Greyling C, Maulit JA, Parry S, Robinson D, Smith S, Street A, et al. Lessons from the faith-driven response to the West Africa Ebola epidemic [Internet]. Rev Faith Int Aff. 2016 Jul;14(3):118–23. https://doi.org/10.1080/15570274.2016.1215829.

75. Wijesinghe MS, Ariyaratne VS, Gunawardana BM, Rajapaksha RM, Weerasinghe WM, Gomez P, et al. Role of religious leaders in COVID-19 prevention: a community-level prevention model in Sri Lanka [Internet]. J Relig Health. 2022 Feb;61(1):687–702. https://doi.org/10.1007/s10943-021-01463-8 PMID:34812996.

76. Allen L, Hatala A, Ijaz S, Courchene ED, Bushie EB. Indigenous-led health care partnerships in Canada [Internet]. CMAJ. 2020 Mar;192(9):E208–16. https://doi.org/10.1503/cmaj.190728 PMID:32122977.

77. Pickering K, Galappaththi EK, Ford JD, Singh C, Zavaleta-Cortijo C, Hyams K, et al.; COVID-Observatories Team. Indigenous peoples and the COVID-19 pandemic: a systematic scoping review [Internet]. Environ Res Lett. 2023 Mar;18(3):033001. https://doi.org/10.1088/1748-9326/acb804 PMID:36798651.

78. Zavaleta-Cortijo C, Ford JD, Galappaththi EK, Namanya DB, Nkwinti N, George B, et al.; COVID Observatories Team. Indigenous knowledge, community resilience, and health emergency preparedness [Internet]. Lancet Planet Health. 2023 Aug;7(8):e641–3. https://doi.org/10.1016/S2542-5196(23)00140-7 PMID:37558343.

CHAPTER 33

SUCCESSFUL RISK COMMUNICATION AND COMMUNITY ENGAGEMENT

by Wai Jia Tam and Rachel Peh

Communication and community engagement form a key, yet sometimes neglected, pillar in public health emergency response. The emergency response community has created a methodology and professional practice here which goes by the acronym RCCE, which stands for Risk Communication and Community Engagement. While previously under-recognised, RCCE practice was pushed to the forefront by the COVID-19 pandemic, becoming a key response pillar equal to that of surveillance or infection prevention and control (IPC) in some contexts. However, more can be done. Effective RCCE plays a crucial role in breaking the chains of transmission and mitigating the impact of a pandemic by targeting people's behaviour and willingness to follow public health and social measures. In this chapter, we give an overview of the objectives and functions of RCCE during an emergency. Guidelines to the components of effective and successful RCCE along with challenges to its implementation will also be discussed.

INTRODUCTION

RCCE is one of the key pillars identified by the World Health Organization (WHO) in responding to a public health emergency of international concern (1). Nonetheless, the definition, importance, and application of RCCE are not universally understood or accepted by all (2–3). Due to the breadth of capacities required from the ground to the highest levels of leadership, as well as the complex nature of working with affected populations, the applications, skills, and implementation of RCCE will vary country to country. Practising RCCE effectively is challenging. Ultimately, the uneven application of these skills at country levels may result in different outcomes.

Purists argue that community engagement should be an overarching goal instead of being framed as parallel to or a sub-component of risk communication (3). Others use the term interchangeably with risk communication. In recent years, greater distinction has been made between risk communication and community engagement to highlight the importance of community engagement as a concept deserving of its own attention (2). RCCE thus combines two distinct but interrelated approaches to supporting communities to adopt safe behaviours and take community action in support of ending disease transmission (2).

The use of emergency risk communication in public health response dates to the early 1990s and the management of brownfield risks, the risks to health from heavily polluted areas, among local populations in the U.S. (4–5). Since then, the field has grown in breadth and depth and now encompasses the use of media, social media, influencers, social and behavioural sciences, infodemics, and most importantly, community engagement. The capacities required of RCCE often exceed the skills of small response teams in public health institutions resulting in an uneven and inconsistent application of the emergency function.

In 2009, a WHO consultation concluded that there was a general lack of appreciation of the behavioural imperative underlying responses to public health emergencies, even though human behaviour drives much of epidemic emergence, transmission, and complications (2). Since then, an interagency guide on communication for behavioural impact during an outbreak response has been developed by the WHO, and recognition of RCCE has increased in prominence, as reflected in a range of international guidelines and agreements (1,6–8). Additional guidance published by the WHO in late 2017 provided countries with "overarching, evidence-based guidance on how risk communication should be practised in an emergency". The guidance also identified numerous gaps in knowledge and unresolved research priorities. Many of these deficits showed up when it came time to understand the lessons learned from the COVID-19 pandemic (9).

Historically, or at least prior to the COVID-19 pandemic response, RCCE efforts were underrated and under-resourced. They were treated as supplementary activities during emergencies rather than core components of outbreak response, since components such as epidemiology and case management tend to attract outbreak managers' attention, especially if managers are less experienced in the dynamics of outbreak response (3). Thus, RCCE, like previous communications approaches, can suffer from delayed implementation and inadequate investment. Often, funding supports ad hoc reactionary interventions rather than sustained outbreak control measures (10). The COVID-19 response saw much more continuity in terms of the presence of RCCE as a key pillar of the response at WHO global, regional, and country levels, as well as national emergency operations.

During public health emergencies, people need to know the risks posed to their health and the actions available to them to protect themselves (9). Access to such information allows people to make informed decisions for themselves and their families (9). In times of uncertainty, communication needs to occur regularly, frequently, transparently in various languages and formats, from a variety of relatable messengers, and via media that are contextually appropriate and accessible for all groups in a community (11–13). This is why RCCE is so critical (14–16).

What is risk communication?

Risk communication refers to an ongoing exchange of information based on the disciplines of organisational and message development, audience research and relations, message delivery, and media relations (5). It helps ensure the exchange of accurate information among scientists, healthcare workers and authorities, responders, and the population at risk. The goal is to improve knowledge and understanding of the disease (modes of spread, signs and symptoms, preventative and treatment measures) and adopt appropriate protective or treatment behaviours (1). Simply put, it is two-way and multidirectional communication and engagement with affected populations so they can make informed decisions on how to protect themselves and their loved ones (17).

In the context of the COVID-19 pandemic, this included the range of communication actions required through the preparedness, response, and recovery phases in order to encourage informed decision-making, protective behaviour change, and the maintenance of trust (17).

Various deep-seated cognitive biases make understanding and planning for different kinds of risks challenging as people tend to take cognitive shortcuts in dealing with risk and uncertainty (18). Communication needs to take these responses into account, especially when the hazards involved are potentially life-threatening, exotic or unfamiliar, acute, and/or cause permanent damage (19–21).

What is community engagement?

Community engagement is a critical component of civil society, international development practice, and humanitarian assistance. It brings together all populations that are affiliated by geographic proximity, special interests, and similar risk situations or circumstances to work collaboratively in addressing issues affecting their health (1,22). It is based on the simple premise that communities should be listened to and have a meaningful role in decision-making and co-ownership of the solutions, processes, and issues that affect them (7). In more recent times, social science literature has shown how overly simplistic notions of community can lead to ineffective policies and harm vulnerable populations (23). Understanding social dynamics, and the nuanced complexities of social hierarchies and politics, is essential to designing robust interventions. To truly engage communities and understand their complex social, political, and economic interests, anthropologists with specialist knowledge of local people and contexts can be important allies in forming and implementing public health policies (23).

What is RCCE?

Today, RCCE refers to "the processes and approaches to systematically consult, engage, and communicate with communities who are at risk, or whose practices affect risk" (24–25).

RCCE is essential for surveillance, case reporting, contact tracing, information-sharing, public health interventions, IPC efforts, promoting mental health and well-being, and harnessing local support for logistical and operational needs in the outbreak response (26). RCCE has specific actions associated with all phases of emergency response including prevention, preparedness, readiness, response, and recovery. It is one of the more complex emergency pillars as it directly relates to affected populations and their risk perceptions while enabling all other response pillars (e.g., IPC, clinical care, surveillance, vaccination, etc.) to gather data and meet population information needs more effectively.

The aim of RCCE is to urge, enable, and include stakeholders in the prevention of and response to public health emergencies, including natural or man-made disasters, by adapting communication to community realities (1). For many infectious diseases, RCCE enables stakeholders to work hand-in-hand to ensure healthy behaviours and reduce the risk of transmitting and spreading disease (17).

Proactively communicating what is known and unknown, and what is being done to learn, saves lives and reduces adverse consequences. In addition to protecting health, RCCE can also preserve economies and protect livelihoods by minimising social disruptions (26). At its best, effective RCCE builds community trust in the outbreak response, alleviates confusion among the public, and increases the chances that health advice will be adhered to, thus minimising rumours or actions that undermine outbreak control (26). Ultimately, effective RCCE results in communities that are informed, engaged, and empowered to protect themselves.

> **24/7 COVID-19 hotline operated by Azerbaijan's State Agency and Mandatory Health Insurance (SAMHI)**
>
> In March 2020, SAMHI set up a COVID-19 hotline to offer information on mandatory health insurance and other related issues, support lines, and outpatient services. The hotline enabled two-way communication on COVID-19 and built trust between health authorities and the public. All calls were free and there was increasing public satisfaction with the services provided by the call centre. It also aided in contact tracing and case finding, and enabled the rapid referral of suspected COVID-19 cases, or those with other serious health conditions, to health facilities for necessary and timely treatment (27).

RCCE IN MARGINALISED COMMUNITIES

RCCE among vulnerable groups deserves special attention. In the acute phase of an outbreak, the identification of infectious clusters, superspreaders, and community outbreaks often causes widespread fear among the public, resulting in social stigmatisation and discrimination against certain groups (14). Those from marginalised communities may experience multiple intersecting stigmas, negatively impacting social justice which comprises agency (the capacity of individuals to act independently and make their own free choices), respect, and association (the capacity to connect and participate) (16). Ultimately, this leads to hazardous public health consequences, such as the delayed presentation of symptomatic patients to healthcare services and under-detection of infectious individuals (28). This can impact the general community. Over the years, RCCE among marginalised communities has attracted greater attention due to the real and widespread risks posed (29).

> **No one should be left behind: lessons from Singapore**
>
> In August 2020, Singapore reported 55,661 laboratory-confirmed cases of COVID-19 in a population of 5.7 million (30–31). Low-wage migrant workers living in high-density accommodation comprised 94.6 per cent of the cases (31–32). Initially, health messaging to migrant workers was overlooked, uncoordinated, and unidirectional. Later, an organic RCCE working group comprising health workers and non-profit staff ensured health messages were translated, pictorial, culturally sensitive, contextual, and delivered with the help of migrant worker leaders. The RCCE working group's efforts eventually evolved into a centralised, coordinated nationwide strategy, improving trust and social cohesion among migrant workers. Within four months, new COVID-19 cases reduced from approximately 100 laboratory-confirmed cases each day to zero (33–36).

WHAT EFFECTIVE RCCE LOOKS LIKE

The WHO's pandemic strategy outlines how RCCE should be nationally-led but community-centred, participatory, trust-nurturing, and transparent. For professionals responding to an outbreak, this may be a tall order, especially if they do not have longstanding ties to or an in-depth understanding of the communities they are trying to assist.

RCCE should be integrated and coordinated. It should also be inclusive and accountable in order to promote trust and social cohesion to reduce the negative consequences of infectious disease (33). It should be two-way communication, accurate, and standardised, yet tailored to the target community and delivered in a timely manner through familiar and trusted communication channels or influencers. This means that understanding the community's demographics, literacy level, access to information, and beliefs in health and healthcare is crucial to preparedness. Market segmentation research that provides information on specific subgroups can assist in tracking concerns, fears, and rumours. Delivery must be multimodal and provided by selected key individuals including political, religious, and cultural leaders, scientists, and other trusted influencers (33). This emphasises the need for ground-up, participatory approaches to RCCE, for efforts to be adaptive, localised, sustainable, empowering, and impactful. These would be demanding standards of communication for any institution in the best times, more so during an emergency, but the importance of RCCE demands nothing less.

RCCE requires integration across all pillars of outbreak response

RCCE aims to assist leaders and emergency response personnel to listen to and work with affected communities while also enabling other response pillars to keep communities at the forefront of their responses. RCCE, when implemented in an integrative manner, can complement, support, encourage, and accelerate action by filling information gaps and providing resources and tools for taking action (33). When enabled early, it strengthens preparedness. Without it, the response struggles. Establishing multidisciplinary crisis communications teams can improve coordination among government, private sectors, non-governmental organisations, and individuals, leading to the streamlining of efforts or adaptation of a single harmonised campaign that furthers message dissemination and uptake (34).

When integrated across other biomedical response pillars in humanitarian response efforts, community engagement activities can create strong functional linkages between community-level prevention and other aspects of the response, enhancing their effectiveness (2). Biomedical solutions can only go so far without the support of communities, especially in the context of COVID-19 where the solutions are currently solely social and behavioural (6). Without two-way communication platforms between response actors and communities, misinformation, confusion, and mistrust can undermine efforts to save lives. There is great opportunity now for RCCE to be integrated collaboratively into the different response pillars (2,6,13).

RCCE relies on trust

A key to the effective implementation of public health measures is earning and maintaining trust between communities and governing authorities. Trust is a reflection of positive perception about the actions of an individual or an organisation that shapes behaviour. In outbreaks, trust in three types of actors is relevant for behavioural change (3):
- the government that imposes changes
- fellow citizens whose cooperation is needed
- scientists who provide the evidence for change

> **Trust is key: lessons from Africa**
>
> The role of trust in effective RCCE cannot be overstated. A large representative survey in Liberia during the 2014–2015 Ebola outbreak showed that people who expressed low trust in the government ignored precautions against Ebola in their homes and were reluctant to follow Ebola control policies. Results suggested that respondents who refused to comply did so because they did not trust the capacity or integrity of government institutions to slow the spread of Ebola. This was also observed during the Ebola epidemic in eastern Democratic Republic of the Congo (DRC). There was resistance to control efforts due to mistrust and suspicion over the response team's financial motivations (37). Furthermore, a large study conducted in 2021, which aimed to catalogue RCCE strategies in 13 African countries threatened by COVID-19, revealed that one of the most significant challenges surrounded distrust in government (15).

In preparation for a health emergency, it is necessary for countries to establish RCCE operations (38). RCCE can be the basis for the quick activation of other outbreak response strategies. Countries with an RCCE plan, stakeholders mapped out, and trained RCCE staff are able to swiftly respond during a health emergency, engaging in two-way communication that addresses misunderstandings and frequently asked questions, and coordinating collaboration among response partners for technical health operations and control measures. Furthermore, countries with strong pre-existing networks of community engagement can anticipate community support during an outbreak emergency. This enables a resilient community that will attenuate the harm of a health emergency (3).

RCCE requires quality standards and indicators
The Minimum Quality Standards and Indicators for Community Engagement were developed to guide the efforts of stakeholders in establishing an enabling environment where community engagement is intentional and structured (7).

Measuring the success of RCCE
The Joint External Evaluation (JEE), which assesses a nation's core capacities under the International Health Regulations (IHR) structure, includes measures of RCCE preparedness. The JEE creates a platform that allows countries to identify the most urgent needs within their health security system and prioritise opportunities for enhanced preparedness, operational readiness, response, and action, and to engage with stakeholders effectively. JEE priorities and the development of a national action plan can help ensure operational readiness in countries with urgent needs.

Ultimately, the desired impact of RCCE is for responsible entities to actively listen, respond to concerns of the public, effectively engage the public, and communicate through media, social media, mass awareness campaigns, health promotion, social mobilisation, and stakeholder engagement, with the end goal of mitigating the potential negative impact of health hazards (35).

PART A: Core community engagement standards	PART B: Standards supporting implementation
1. Participation	7. Informed design
2. Empowerment and ownership	8. Planning and preparation
3. Inclusion	9. Managing activities
4. Two-way communication	10. Monitoring, evaluation, and learning
5. Adaptability and localisation	
6. Building on local capacity	
PART C: Standards supporting coordination and integration	**PART D:** Standards supporting resource mobilisation
11. Government leadership	14. Human resources and organisational structures
12. Partner coordination	15. Data management
13. Integration	16. Resource mobilisation and budgeting

Table 33.1: Summary of Minimum Quality Standards and Indicators for Community Engagement *(adapted from Minimum Quality Standards and Indicators for Community Engagement by UNICEF, 2020)*

CHALLENGES OF DELIVERING RCCE

RCCE is challenging to implement (3). It is no simple matter to deliver responsive, empathetic, transparent, and consistent messaging in local languages through trusted channels of communication, using community-based networks and key influencers and the building capacity of local entities. Yet these efforts are essential to establish expertise and trust (12–13).

Communicating uncertainty and risk while addressing public concern can lead to a range of outcomes, some of which will be unexpected, including a loss of trust and reputation, economic impacts, and unfortunately, a loss of lives (26). Navigating cultural nuances, preventing the spread of mis- and disinformation amidst an "infodemic", and exploring different and correct modalities of communication are some of the known challenges (41) **(See Chapter 6, Integrated outbreak analytics; See Chapter 34, Infodemics)**.

Using the proposed checklist for components of effective RCCE: a Singapore case study on the COVID-19 outbreak

In 2020, early in the COVID-19 pandemic, the Singapore government implemented a strong, coordinated RCCE response for the general public. Locals could receive official and factual information on COVID-19 via a government phone application called Gov.sg. Epidemiological data,

Successful Risk Communication and Community Engagement

A proposed checklist for the components of effective RCCE
A consensus has emerged over the last decade or more on the components of effective RCCE, as presented in this checklist (22,25,39–40).

Early identification of partners
- Who are the existing stakeholders/partners and what are their roles?
- How are they actively engaging together?
- Has a social network analysis been carried out?
- What is the role of the community?

Programme implementation
- Are the frontline workers trained in RCCE and communication approaches? Are they aware of the policies and processes?
- Is there an understanding of the context and information needs of the target audience? Has a community needs assessment been conducted?
- Who are the community's trusted sources and channels of communication?
- Is the RCCE strategy inclusive of vulnerable communities?
- Are the messages developed together with the community with local solutions?
- Are the RCCE activities data-driven?
- Is information disseminated in a timely, frequent, and regular manner by trusted sources?
- Have community members received feedback or response in a timely manner? Has their feedback been taken into consideration for iterative adjustments to health messages?

Plans and strategies
- What plans, guidelines, and strategies are in place to support RCCE?
- Are there gaps identified with appropriate interventions suggested?
- How can these be implemented in a coordinated, synergistic manner involving various stakeholders?

Coordination structures
- Are there existing coordination structures at the national, provincial, and community levels?
- How does information flow between these structures?
- Is RCCE part of the incident management system (IMS)?

Reporting/documentation
- Are RCCE activities reported and documented at various levels?
- How regularly do partners meet or engage with each other for information sharing?

Figure 33.1: Components for effective RCCE

---

updates on policy measures, and clarifications and corrections of rumours and misinformation were disseminated promptly, widely, and accurately. Given the multiracial context of Singapore, information was made available in various languages, based on individual preferences (42).

What was implemented for Singapore's general population was not quite relevant to the migrant worker community living in dormitories. Language barriers were one issue. RCCE was initially overlooked. Here, we describe the evolution of the implementation of RCCE among migrant workers using the checklist developed, while sharing the real-life challenges and how these were overcome.

Early identification of partners

The failure of early identification of partners resulted in several health institutions scrambling to create health communication resources in different languages and duplicating those efforts. Once this gap was identified, an organic RCCE working group was developed, comprising stakeholders from the three different health system clusters and migrant worker non-profit organisations. The group met regularly (once to twice a week) over videoconference to discuss health communication needs, share on-ground insights and challenges, and synergise and align RCCE efforts.

Plans and strategies

Initially, no clear strategies to support RCCE were in place. However, very quickly, the fact that stakeholders were seeing similar gaps helped streamline these plans over the weekly RCCE working group meetings. These included the need for pictorial collaterals in different languages, as well as resources in different modalities such as printed brochures, posters, podcasts, and videos. Migrant worker social media influencers were soon identified as key stakeholders to join in the discussion of plans and strategies moving forward. The various stakeholders discussed the priorities of the various needs and delegated the tasks accordingly.

Programme implementation

The context and information needs of the target audience and their trusted sources and channels of communication were initially not well understood. However, identifying migrant worker leaders in dormitories, workspaces, and digital spaces and including them as part of the RCCE working group were helpful in understanding the needs of the migrant worker community. A rapid needs assessment was conducted via face-to-face surveys at dormitories with the assistance of migrant worker leaders. Subgroups of migrant worker communities of different nationalities and with different languages were formed over Whatsapp to identify information gaps, incorporate feedback, and co-develop messaging together. This enabled vulnerable communities such as minority groups within the worker community to be included as well.

Coordination structures

Coordination structures at national and community levels were initially unclear. However, as the RCCE working group matured and involved government sector stakeholders, the coordination structures at the national level became clearer, enabling information to flow more smoothly from the government to the community and vice versa. The RCCE working group then became a key component of the IMS, helping to alert the government of new developments on the ground via their newly set-up "Assurance, Care and Engagement (ACE)" team which focused on helping migrant workers.

Reporting/documentation

When the acute part of the outbreak was over, the RCCE activities were reported and documented, then shared with local and regional networks. Partners from the RCCE working group then met on a less frequent (fortnightly) basis to continue to strengthen preparedness and prevention efforts. The RCCE working group's efforts eventually evolved into a centralised, coordinated, nationwide strategy, improving trust and social cohesion among migrant workers.

The checklist gives RCCE practitioners a framework to systematically work through. The early identification of partners, co-development of plans and strategies, in-depth understanding of the community for programme implementation, a recognition and strengthening of coordination structures in place, and the documentation of RCCE activities can help strengthen the RCCE response of even the amateur RCCE practitioner.

There are known strategies to overcome the many challenges (8):
- establishing strong and cohesive RCCE partner coordination at global, regional, and country levels for a more effective response
- communicating easily understood science-based information and recommendations in a timely manner that addresses critical risks and counters misinformation
- accelerating priority research and innovation in social sciences to support the implementation of public health measures and to ensure the participation of at-risk and affected communities to ensure effectiveness and efficiency of the response and accountability for people
- enhancing country-level capacity to roll out effective and coordinated RCCE approaches through the identification of capacity needs, provision of simplified tools and resources, distance-based training and guidance, and rapid deployment of RCCE expertise

At a practical level, governments managing outbreaks can define a RCCE cell within an IMS. The challenge of establishing nimble community feedback mechanisms can be addressed through pre-identified, existing to sense community concerns. The Singapore government's ACE team delivered healthcare messaging, disease surveillance, and connected workers with COVID-19 or mental health symptoms to healthcare and social support resources.

Examples of leveraging existing networks to overcome the challenges of receiving community feedback and community mobilisation during the COVID-19 pandemic
- Local health authorities in northwest Syria adopted a decade-old polio vaccination mobilisation system of local volunteers.
- A medical network across Syria's border in Turkey helped raise COVID-19 awareness, referred patients, and trained health workers.
- Self-help groups of women in India were entrusted to run community kitchens for quarantined people.
- Local women's associations in Yemen (supported by international agencies) trained women in a rural district to produce masks and personal protective equipment.

HOW RCCE HAS EVOLVED AND IS EVOLVING

A pre-COVID-19 assessment of countries' preparedness and response abilities, as per the IHR, highlighted the low prioritisation for RCCE among WHO member countries. In particular, indicator 5.4, which represents "community engagement with the affected communities", had the second lowest average score of the five indicators relevant to RCCE (43). A review by the Independent Panel for Pandemic Preparedness and Response showed varying levels of RCCE efforts among 28 countries for the first year of the pandemic, revealing that with few exceptions, most communities lacked formal community engagement plans as part of their response efforts (44). However, over the course of the COVID-19 outbreak, governments started to prioritise RCCE efforts. While only about 36 per cent of countries reported having an RCCE plan in April 2020, that number increased to 90 per cent six months later (3,6).

Over the course of many more recent large-scale outbreaks and pandemics (e.g., H1N1, Ebola, Zika, and COVID-19), more concerted efforts have been made globally to better define, integrate, and resource RCCE initiatives into outbreak response and to adapt RCCE strategies to local contexts. The revised global RCCE strategy moves from directive unilateral communication, which characterised the early stages of the COVID-19 response, towards people-centred participatory approaches proven to promote trust and social cohesion, reducing the negative impacts of outbreaks (33). One approach for building better participatory systems is to start by assessing communities' knowledge, attitudes, and perceptions about COVID-19. Qualitative and quantitative methods, such as focus group discussions, key informant interviews, and surveys, could be used to obtain feedback and understand what audiences do not understand or their resource needs (8). Information collected helps in the creation and dissemination of knowledge and information. Recent studies show that community cooperation, transparency, and trust fostered can alleviate fear, vulnerability, and uncertainty, and promote adherence to protective measures (14,45). The importance of community engagement to ensure the bilateral exchange of information also came to the fore as an important focus (3).

> **Engaging communities for Ebola outbreak control in Guinea**
>
> The Ebola outbreak in West Africa between 2013 and 2016 showed that community engagement is important. When an outbreak occurred in Guinea's forested region in 2014, self-identified and assumed 'community leaders' (based on their job titles and organisations) were initially selected to help liaise between external response partners and the 'community'. However, international response teams faced resistance from local populations due to the long-running experiences of being stigmatised and oppressed by others during the colonial and post-colonial periods. WHO consultant anthropologist Julienne Anoko tried a different approach by speaking with people from the community to identify who they trusted. A new list of community leaders containing influencers such as traditional practitioners, village birth attendants, and religious leaders was subsequently generated. These community leaders were able to work together with response workers and lessen the resistance of the community (23).

Today, RCCE has moved beyond information conveyance to a practice of building knowledge, trust, and relationships (46). Calls to adopt a community resilience approach to outbreak response are becoming mainstream to ensure investment in community engagement before, during, and after an outbreak (3). Investments are needed to sustain community engagement efforts in building and maintaining trust. This is a continuous process and cannot only happen in times of crisis (6). Furthermore, the need for speed, accuracy, and effectiveness in RCCE implementation has never been greater in light of fresh challenges introduced by the COVID-19 pandemic for RCCE practitioners. Concrete approaches for how to do this quickly, accurately, and effectively include investing into capacity building of RCCE stakeholders, maintaining close ties during preparedness phases, and creating protocols and mechanisms that can be easy to follow during times of crises. These challenges call for expanding existing health communication principles to take into account the challenges of misinformation and the urgent need to improve the communication of risk and uncertainty amidst an increasingly diverse media environment which includes the instantaneous nature of social media (47).

In spite of its history of being overlooked in emergency responses, RCCE continues to gain prominence in pandemic preparedness. In June 2020, the Collective Service, a global partnership bringing together the strengths of the International Federation of Red Cross and Red Crescent Societies (IFRC), UNICEF, and WHO, was established to enhance community engagement efforts (https://www.rcce-collective.net/) (3). More than ever before, RCCE needs able, adaptable leadership to spearhead progress and target ever-changing communication strategies to adapt to different stages of an outbreak.

THE FUTURE OF RCCE

In the future, RCCE interventions which both boost media literacy and teach emotional scepticism will be increasingly important (47). The first refers to the ability to navigate media and better judge the quality of information encountered. The second is aimed at getting people to understand their cognitive biases and mistakes we tend to make in assimilating information (48).

Checklists for RCCE practices must be continually and nimbly adapted, updated, and shared. Efforts to train RCCE experts in public health must be furthered, and their partnerships with governments, media agencies, and advertising companies strengthened. Standardised RCCE concepts need to be integrated into all outbreak response pillars and practices, particularly when targeted at disadvantaged populations (46). Greater efforts to include marginalised groups to uphold privacy, equity, and human rights in a public health response can be made for better health outcomes (29).

In the wake of the COVID-19 response, RCCE should aim to increase trust through strategic communication, co-develop solutions with communities, and maintain RCCE capacity at emergency levels, even in the absence of an emergency (24).

RCCE should also build from the research gaps identified prior to the COVID-19 pandemic while building upon the great strides made during the pandemic response. Clear gaps in research were highlighted in the WHO's most recent global guidance on general practice. Additional research was needed in lower- and middle-income countries across a range of RCCE tenets such as trust, communicating uncertainty, and effective engagement with affected populations. Gaps in understanding of how RCCE could best weave into health emergency response systems were identified through governance and leadership, coordination and information systems, capacity building, and financing. Finally, further studies were needed to better support basic RCCE practices such as strategic communications planning, monitoring, and evaluation, the use of social media, and messaging (9).

Throughout the COVID-19 pandemic, great strides were made in response functions while old lessons learned were relearned. RCCE was a key pillar in global, regional, and national IMS, there was broader access and use of social and behavioural data, partners coordinated for more effective engagement with affected populations, the infodemics work highlighted digital social media mis- and disinformation, and other response pillars such as IPC, clinical care, and vaccine roll-out relied heavily on RCCE mechanisms for a more effective overall response. However, as in every response, we recognise the need to better include communities and affected populations in emergency prevention, preparedness, readiness, response, and recovery. This is now further recognised in the WHO Health Emergency Response architecture which places importance on community protection, indicating a future strengthening of community-level actions.

> **"Effective community protection hinges on the achievement of three objectives (49):**
> - Community engagement, risk communication, and infodemic management to guide priority actions and strengthen community resilience.
> - Population and environmental public health interventions.
> - Multisectoral action to respond to community concerns and ensure community welfare".

REFERENCES:

1. World Health Organization. COVID-19 strategic preparedness and response plan. Geneva; 2021.
2. Bedson J, Jalloh MF, Pedi D, Bah S, Owen K, Oniba A, et al. Community engagement in outbreak response: lessons from the 2014-2016 Ebola outbreak in Sierra Leone. BMJ Glob Health. 2020 Aug;5(8):e002145. https://doi.org/10.1136/bmjgh-2019-002145 PMID:32830128.
3. Abdalla SM, Koya SF, Jamieson M, Verma M, Haldane V, Jung AS, et al. Investing in trust and community resilience: lessons from the early months of the first digital pandemic. BMJ. 2021 Nov;375:e067487. https://doi.org/10.1136/bmj-2021-067487 PMID:34840130.
4. Duffy JG, Omwenga RM. Strategic communications can enhance brownfields public participation. 2002.
5. Glik DC. Risk communication for public health emergencies. Annu Rev Public Health. 2007;28(1):33–54. https://doi.org/10.1146/annurev.publhealth.28.021406.144123 PMID:17222081.
6. Collective Service. About us [cited 26 May 2024]. https://www.rcce-collective.net/about-us/.
7. UNICEF. Minimum quality standards and indicators for community engagement. 2020. https://www.unicef.org/mena/reports/community-engagement-standards.
8. IFRC. UNICEF, WHO. COVID-19 global response risk communication & community engagement (RCCE). Strategy; 2020.
9. World Health Organization. Communicating risk in public health emergencies: a WHO guideline for emergency risk communication (ERC) policy and practice. Geneva; 2017.
10. The Independent Panel for Pandemic Preparedness and Response. Centering communities in pandemic preparedness and response; 2021.
11. United Nations High Commissioner for Refugees. People at the centre: the intersection of age, gender and diversity. Age, Gender and Diversity Accountability Report; 2020.
12. United Nations High Commissioner for Refugees. Risk communication and community engagement (RCCE) – COVID-19; 2020.
13. World Health Organization. COVID-19 Strategic Preparedness and Response Plan: operational planning guidelines to support country preparedness and response; 2020.
14. Menon KU, Goh KT. Transparency and trust: risk communications and the Singapore experience in managing SARS. J Commun Manag (Lond). 2005;9(4):375–83. https://doi.org/10.1108/13632540510621614.
15. Adebisi YA, Rabe A, Lucero-Prisno Iii DE. Risk communication and community engagement strategies for COVID-19 in 13 African countries. Health Promot Perspect. 2021 May;11(2):137–47. https://doi.org/10.34172/hpp.2021.18 PMID:34195037.
16. World Health Organization. Risk communication and community engagement (RCCE) considerations: Ebola response in the Democratic Republic of the Congo. Geneva; 2018.
17. Pan American Health Organization. COVID-19 risk communication and community engagement (RCCE). Planning Template; 2020.
18. Madison AA, Way BM, Beauchaine TP, Kiecolt-Glaser JK. Risk assessment and heuristics: how cognitive shortcuts can fuel the spread of COVID-19. Brain Behav Immun. 2021 May;94:6–7. https://doi.org/10.1016/j.bbi.2021.02.023 PMID:33647433.
19. Sandman PM. Risk communication: facing public outrage. Manage Commun Q. 1988;2(2):235–8. https://doi.org/10.1177/0893318988002002006.
20. Fischhoff B. Risk perception and communication unplugged: twenty years of process. Risk Anal. 1995 Apr;15(2):137–45. https://doi.org/10.1111/j.1539-6924.1995.tb00308.x PMID:7597253.
21. Slovic P. Trust, emotion, sex, politics, and science: surveying the risk-assessment battlefield. Risk Anal. 1999 Aug;19(4):689–701. https://doi.org/10.1111/j.1539-6924.1999.tb00439.x PMID:10765431.

22. Gonah L. Key considerations for successful risk communication and community engagement (RCCE) programmes during COVID-19 pandemic and other public health emergencies. Ann Glob Health. 2020 Nov;86(1):146. https://doi.org/10.5334/aogh.3119 PMID:33262935.
23. Wilkinson A, Parker M, Martineau F, Leach M. Engaging 'communities': anthropological insights from the West African Ebola epidemic. Philos Trans R Soc Lond B Biol Sci. 2017 May;372(1721):372. https://doi.org/10.1098/rstb.2016.0305 PMID:28396476.
24. World Health Organization. WHO COVID-19 policy brief: building trust through risk communication and community engagement; 2022.
25. FAO. Guidance note: Risk communication and community engagement: Coronavirus disease 2019 (COVID-19) pandemic. Rome; 2020.
26. World Health Organization. Risk communication and community engagement (RCCE) readiness and response to the 2019 novel coronavirus (2019-nCoV): interim guidance; 2020.
27. World Health Organization Regional Office for Europe. Risk communication and community engagement: a compendium of case studies in times of COVID-19. Copenhagen: WHO Regional Office for Europe; 2022.
28. Sotgiu G, Dobler CC. Social stigma in the time of coronavirus disease 2019. Eur Respir J. 2020 Aug;56(2):2002461. https://doi.org/10.1183/13993003.02461-2020 PMID:32631833.
29. Haldane V, Jung AS, De Foo C, Bonk M, Jamieson M, Wu S, et al. Strengthening the basics: public health responses to prevent the next pandemic. BMJ. 2021 Nov;375:e067510. https://doi.org/10.1136/bmj-2021-067510 PMID:34840134.
30. John Hopkins University of Medicine Coronavirus Resource Center. COVID-19 Dashboard by the Center for Systems Science and Engineering (CSSE) at Johns Hopkins University (JHU) 2020 [16 July 2022]. https://coronavirus.jhu.edu/map.html.
31. Yi H, Ng ST, Farwin A, Pei Ting Low A, Chang CM, Lim J. Health equity considerations in COVID-19: geospatial network analysis of the COVID-19 outbreak in the migrant population in Singapore. J Travel Med. 2021 Feb;28(2):taaa159. https://doi.org/10.1093/jtm/taaa159 PMID:32894286.
32. Singapore Ministry of Health. Updates on COVID-19 local situation report 2020 [cited 16 July 2022]. https://www.moh.gov.sg/covid-19/past-updates.
33. World Health Organization. COVID-19 global risk communication and community engagement strategy; 2020.
34. Ihekweazu V, Ejibe U, Kaduru C, Disu Y, Oyebanji O, Oguanuo E, et al. Implementing an emergency risk communication campaign in response to the COVID-19 pandemic in Nigeria: lessons learned. BMJ Glob Health. 2022 Jun;7(6):e008846. https://doi.org/10.1136/bmjgh-2022-008846 PMID:35675971.
35. World Health Organization. Joint external evaluation tool: Internal Health Regulations (2005). Geneva; 2022.
36. Phua RI. FOCUS: The long, challenging journey to bring COVID-19 under control in migrant worker dormitories. Channel News Asia. 2020. Accessed but no longer available from: https://www.channelnewsasia.com/news/singapore/in-focus-covid19-singapore-migrant-worker-dormitories-lockdown-13081210 in October 2021.
37. Masumbuko Claude K, Underschultz J, Hawkes MT. Social resistance drives persistent transmission of Ebola virus disease in Eastern Democratic Republic of Congo: a mixed-methods study. PLoS One. 2019 Sep;14(9):e0223104. https://doi.org/10.1371/journal.pone.0223104 PMID:31557243.
38. Dick L, Moodie J, Greiner AL. Are we ready? Operationalising risk communication and community engagement programming for public health emergencies. BMJ Glob Health. 2022 Mar;7(3):e008486. https://doi.org/10.1136/bmjgh-2022-008486 PMID:35318265.
39. Zhang Y, Tambo E, Djuikoue IC, Tazemda GK, Fotsing MF, Zhou XN. Early stage risk communication and community engagement (RCCE) strategies and measures against the coronavirus disease 2019 (COVID-19) pandemic crisis. Glob Health J. 2021 Mar;5(1):44–50. https://doi.org/10.1186/s12992-021-00694-4 PMID:33850632.
40. International Rescue Committee. Risk communications & community engagement 2021 [cited 2 August 2023]. https://rcce.rescue.org/.
41. World Health Organization. Managing the COVID-19 infodemic: promoting healthy behaviours and mitigating the harm from misinformation and disinformation - Joint statement by WHO, UN, UNICEF, UNDP, UNESCO, UNAIDS, ITU, UN Global Pulse, and IFRC 2020 [cited 29 July 2022].

42. Gov.sg. Gov.sg on WhatsApp: how to sign up [6 November 2022]. https://www.gov.sg/article/govsg-on-whatsapp.
43. International Federation of Red Cross and Red Crescent Societies. From words to action: towards a community-centred approach to preparedness and response in health emergencies; 2019.
44. Haldane V, De Foo C, Abdalla SM, Jung AS, Tan M, Wu S, et al. Health systems resilience in managing the COVID-19 pandemic: lessons from 28 countries. Nat Med. 2021 Jun;27(6):964–80. https://doi.org/10.1038/s41591-021-01381-y PMID:34002090.
45. Blair RA, Morse BS, Tsai LL. Public health and public trust: survey evidence from the Ebola Virus Disease epidemic in Liberia. Soc Sci Med. 2017 Jan;172:89–97. https://doi.org/10.1016/j.socscimed.2016.11.016 PMID:27914936.
46. Dickmann P, Abraham T, Sarkar S, Wysocki P, Cecconi S, Apfel F, et al. Risk communication as a core public health competence in infectious disease management: development of the ECDC training curriculum and programme. Euro Surveill. 2016;21(14). https://doi.org/10.2807/1560-7917.ES.2016.21.14.30188 PMID:27103616.
47. Ratzan SC, Sommariva S, Rauh L. Enhancing global health communication during a crisis: lessons from the COVID-19 pandemic. Public Health Res Pract. 2020 Jun;30(2):3022010. https://doi.org/10.17061/phrp3022010 PMID:32601655.
48. Wardle C. Fake news. It's complicated. First Draft 2017 [cited 23 Jan 2023]. https://firstdraftnews.org/articles/fake-news-complicated/.
49. World Health Organization. Strengthening health emergency prevention, preparedness, response and resilience. Geneva; 2023.

*Special thanks to Angela Omondi and Cynthia Wamwayi.

CHAPTER 34

INFODEMICS AND INFORMATION MANAGEMENT

by Sarah Hess, Sylvie Briand, Tim Nguyen, Elisabeth Wilhelm, and Tina D. Purnat

> *"An infodemic is an overabundance of information, accurate or not, in the digital and physical space, accompanying an acute health event such as an outbreak or epidemic"* (1).

INTRODUCTION

Each epidemic and pandemic is accompanied by an infodemic. An infodemic refers to an overabundance of information that includes accurate information, mis- and disinformation, and the dynamic contexts within which this information is generated, sought out, and shared during an epidemic.

Infodemics are not a new phenomenon and have been witnessed during previous disease outbreaks including Zika, Ebola (2), polio, and measles (3). For example, during the yellow fever epidemic in Angola in 2016, there were rumours that one could not drink alcohol following vaccination or that the vaccine might result in infertility. This negatively impacted vaccine coverage, especially among young men (4). By working with traditional leaders to listen to people's concerns and provide reliable information about the vaccine, gradually these false beliefs were changed.

The COVID-19 pandemic, however, presents an unrivalled example of an infodemic. There was an exponential increase in the generation of scientific evidence and information that was distributed widely in both preprint and publication versions, making the quality of information more difficult to assess. In addition, numerous experts and scientists aired their views and opinions regarding science and public health guidance, stimulating a polarised discourse around many pertinent subjects, both off- and online. This was accompanied by an increase in media coverage, with highly sensationalised and potentially manipulative content. Credible health information was 'lost in the noise', and in many settings, the questions and concerns of individuals and communities went unaddressed, creating further space for rumours and myths.

THE NEW INFORMATION ECOSYSTEM

Each individual experience of an infodemic is different as it is influenced by the information ecosystem within which a person lives—the information ecosystem refers to the complex dynamic infrastructure, sources, and relationships through which information flows and reaches an individual (5). This includes both the digital and physical information environments, and a number of structural and behavioural factors such as an individual's access to and interactions with the health system, their health behaviours, information-seeking behaviours, and barriers that can affect access to information. All of these factors shape an information ecosystem.

When there is an epidemic, it is natural that with an increase in uncertainty and fear, people seek information differently by searching for different sources, talking to others about the disease and its impact, and listening to opinions and thoughts from peers, experts, and community leaders (6). People also tend to generate and share information more. The change in information-seeking behaviour that is experienced at the individual level is reflected in changes in the overall information ecosystem. New sources of health information emerge and existing sources transform. Many outlets may disseminate accurate information, misinformation, disinformation, and outdated information simultaneously. This makes it difficult for a person to identify trustworthy sources, absorb and process the information, and make informed decisions to protect their health. Furthermore, during an epidemic, an individual's perception of risk may be altered, which further impacts their acceptance of and response to health information (7–10). Responses to an infodemic often focus on reducing mis- and disinformation. However, a more effective approach is to take into consideration the entire information ecosystem, including how it evolves during times of crisis, and develop a comprehensive strategy to manage the infodemic.

The individual experience of an infodemic

The following are common to most experiences during a health-related infodemic:

A person has challenges accessing credible, accurate health information.

Access to information is not just influenced by exposure to information but also by a person's digital literacy, digital connectivity, language, certain disabilities, and certain structural barriers. Previous experience in the health system, trust in authorities, and the opinions and actions of their family, friends, or community leaders also play a role.

A person has challenges discerning low-quality from higher quality health information.

This is also linked to different literacies (digital, health, media, and information literacy), all of which impact an individual's ability to navigate the large volume of information within the information ecosystem and differentiate between different types of health information.

A person does not always know what health information is relevant to their situation.

The science and guidance evolve during an epidemic. If guidance is not updated regularly, tailored to different situations, and communicated clearly, individuals and communities may be confused and begin to mistrust the science or authorities.

Individual and community information-seeking and health-seeking needs change constantly.

Epidemics are dynamic, and information and science evolve rapidly—therefore, the questions, concerns, narratives, information voids, and circulating mis- and disinformation change too.

A person has challenges to make health decisions for themselves and their families with the information available to them.

There are many factors that influence a person's access to information and their subsequent actions based on that information.

Science and evidence-generation during epidemics

During epidemics, the volume and speed with which scientific evidence is generated, analysed, published, and shared increases exponentially. During the first six months of the COVID-19 pandemic, more than 20,000 articles related to COVID-19 were published (11). Many publications were of suboptimal quality and lacked scientific rigour, leading to misinterpretation of results, confusion, and diminishing trust in science. While the rapid and transparent sharing of scientific information on open access platforms is positive, the speed of publication must not happen at the expense of rigour (for example, peer review and editorial validation). In addition, efforts must be made to bridge the gap between the scientific community and the public's understanding of how scientific evidence is generated and why it might change. For example, an article published in a reputable journal on the use of hydroxychloroquine as a treatment for COVID-19 (12) was retracted and rumours ensued, stating that scientific information was being manipulated by health authorities.

Furthermore, even when high-quality scientific work is published, intentional efforts are needed to translate the science into different contexts and cultures in order to make it relevant and actionable. This can be supported by interventions to build scientific literacy before and during the crisis, as this will enable an understanding of the iterative process of evidence generation, interpretation, and evaluation, which, in turn, helps to build trust in science and resilience to misinformation (13). Scientific literacy usually starts with a well-functioning education system where critical thinking skills are built from an early age. However, during an epidemic or pandemic, efforts to build scientific literacy can include working with science and health journalists or identified social media influencers who can support ongoing science translation efforts, or providing communication training to scientists and other health professionals who are exposed to the public. Scientific literacy is one of many literacies (health, digital, media, and information) that influences the individual's ability to process, understand, and act on information.

IMPACT OF AN INFODEMIC

An infodemic can cause direct harm to public health. For example, early in the COVID-19 pandemic, misinformation stated that methanol was a treatment, resulting in a large number of deaths in Iran (14).

It can also negatively impact the public health response to the epidemic by undermining trust in interventions (e.g., vaccination, wearing masks) and increasing mistrust in health authorities, the government, or the scientific community. Ultimately, the polarisation and politicisation of public health information and action can undermine social cohesiveness, the repercussions of which can be long lasting.

It is possible to avoid these harms if certain elements of an infodemic are understood so that the situations within which they occur can be addressed. **Figure 34.1** details the different elements of an infodemic, which increase in the potential to cause harm (from left to right).

Situations where misinformation, disinformation, and narratives are circulating are situations with the most potential to cause harm. Most people who share misinformation are not aware that it is misinformation; however, misinformation is often packaged in emotionally compelling ways and in formats that are easy to share. Disinformation is often motivated by economic or political profit and is reshared by people who either believe it or identify with a particular cause. Addressing disinformation requires a more comprehensive approach that may go beyond the health system or legal or consumer protection interventions. As more people become concerned about a specific topic, the discussion that is generated can become a narrative which can be characterised by an organised set of mutually reinforcing information elements. Narratives are trending topics discussed offline, online, and in the media, and while they may grow from information voids, and mis- and disinformation, they can also be influenced by social, political, and economic factors.

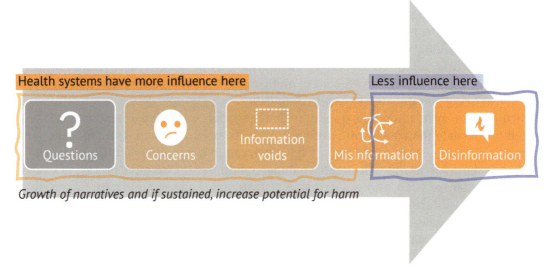

Figure 34.1: Different elements of an infodemic
(adapted from Purnat TD, Nguyen T, Briand S, editors. Managing infodemics in the 21st century: addressing new public health challenges in the information ecosystem [Internet]. Cham: Springer International Publishing; 2023 [cited 2023 Oct 15]. https://link.springer.com/10.1007/978-3-031-27789-4)

INFODEMIC MANAGEMENT – THE FOUR ESSENTIAL COMPONENTS

Pandemics and epidemics are evolving situations characterised by high levels of uncertainty and variable levels of societal and individual-level disruption, from the disease itself, or from the interventions put in place to stop transmission. During epidemics, people are asked to rapidly change behaviours for a limited time period to protect their individual health and that of their community. If there is limited trust in the authorities or in the scientific communication, individuals and communities may not be inclined to change behaviours and practices. Infodemic management recognises that trust is a valuable social capital that must be nurtured. However, trust is complex; it can take a long time to build but can be destroyed very quickly. Successful infodemic management requires multi-stakeholder engagement (15) and a comprehensive understanding of infodemics, the overall information ecosystem, and its interdependency with epidemics (16–17). It also requires that important aspects of trust are considered equally. An enhanced approach to managing an infodemic is based on three important shifts:
- It takes into consideration the entire information ecosystem of individuals and communities.

- It always starts with listening to individual and community concerns (rather than an approach that involves top-down dissemination of messages from "experts" to passive recipients).
- It focuses on the meaningful engagement of communities to co-develop guidance and solutions to mitigate the impact of an epidemic (**See Chapter 33, RCCE**).

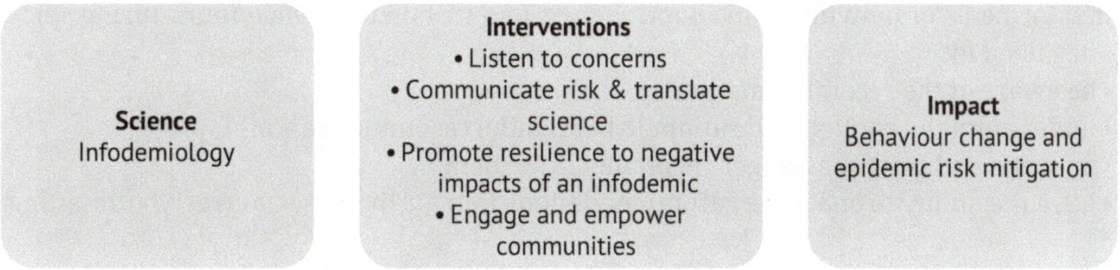

Science
Infodemiology

Interventions
- Listen to concerns
- Communicate risk & translate science
- Promote resilience to negative impacts of an infodemic
- Engage and empower communities

Impact
Behaviour change and epidemic risk mitigation

Figure 34.2: Infodemic management—from science to interventions—achieving impactful behaviour change and epidemic risk mitigation
(adapted from "WHO competency framework: building a response workforce to manage infodemics". https://www.who.int/publications-detail-redirect/9789240035287)

Listen to concerns

Listening increases understanding of the concerns of communities, the contexts within which they live, and their experience and knowledge related to the outbreak or epidemic. Listening is the first step towards formulating interventions, guidance, and communication in a way that is more relevant, implementable, and acceptable to communities. In the current information ecosystem, much listening can occur on social media platforms, and incorporating sentiment analysis to social digital listening at scale (18) can generate useful insights. Sentiment is emotion portrayed in social media or media content, which can be an indicator of popular feeling towards a health topic or issue. Sentiment analysis can contribute to the production of infodemic insights and recommendations. Other offline or interpersonal platforms for listening can be built into physical spaces such as workplaces, health or community centres, places of worship, or schools. For social listening to be useful and effective, however, it needs to happen in real time and must also be grounded in an analytical framework (19) that makes it possible to rapidly operationalise the knowledge that is generated. In general, during epidemics, questions can be grouped into four categories:
- the disease (its symptoms, the sequelae)
- the cause and aetiology of the disease (e.g., the virus) and explanation of the disease (why me, why us?)
- treatments
- epidemic response interventions (personal protective equipment, vaccines, masks etc.)

Grouping questions into a limited number of categories facilitates social listening and faster reactive risk communication. Health authorities can simultaneously prepare communications that are tailored and encompassing.

Communicate risk and translate science

Risk communication is a core capacity within the monitoring and evaluation framework of the International Health Regulations (20) (**See Chapter 33, RCCE**). Regular, transparent communication that acknowledges uncertainty is essential to reassure communities and keep them informed. For individuals to adopt, change, and sustain new behaviours during epidemics, they need to:
- be aware of the recommendations
- understand the context and rationale behind the recommendations
- trust the authority/messenger recommending them
- have the ability to enact the recommendations in their living/social/work/faith setting

Science translation is challenging in epidemics where scientific understanding evolves quickly and is generated rapidly, often leading to changes in guidance. Health workers, in addition to the vital services they deliver, can play a critical role in translating science, allaying fears, and understanding individual and community information needs during epidemics (21–23).

Promote resilience to negative impacts of the infodemic

To build resilience to misinformation at an individual level, it is crucial to:
- strengthen an individual's ability to distinguish between accurate and inaccurate information
- recognise media manipulation
- successfully debunk misinformation with friends and family

Building resilience to misinformation takes time and requires investment during preparedness, prior to an outbreak. During an epidemic, people tend to seek information actively, thereby increasing their exposure to all types of information. In addition, fear and uncertainty may impair a person's ability to analyse information objectively. Strengthening health and digital literacy is an important and often undervalued component of infodemic management that can enhance resilience to misinformation. At a community level, resilience to mis- and disinformation requires structural approaches. A resilient community has both access and the ability to disseminate credible, accurate information that is tailored and acceptable to the population. A resilient community also has a localised ability to fact check claims, has access to trusted messengers who have been trained in effective infodemic management principles, and has a feedback loop with the health system to share rumours, questions, and concerns, and elicit rapid responses.

Engage and empower communities

Active engagement of communities is essential to epidemic response. In the current information ecosystem, the concept of communities is evolving. In localised epidemics, geographical communities are an important focus. However, in the current hyperconnected world, each individual belongs to multiple communities, including:

- traditional communities (neighbours, friends, family)
- virtual communities (social media platforms and networks)
- communities defined by similar vocations or interests (faith, sport, workplace)

These different communities may be represented by leaders who are often a trusted voice; by engaging trusted voices within communities to both feedback on concerns and needs and help deliver recommendations, it is possible to make recommendations more acceptable and accessible to local communities. Community engagement in the 21st century must account for this new network structure. Without the knowledge, expertise, and experience of these networks feeding into the 'operationalisation' of scientific knowledge and technical guidance, there is a risk that it remains too technical or its implementation is not feasible. It is also important to ensure that certain groups such as migrants, minority language communities, and hard-to-reach populations are identified and supported through intentional and respectful efforts to facilitate listening, increase access to credible health information, and build resilience to misinformation. Often, peer-to-peer approaches (24) are effective in these situations. For example, engaging religious leaders from within local communities to feedback on community concerns and co-develop public health messaging that resonates with their constituents, or increasing the capacities and resources of healthcare providers and community health workers to engage, converse with, and feedback on behalf of patients.

Partnerships between national governments, religious leaders, and faith-based organisations to provide accurate, culturally-sensitive information, and counter vaccine hesitancy during the COVID-19 pandemic

There were many examples during the COVID-19 pandemic where religious leaders and faith-based organisations worked alongside national authorities to provide tailored, accurate information to communities (25). In Zimbabwe, a National Miscommunication and Community Engagement Committee was established with faith-based organisations as close collaborators. The group co-developed strategies and educational materials to address the false information that was circulating. One member of the Committee was the Apostolic Women Empowerment Trust or AWET. AWET worked with village heads and religious leaders to raise awareness of COVID-19 in Muslim, Christian, Apostolic, and African religious communities, and trained 3,744 behaviour change facilitators, 715 counsellors, 1,570 traditional faith leaders, and 850 faith leaders in countering COVID-19 misinformation. Religious leaders and faith-based organisations are embedded within communities and trusted and relied upon during crises, and are therefore key partners in increasing access to accurate information and countering misinformation during epidemics and pandemics.

INFODEMIOLOGY – AN EMERGING SCIENTIFIC DISCIPLINE

Infodemiology is an emerging scientific discipline underpinning infodemic management, drawing on concepts from data science, epidemiology, physics, chemistry, anthropology, behavioural sciences, sociology, psychology, philosophy, political science, and communica-

tion (26). Infodemiology produces the evidence necessary to improve infodemic management by deepening the knowledge base regarding the nature of infodemics. For instance, infodemiology will answer the following critical questions:
- How can exposure to information be measured?
- How does an individual's information diet influence behaviours?
- How can the effectiveness of infodemic management strategies, interventions, and policies be evaluated and their impact be measured?
- What are the diverse impacts of the potentially harmful situations within an infodemic?
- What makes some individuals and communities more resilient to misinformation than others?

The global research agenda for infodemiology is rapidly building the evidence base needed to guide future interventions on infodemic management. However, there is still much to learn about dynamic information ecosystems, how individuals and communities communicate during acute health events, and subsequent behaviours.

CONCLUSION

Infodemic management should be considered an intervention of equal importance to other epidemic response interventions such as the development of medical countermeasures.

As the world recovers from the COVID-19 pandemic, there is a growing acknowledgement of the importance of preparedness for the next pandemic. Infodemic management preparedness must be a critical component of broader pandemic preparedness efforts. Infodemic preparedness needs to be established at global, regional, national, and subnational levels. It requires strategic action plans that include relevant stakeholders, the establishment of surveillance and monitoring systems, and the creation of interventions for various scenarios that could arise in future crises. In this sense, infodemic management is similar to all aspects of outbreak response in that effective management requires comprehensive preparedness.

REFERENCES:

1. World Health Organization. Infodemic. https://www.who.int/health-topics/infodemic#tab=tab_1.
2. World Health Organization. (2019) Ebola - Democratic Republic of the Congo. https://www.who.int/emergencies/disease-outbreak-news/item/23-may-2019-ebola-drc-en.
3. Datta SS, O'Connor PM, Jankovic D, Muscat M, Ben Mamou MC, Singh S, et al. Progress and challenges in measles and rubella elimination in the WHO European Region. Vaccine. 2018 Aug;36(36):5408–15. https://doi.org/10.1016/j.vaccine.2017.06.042 PMID:28651838.
4. In Angola, keeping yellow fever cases at zero. https://www.unicef.org/stories/angola-keeping-yellow-fever-cases-zero.
5. Wardle C, Derakhshan H (2017). Information disorder: toward an interdisciplinary framework for research and policy making. https://rm.coe.int/information-disorder-report-version-august-2018/16808c9c77.
6. Seeger MW, Reynolds B, Sellnow TL (2020). Crisis and emergency risk communication in health contexts: applying the CDC model to pandemic influenza. In: Heath RL, O'Hair HD (eds) Handbook of Risk and Crisis Communication. Routledge, pp. 493–506. https://doi.org/10.4324/9781003070726.
7. Bhuiya T, Klares Iii R, Conte MA, Cervia JS. Predictors of misperceptions, risk perceptions, and personal risk perceptions about COVID-19 by country, education and income. J Investig Med. 2021 Dec;69(8):1473–8. https://doi.org/10.1136/jim-2021-001835 PMID:34380630.
8. Erchick DJ, Zapf AJ, Baral P, Edwards J, Mehta SH, Solomon SS, et al. COVID-19 risk perceptions of social interaction and essential activities and inequity in the USA: results from a nationally representative survey. BMJ Open. 2022 Feb;12(2):e051882. https://doi.org/10.1136/bmjopen-2021-051882 PMID:35131820.

9. Patterson NJ, Paz-Soldan VA, Oberhelman R, Moses L, Madkour A, Miles TT. Exploring perceived risk for COVID-19 and its role in protective behavior and COVID-19 vaccine hesitancy: a qualitative study after the first wave. BMC Public Health. 2022 Mar;22(1):503. https://doi.org/10.1186/s12889-022-12900-y PMID:35292002.

10. Priesemann V, Balling R, Bauer S, Beutels P, Valdez AC, Cuschieri S, et al. Towards a European strategy to address the COVID-19 pandemic. Lancet. 2021 Sep;398(10303):838–9. https://doi.org/10.1016/S0140-6736(21)01808-0 PMID:34384539.

11. Teixeira da Silva JA, Tsigaris P, Erfanmanesh M. Publishing volumes in major databases related to Covid-19. Scientometrics. 2021;126(1):831–42. https://doi.org/10.1007/s11192-020-03675-3 PMID:32904414.

12. Mehra MR, Desaii SS, Ruschitzka F, Patel AN (2020). RETRACTED: Hydroxychloroquine or chloroquine with or without a macrolide for treatment of COVID-19: a multinational registry analysis. The Lancet (Retraction published 2020). https://doi.org/10.1016/S0140-6736(20)31180-6.

13. World Health Organization. An ad hoc WHO technical consultation managing the COVID-19 infodemic: call for action. https://www.who.int/publications/i/item/9789240010314.

14. Sefidbakht S, Lotfi M, Jalli R, Moghadami M, Sabetian G, Iranpour P. Methanol toxicity outbreak: when fear of COVID-19 goes viral. Emerg Med J. 2020 Jul;37(7):416. https://emj.bmj.com/content/37/7/416#ref-5 https://doi.org/10.1136/emermed-2020-209886 PMID:32414710.

15. World Health Organization. (2021d). WHO public health research agenda for managing infodemics. https://www.who.int/publications/i/item/9789240019508.

16. Rubinelli S, Purnat TD, Wilhelm E, Traicoff D, Namageyo-Funa A, Thomson A, et al. WHO competency framework for health authorities and institutions to manage infodemics: its development and features. Hum Resour Health. 2022 May;20(1):35. https://doi.org/10.1186/s12960-022-00733-0 PMID:35525924.

17. World Health Organization. (2020b). Call for action: managing the infodemic. https://www.who.int/news/item/11-12-2020-call-for-action-managing-the-infodemic.

18. WHO-EARS EARS - Early AI-supported response with social listening. https://www.who-ea.

19. World Health Organization. Organisation mondiale de la Santé (2022). Delivering actionable infodemic insights and recommendations for the COVID-19 pandemic response –Fournir des données d'observation de l'infodémie et des recommandations exploitables pour la riposte à la pandémie de COVID-19. Weekly Epidemiological Record = Relevé épidémiologique hebdomadaire, 97(27):313-324. https://apps.who.int/iris/handle/10665/359145.

20. World Health Organization. (2005). International Health Regulations (3rd ed). https://www.who.int/publications/i/item/9789241580496.

21. OpenWHO. Infodemic management 101. https://openwho.org/courses/infodemic-management-101.

22. World Health Organization. (2022a). Call for applicants for comprehensive training for promotion of vaccine demand to maintain and restore routine immunization and promote COVID-19 vaccination. https://www.who.int/news-room/articles-detail/call-for-applicants-for-comprehensive-training-for-promotion-of-vaccine-demand-to-maintain-and-restore-routine-immunization-and-promote-COVID-19-vaccination.

23. World Health Organization. (2022b). Fifth Virtual WHO Infodemic Management Conference, 2, 4, 9 and 11 November 2021: meeting report: steps towards measuring the burden of infodemics. https://apps.who.int/iris/handle/10665/353410.

24. Finding the signal through the noise. A landscape review and framework to enhance the effective use of digital social listening for immunisation demand generation. https://www.gavi.org/sites/default/files/2021-06/Finding-the-Signal-Through-the-Noise.pdf.

25. Report of the WHO and Religions for Peace global conference: strengthening national responses to health emergencies, October–December 2021 [Internet]. [cited 2023 Oct 15]. https://www.who.int/publications-detail-redirect/9789240054035.

26. World Health Organization. (2020a). 1st Infodemiology Conference. https://www.who.int/teams/epi-win/infodemic-management/1st-who-infodemiology-conference.

CHAPTER 35

WORKING WITH COMMUNITIES AND VOLUNTEERS

by Sylvia Phua and Gwendolen Eamer

Outbreaks start in communities and are controlled by communities. Affected communities, volunteers, and local health and social workers are central to the rapid and effective resolution of the health emergency. Early and sustained implementation of public health measures is not possible without the full participation and engagement of communities and volunteers. This chapter highlights the importance of the role of community-based organisations and volunteers in outbreak response and covers key issues such as how to maximise the capacities and skills of affected communities, the different ways to harness community skills and resources, and adaptations that might be required to manage differences in and between different community groups.

INTRODUCTION

Infectious disease epidemics can cause major public health crises. Government officials and public health experts have the responsibility to formulate and implement plans to tackle such epidemics. This involves coming up with a public health plan comprising feasible disease control actions. Often, these plans are solely focused on health system capacities and disregard the important role of affected communities, volunteers, and local health and social workers. This may doom them to failure. It is critical that epidemic response plans are developed together with the communities affected by the epidemic. Experience has proven that the effective management of epidemics requires the active participation of those who are affected, including adaptation for the specific capacities, vulnerabilities, and cultural and social needs of the affected majority and minority populations (1). The affected communities themselves—including volunteers, local workers, community-based organisations, local leaders, and community representatives—are key stakeholders in the management of an epidemic. They are not only crucial to ensure the "acceptance" of epidemic control measures, but also provide crucial resources to achieve the disease control objectives.

ADAPTING STANDARD GUIDANCE TO LOCAL CONTEXTS

The global COVID-19 pandemic has wrought destruction in people's lives and livelihoods and had devastating and far-reaching consequences for health and social systems as well as the economy. Lessons learned from COVID-19 and other epidemic responses point to the need to develop a comprehensive approach to epidemic response at all levels, including the community. Key elements of a successful public health response include the early engagement of all stakeholders starting with the affected community, clear and accountable epidemic response governance, and adequate resourcing.

Standard international guidance for epidemic response is, by definition, generic. It cannot account for the myriad of local circumstances, sensitivities, capacities, and resources present in each community. Therefore, plans need to be adapted early in the process of a specific response so that they reflect the reality of the communities affected by the epidemic. The impact of epidemic control guidelines and plans is severely degraded when they are not translated into actions and approaches that are relevant and acceptable to, and achievable by, the affected communities. At worst, the lack of involvement of communities may jeopardise the effectiveness of such plans and worsen the epidemic. Failure to appropriately adapt to and build on the capacities of the affected communities causes detrimental yet preventable consequences, while failing to make use of valuable resources and capacities that can help control transmission. In order to break the chain of infection transmission as early as possible, public health responders must identify and roll out infection control measures with the consultation and leadership of affected communities (2).

In addition to meaningfully consulting the affected communities to design epidemic response approaches, the responding authorities must also engage them in identifying, preventing, and mitigating the negative consequences of epidemic control measures. Failure to properly anticipate and mitigate these impacts can have significant negative consequences for short- and long-term health and social issues in the community, well beyond the epidemic. These negative impacts, and the heavy socioeconomic burden that epidemic control measures may impose in communities, may eventually become unbearable and can cause the response plan to fail. Uncertainty and a lack of information about epidemic control measures, their predicted impacts and social costs, and what is being done to mitigate those negative impacts can generate anger and distrust in the community. The relevant community stakeholders must be empowered to act locally to meaningfully adapt epidemic control measures to meet local realities.

Without exception, epidemic control measures rely heavily on a community's understanding, cooperation, and active participation. Epidemic response often imposes on communities some sacrifices and losses for the common good (i.e., controlling the epidemic). Community understanding and involvement in decision-making should be pre-empted and well emphasised. Stakeholders should build response planning around the systematic and meaningful involvement of affected communities to ensure a common understanding that all are tackling this epidemic together. Divisions in and between communities are important to understand and anticipate, and discussions of such issues need to come into building this common understanding. Communities that are not geographically bound, or do not have clear governing bodies, may be neglected by higher authorities, while communities of belonging—for example, those based on identity or values, rather than geography—are sometimes harder to define, and are often missed when identifying stakeholders in epidemic response. As such, involving all affected communities early and effectively is crucial for the management of epidemics.

In addition, epidemic responders must not only involve community stakeholders, but also support or build on local systems that allow for the early mobilisation of local resources for better epidemic control. Early mobilisation involves not only systematically identifying local resources (e.g., human, social, logistical), but also planning for the procurement and distribution of needed resources to support those local capacities to carry out both their regular activities and their epidemic response activities safely. Volunteer- and community-based organisations are frequently forgotten in procurement planning, placing those critical frontline workers at heightened risk or undermining the effectiveness of their activities.

UNDERSTANDING COMMUNITY PRIORITIES AND BARRIERS

A public health response to an epidemic involves a delicate process of identifying cases and implementing control measures, while co-developing these measures with the affected public. Community engagement must go far beyond sharing information about the epidemic disease, and rather focus on identifying local vulnerabilities and capacities, co-designing responses and mitigation measures with the affected people, and empowering local actors to act meaningfully. Participatory approaches to epidemic response planning can help identify both local capacities that can be harnessed to respond to a developing health emergency, as well as barriers to the implementation of planned control measures.

Truly participatory planning requires the humility and flexibility of the responding authorities to acknowledge the affected community's own agency and knowledge of its needs and capacities. In addition to co-designing any epidemic-control programming, communities also need to be continually consulted as their needs and barriers will continue to evolve throughout the response. Participatory planning is therefore not a one-time kick-off event, but rather an ongoing process wherein the affected population can meaningfully contribute to the overall strategic direction of the response itself.

Building trust

A lack of trust in the authorities, and health services in particular, is a key driver of epidemics and a major obstacle to their control. Multiple studies suggest that trust—both interpersonal (i.e., social cohesion) and in government (i.e., public trust)—was one of the best predictors of a country's success or failure in managing the COVID-19 pandemic. Higher levels of trust were associated with lower infection rates and a higher uptake of vaccines where they were available (3). While trust is multifaceted, one determinant is that many populations see governments as discredited due to the perception of having largely failed to tackle ongoing issues such as the climate crisis or high levels of economic inequality (4). Compounding this, marginalised communities frequently have the least trust in authorities, often seeing them as placing demands on their communities rather than providing them with needed and appropriate services (5). This marginalisation and distrust intersect, creating conditions in which marginalised communities often face higher exposure to epidemics while having the least resources or trust in the authorities to appropriately respond (6).

People tend to trust neighbours and members of their own communities with shared backgrounds and lived experiences. Many challenges can be addressed by empowering and equipping local actors to respond within their own communities. However, many communities and local actors lack the support, funding, and training needed to handle an epidemic, nor do they know with whom to coordinate (6). Responding authorities should proactively engage local actors and plan to support them throughout the course of the epidemic, including through training, equipment, and support for coordination.

Public health workers may not be burdened with the responsibility to increase trust in national and local authorities or social cohesion. However, a thorough understanding of how a lack of trust may affect epidemic response plans is necessary to anticipate the potential pitfalls of these plans and co-develop strategies and community-based activities to counteract them.

Responding to epidemics while ensuring continuity of services (synergies)

During the acute phase of epidemic response, a large part of the health system is redirected to treating cases and controlling the epidemic. While intended to reduce epidemic-related morbidity and mortality, this can have a pernicious and widespread impact on access to health and social services far beyond access to treatment for the epidemic illness (7–10) (**See Chapter 23, Essential services**). Epidemics can reduce access to and the availability of all types of local health services. During the acute phases of the COVID-19 pandemic, in many communities, particularly those that did not have an on-site health centre, people who became ill from COVID-19 or other diseases had no one to turn to. In other settings, the local health services became overwhelmed by the huge demand for COVID-19 assistance. Many health services temporarily interrupted other critical services such as elective surgery, maternal and newborn infant care, routine vaccination, and the management of chronic illnesses (11).

The horizontal integration of community-based actors and volunteers into health service planning and delivery should extend beyond the epidemic disease in question in order to more broadly address questions of access to, and quality and availability of, essential health services. This includes facilitating the affected communities' ability to prioritise health interventions. Responding authorities should consider bundling epidemic response activities with other essential health services to ensure that access to basic services is maintained, communities do not experience a real or perceived mismatch between their principal health concerns and needs, and the authorities' focus on the epidemic disease in question. They should also develop and implement specific plans to ensure the continuity of key preventative and lifesaving services at the community level such as obstetric care, immunisation, and emergency services, among others.

While working to address secondary health system impacts of epidemics and efforts to respond to them, emergency authorities and community leaders should also address the social and economic impacts of both the epidemic and measures intended to control it. This should include targeted interventions to ensure that the affected community's most vulnerable people do not suffer unintended consequences of public health and social measures that may cut them off from essential services, their livelihoods, or their ability to meet basic needs. Local community-based organisations and volunteers may be very well placed to identify these communities and be engaged to deliver services to ensure their continued well-being during epidemic-related disruptions.

HARNESSING THE AFFECTED COMMUNITY'S SKILLS THROUGH LOCAL ACTION

Community volunteers and community-based organisations can directly participate in epidemic response efforts through health and workforce extension activities, including through task shifting, along with administrative and support services, and community engagement work. Highly skilled volunteers and those with relevant professional skills should be identified early for mobilisation at the appropriate level of the response. Key lessons learned from health systems research point to the need for these volunteers or community health workers to be officially recognised and tasked by the health and social care systems; parallel systems are likely to result in these critical workers being underutilised (12).

> **The community perspective**
>
> Community stakeholders may wish to understand from emergency response authorities the areas of work in which volunteers and local health and social workers may have the greatest impact and consider specific plans to integrate them into existing and newly implemented health systems and structures, including plans for their supervision by qualified personnel. Community leaders may wish to proactively establish relationships with public health authorities prior to emergency situations. They may want to think about how communication in a health emergency could be best handled within existing community structures. Public health authorities, for their part, will want to understand the coordination mechanisms within each affected or at-risk community and have visibility on local response plans and capacities. Establishing these relationships early—ideally before a crisis—facilitates the rapid inclusion of community-based actors and community capacities in responses.

Organised volunteers tend to be able to focus and carry out tasks more effectively than spontaneous or crowd-sourced volunteers (13). Community-based organisations, such as the National Red Cross or Red Crescent Societies and other local actors, are critical partners in training, equipping, directing, and managing community volunteers and workers. Public health authorities should develop response plans before, during, and after epidemics, ensuring that local organisations with the capacity to organise volunteers are systematically included in planning and response, and that coordination mechanisms are in place and clear to all.

> **Working with communities to manage mpox**
>
> As mpox cases in the U.S. rapidly escalated in 2022, initial clusters were associated with large gatherings involving sex, and concentrated among men who have sex with men, along with transgender communities (14–15). Government responses were not meeting the needs for testing and case management (16). In response, a group of queer and transgender activists (academics and non-academics alike) formed the Rapid Epidemiologic Study of Prevalence, Network, and Demographics of Mpox Infection (RESPND-MI) which:
> - measured the outbreak's demographics and spatial epidemiology
> - addressed gaps in mpox vaccine and treatment access, drawing from their understanding of the dynamics of group sex within their communities
>
> Pulling from approaches used in the Global South, this community-led response centred on community empowerment, leadership, and accountability. The study team self-organised into three working groups (administration, technical, and external affairs) with collective decision-making. External affairs led a community forum with stakeholders—including activists, governments, community-based organisations, clinicians, researchers, and others—which led to improved service delivery by increasing the appropriateness of the interventions for the transgender community, and influenced the study design to ensure sexual practices were not stigmatised. The forum also

evolved into a coordination mechanism to identify and address needs, with outputs including a vaccination locator (16), sex-positive safer-sex guidance (17), and a policy brief (18). A strong focus on accountability led to data collection to ensure that public health agencies were effectively serving the affected communities (19–20); this was central to the objective of influencing how government served queer and transgender communities. This demonstrates the critical importance of shifting decision-making power towards affected people, and community-based organisations driving accountability of government responses (21).

To hold authorities responsible, primary investigators and co-investigators of the RESPND-MI study team:
- spoke out in mainstream media
- published thought leadership such as open letters and policy briefs
- attended calls with city, state, and federal public health agencies
- organised (and participated in) protests
- disseminated lessons learned at convenings with city, state, and federal public health agencies

The key lessons learned in this space were that:
- city, state, and federal public health agencies were unprepared for a public health emergency even after the COVID-19 pandemic
- it is possible to rapidly mobilise vulnerable populations in community-based participatory research during a public health emergency
- it is useful for public health agencies in the Global North to reference models in the Global South during a public health emergency
- bureaucracy and the infrastructure of health financing are barriers during a public health emergency
- we cannot disseminate a limited supply of vaccine without understanding the social networks of vulnerable populations, particularly when we need to prioritise doses while ensuring equity (RESPND-MI team)

Task shifting

In the context of an epidemic and a surge in demand on the health system, the strategic use of temporary task shifting—not just in the direct provision of care but also in administration, procurement, social care, health promotion, and other areas—can improve both the quality and quantity of health and epidemic control services provided. Volunteers have a long history of being successfully used to shift critical pillars of epidemic response towards community-based action. One example is the use of local volunteers to run Oral Rehydration Points for the management of mild and moderate cholera cases at the community level. This shifting of basic case management through oral rehydration therapy to volunteers trained to deliver this service within walking distance of patients' homes allows for the early recognition and referral of severe cases requiring clinical support and reduces the burden on clinical teams by treating mild and moderate cases outside of the official health system. Contact tracing, which requires significant human resources, and community-based surveillance for epidemic diseases, are two other areas where trained and supervised volunteers can provide significant value to the health system, allowing professional health workers to focus on tasks that require a higher degree of training.

Social care and basic health services for people in isolation, ill at home, or in quarantine can also be provided by laypeople within the framework of good supervision and clearly defined parameters for referral or escalation to a professional. Meanwhile, health promotion and communication regarding risk and behaviour change may be even more successful when delivered by people within the community who share backgrounds or lived experiences with those whose behaviours they seek to inform. All these are clear examples of task shifting in the context of epidemic response, and all require organised training and strong supervisory and referral structures, provided through and in alignment with the official health system.

> **Case study: task shifting to Red Cross and Red Crescent community volunteers**
>
> Trained Red Cross and Red Crescent volunteers regularly take on technical epidemic-control or response activities, freeing highly qualified health workers in the local health system to focus on higher levels of care. In cholera outbreaks, thousands of Red Cross and Red Crescent volunteers across cholera-endemic countries are trained to rapidly scale up Oral Rehydration Points, which allow people suffering from mild-to-moderate cholera to receive oral rehydration therapy in their own communities, reducing the burden on cholera treatment centres and allowing for earlier intervention, preventing many cases from becoming severe.
>
> During epidemics of Ebola and Marburg virus disease, volunteers with intensive training and structured supervision can provide the entirety of the service to ensure people who have died as suspect and confirmed cases are buried safely, without the risk of further transmission of the virus, while adapting to local social, cultural, and religious norms.
>
> Local branches of many National Red Cross and Red Crescent Societies helped extend COVID-19 testing services into affected communities, allowing more highly trained medical professionals to focus on providing acute and preventative care in an overburdened health system. This simultaneously relieved the healthcare system by removing the need to conduct screening and ensured as many people as possible received health care when they developed COVID-19. Similarly, many National Red Cross and Red Crescent Societies set up telephone hotlines to provide mental health and psychosocial support during the pandemic. In 2020 alone, the Ecuadorian Red Cross provided mental health and psychosocial support services to 8,677 people (22).

What do volunteers and community-based organisations need?

Supportive supervision is critical to harnessing the power of community-based volunteers and local organisations, along with proper in-service training and a functional logistical pipeline to ensure they can carry out their tasks safely and effectively (23). Response authorities should plan to horizontally integrate volunteers and community health workers into existing or epidemic-specific programming, and clearly define volunteers' roles and responsibilities. Volunteers and other local actors also need clear structures in which they can influence decision-makers, to ensure that epidemic control programmes continue to adapt to changing needs. As members of the affected communities at the grassroots level and the response mechanism, local volunteers can be a critical bridge between strategy and implementation reality, but only if the response is structured in such a way that their experience on the ground can meaningfully change the response itself.

At the systems level, research on COVID-19 found that in many countries, local actors were neglected by the authorities charged with leading the pandemic response (24); they found themselves working in partial isolation from health systems and other, officially mandated, responders. Policy and legal frameworks that underpinned the response did not address the role of local actors, making it difficult for them to appropriately coordinate and leverage their local reach. National Red Cross and Red Crescent Societies reported that close coordination with the authorities significantly enabled their response, allowing them to scale up the most relevant services, which were more likely to be complementary to those provided by public authorities and other agencies (25). Early investment—ideally before an epidemic occurs, but otherwise in the very early days of response—in the policies, coordination structures, and relationships between authorities and local actors is critical to effectively harness the power of community-based actors and volunteers.

> **Duty of care extends to volunteers**
>
> As with professional health and emergency response personnel, volunteers may face significant risks of mental health challenges, stigma, or burnout. Safe and dignified burials volunteers in West Africa reported experiencing stigma, exclusion from family and community activities, and mental health impacts that lasted beyond the Ebola epidemic. The Community-Led Ebola Action (CLEA) led to good outcomes with communities reporting early on Ebola deaths and reaching out for proper burial methods (26–27). Therefore, it is critical that the duty of care is planned for, and that resources are dedicated to prevent, detect, and respond to the negative mental health and social impacts of volunteers responding to outbreaks.
>
> Reliance on volunteers for epidemic response also entails a duty to care for their social, mental, and physical well-being. In addition to the structures needed to provide safe services, responding authorities must ensure that support systems are in place to prevent, mitigate, and respond to negative impacts on frontline responders, including volunteers. Volunteers working in epidemics may be confronted with potentially traumatic events, as well as face long-lasting social consequences for their service, including stigma and discrimination. Activities to prevent these consequences can be carried out at the community level, for example, working with the affected communities to celebrate and recognise the contributions of community members volunteering their time, or education to improve understanding of any risks posed by volunteering or volunteers. At the individual level, authorities should ensure that appropriate mental health and social support are available to volunteers and community-based workers. This can be done by providing psychological first aid through (resourced and supported) peer support groups, access to appropriate mental health referrals and care, and other resources (28).

What motivates volunteers?

The demands on volunteers can be high during an epidemic response. As such, emergency response authorities must plan, from the beginning, for ways to keep volunteers engaged and motivated. For many volunteers, motivation stems from a sense of moral responsibility, social recognition, and doing good (29). Positive reinforcement by community members can be critical for sustaining volunteers' commitment and can offer a social form of repayment for the services provided. Different models exist for community-led remuneration or the incentivisation of volunteers and other community health workers. Epidemic response authorities should identify incentives that appropriately value the inputs of the volunteers (30).

Ethical considerations of volunteering

Response authorities should be explicitly aware of and plan to mitigate the potential ethical pitfalls or considerations when relying on local actors and volunteers. The sustainability of volunteer engagement in a long-lasting epidemic must be planned for, and the ethics of prolonged volunteering without remuneration must be considered. The availability of full-time or consistent volunteers, while often helpful from a programming continuity perspective, is also likely to reflect community structures, where those with the fewest resources—often from vulnerable or marginalised communities—are least able to volunteer for non-remunerated work. Without the conscious engagement of vulnerable and marginalised groups, responders risk mirroring societal power structures that continue to have specific groups under-represented, unseen, and unserved by the epidemic response. Likewise, women are over-represented in unpaid and volunteer work (24,27).

The limits of task shifting to unpaid workers must also be recognised and structures put in place to ensure that formerly paid work is not permanently transitioned to unpaid work even after the epidemic response has stabilised or ended. In addition, local workers and volunteers should abide by the same ethical mandates as regular health workers in relation to, among others, confidentiality and respect for the autonomy of patients and their families. In many cases, this may require explicit systems development, training, and education by health authorities, as volunteers coming from non-health or non-regulated professions generally do not have an innate knowledge of these aspects of health services.

PLANNING FOR DIVERSITY, EQUITY, AND INCLUSION

Disease epidemics both drive and thrive on inequity. Systematically addressing equity is an imperative from both an ethical and a disease control perspective. Vulnerable and marginalised communities often bear the brunt of epidemics and have the least adapted or appropriate programming available to assist them. Responding authorities and communities should prioritise identifying and supporting local actors who have the trust of and can access and work with these communities (or disadvantaged groups within communities) and adapt programming to meet their specific needs and circumstances. In addition, responders, both authorities and local actors, should ensure that volunteers appropriately reflect the makeup of society in the area where they are responding.

Foreseeable challenges include preventing discrimination against minorities and the inclusion of these minorities in public health plans (31). Responding authorities should prioritise the early identification of vulnerable or marginalised communities who might face specific barriers to behaviour change or access to preventive or curative services. This includes community engagement and accountability approaches that are culturally appropriate, gender-sensitive, and accessible to people with disabilities, which allow those communities to proactively identify their needs and suggest adaptations. Authorities must go beyond "engaging" these communities to focus on adapting services to meet their needs. For a variety of legal, cultural, and trust issues, this may entail engaging organisations that stem from or work with these populations to deliver the services at an arm's length from the authorities.

> **Using local actors to reach people excluded from the health system**
>
> In the U.K., the British Red Cross Refugee Support Team worked closely with people seeking asylum, many of whom faced barriers to accessing COVID-19–related health services. The Red Cross produced informational material in 20 languages and ensured that they were relevant to members of the community. They also supported pop-up vaccination clinics for people who did not have access to the health system (25). In the Maldives, the Maldivian Red Crescent supported the vaccination of unregistered migrants who likewise could not access the country's vaccination programme through regular channels.

ADAPTING TO MEET CULTURAL AND SOCIAL DIFFERENCES

Disease epidemics across the globe have clearly demonstrated the impact of cultural and social differences and trust between (and within) affected communities and those designated to respond. Bridging this gap is critical to effective epidemic response. Public health and emergency response authorities have a key coordinating and convening role to play early in and throughout the epidemic response to ensure that the various components of the affected communities—different ethnic, social, and religious majorities and minorities—are consulted and that prevention and response activities are adapted to their specific needs.

The implementation of public health measures can be challenging given that not all measures can be accepted or executed by the community. Community stakeholders can act as the bridge between public health officials and the affected community, so long as response authorities create systems that allow for the adaptation of strategies and tactics based on community needs and preferences, and that cultural and social needs are documented and systematically accounted for.

A one-size-fits-all epidemic response plan is, at best, adapted to the needs and realities of the majority or dominant population, and may systematically exclude those whose cultural practices, resources, or other factors do not align with the envisioned response. Whether they be indigenous communities, people living in remote or hard-to-access areas, linguistic minorities, or the chronically unhoused, groups who experience entrenched marginalisation require specifically adapted and co-designed interventions. These interventions may require additional resources compared to the response plan targeting the majority population, and the allocation of resources, along with the selection of interventions itself, must be done with the consultation and agreement of members and representatives of the minority communities. This process of culturally appropriate adaptation must occur at the level of the fundamentals of epidemic response, and not merely as a cultural adaptation of the majority plan. One size does not fit all, and response managers should be prepared for the joint planning required as well as the variations in implementation needed for successful response in a heterogeneous society.

Humans and the ecosystem are tightly connected. In certain cultures, the interaction between humans and animals should be considered to anticipate possible zoonotic infections and initiate surveillance and prevention methods. Farming practices and environmental changes are also potential sources of epidemics and the affected communities should be alerted and engaged to identify feasible alternatives to higher risk behaviours (**See Chapter 13, One Health**).

Community behaviours and cultural practices should also be studied carefully to understand the potential impacts of standardised epidemic control approaches. Certain public health measures may not be feasible for some or may require collaboration between cultural leaders and technical experts to adapt public health or epidemic control practices or activities to meet cultural needs or expectations. Any possible conflicts between cultural needs and public health objectives should be explicitly addressed and emphasised for measures to be executed. Similarly, cultural practices should be identified to ensure there are no contraindications to public health measures for epidemic response. For example, traditional burial practices were one of the key drivers of transmission in the Ebola epidemic in West Africa. Cultural practices that drive transmission or may contradict generalised public health measures should be identified—systematically, intentionally, and quickly—and interventions or workarounds planned to ensure efforts of the epidemic response do not go to waste.

Traditional cultural practices are difficult to change or ban. It may seem disrespectful to the community in question when public health officials state that their cultural practices have a negative impact on the community's well-being. Therefore, additional efforts are required to establish a common understanding between public health officials and the community without being forceful or offensive. Engaging these communities provides a platform for negotiation for the modification of cultural practices—and response practices!—for the better of the communities in an epidemic response.

Indigenous-led responses to COVID-19: examples from the Americas

Community-led approaches can counteract the systemic discrimination indigenous communities may face, while rolling out effective epidemic countermeasures. Many indigenous communities implemented COVID-19 shielding, quarantine, or access control that were distinct from those of the surrounding non-indigenous population. For example, the Siekopai population in Ecuador shielded Elders by taking them into the jungle following the death of a single suspect case (32).

Alongside these approaches, many indigenous governments—whether traditional or state-sanctioned—provided social support to those whose livelihoods were most impacted by the collectively-decided restrictions. In Canada, the Innu community of Uashat took emergency measures and implemented approaches to mitigate their negative impacts, including establishing a psychological care plan for social workers and people experiencing social isolation. The integration of traditional shamanic medicine and spiritual practices into Western medicine-backed approaches also proved critical to uptake and ownership. In Bolivia, indigenous communities promoted the use of traditional antiviral plants alongside Western medicine, with the Kallawaya people, traditional doctors, and the Vice-Ministry of Traditional Medicine and Interculturality co-creating approaches to improve symptoms. The Uashat community held socially distanced

> sacred fires to strengthen community cohesion and support, while various indigenous groups integrated shamanic practitioners, midwives, and other traditional care providers into home-based care for COVID-19 and to extend other health services impacted by the pandemic (33).
>
> Finally, the U.S. government devolved vaccine distribution decision-making to Native American communities for their own populations. This resulted in a higher vaccination uptake in indigenous communities than any other group in the U.S. population during the first half of 2020. Community leaders ascribe this success to community-led ownership of the process and traditional values of respect for Elders, "community first" philosophies, and a willingness to trust science when it was communicated by members of their own communities (34).

SUPPORTING LOCAL ACTORS TO LEAD TRANSITION AND RECOVERY

Community-led action and volunteerism should not stop when the epidemic is over (1). It is important that emergency response authorities plan for and make technical and financial resources available to support community stakeholders, local organisations, and volunteers in their efforts to build and maintain sustainable actions to prevent, detect, and rapidly respond to future epidemics. For example, while scaling down a community-led epidemic response, community structures and volunteers can transition to activities aimed at preventing or rapidly detecting the next epidemic. It is also crucial to always identify learning points from previous epidemics and reflect on how to make a better epidemic response plan with the affected communities. By constantly reviewing the needs and input of the community, practical solutions can be created and implemented as the communities are within reach due to the continuity of involvement. This should be a cornerstone of health emergencies preparedness at the local level and be systematically included in national action plans for health security.

As communities face increasing hazards related to the climate crisis, epidemic disease outbreaks, and the risk of natural disasters, there is an increase in the experience of overlapping or compounding emergencies, or multiple emergencies in rapid succession. When emergencies overlap or occur consecutively, community resilience is consistently undermined. A forward-looking recovery plan should empower local actors to address community needs from a multi-hazard perspective that includes animal and environmental health so that recovery from an epidemic supports preparedness for a multitude of hazards in the future.

> **Case study: coordination between public health authorities and community-based volunteers in Kenya helped stop Anthrax outbreak**
>
> On 15 August 2019, a Kenya Red Cross Society volunteer received some concerning news. A herder and two students in the town of Narok, near the Maasai Mara National Reserve, had become ill after eating beef and were diagnosed with anthrax. The volunteer was trained in the Red Cross' community-based surveillance system and quickly sent an SMS through the system, informing their supervisor. This message was passed to government human and animal health authorities

and the national surveillance system, triggering an investigation by the authorities and the rapid vaccination of more than 24,000 cattle and sheep.

Responding authorities and the Red Cross knew they needed the active participation and trust of the herders, so they convened a traditional community dialogue session with the affected communities. School teachers were engaged and taught to screen children for infection and how to report possible cases to local health authorities or Red Cross volunteers. Volunteers carried out activities to raise awareness, including radio broadcasts, household visits, and group education sessions in the affected communities. These improved the people's knowledge of how to safely dispose of animal carcasses and report unusual illnesses in their animals. The outreach was successful, with even community members who were previously sceptical of the risks of anthrax recognising the importance of prevention measures. Just over a month after the incident was first reported by the Red Cross volunteer, the authorities deemed the situation under control, with four cases in humans and one death. The community emerged with stronger links to public authorities for human and animal health, and better preparedness for a future outbreak (35).

CONCLUSION

Epidemic response entails deep collaboration between public health authorities and affected communities, and this means working with volunteers and local organisations from within those communities. Response measures should be co-created and co-owned between public health authorities and the communities experiencing the epidemic. Community participation must go far beyond information sharing to include participatory assessment and planning processes, not just once but throughout the response, with epidemic control measures adapted to meet the affected community's changing needs and capacities, including ensuring the continuity of health and social services.

Community-based actors must be systematically incorporated into coordination, integrating horizontally into the health system and epidemic response mechanisms. Community-based actors can be a particular value-add in providing services to marginalised and hard-to-reach communities who may be systematically excluded—whether intentionally or not—from public authorities' plans and actions. The onus must be on expert epidemic responders and public authorities to reach out to local actors and facilitate their integration into response mechanisms and to ensure that response planning and implementation is receptive to and adapts based on the feedback, gaps, challenges, and opportunities identified by local actors. Finally, local actors must remain central to transition and recovery activities and be supported to contribute to and lead the next cycle of local multi-hazard preparedness efforts. This will build community resilience to future shocks.

REFERENCES:

1. Gilmore B, Ndejjo R, Tchetchia A, et al. Community engagement for COVID-19 prevention and control: a rapid evidence synthesis. BMJ Global Health. 2020. https://gh.bmj.com/content/5/10/e003188#T2 https://doi.org/10.1136/bmjgh-2020-003188. PMID: 33051285.
2. Tabari P, Amini M, Moghadami M, Moosavi M. International public health responses to COVID-19 outbreak: a rapid review. Iran J Med Sci. 2020 May;45(3):157–69. https://www.ncbi.nlm.nih.gov/pmc/articles/PMC7253494/ https://doi.org/10.30476/ijms.2020.85810.1537 PMID:32546882.

3. Bollyky TJ, Hulland EN, Barber RM, Collins JK, Kiernan S, Moses M, et al.; COVID-19 National Preparedness Collaborators. Pandemic preparedness and COVID-19: an exploratory analysis of infection and fatality rates, and contextual factors associated with preparedness in 177 countries, from Jan 1, 2020, to Sept 30, 2021. Lancet. 2022 Apr;399(10334):1489–512. https://doi.org/10.1016/S0140-6736(22)00172-6 PMID:35120592.
4. Edelman. 2022 Edelman Trust Barometer: the cycle of distrust. Daniel J Edelman Holdings Inc. https://www.edelman.com/trust/2022-trust-barometer.
5. Bavel JJ, et al. Using social and behavioural science to support COVID-19 pandemic. 2020 April. https://www.nature.com/articles/s41562-020-0884-z https://doi.org/10.1038/s41562-020-0884-z.
6. IFRC. World Disasters Report 2022. 2023 January. https://www.ifrc.org/document/world-disasters-report-2022.
7. Wilhelm JA, Helleringer S. Utilization of non-Ebola health care services during Ebola outbreaks: a systematic review and meta-analysis. J Glob Health. 2019 Jun;9(1):010406. https://doi.org/10.7189/jogh.09.010406 PMID:30701070.
8. Ribacke KJ, et al. Effects of the West Africa Ebola virus disease on health-care utilisation – a systematic review. Front Public Health. 2016. Vol 4 No 222. https://www.frontiersin.org/articles/10.3389/fpubh.2016.00222/full.
9. World Health Organization. Essential health services face continued disruption during COVID-19 pandemic. 2022 February. https://www.who.int/news/item/07-02-2022-essential-health-services-face-continued-disruption-during-covid-19-pandemic.
10. Moynihan R, et al. Impact of COVID-19 pandemic on utilisation of healthcare services: a systemic review. BMJ. 2021;11(3). https://bmjopen.bmj.com/content/11/3/e045343.
11. World Disaster Report. 2022. https://www.ifrc.org/sites/default/files/2023-01/20230130_2022_WDR_Chapter2.pdf.
12. Najafizada SA, et al. Community health workers in Canada and other high-income countries: a scoping review and research gaps. Canadian journal of public health= Revue canadienne de sante publique. 2015. Vol 106 No 3. https://pubmed.ncbi.nlm.nih.gov/26125243/ https://doi.org/10.17269/CJPH.106.4747.
13. Zhang A, Zhang K, Li W, Wang Y, Li Y, Zhang L. Optimising self-organised volunteer efforts in response to the COVID-19 pandemic. Humanit Soc Sci Commun. 2022;9(134):134. https://www.nature.com/articles/s41599-022-01127-2 https://doi.org/10.1057/s41599-022-01127-2.
14. Minhaj FS, Ogale YP, Whitehill F, Schultz J, Foote M, Davidson W, et al.; Monkeypox Response Team 2022. Monkeypox outbreak—nine states, May 2022. MMWR Morb Mortal Wkly Rep. 2022 Jun;71(23):764–9. https://doi.org/10.15585/mmwr.mm7123e1 PMID:35679181.
15. Blackburn D, Roth NM, Gold JA, Pao LZ, Olansky E, Torrone EA, et al. Epidemiologic and clinical features of mpox in transgender and gender-diverse adults—United States, May-November 2022. MMWR Morb Mortal Wkly Rep. 2022 Dec;71(5152):1605–9. https://doi.org/10.15585/mmwr.mm715152a1 PMID:36580418.
16. Krellenstein J, Osmundson J, Makofane K. Opinion | To fight monkeypox, remember the lessons of Covid and H.I.V. The New York Times. 29 May 2022. https://www.nytimes.com/2022/05/29/opinion/monkeypox-covid-and-hiv.html. Accessed 8 Jun 2022.
17. Diamond N, Osmundson J, Roth G. Six ways we can have safer sex in the time of monkeypox. POZ. 21 Jul 2022. https://www.poz.com/article/six-ways-can-safer-sex-time-monkeypox. Accessed 16 Mar 2023.
18. Barnes-Balenciaga J, Cahill S, Carneiro PB, Carpino T, Diamond N, Feng Z. (Jack), et al. An open letter to the Biden administration on monkeypox. 8 Aug 2022. https://harvardpublichealth.org/equity/an-open-letter-to-the-biden-administration-on-monkeypox/. Accessed 16 Mar 2023.
19. UNAIDS. Establishing community-led monitoring of HIV services. Geneva, Switzerland: UNAIDS; 2021. https://www.unaids.org/sites/default/files/media_asset/establishing-community-led-monitoring-hiv-services_en.pdf.
20. O'Neil Institute, Treatment Action Campaign (TAC), Health Gap, International Treatment Preparedness Coalition (ITPC), International Community of Women Living with HIV Eastern Africa, Sexual Minorities Uganda (SMUG), et al. Community-Led Monitoring of Health Services: Building Accountability for HIV Service Quality.
21. Roth G, Barnes-Balenciaga J, Osmundson J, Smith MD, Tran NK, Diamond N, et al. Global North learning from Global South: a community-led response to mpox in New York City. PLOS Glob Public Health. 2023 Jun;3(6):e0002042. https://doi.org/10.1371/journal.pgph.0002042 PMID:37379259.
22. IFRC Psychosocial Centre, 2020. https://pscentre.org/.

23. Woldie M, Feyissa GT, Admasu B, Hassen K, Mitchell K, Mayhew S, et al. Community health volunteers could help improve access to and use of essential health services by communities in LMICs: an umbrella review. Health Policy Plan. 2018 Dec;33(10):1128–43. https://doi.org/10.1093/heapol/czy094 PMID:30590543.

24. IPPPR (The Independent Panel for Pandemic Preparedness & Response). Centering communities in pandemic preparedness and response. 2021. Vol 10. https://theindependentpanel.org/wp-content/uploads/2021/05/Background-paper-10-community-involvement.pdf.

25. Johnston A. Analysis of learning from IFRC COVID-19 response. International Federation of Red Cross and Red Crescent Societies. 2022. Available from IFRC upon request.

26. Wilkinson A, Parker M, Martineau F, Leach M. Engaging 'communities': anthropological insights from the West African Ebola epidemic. Philosophical Transactions of the Royal Society B: Biological Sciences. 2017. Vol 372 No 1721. https://royalsocietypublishing.org/doi/full/10.1098/rstb.2016.0305 https://doi.org/10.1098/rstb.2016.0305.

27. Bhaumik S, Moola S, Tyagi J, Nambiar D, Kakoti M. Community health workers for pandemic response: a rapid evidence synthesis. BMJ Glob Health. 2020 Jun;5(6):e002769. https://doi.org/10.1136/bmjgh-2020-002769 PMID:32522738.

28. Lamoure G, Juilliard H. ALNAP lessons paper: responding to Ebola epidemics. 2020 December. https://www.alnap.org/help-library/alnap-lessons-paper-responding-to-ebola-epidemics.

29. Kpanake et al. Human Resources for Health. 2019. Vol 17 No 81. https://d-nb.info/1205637664/34.

30. Frida et al. 2016. Health Policy and Planning, Volume 31. Issue 2. 2016. https://academic.oup.com/heapol/article/31/2/205/2355511.

31. Bedford J, Farrar J, Ihekweazu C, et al. A new twenty-first century science for effective epidemic response. Nature. 2019. Vol 575 No 130–136. https://www.nature.com/articles/s41586-019-1717-y https://doi.org/10.1038/s41586-019-1717-y.

32. FILAC, & FIAY. (2020). Los Pueblos Indígenas ante la pandemia del COVID-19. http://indigenascovid19.red/wp-content/uploads/2020/05/FILAC_FIAY_primer-informe-PI_COVID19.pdf.

33. SSHAP. Key considerations: Indigenous peoples in COVID-19 response and recovery. https://www.socialscienceinaction.org/resources/key-considerations-indigenous-peoples-in-covid-19-response-and-recovery/.

34. Silberner J. Covid-19: how Native Americans led the way in the US vaccination effort. BMJ. 2021 Sep;374(2168):n2168. https://doi.org/10.1136/bmj.n2168 PMID:34535445.

35. IFRC. Resolve to Save Lives. 2021 July. https://www.ifrc.org/document/case-study-anthrax-kenya.

CHAPTER 36

LEARNING THE LESSONS: RECOVERY AND REVIEW

by Jen O. Lim, Ebere Okereke, Magda Robalo, and Renu Bindra

The recovery phase of an infectious disease emergency is rarely a linear process, but it represents an opportunity to 'build back better'. In this chapter, we focus on efforts to restore a community's health system, recognising that recovery also refers to restoring (and improving) all emergency-affected systems and structures. Restoration of health system functions needs to be done while still controlling the disease, addressing the inequalities and disproportionate impacts that the emergency has revealed, and beginning the process of effective reviews that will feedback into future preparedness efforts.

INTRODUCTION

The recovery phase of the emergency cycle, as defined by the World Health Organization (WHO), involves "restoring or improving — livelihoods and health, as well as economic, physical, social, cultural, and environmental assets, systems, and activities [in an emergency-affected community or society], aligning with the principles of sustainable development and 'build back better'" (1).

The study of how societies can recover effectively from infectious disease emergencies receives relatively little attention, and there is a significant risk that national and multinational organisations in the throes of a health emergency may overlook this key phase of the emergency management cycle. Progression from response to recovery and through the recovery phase is unlikely to be linear and unidirectional. Further outbreaks and emergencies during recovery can complicate the situation, while developments in our knowledge and management of the infectious disease can change our understanding of what the recovery phase should look like.

In this chapter, we focus on one crucial aspect of the broad scope of recovery as defined by the WHO, the recovery of health systems. To do this, we have developed a framework consisting of four broad objectives:
- resuming the provision of health services
- maintaining control of the infectious disease even as urgency recedes
- addressing inequalities and the needs of disproportionately affected groups
- undertaking effective reviews that contribute to learning and future preparedness

These four objectives are actualised by three principles, which should be applied across all objectives and underlie policy and operational considerations during recovery:
• capitalise on opportunities to improve health
• always consider local contexts and their implications on policy goals and effectiveness
• support the well-being of health workers

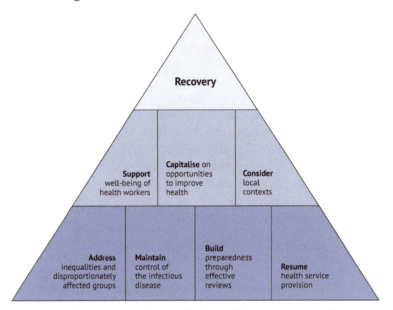

Figure 36.1: A framework for recovery from infectious disease emergencies

RESUMPTION OF HEALTH SERVICE PROVISION

The resumption of health service provision during recovery is crucial for the restoration and improvement of health and well-being. This is related to, but distinct from, the maintenance of essential health services during the response phase (**See Chapter 23, Essential services**). Approaches to aid the resumption of health service provision fall under several broad areas.

Reducing the risk of transmission in health facilities

The risk of further disease transmission in health facilities is likely elevated in the recovery period as preventive measures are lifted, posing a potential impediment for a return to 'business as usual'. Outbreaks of infectious diseases distinct from the cause of the primary emergency can also occur, and indeed may be more likely due to the stress placed upon health, social, and economic systems. Further infectious disease outbreaks can severely impede health service provision as resources have to be redirected and healthcare staff may themselves be affected. Patients are also less likely to attend health centres if there is a perceived risk of infection.

The risk of transmission in health facilities may need to be re-addressed for the recovery phase, including through the modification of physical facilities. Walls, screens, and doors can be installed to delineate "high-risk" and "low-risk" areas, with buffer zones for activities such as the removal of personal protective equipment (PPE), and areas used by healthcare workers (HCWs) can be separated from those used by patients and other visitors. Waiting rooms can be reconfigured or expanded, and processes such as patient registration or checking out can also be conducted virtually to facilitate physical distancing (2–3). Another possible approach is to do away entirely with waiting rooms, either by scheduling patients to arrive precisely on time for their appointments or encouraging them to wait in cars if suitable parking facilities are available. Improving the ventilation of high-risk areas should be considered if airborne transmission of the pathogen is suspected. This can involve setting up negative pressure rooms, but simpler approaches such as carrying out aerosol-generating procedures near windows may also be helpful in resource- and time-constrained settings (4). Some of these interventions may already have been carried out in the response phase. An assessment of their effectiveness, including any adverse impacts on service capacity, quality, or equity, should be undertaken to actions taken during recovery. If planned and executed well, changes made during recovery can lay the foundation for preparedness for the next emergency.

Workforce management and training

In recovery, health systems must address backlogs of elective clinical work even while dealing with long-term health sequelae of the infectious disease outbreak. It is crucial to ensure that all HCWs are equipped with the skills, knowledge, and support required for the resumption of health services during the recovery phase. Given the challenges of recovery, it is not too late for training in infection prevention and control (IPC) measures, epidemiological data collection, and skills required to address community-specific priorities (4–5).

Extending operating hours or running weekend clinics, theatres, and radiology and pathology services can also directly increase the number of patients served (2,6–7), although human resources and funding constraints may limit the practicality of this in the longer term. In addition, health leaders and administrators should actively review performance and make contingencies for surge capacity to deal with further outbreaks or other emergencies.

Engagement with communities, healthcare staff, and other stakeholders

Engagement with local communities and other national and international actors is important for ensuring that recovery plans adequately address local needs and priorities which may change over time. Furthermore, reassuring communities about infection control measures implemented in hospitals and other health centres is crucial for overcoming hesitancy in seeking medical care. Regular and clear communication between healthcare staff is also required to convey changes in processes and ensure that logistical support meets demand (2).

Improvement of supply chains and health system logistics

Recovery is a highly dynamic phase which often involves repeated local infectious disease outbreaks and associated social and economic challenges. The emergency may have revealed weaknesses in infrastructure and the inadequacy of logistical planning and networks. While it is difficult to build infrastructure like bridges, roads, and storage facilities, or to improve cold chains for distribution of vaccines and medication in this phase, such improvements may nonetheless be needed to enable regular health service provision. Because of the risk of ongoing outbreak-related disruption in the recovery phase, such projects should ideally be carried out as part of preparedness measures in the pre-outbreak period, though this is often impeded by financial costs and limitations in understanding the weaknesses of health system logistics (8). Supplies of certain medications, PPE, and blood for transfusions are also likely to be constrained during and after an infectious disease emergency, and this may impede the resumption of health services (9).

> **Cholera response**
>
> The recovery phase following an infectious disease outbreak can interact with outbreaks of other infectious diseases. For example, countries in Western and Central Africa experienced a surge of cholera cases in the aftermath of an Ebola epidemic in 2017. Such situations are complicated by the adverse impact that the acute response to the preceding epidemic may have had on care for patients with other infectious diseases (10–11).

Prioritisation of services and research activity

Higher-level actors should facilitate coordinated initiatives to improve health service provision in particular areas of concern, while allowing local bodies the flexibility to address local needs. Modelling and epidemiological studies can reveal services for which rapid resumption is critical for reducing mortality (9,12). Examples of areas which regional and national health systems have chosen to focus on during recovery include cancer diagnosis and care, catching up with childhood vaccinations, prevention of malnutrition, and management of chronic diseases. Research priorities should also be reviewed to re-evaluate underlying cost-benefit assumptions which may have changed over the course of the emergency, and to free up resources for more pertinent needs where appropriate. Considerations relevant to research activity prioritisation include the severity of the associated disease, patient needs, demands on human and financial resources, and the potential for reducing in-person visits to health centres to decrease the risk of infectious disease transmission (2).

Objective	Possible approaches
Reducing risk of transmission in health facilities	• Modifications to health facilities • Digitalisation of administrative processes • Appropriate use of PPE • Adjustments to visitor policies • Regular asymptomatic testing for HCWs • Adjustments to treatments and appointment rescheduling to reduce health facility crowding • Use of telehealth and virtual consultations where appropriate
Workforce management and training	• Training in competencies required to address local healthcare needs • Extending operating hours and/or running weekend clinics • Training in infection control and community relationship-building skills • Offering flexible working arrangements to improve staff well-being and retention

Objective	Possible approaches
Communication with communities, healthcare staff, and other stakeholders	• Health promotion and awareness creation • Identification of local needs and priorities • Contact and follow up of at-risk and underserved groups • Reassure patients about the safety of attending health facilities
Improve supply chains and logistical networks	• Enhance communication, planning, and procurement processes to ensure sufficient supply of PPE, medication, blood, and oxygen supplies • Building of logistics and storage facilities
Prioritisation of services and research activity	• Modelling impact of service resumption on mortality • Review research programmes and balance these against health service demands • Local community input on prioritisation of services

Table 36.1: Possible approaches to support effective resumption of health service provision during the recovery phase
The appropriateness of these approaches is pathogen- and context-dependent—this should not be interpreted as a checklist of policies to implement.

MAINTAINING CONTROL OF THE INFECTIOUS DISEASE

Although infectious disease emergencies would ideally conclude with complete eradication of the disease in question, this is historically a rare outcome and unrealistic in most circumstances. It would thus be unwise to assume that vaccination or other measures will be successful in fully eradicating any novel infectious disease. There is thus a need for health leaders and policymakers to plan for dealing with the disease in the long term. This is best done with a full understanding of the socioeconomic impact of public health measures on the community, and the community's capacity to implement and adhere to public health policies and other measures.

Transmission control measures should be locally stratified in recovery

The impact and utility of community transmission control measures including vaccination, testing, school closures, isolation requirements, and restrictions on public gatherings and business and social activities have been discussed elsewhere in this book. Some of these measures may maintain a degree of usefulness at preventing and controlling infectious disease transmission sufficient to justify their use in the recovery phase, although this should be reassessed based on pathogen and population factors such as the prevalence of vaccination or infection-derived immunity.

The substantial financial and human costs involved in these transmission control measures mean that they should be relaxed to a baseline level in the recovery phase and dynamically stepped up or down to control local outbreaks where appropriate (13). Risk-based stratification of transmission control measures across different communities is important for supporting sustainable and dynamic infectious disease control and preventing potential spillover events, whilst facilitating a timely return towards a 'new normal' for as many people as possible (14).

Data collection and monitoring capacities required during recovery

Monitoring pathogen transmission and evolution is important for informing decisions about public health measures and resource allocation but plays a somewhat different role during response and recovery. The focus of testing in the recovery phase, from a health systems perspective, shifts from diagnosis for clinical and public health purposes to monitoring community prevalence, particularly if the availability of vaccines or effective treatments reduces the utility of early diagnosis. Such studies can also improve our understanding of symptoms associated with infection and the proportions of symptomatic and asymptomatic infections, which may vary over time based on pathogen and host factors (15). It is important to ensure that accessibility barriers, such as testing costs, do not limit the ability to maintain surveillance activities during the recovery phase.

Surveillance strategy	Advantages	Disadvantages
Community sampling and testing (e.g., sentinel surveillance)	• Data on test sensitivity and specificity allows the overall degree of uncertainty to be inferred • Can be used to monitor trends among specific groups of people	• Relatively expensive • Willing participants can be difficult to find
Wastewater sampling	• Generally inexpensive • Sensitivity to certain pathogens may be high – detection by wastewater sampling can precede detection by traditional clinician report-based monitoring systems	• Lack of systematic studies on pathogen-specific sensitivity • Cannot examine trends among communities that are not spatially associated, such as members of specific ethnic groups or age cohorts (9)

Table 36.2: General strengths and weaknesses of two examples of surveillance strategies
There is significant technical and procedural complexity involved in the use of these tests for surveillance programmes (See Chapter 20, Diagnostics).

Genomic sequencing (**See Chapter 21, Genomics**) is another important tool for the surveillance of pathogens and is of use in the recovery phase for detecting emerging variants which may be more transmissible or virulent, or more able to escape population-level immunity (16). However, the SARS-CoV-2 pandemic revealed that marked regional differences in sequencing availability exist along economic lines. Furthermore, much sequencing data is not shared on publicly available repositories (17). These issues must be addressed to fully realise the potential of genomic surveillance for detecting and tracking emerging variants globally. Other methods of disease surveillance include sentinel surveillance, wastewater testing, and event-based and indicator-based surveillance. Their relative appropriateness in the recovery phase is dependent on factors including prevalence, degree of health-seeking behaviour, quality of data collection systems, and cost.

Monitoring the state and capacity of health systems is just as important as monitoring the evolution and spread of pathogens. Reliable and up-to-date data on hospitalisations, deaths, intensive therapy unit occupancy rates, supplies of critical medications, and workforce capacity and capabilities are necessary for health leaders and policymakers to make informed decisions. Equally critical will be planned and proactive application of behavioural science approaches to ensure a good understanding of evolving community attitudes and perceptions.

ADDRESSING INEQUALITIES

The burden of infectious diseases has consistently fallen heaviest upon underprivileged communities. Greater pre-existing inequality has been associated with increased mortality, both among deprived communities and at the national level between countries (18–20). Contributing factors include poorer access to and provision of health care, pre-existing health, economic, and educational disparities, and less extensive social support networks. Public health and social measures adopted to suppress disease transmission during the response phase can also disproportionately affect certain groups of people and widen existing inequalities. School closures, for example, have a greater impact on disadvantaged children for reasons that may include interruptions in the provision of free school meals, reduced opportunities for safeguarding interventions, and differences in accessibility of online learning resources and private tuition (19,21). Other groups that may be disproportionately affected over the course of an infectious disease outbreak include ethnic minorities, people with disabilities, the elderly, the homeless, and migrants. Elderly care homes, refugee camps, slums, crowded factories, prisons, and migrant centres and dormitories are all possible settings where transmission may be elevated.

It is important to bear these considerations in mind throughout all stages of the emergency cycle, but this is especially important in the recovery phase where the relatively stable situation allows data-driven assessments to be made of inequalities arising from the outbreak and response measures. An effective emergency response system should include mechanisms for collating information about the impact of the emergency on marginalised and underserved groups in the population. Analysis of such information should inform areas of focus and prioritisation of recovery objectives.

Prioritisation between different areas of recovery

The recovery phase is certainly a key period for seeking to correct inequalities and mitigate the effects of the outbreak on disadvantaged groups. However, the objectives of recovery detailed thus far all require large-scale, resource-intensive approaches for them to be comprehensively addressed. The question of prioritisation between competing health, economic, and social priorities is fundamentally one for governments to address. However, it would be inaccurate to see goals in these areas as mutually exclusive. Improvements in the health of communities can contribute significantly to economic and social recovery, and vice versa. Health policymakers should interact closely with leaders from other fields to develop interventions and reforms that can achieve broad gains across different areas as part of a "health in all policies" approach (22).

UNDERTAKING EFFECTIVE REVIEWS

Reviews of health system preparedness and response to infectious disease emergencies are by no means exclusive to the recovery phase. However, the recovery phase is an opportune period for organisations to examine their preparations for and response to emergencies, and to apply lessons learnt with the goal of improving preparedness and building resilience for the future. Such reviews should not be limited to the health sector as infectious disease emergencies impact all aspects of social and economic development, and preparedness and response efforts are also influenced by political factors. National reviews should be conducted and fully owned by governments, even if they are supported by the WHO or other partners, and should be undertaken on a whole-of-government and whole-of-society basis. Whether conducted at national, other governmental levels, or by non-governmental organisations, leaders need to own the review process, agree with the methodology, make it as transparent as possible, and provide appropriate resources. Ownership and full engagement from the top are necessary if reviews are to accurately identify learning points and lead to real improvements.

Types of reviews

Multiple forms of reviews are applicable to health emergencies. After-action reviews are mainly conducted during recovery and examine actions taken during and prior to the response phase to identify best practice, areas for improvement, and lessons learnt (25). These are distinct from intra-action reviews carried out during the response phase, which focus more on applying lessons learnt to improve the contemporaneous emergency response. Issues and areas for improvement uncovered by intra-action reviews can also inform the planning and implementation of recovery efforts. The WHO produces guidance on how to undertake these types of reviews, and itself regularly conducts joint operational reviews (26). These operational reviews are distinguishable from other types of reviews in that they are WHO-led, typically occur during or towards the end of the response phase, and seek to ensure that the efforts of the WHO at all levels are effectively aligned with national ministries of health in achieving objectives as planned.

Reviews may be conducted informally, for example as part of a debrief session, or formally with a more structured process usually overseen by someone outside the team directly involved in the action. The precise manner in which an after-action review is conducted can be varied to suit the context, resources, and time available. The general aim is to facilitate the exchange of observations, ideas, feedback, and other data, with a focus on identifying lessons and proposing recommendations for future practice. Options for accomplishing this include interviews, focus group discussions, surveys, and workshops, which should be conducted as soon as possible after the event or outbreak (26).

Informing future preparedness

Learning should occur at all levels, from individuals to organisations, nationally and globally. Meaningful engagement with the review process, transparency, and effective follow-up are key components of effective reviews that can contribute to learning across multiple levels.

Engagement with the review process is greatly supported by fostering a 'no-blame' culture, as people may refrain from engaging candidly if they feel it may result in them suffering personal repercussions. After-action reviews serve to identify lessons and ways to improve, and should not be an evaluation of any individual's performance nor a means of apportioning blame (26). This also helps ensure that the results of reviews—particularly formal ones—are shared widely to spread learning and increase public confidence. A 'no-blame' approach has been successfully used to promote organisational learning at the sector level in the aviation industry (27), and is also conducive to learning because incidents (near-miss or otherwise) linked to human error often have underlying system failures (28).

Reviews cannot produce full solutions to the complex issues faced in outbreak preparedness and response, and reviewers should not aim for them to do so. Rather, reviews should seek to provide recommendations for improvements which, if appropriately translated into policy, can serve as the basis for further evaluation and learning. In this way, reviews contribute to organisational learning through an incremental and iterative process. Several practices have been suggested to improve the application of lessons learnt from reviews. Reviews should have clearly defined objectives, frameworks, guidelines, and tools underlying the process to facilitate the generation of clear recommendations for improvement and follow-up actions (24). Follow-up actions typically involve the direct implementation of a recommendation or the monitoring and oversight of its implementation, the latter being more likely if broad changes at the organisational level and senior leadership decision-making are required. In such cases, the reviewing group or another body should be empowered with sufficient resources to monitor the implementation of recommendations of the review. Subsequent communication and implementation of recommendations may be aided by identifying a point of contact and timeframes for feedback for each follow-up action (29).

The early part of the recovery phase is a key period for after-action reviews to be initiated and conducted. These should be conducted at multiple levels, openly and honestly, and with appropriate follow-up measures to effectively contribute to learning and long-term preparedness.

Effective reviews improve preparedness – Ebola outbreaks in the DRC

Following several outbreaks of Ebola virus disease (EBOD) from 2018–2021, the Ministry of Health of the Democratic Republic of the Congo (DRC) conducted an after-action review with the support of the WHO, drawing data from multiple sources including a literature review, interviews, online surveys, and focus group discussions. This led to improvements in various areas including leadership, IPC, coordination, and disease surveillance, which may have contributed to a better response to the subsequent EBOD outbreak (23). This is not always the case. Several multinational organisation offices in neighbouring countries did not carry out timely after-action reviews following the same outbreaks, in part due to complications arising from the developing SARS-CoV-2 pandemic. This area for improvement was itself identified in a stocktake exercise designed to identify best practices and challenges to improve preparedness (24).

PRINCIPLES FOR RECOVERY

The planning and execution of policies aimed at achieving any of the four broad objectives for recovery of health systems should be guided by several key principles to ensure that recovery is effective and provides health systems with enhanced resilience for future stresses.

Capitalising on opportunities to improve health

Technological developments can provide new, more effective means of achieving desired outcomes in recovery and beyond. For example, technological advancements can allow for mobile applications and software to aid in the collection and monitoring of infectious disease-related epidemiological data (8). Technological developments may also provide much-needed tools to collect, integrate, and track data on the longer term effects of an outbreak, such as information on developmental delays in children (30). In addition, advances in tele-health may offer cost-effective means of addressing health service backlogs while reducing the risk of transmission in crowded health facilities, although this may be more limited in rural or resource-constrained settings.

The recovery phase is a key period for considering how technological advancements should be used to improve health in the long term. Doing this effectively requires an understanding that recovery involves societies moving towards a 'new normal' which may look quite different from the pre-emergency situation, with ample room to accommodate new methods and platforms. However, underlying evidence must be carefully evaluated from the outset, with a particular focus on assessing the potential of new processes to exacerbate inequalities in healthcare and the suitability of such processes for particular groups of patients.

Not all opportunities to improve health in the wake of an infectious disease emergency are technology related. Disruption to everyday life and habits during outbreaks can open the door to interventions that promote lasting improvements in health, such as by discouraging the use of carbon-emitting motor vehicles in cities and adjusting policies to support environmental improvements, as proposed by the WHO in the aftermath of the SARS-CoV-2 pandemic (31). Large-scale vaccination campaigns can also be 'piggybacked' on to reach underserved members of the community, while greater health literacy and community involvement can be leveraged to address other health issues such as malnutrition and diabetes (32).

Consideration of local contexts

In recovery, as in the response phase, consideration of local social, political, economic, and cultural contexts is important to ensure that policies are effective at addressing the needs of local communities. This requires close engagement with local communities and stakeholders, as well as the understanding that careful consideration is required before the evidential bases for policies established by research in one country or community are extrapolated to other communities.

Important points for health leaders and policymakers to consider during recovery include the prevalence of misinformation, levels of public trust in health-related institutions, and attitudes towards disease survivors and their families. A deeper understanding of the nuanced social context can often help to address problems during recovery. For example, community-based care for orphans following an outbreak may be impeded by resource constraints, stigmatisation, and discrimination, or all of the above (33). A focused approach tailored to local contexts is thus required.

Support for the welfare and well-being of health and social care workers

Prioritisation of the welfare and well-being of health and social care workers, including both formal employees and volunteers, should be a feature across all policies adopted as part of emergency response and recovery. Factors which contribute to this include good workforce planning, fair remuneration, and flexibility in terms of working arrangements (2). The psychosocial and mental well-being of health and social care workers can be supported in greater detail (**See Chapter 31, Mental health**).

CONCLUSION

Given the immediate stresses of the emergency response, the recovery phase of the emergency cycle is often overlooked by both researchers and policymakers. The framework for recovery outlined in this chapter will hopefully be helpful when considering issues in this highly complex field. Most of the practical points raised in this chapter have been presented from the perspective of clinicians and public health leaders. Of course, much more can be written about recovery from economic, social, cultural, and environmental perspectives. Many of the underlying considerations of our framework, such as the need to address inequalities and conduct reviews that contribute to learning, are very relevant to non-health organisations as well. Indeed, a coherent and coordinated multisectoral and multidisciplinary approach is required to achieve an effective recovery that will stand societies in good stead for the future.

REFERENCES:

1. Health Emergency Risk Management [Internet]. 2019. https://apps.who.int/iris/bitstream/handle/10665/340893/WHO-EURO-2019-2378-42133-58035-eng.pdf.
2. Cinar P, Bold R, Bosslet BA, Bota DA, Burgess D, Chew HK, et al. Planning for post-pandemic cancer care delivery: recovery or opportunity for redesign? [Internet]. CA Cancer J Clin. 2021 Jan;71(1):34–46. https://doi.org/10.3322/caac.21644 PMID:32997807.
3. Ndede PO, Senkungu JK, Shakpeh JK, Jones TE, Sky R, McDonnell S. Health services and infrastructure recovery of a major public hospital in Liberia during the 2014–2016 Ebola epidemic [Internet]. Disaster Med Public Health Prep. 2019 Aug;13(4):767–73. https://doi.org/10.1017/dmp.2018.124 PMID:31526416.
4. You J, Mao Q. An improved ward architecture for treatment of patients with Ebola virus disease in Liberia [Internet]. Am J Trop Med Hyg. 2016 Apr;94(4):701–3. https://doi.org/10.4269/ajtmh.15-0209 PMID:26755568.
5. Kodish SR, Simen-Kapeu A, Beauliere JM, Ngnie-Teta I, Jalloh MB, Pyne-Bailey S, et al. Consensus building around nutrition lessons from the 2014-16 Ebola virus disease outbreak in Guinea and Sierra Leone [Internet]. Health Policy Plan. 2019 Mar;34(2):83–91. https://doi.org/10.1093/heapol/czy108 PMID:30753437.
6. Stein J, Visco CJ, Barbuto S. Rehabilitation medicine response to the COVID-19 pandemic [Internet]. Am J Phys Med Rehabil. 2020 Jul;99(7):573–9. https://doi.org/10.1097/PHM.0000000000001470 PMID:32433243.
7. Doubova SV, Arsenault C, Contreras-Sánchez SE, Borrayo-Sánchez G, Leslie HH. The road to recovery: an interrupted time series analysis of policy intervention to restore essential health services in Mexico during the COVID-19 pandemic [Internet]. J Glob Health. 2022 Jul;12:05033. https://doi.org/10.7189/jogh.12.05033 PMID:35866236.
8. Clarke A, Blidi N, Yokie J, Momolu M, Agbo C, Tuopileyi R, et al. Strengthening immunization service delivery post Ebola virus disease (EVD) outbreak in Liberia 2015-2017 [Internet]. Pan Afr Med J. 2019 May;33 Suppl 2:5. https://doi.org/10.11604/pamj.supp.2019.33.2.17116 PMID:31402965.
9. Barie PS, Ho VP, Hunter CJ, Kaufman EJ, Narayan M, Pieracci FM, et al. Surgical infection society guidance for restoration of surgical services during the coronavirus disease-2019 pandemic [Internet]. Surg Infect (Larchmt). 2021 Oct;22(8):818–27. https://doi.org/10.1089/sur.2020.421 PMID:33635145.
10. Cholera Outbreaks in Central and West Africa: 2017 Regional Update - Week 52 [Internet]. 2018. https://reliefweb.int/report/democratic-republic-congo/cholera-outbreaks-central-and-west-africa-2017-regional-update-19.
11. Parpia AS, Ndeffo-Mbah ML, Wenzel NS, Galvani AP. Effects of response to 2014–2015 Ebola outbreak on deaths from malaria, HIV/AIDS, and tuberculosis, West Africa [Internet]. Emerg Infect Dis. 2016 Mar;22(3):433–41. https://doi.org/10.3201/eid2203.150977 PMID:26886846.
12. Sud A, Torr B, Jones ME, Broggio J, Scott S, Loveday C, et al. Effect of delays in the 2-week-wait cancer referral pathway during the COVID-19 pandemic on cancer survival in the UK: a modelling study [Internet]. Lancet Oncol. 2020 Aug;21(8):1035–44. https://doi.org/10.1016/S1470-2045(20)30392-2 PMID:32702311.

13. Chen S, Zhang P, Zhang Y, Fung H, Han Y, Law CK, et al. Coordinated management of COVID-19 response: lessons from whole-of-society and whole-of-health strategies in Wuhan, China [Internet]. Front Public Health. 2021 Aug;9:664214. https://doi.org/10.3389/fpubh.2021.664214 PMID:34414153.
14. Trump BD, Bridges TS, Cegan JC, Cibulsky SM, Greer SL, Jarman H, et al. An analytical perspective on pandemic recovery [Internet]. Health Secur. 2020;18(3):250–6. https://doi.org/10.1089/hs.2020.0057 PMID:32525747.
15. Elliott J, Whitaker M, Bodinier B, Eales O, Riley S, Ward H, et al. Predictive symptoms for COVID-19 in the community: REACT-1 study of over 1 million people. PLoS Med [Internet]. 2021 Sep 28;18(9):e1003777. https://doi.org/10.1371/journal.pmed.1003777 PMID: 34582457.
16. Disease Prevention EC. Control. COVID-19 surveillance guidance [Internet]. Stockholm; 2021. https://www.ecdc.europa.eu/en/publications-data/covid-19-surveillance-guidance.
17. Chen Z, Azman AS, Chen X, Zou J, Tian Y, Sun R, et al. Global landscape of SARS-CoV-2 genomic surveillance and data sharing [Internet]. Nat Genet. 2022 Apr;54(4):499–507. https://doi.org/10.1038/s41588-022-01033-y PMID:35347305.
18. Sydenstricker E. The incidence of influenza among persons of different economic status during the epidemic of 1918. Public Health Reports (1896-1970) [Internet]. 1931;46(4):154. https://doi.org/10.2307/4579923.
19. Marmot M, Allen J, Goldblatt P, Herd E, Morrison J. Build back fairer: the COVID-19 Marmot review [Internet]. Institute of Health Equity; 2020. https://www.instituteofhealthequity.org/resources-reports/build-back-fairer-the-covid-19-marmot-review.
20. Lowcock EC, Rosella LC, Foisy J, McGeer A, Crowcroft N. The social determinants of health and pandemic H1N1 2009 influenza severity [Internet]. Am J Public Health. 2012 Aug;102(8):e51–8. https://doi.org/10.2105/AJPH.2012.300814 PMID:22698024.
21. Hefferon C, Taylor C, Bennett D, Falconer C, Campbell M, Williams JG, et al. Priorities for the child public health response to the COVID-19 pandemic recovery in England [Internet]. Arch Dis Child. 2021 Jun;106(6):533–8. https://doi.org/10.1136/archdischild-2020-320214 PMID:33298551.
22. McCartney G, Douglas M, Taulbut M, Katikireddi SV, McKee M. Tackling population health challenges as we build back from the pandemic [Internet]. BMJ. 2021 Dec;375:e066232. https://doi.org/10.1136/bmj-2021-066232 PMID:34876411.
23. World Health Organization. After Action Review of the Ebola outbreak in the Democratic Republic of Congo [Internet]. 2021. https://www.who.int/about/accountability/results/who-results-report-2020-mtr/country-story/2021/democratic-republic-of-congo.
24. Eastern UN, Office SA. Ebola Virus Disease UNICEF Eastern and Southern Africa Regional Office Preparedness and Response in Priority Eastern and Southern Africa Countries 2018–2020 [Internet]. 2020. https://www.unicef.org/esa/reports/ebola-virus-disease.
25. The Global Practice of After Action Review [Internet]. 2019. https://www.who.int/publications/i/item/WHO-WHE-CPI-2019.9.
26. World Health Organization. Guidance for Conducting a Country Covid-19 Intra-Action Review (IAR [Internet]. 2020. https://www.who.int/publications/i/item/WHO-2019-nCoV-Country_IAR-2020.1.
27. Provera B, Montefusco A, Canato AA. A 'no blame' approach to organizational learning [Internet]. Br J Manage. 2010 Nov;21(4):1057–74. https://doi.org/10.1111/j.1467-8551.2008.00599.x.
28. Elmqvist KO, Rigaudy MT, Vink JP. Creating a no-blame culture through medical education: a UK perspective. J Multidiscip Healthc. 2016 Aug;9:345–6. https://doi.org/10.2147/JMDH.S111813 PMID:27540298.
29. Serrat OD. Conducting After-Action Reviews and Retrospects. Knowledge Solutions [Internet]. 2008. https://www.adb.org/publications/conducting-after-action-reviews-and-retrospects.
30. Côté SM, Geoffroy MC, Haeck C, Ouellet-Morin I, Larose S, Chadi N, et al. Understanding and attenuating pandemic-related disruptions: a plan to reduce inequalities in child development [Internet]. Can J Public Health. 2022 Feb;113(1):23–35. https://doi.org/10.17269/s41997-021-00584-7 PMID:35089591.
31. World Health Organization. WHO Manifesto for a healthy recovery from COVID-19 [Internet]. 2020. https://www.who.int/news-room/feature-stories/detail/who-manifesto-for-a-healthy-recovery-from-covid-19.
32. Sacco PL, De Domenico M. Public health challenges and opportunities after COVID-19. Bull World Health Organ. 2021 Jul;99(7):529–35. https://doi.org/10.2471/BLT.20.267757 PMID:34248225.
33. Abramowitz SA, McLean KE, McKune SL, Bardosh KL, Fallah M, Monger J, et al. Community-centered responses to Ebola in urban Liberia: the view from below [Internet]. PLoS Negl Trop Dis. 2015 Apr;9(4):e0003706. https://doi.org/10.1371/journal.pntd.0003706 PMID:25856072.

CHAPTER 37

CAPACITY BUILDING THROUGH STAKEHOLDER TRAINING

by Renée Christensen, Paul Effler, Ashley Greiner, and Sharon Salmon

An adequately trained multidisciplinary workforce is essential to the success of any outbreak response and therefore fundamental in long-term preparedness efforts. In recognition of the critically important role that training plays in a public health emergency response, international organisations, public health institutes, and governments around the world continue to invest in designing and delivering outbreak response trainings. However, these trainings can vary in quality and utility. In this chapter, we explore the different contexts of outbreak response training and present the best practice approaches for designing and delivering outbreak and public health emergency response trainings to the highest standards.

INTRODUCTION

A trained multidisciplinary workforce is essential to the success of any outbreak response. Recognising the need to have ample capacity to respond promptly and effectively to public health risks, as detailed in the International Health Regulations (2005) (1), public health institutions and emergency response agencies around the world continue to invest in building a well-trained and interoperable public health emergency workforce. Lessons learned from a diversity of outbreak responses have indicated the need for specific multidisciplinary workforce competencies including key technical skills, foundational or soft skills, and leadership skills, to efficiently and effectively respond to the demanding and quickly evolving needs during an outbreak response. Whether designing a technical specialty training—such as Field Epidemiology Training Programmes (FETPs) (2), Rapid Response Team training (3), or disease-specific training (4)—or a course designed to enhance cross-cutting foundational skills required for successful multidisciplinary outbreak response (5), all should be tailored to meet the specific learning needs of each target audience. They should be designed, delivered, and evaluated following adult learning best practices most appropriate to the training delivery context.

THE DIFFERENT CONTEXTS OF OUTBREAK RESPONSE TRAINING

For the purposes of this chapter, outbreak response training refers to targeted learning interventions designed to build a specific skill or ability of a public health professional for adaptation and application in an outbreak response setting. Different from a formal academic programme, such as an undergraduate or postgraduate degree or diploma, outbreak response training programmes generally consist of one or more hands-on practical learning opportunities designed to complement the learner's academic qualifications and technical expertise.

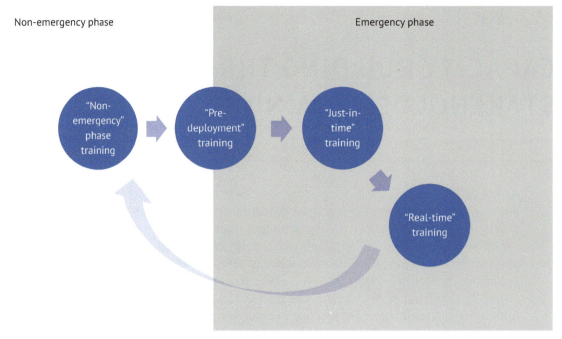

Figure 37.1: Contexts for outbreak response training

Depending upon the needs and content, outbreak response training generally takes place during four different contexts as illustrated in **Figure 37.1**. It can be initiated during:
- the non-emergency phase
- "pre-deployment" (**See "Non-emergency" phase training** in **Table 37.1**) which can be outside or within an emergency phase
- the early stage of a response "just-in-time" training
- an ongoing response "real-time" training (**See "Real-time" training** below)

	"Non-emergency" phase training	"Pre-deployment" training"	"Just-in-time" training	"Real-time" training
When does the training take place?	When there is no ongoing emergency response.	Usually in the non-emergency phase. Can also take place in the early stages of the emergency response phase.	Usually during the early stages of the emergency response phase.	Anytime during the emergency response phase.
Context	• This is the ideal stage for an outbreak response training to take place, with adequate time and space to design and deliver quality training.	• Generally, a standardised training for select public health experts who are likely to deploy to a future outbreak response (7–8).	• Generally, a bespoke training tailored to the specific emergency occurring (9).	• Generally, a knowledge or skill-based training designed and developed urgently with the purpose of immediately addressing specific gaps (e.g., often

"Non-emergency" phase training	"Pre-deployment" training	"Just-in-time" training	"Real-time" training
• Training types may include preparedness and/or readiness training for a known public health emergency threat, or a refresher training for seasoned responders (3). May also include exercises—either simulation or tabletop—to practise and/or test relevant competencies, or a new/revised training designed to address lessons learned from a previous outbreak response (6).	• This may include members of local provincial, national, or international rapid response teams, or surge capacity response rosters. • In large-scale emergency responses or protracted crises, pre-deployment training may also occur during the emergency response phase to train new responders before they join the ongoing emergency response. In this case, the pre-deployment training may also be referred to as "just-in-time" training.	• This may include training on a particular disease or specialised technical skill, or capacity required for the specific response. • In large-scale emergency responses, or protracted crises with a high turnover of staff, this may also include pre-deployment training for additional surge capacity.	skills-based training targeted to healthcare workers), the scope of which may continue to change over the course of the emergency response as the information and/or needs continue to change (4).

Table 37.1: Description of the contexts for outbreak response training

DESIGNING OUTBREAK RESPONSE TRAINING

Regardless of the type of outbreak response training being developed, it is essential that it be founded on public health emergency training best practices and adult learning theories. This approach can be used to define the learning priorities and activities (10), while helping to ensure learning outcomes are measurable and the learning intervention remains flexible and adaptable to the training environment.

Effective outbreak response training is framed on the key adult learning principles of andragogy, which is based on learner-led and learner-centred instruction (10). Expanding beyond traditional pedagogical teacher-centred approaches, which are often employed in formal education settings for less-experienced learners, andragogy principles recognise that adult learners bring with them their own knowledge and experience that shape their way of thinking and performing, as well as their motivation and readiness for learning (11). As such, outbreak response trainings following andragogy methodologies are designed to take into consideration personal learning style and tend to be more self-directed and collaborative while emphasising experiential learning (i.e., learning by doing and limiting/excluding didactic presentations) (12).

Another key feature of quality outbreak response training programmes is that they are often competency based. Competency refers to a person's capability to integrate and apply select knowledge, skills, and attitudes necessary to successfully perform a specific task in a given context (13). Recognised as a best practice approach to outbreak response training, many international organisations including the Global Outbreak Alert and Response Network (GOARN), the U.S. Centers for Disease Control and Prevention (U.S. CDC), the African Union's Africa Centres for Disease Control and Prevention, and numerous FETPs have developed competency-based training programmes (3,5,14) with bespoke curricula intended to build and assess specific competencies expected of public health emergency responders.

Given the diversity of roles needed during an outbreak response, ensuring a multidisciplinary perspective in any technical training is key. In addition to typical responder roles (e.g., epidemiologist, case manager, etc.), delineating the specific skills needed in an outbreak is critical to ensuring a curriculum that comprehensively addresses the common demands in an outbreak response. For example, epidemiologists' skill sets may range from in-depth statistical analyses, to setting up an emergency surveillance system, to conducting household surveys. Thus, designing a cross-cutting training programme to fulfil common field emergency epidemiology skills (e.g., data management, contact tracing, emergency surveillance, etc.) will be more useful than a training programme on general epidemiology.

Real-time training: Ebola virus disease (EBOD) care for the community in Liberia

In Liberia in September 2014, EBOD cases sharply increased causing an alarming concern regarding hospital and treatment centre bed availability. It was inevitable that infected individuals would need to be cared for at home or in community care centres, which were established in otherwise non-functioning hospitals, schools, and sporting arenas.

Led by the Liberian Ministry of Health and Social Welfare, a community infection prevention and control (IPC) strategy was developed. The strategy would identify community volunteers who would go from house to house, providing education and checking for ill people.

To support the community volunteers, a training programme was developed. Training guides included graphics and texts explaining how to minimise household transmission when an ill person was there. Around 250 trainers from various religious and non-governmental organisations were initially trained. They, in turn, trained and oversaw the community volunteers with the capacity of reaching the Liberian population at large. Training was provided by influential community leaders and included practical sessions to demonstrate chlorine concentrations for environment disinfection, handwashing, and hand protection when gloves are unavailable. To expect the community to use hospital-grade personal protective equipment (PPE) is unrealistic. Wearing PPE can become dangerous because of dehydration and overheating in the community living environment in Liberia, and to remove it safely is difficult. Practical training with locally-adapted solutions to educate and protect the community was paramount.

Non-emergency phase training provided by GOARN

For over 20 years, GOARN has been a leader in the coordination of international outbreak response. The cumulative experience of GOARN's extensive engagement in public health response has highlighted the need to complement the significant levels of existing technical expertise with additional foundational or soft skill competencies for effective multidisciplinary outbreak response.

Building upon the many highly regarded and longstanding technical training programmes, over the last decade, the World Health Organization (WHO) and other GOARN partners from across the globe collaborated to create and implement an evolving soft skill competency-based GOARN Capacity Building and Training Programme. This uniquely collaborative and needs-driven programme, collectively purpose-built by many of the world's leading public health institutions, is a robust multifaceted three-tiered programme that aims to prepare individuals from all public health disciplines to work effectively in the field in support of outbreak responses.

Tier 1 of the programme introduces the basic essentials for pre-deployment through a series of online self-directed courses, as well as more advanced 1–2-day classroom-based workshops and in-service public health courses such as FETPs. Tier 2 is an immersive, long-standing, 5-day outbreak response scenario-driven simulation exercise that serves as a field adaptation training, intensively exploring the realities and challenges of working in an international multidisciplinary outbreak response team trying to stop an evolving outbreak and designed to build the critical soft skill core competencies required of international outbreak responders. Tier 3 includes specialised outbreak response leadership training for highly experienced responders to build the individual and collective leadership and crisis management skills of deployees to act as influential and trusted leaders during public health emergencies.

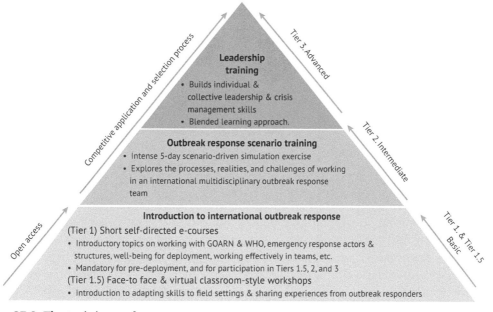

Figure 37.2: The training cycle

While many training programmes focus on addressing these technical competencies for specific public health and emergency functions, there is increasing recognition of the critical importance of complementing outbreak responders' technical expertise with additional foundational or soft skill competencies, including how to communicate effectively, foster teamwork, demonstrate flexibility in quickly evolving situations, and respect individual and cultural diversity (5). Refer to "**Non-emergency phase training**" for an example of a soft skill competency-based outbreak response training programme developed by GOARN (5,15) and "**Crafting SMART learning outcomes**" for a competency-based example with corresponding behavioural indicators and subsequent learning outcomes for use in a training.

DESIGNING NEEDS-BASED OUTBREAK RESPONSE TRAINING

The practice of creating and implementing outbreak response training is a cyclical process that progresses through an analysis of learning needs, designing, developing, delivering, and evaluating the training, followed by revision as required based on the training evaluation and emerging learning needs.

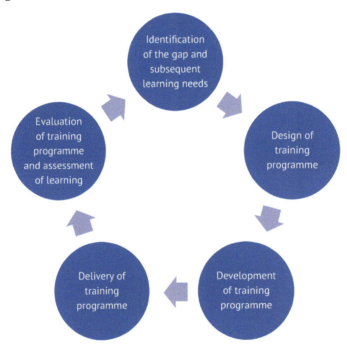

Figure 37.3: The training cycle

Once a gap in response capacity has been identified and a training intervention is determined to be the best way to fill the gap, learning needs can be identified and desired outcomes can be developed. A learning outcome is a statement of what the learner is expected to gain—knowledge, skill, attitude, or behaviour—as a result of the learning process. In this first step, it is important to distinguish between a "training aim" and a "learning outcome". A training aim refers to the purpose of a course to the overall goal you want to accomplish in your outbreak response training. It is usually a broad statement of what will be achieved and is used to concisely describe the course. A learning outcome is a breakdown of this aim that is actionable and measurable. It is the sum of all these learning outcomes that will contribute to participants meeting the aim of the outbreak response training course. The importance of crafting needs-based and SMART (Specific, Measurable, Achievable, Relevant, and Timely) learning outcomes cannot be overstated. Well-written learning outcomes tell the trainers what they will teach, the participants what they will learn, and any observers/donors what will be accomplished in the training programme. In general, there are four components of a learning outcome:

- **Audience (A)** – the learners of the training activity. Often referred to as participants or students.
- **Behaviour (B)** – what will the audience be able to do as a result of their participation in the training activity? This should be clearly observable and measurable behaviour.
- **Condition (C)** – the circumstances or context in which the learning will occur. This can be a training session, training event, activity, etc.
- **Degree of achievement (D)** – the standard of which the behaviour will be performed.

The Behaviour, or action verb, is the most important element of a learning outcome and can never be omitted, as it states precisely what the participant will be able to do after the instructional activity. These verbs are categorised by domains of learning and various hierarchies, such as Bloom's Taxonomy (16). Typically, learning outcomes are written in the order of **CABD**. As the Condition and the Audience of a training event are usually the same for each session, often the learning outcomes of a session are phrased as "At the end of this training session, participants will be able to...", with a list of a few bullet points following that include the measurable verb Behaviour and a corresponding Degree of achievement. Once the learning needs and outcomes have been defined, the outbreak response training programme curriculum can be designed, and a training course subsequently developed and delivered.

Table 37.2 provides examples of crafting SMART learning outcomes associated with building and assessing competencies and their behavioural indicators.

Using the CABD approach to build and assess specific competencies and behavioural indicators		
The relationship between competency, behavioural indicators, and sample learning outcomes is illustrated below. Mastery of the learning outcomes combines to demonstrate confidence that the participant will be able to exhibit the relevant behavioural indicators of a desired competency.		
Example of competency	**Example of behavioural indicators for this competency**	**Example of SMART learning outcomes crafted to build and assess mastery of the associated behavioural indicators for this competency**
	By the end of this training, participants will be able to:	
Respecting and promoting individual and cultural differences	Understand and respect cultural and gender issues and apply this to daily work and decision-making.	**Examine** an outbreak or health emergency response for cultural and gender issues. **Draft** interventions to mitigate cultural and gender issues as part of outbreak or public health emergency response.

Example of competency	Example of behavioural indicators for this competency	Example of SMART learning outcomes crafted to build and assess mastery of the associated behavioural indicators for this competency
	Relate and work well with people of different cultures, genders, and backgrounds.	**Recognise** common traits between people of different cultures, genders, and backgrounds. **Exhibit** the ability to work well with people of different cultures, genders, and backgrounds in response to an outbreak or public health emergency.
	Examine own behaviour and attitudes to avoid stereotypical responses.	**Reflect** on one's own behaviour, considering how others could interpret words or actions. **Demonstrate** awareness of the perspectives of others, through both verbal and non-verbal actions.
	Draw on diversity of skills, backgrounds, and knowledge of people to achieve more effective results.	**Explain** the benefits of combining the diversity of skills, backgrounds, and knowledge of people to achieve more effective results. **Formulate** interventions to outbreak and public health emergency response that draw upon the diversity of skills, backgrounds, and knowledge of relevant stakeholders.

Table 37.2: Crafting SMART learning outcomes for building and assessing competencies

The final step of the training cycle is evaluation. This essential activity measures the overall success of a training and is needed to ensure that learning outcomes are appropriate and have indeed been achieved. The evaluation provides feedback on how the training course was received by participants, the extent of their learning and retention, the appropriateness and effectiveness of the instructional processes, and the impact of the training course on the participants and their institutions or workplaces, and further identifies areas that are either missing or needing revision. A commonly applied and widely recognised evaluation framework used by major public health institutions leading outbreak response training is the Kirkpatrick model (5,17). The four levels of training evaluation in the Kirkpatrick model are formative, and summative assessments applied before, during, and after a learning intervention are intended to assess the effectiveness of the training, and can help inform what value it adds to outbreak response capacity. As depicted in **Figure 37.4**, while each level of evaluation adds greater insight into the value and impact of the training, it also becomes more complex in methodology to undertake.

As the training cycle continues, it is essential that any recommendations captured during evaluations are continually incorporated into the outbreak response course for future iterations, along with efforts to address any gaps identified or lessons learned from other public health preparedness and response assessments, including relevant After-Action Reviews (3,18) or Joint External Evaluations (1). Furthermore, for outbreak response training, ongoing identification of gaps and subsequent learning needs analyses should take advantage of opportunities before a crisis, for example by "testing" competencies in a planned exercise as a skills-drill, tabletop, or full-scale simulation. During ongoing or protracted emergencies, respectively, capacity gaps and learning needs analysis can continue to be undertaken through post-deployment responder briefs (if applicable) or intra-action reviews which may offer useful insight into real-time training content as well.

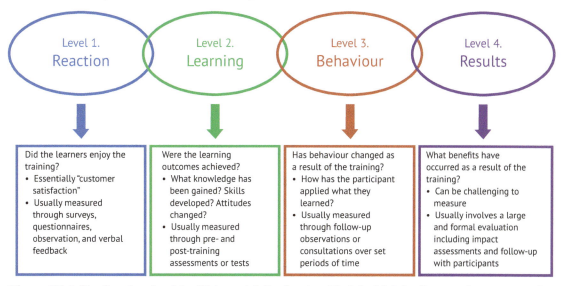

Figure 37.4: The four levels of the Kirkpatrick Evaluation Model which is often used to measure the success of outbreak response training

SELECTING TRAINING MODALITIES

There are many factors to consider when selecting the most appropriate instructional design approaches and teaching and learning modalities when developing an outbreak response training package. Following the best practices of adult learning as described above, an effective outbreak response training package needs to cater to the various preferred learning styles of the participants' (e.g., visual, auditory, kinaesthetic, etc.), encourage learner autonomy, appeal to the participants motivation for learning, and utilise and build upon the knowledge and experience the participants bring to the training as public health professionals. At the same time, this needs to be balanced with the reality of resources available to design and deliver the training. Different modalities, and combinations of modalities, will be best suited for use in different outbreak response trainings depending on the following:
- the available financial and human resources
- the electronic resources and information technology available
- the timeframe for both design and delivery of the training
- the scale and reach of participants needing to be trained
- the availability of participants to attend the training
- the ability to source/prepare necessary training faculties

- the desired frequency of the training
- the operational context of the training (i.e., non-emergency vs emergency phase, low- or high-resource setting, etc.)

Table 37.3 provides an overview of commonly employed training modalities along with their advantages and limitations for use in outbreak response training.

TRACKING AND TRAINING AND GRADUATES

Training of the emergency workforce alone is not sufficient to be prepared for an outbreak response. Developing a system to record, track, and update a trained *and* rostered workforce is critical to quickly identify staff with the necessary skills to address the specific outbreak or public health emergency. Tracking training, dates, skills, and evaluative elements, possibly in a searchable database, should be considered as part of the critical operations to ensure training translates into a ready workforce that can be quickly activated during an emergency.

Additionally, outbreak response training is often a key activity that the emergency workforce delivers in response to a variety of multisectoral stakeholders including healthcare workers, community representatives, etc. Tracking the delivery of these trainings, particularly who was trained and from what institutions, can help enable training the trainer models and leveraging that workforce in future public health emergencies, along with identifying gaps in the different workforces that can be targeted and addressed during the non-emergency phase in particular.

CONCLUSION

Quality training of public health emergency response personnel plays a critically important role in enhancing the effectiveness of an outbreak response. It is therefore imperative that key principles of adult learning (andragogy) and best practices in instructional design are incorporated in the development and delivery of future outbreak response training packages. Adopting this approach will help maximise their impact and ultimately assist in demonstrating the value of training to enhance local, national, and global public health emergency response capacity.

Key takeaways for consideration when designing and delivering outbreak response training are:
- Follow best practices of adult learning and where possible, avoid didactic learning instruction.
- Keep in mind the context and practicalities for the delivery of the outbreak response training.
- Know your target audience. What are their educational, resource, and literacy levels, as well as time and other constraints? Ensure that their participation in the outbreak response training is indeed the best use of their time (particularly in the emergency phase).
- Consider the need and appropriate use of incentives for engaging training participants in specific contexts (e.g., transportation to/from training venue, meals, accommodation, per diems, etc.) which may or may not be suitable depending upon the local culture and institutional policies of stakeholders delivering or supporting the training.

	What is it?	How is it delivered?	Advantages	Limitations	Contexts of use
Online training (e-learning)	Training that takes place virtually over a computer, smartphone, or other device.	• Usually delivered remotely through a type of learning management system, learner experience platform, or massive open online course platform. • Can be self-directed asynchronous learning (self-directed courses) or instructor-led synchronous learning (real-time facilitated learning).	• Can reach a much larger and dispersed audience. • Cost-effective, repeatable, and allows instant updating of content. • Useful training modality when travel is not possible. • Asynchronous training allows maximum flexibility for learners. • Synchronous learning can enable interaction and collaboration between the instructor, learner, and peers.	• Limited social interaction between instructor, learners, and peers. • Risk of online learning fatigue and lack of learning retention. • Requires learners to have access to online technology. • Most appropriate for knowledge-based content, considered less effective for training technical and/or soft skills.	• Commonly used across nearly all types and contexts of outbreak response training, in its entirety or part of a blended training programme (see below). • Asynchronous microlearning can be effectively used to provide up-to-date guidance and knowledge-based learning in real-time during rapidly changing emergencies (4).
Face-to-face learning	Training that takes place with instructors and learners in the same place at the same time.	• Usually delivered in a classroom setting in the form of a workshop or simulation exercise.	• Facilitates strong social interactions between instructor, learners, and peers. • Enables flexibility of the instructor to adapt as needed. • Can cater to more learning styles and facilitates additional learning and assessment through the use of body language, voice, etc.	• Can be costly to implement. • Lack of flexibility for the timing of attendance and pace of learning.	• Commonly used in training during non-crisis periods, and as part of a blended training programme (see below). • Also used frequently for training on specific technical skills, often at the local level during the emergency phase.

	What is it?	How is it delivered?	Advantages	Limitations	Contexts of use
Blended learning	Combination of self-directed and instructor-led training modalities.	• Most generally occur with asynchronous e-learning tasks followed by face-to-face or virtual instructor-led training.	• Use of different modalities appeals to more preferred learning styles and can facilitate learning reinforcement and retention. • Can also be cost-effective, reducing face-to-face training time.	• Can have a tendency to overload learners with online self-directed training before the instructor-led component (See limitations of online training and face-to-face learning).	• Commonly used across outbreak response trainings. • May be used less in time-poor settings such as training during an emergency phase.
Simulation exercises (SimEx)	Scenarios are used to simulate specific situations and assess how a learner responds.	• Can be face-to-face with roleplayers or implemented remotely using a virtual simulation platform. • Outbreak response trainings also often use tabletop exercises which involve discussions of scenarios and case studies without roleplay.	• As a form of experiential learning, the SimEx modality is highly effective at teaching and assessing a wide range of skills in a safe and controlled environment. • It fosters teamwork and is generally appealing and engaging to adult learners.	• Can be costly to implement and may require large numbers of role players. • The "reality" of the scenario or simulation setting can be challenging to create. • Requires faculty to have sound debriefing skills, as that is where the critical learning takes place.	• Used often in non-crisis periods to test outbreak response systems and procedures, as well as in pre-deployment and team building trainings. • Also used in the emergency phase as an effective means to train and test specific technical skills required for the response (19). • Also often referred to as skills stations or drills.

	What is it?	How is it delivered?	Advantages	Limitations	Contexts of use
Serious gaming	Interactive game instructionally designed for education purposes.	• Can be online in a player versus environment or player versus player format. • Can also be in an offline format.	• Serious gaming is increasingly being regarded as one of the most effective and motivating tools for learning (20). • Learner has flexible access, receives rapid feedback, and has the opportunity to improve and apply learning repetitively. • Online serious games also have the capacity to reach many learners.	• Expensive and time-consuming to create. • Online serious gaming requires the learner to have adequate access to online technology.	• Aspects of gamification are commonly included in outbreak response training. • However, online serious gaming is a relatively new modality, with international networks like GOARN exploring usage for widespread outbreak response training (5).
Virtual/ augmented reality	Interactive experiences in a computer-generated environment (virtual reality) or combination of real-world and computer-generated content (augmented reality).	• Virtual reality requires the use of a specialised headset to create a computer-generated 3D environment. • Augmented reality adds interactive digital elements to the real-work environment through use of a smartphone, tablet, or headset.	• Highly interactive, engaging, motivating, and replicable. • Well suited for developing and testing an array of technical and soft skills, and for application to simulation exercises (in particular, skills training in a safe and controlled environment).	• Expensive to build and requires the use of technology devices such as smartphones, tablets, and headsets.	• Relatively new modality being used primarily in non-crisis periods for specific public health emergency function skills trainings (e.g., emergency medicine or IPC practices). • Forecast for future use in real time during emergencies (21).

What is it?	How is it delivered?	Advantages	Limitations	Contexts of use
Training of trainers (ToT)/ cascading learning	Training courses designed and delivered to train and capacitate future trainers to deliver a specific training course.	Master ToT generally delivered (either online, face-to-face, or blended), then cascaded down for the ToT graduates to then deliver the course they were trained to teach at the local levels.	• Cost-effective to simultaneously train multiple future faculties for training delivery. • Effective ToT can ensure the sustainability of a training course for ongoing and scaling up implementation.	• Often challenges with the quality of ToT, suitability of the ToT participants, and the ability of the ToT graduates to confidently and effectively deliver trainings.	• This modality is often used during the emergency phase, in order to cascade specific knowledge or skills required for the outbreak response (e.g., IPC practices) (22).

Table 37.3: Summary of training modalities commonly employed in outbreak response training

- Know your training environment. Will the training be delivered in a high- or low-resource setting? Are there likely to be interruptions to the electricity or internet? Select training modalities accordingly.
- Take advantage of the non-emergency phase and time between outbreaks. Consider if practical to prepare or conduct outbreak response trainings *before* the emergency phase occurs.
- Consider the creation of training content, packages, or toolkits that can be used in the emergency phase and easily adapted to local contexts.
- Be strategic and specific with the purpose of your training and the desired learning outcomes. In outbreak response training, one size does not fit all. Make a training too broad in the attempt to make it fit for everyone and the training is likely to become fit for no one.
- Don't reinvent the wheel. Leverage open-source materials and collaborate with other outbreak response training partners to share materials and resources where relevant.
- Ensure the full training cycle is followed, actively incorporating lessons learned from training evaluations and other assessments into future iterations to ensure ongoing quality and relevance of outbreak response training.

REFERENCES:

1. World Health Organization. IHR (2005) Monitoring and Evaluation framework, Joint External Evaluation tool (JEE tool) Reporting Template. Geneva: The Organization; 2016.
2. Jones DS, Dicker RC, Fontaine RE, Boore AL, Omolo JO, Ashgar RJ, et al. Building global epidemiology and response capacity with field epidemiology training programs. Emerg Infect Dis. 2017 Dec;23(13):S158–65. https://doi.org/10.3201/eid2313.170509 PMID:29155658.
3. Greiner AL, Stehling-Ariza T, Bugli D, Hoffman A, Giese C, Moorhouse L, et al. Challenges in public health rapid response team management. Health Secur. 2020 Jan;18 S1:S8–13. https://doi.org/10.1089/hs.2019.0060 PMID:32004121.
4. Utunen H, George R, Ndiaye N, Tokar A, Attias M, Gamhewage G. Delivering WHO's life-saving information in real-time during a pandemic through an online learning platform: evidence from global use. Stud Health Technol Inform. 2021 May;281:969–73. https://doi.org/10.3233/SHTI210322 PMID:34042817.
5. Christensen R, Fisher D, Salmon S, Drury P, Effler P. Training for outbreak response through the Global Outbreak Alert and Response Network. BMC Med. 2021 May;19(1):123. https://doi.org/10.1186/s12916-021-01996-5 PMID:33985496.
6. Stoto MA, Nelson C, Piltch-Loeb R, Mayigane LN, Copper F, Chungong S. Getting the most from after action reviews to improve global health security. Global Health. 2019; 10;15(1):58. https://doi.org/10.1186/s12992-019-0500-z.
7. Health Focus GmbH and World Health Organization (WHO), Review of the role of training in the WHO Ebola emergency response Final Report, December 2015.
8. Jacquet GA, Obi CC, Chang MP, Bayram JD. Availability and diversity of training programs for responders to international disasters and complex humanitarian emergencies. PLoS Curr. 2014 Jun;6(6):ecurrents.dis.626ae97e629eccd4756f20de04a20823. https://doi.org/10.1371/currents.dis.626ae97e629eccd4756f20de04a20823 PMID:24987573.
9. Weiner D, Rosman A. Just-in-time training for disaster response in the austere environment. Clin Pediatr Emerg Med. 2019;20(2):95–110. https://doi.org/10.1016/j.cpem.2019.07.001.
10. Mahan JD, Stein DS. Teaching adults-best practices that leverage the emerging understanding of the neurobiology of learning. Curr Probl Pediatr Adolesc Health Care. 2014 Jul;44(6):141–9. https://doi.org/10.1016/j.cppeds.2014.01.003 PMID:24981663.
11. Alinier G, Oriot D. Simulation-based education: deceiving learners with good intent. Adv Simul (Lond). 2022 Mar;7(1):8. https://doi.org/10.1186/s41077-022-00206-3 PMID:35303963.

12. Taylor DC, Hamdy H. Adult learning theories: implications for learning and teaching in medical education: AMEE Guide No. 83. Med Teach. 2013 Nov;35(11):e1561–72. https://doi.org/10.3109/0142159X.2013.828153 PMID:24004029.

13. Pirie J, Fayyaz J, Gharib M, Simone L, Glanfield C, Kempinska A. Development and implementation of a novel, mandatory competency-based medical education simulation program for pediatric emergency medicine faculty. Adv Simul (Lond). 2021 May;6(1):17. https://doi.org/10.1186/s41077-021-00170-4 PMID:33957994.

14. Traicoff DA, et al. Replicating success: developing a standard FETP curriculum. Public Health Rep. 2008;123(Suppl 1):28–34. 109. https://doi.org/10.1177/00333549081230S109.

15. Mackenzie JS, Drury P, Arthur RR, Ryan MJ, Grein T, Slattery R, et al. The Global Outbreak Alert and Response Network. Glob Public Health. 2014;9(9):1023–39. https://doi.org/10.1080/17441692.2014.951870 PMID:25186571.

16. Adams NE. Bloom's taxonomy of cognitive learning objectives. J Med Libr Assoc. 2015 Jul;103(3):152–3. https://doi.org/10.3163/1536-5050.103.3.010 PMID:26213509.

17. Ripoll-Gallardo A, Ragazzoni L, Mazzanti E, Meneghetti G, Franc JM, Costa A, et al. Residents working with Médecins Sans Frontières: training and pilot evaluation. Scand J Trauma Resusc Emerg Med. 2020 Aug;28(1):86. https://doi.org/10.1186/s13049-020-00778-x PMID:32843062.

18. Parker GW. Best practices for after-action review: turning lessons observed into lessons learned for preparedness policy. Rev Sci Tech. 2020 Aug;39(2):579–90. https://doi.org/10.20506/rst.39.2.3108 PMID:33046918.

19. Lum LH, Badaruddin H, Salmon S, Cutter J, Lim AY, Fisher D. Pandemic preparedness: nationally-led simulation to test hospital systems. Ann Acad Med Singap. 2016 Aug;45(8):332–7. https://doi.org/10.47102/annals-acadmedsg.V45N8p332 PMID:27683737.

20. Faizan A, Norlaila D, Junaidah J, Mahathir M, Noor Y, Ahmad N, et al. Mohamad Azmi. The application of online games as learning tools in education. In. 2016 International Communication, Education, Language & Social Science Conference, 2016 July 23-24, Kuala Lumpar, Malaysia.

21. Munzer BW, Khan MM, Shipman B, Mahajan P. Augmented reality in emergency medicine: a scoping review. J Med Internet Res [Internet]. 2019 Apr 17;21(4):e12368. http://dx.doi.org/10.2196/12368

22. Eardley W, Bowley D, Hunt P, Round J, Tarmey N, Williams A. Education and Ebola: initiating the cascade of emergency healthcare training. J R Army Med Corps. 2016 Jun;162(3):203–6. https://doi.org/10.1136/jramc-2014-000394 PMID:25645696.

CHAPTER 38

TILL THE NEXT PANDEMIC: NATIONAL PREPAREDNESS

by Danielle A. Thies, Carlos Navarro Colorado, and Ali S. Khan

The COVID-19 pandemic represented an acute catastrophic emergency that threatened global health security, disrupted societies, and has continued repercussions with established endemic disease, complications of long COVID, and distrust of public health. One central theme has emerged—countries were more successful in managing the COVID-19 pandemic if they responded quickly and aggressively to the outbreak and if they had both political and social trust within their borders. The evidence shows that the countries that best handled the pandemic were not necessarily wealthy or democratic. The response hinged on strong and competent leadership which focused on strengthening the community through commitment and sacrifice for the greater good. The political leaders who immediately took action and conferred with the leading health experts to direct public policy and build public trust tended to best handle the COVID-19 pandemic while minimising economic impact.

Future adequate responses will require renewed attention to pandemic preparedness as well as new ways to think about pandemic preparedness based on the lessons learned from COVID-19. Priorities are clear and lessons have been learned.

All countries must individually and collectively improve their preparedness in order to have a better response to future events. These improvements need to be deliberative by heads of state and are more likely to happen with clear national leadership, such as a dedicated national public health authority with sustained resources at the national level and the responsibility, budgetary authority, and accountability to drive preparedness across the whole-of-government and civil society, including the private sector.

INTRODUCTION

One century apart, the influenza pandemic of 1918 and the COVID-19 pandemic represent two of the most catastrophic acute emergencies that have threatened our global health security. In the interim, there have been additional pandemics due to HIV, Zika, dengue, SARS-CoV-2, and influenza, and multiple regional outbreaks suggesting that, collectively, the spillover of zoonotic pathogens, local clusters, and outbreaks has been inevitable despite national health preparedness efforts.

As we review this most recent pandemic, one central theme has emerged—countries were more successful in combating the COVID-19 pandemic if they responded quickly and aggressively to the outbreak, and if they had low corruption and high levels of political and social trust within their borders (1–3). For these pandemics that bookend the 20th century, the science of sanitation and hygiene, the principles of disease transmission, and the benefits of social distancing, wearing masks, cough etiquette, and self-isolation were nothing new. And yet, both pandemics featured mistrust in the government and scientists, refusal to wear masks, irrational ideas of disease and home remedies, hesitation to be vaccinated, and ill-advised use of drugs such as hydroxychloroquine and cleaning solutions as common elements (4).

In addition to the significant loss of life and suffering during the COVID-19 pandemic, a new generation was confronted with the reality that the social, political, educational, and economic impact of a pandemic can far outweigh and overshadow its physical and mental health impact. In a world reliant on intertwined supply chains and the movement of foreign exchange, the impact of mass shutdowns and social distancing measures can overshadow the health effects at national and global levels, well beyond the local reverberations. The same holds true for the impact on children's education (5–6).

Arguably, these restrictive measures were an unfortunate outcome of not "adequately anticipating, prioritizing and funding pandemic preparedness" (7). The COVID-19 pandemic also exposed gross inequities in public health, not just between countries and their varying ability to obtain personal protective equipment (PPE) or vaccines, but also within countries among under-resourced communities. Future adequate responses will require renewed attention to pandemic preparedness and new ways to think about pandemic preparedness based on the lessons learned from COVID-19.

REAL-WORLD EVIDENCE AS LESSONS FOR FUTURE PREPAREDNESS

Not unlike prior global pandemics or regional outbreaks, with severe acute respiratory syndrome (SARS) as a sole inspirational outlier, the global death toll of COVID-19 and ongoing toll were due to a set of cascading national and multilateral failures. These include failures in prevention, rationality, transparency, following established public health practice, operational cooperation, and international solidarity (8). However, it is difficult to neatly characterise countries that did well versus those that did not without accounting for the time of the assessment and the choice of metrics of an excellent response. While collective excess mortality may appear to be the ideal metric to measure the effectiveness of the response, there are other more comprehensive measures, such as the Bloomberg Resilience Index, that include reopening progress, vaccine doses per 100, lockdown severity, flight capacity, vaccinated travel routes, COVID-19 status rating based on monthly cases per 100,000, monthly fatality rate, and total death per one million, as well as quality of life indicators including community mobility, gross domestic product (GDP) growth forecast, universal health coverage (UHC), and the human development index (9). Similarly, countries such as China which did extremely well in limiting excess mortality in the early two years of the pandemic—at great societal cost—did poorly when the country abandoned all public health measures without ensuring universal vaccination with an effective vaccine, leading to one million deaths within months (10).

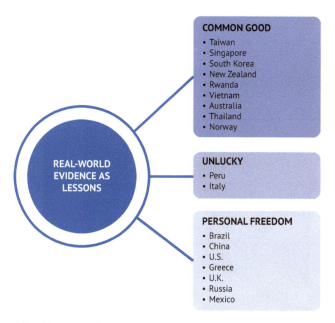

Figure 38.1: Real-world evidence as lessons
Nine countries categorised as "Common Good", two countries categorised as "Unlucky", and seven countries categorised as "Personal Freedom" (1,3,8–12).

Recognising that measuring the response from real-world evidence is very dynamic in nature, the following are some observations based on excess mortality and emerging data that demonstrate that an effective response that limits cases in a community can lead to minimal disruptions in commercial activities and learning.

Common good

As seen in **Figure 38.1** and **Figure 38.6**, there are plenty of data on the outcomes of COVID-19 by country (1,3,11–15). The evidence clearly shows that the countries that best handled the pandemic were not necessarily wealthy or democratic. The response hinged on strong and competent leadership which focused on strengthening the community through commitment and sacrifice for the common good. There is a strong correlation between the political leaders who immediately took action and conferred with the leading health experts to direct public policy and had high levels of government and social trust, as well as lower levels of government corruption, with lower COVID-19 infection rates around the world (1,3,12,16).

Personal freedom

A common theme from countries that had poor outcomes from the COVID-19 pandemic is leaders, often authoritarian, who denied the effects and severity of the coronavirus and were dismissive of public health measures and science in general. They often delayed their responses to COVID-19 because they could not face the reality of the looming pandemic or erroneously believed that saving lives was incompatible with protecting the economy.

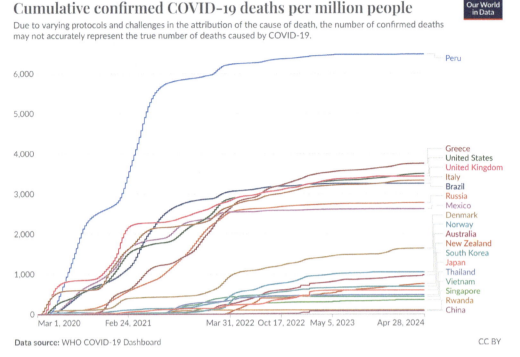

Figure 38.2: Cumulative confirmed COVID-19 deaths per million people in selected countries from **Figure 38.1** and **Figure 38.6** (16)

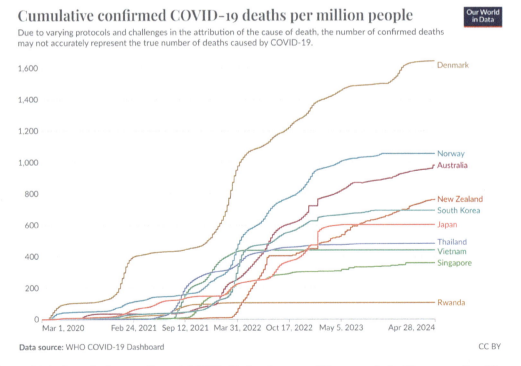

Figure 38.3: Cumulative confirmed COVID-19 deaths per million people in "Common Good" countries (16)

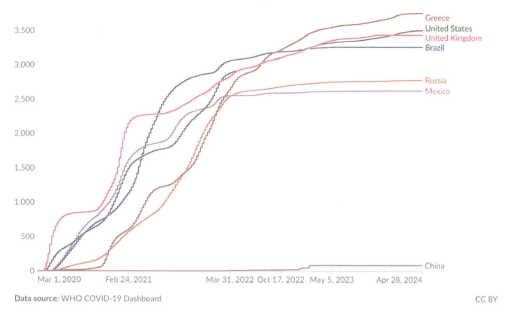

Figure 38.4: Cumulative confirmed COVID-19 deaths per million people in "Personal Freedom" countries (16)

An interesting case study is the national policies of Sweden which are often touted as following the common good approach.

> **Sweden and the Nordic countries**
>
> In an effort to protect its economy, Sweden promoted less restrictive COVID-19 measures and did not call for national lockdowns. As seen in **Figure 38.5**, Sweden surpassed all other Nordic countries in COVID-19 deaths per million people. Moreover, there was no clear benefit to its economy, at least in the short term (17–18).

The U.S. also presents an interesting case study. From the beginning of February to the end of March 2020, U.S. President Donald Trump publicly minimised the threat of COVID-19 by comparing it to the flu at least 15 times (15), the sort of risk minimisation that led to poorer outcomes in many countries, including the U.S. and Brazil. However, while American leadership failed in this dimension, the U.S. led the world in ingenuity. Operation Warp Speed was a highly successful vaccine initiative fuelled by US$ 14 billion from the federal government with no guarantees of success. This allowed for the creation and approval of innovative COVID-19 vaccines which became available within a year of the start of the pandemic (19–20) and saved millions of lives in the U.S. and worldwide (21). Incidentally, the

U.S. topped the COVID Resilience Ranking with its initial and rapid vaccination campaign. There is now a call for a similar initiative against long COVID which could lead to a better understanding of its risk factors (22). The effects of long COVID continue to impact millions of people in the U.S. As of January 2023, an estimated 65 million people worldwide may have long COVID (23).

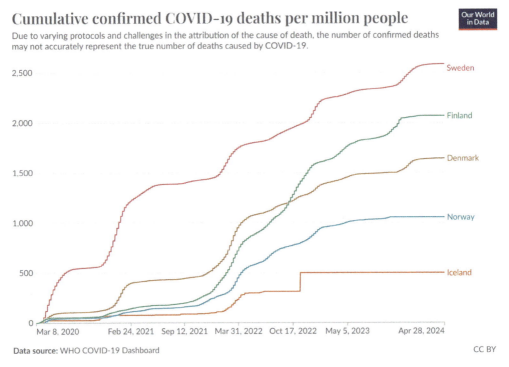

Figure 38.5: Cumulative confirmed COVID-19 deaths per million people in the Nordic countries (16)

Unlucky

This category includes countries that had extensive transmission, usually following a superspreading and supermixing event, often early in the outbreak (e.g., Italy in conjunction with a Champion's league football match). Peru was also very unfortunate when COVID-19 infected a very large, isolated population in an area with few hospitals and lack of oxygen supplies, coupled with a delay in instituting public health measures. Measures like lockdowns are impossible to implement in countries with a large informal workforce and no government unemployment pay. Conversely, there may have been many countries that were "lucky" despite a lack of preparedness due to demographics (e.g., a younger, healthier population) and societal factors (e.g., few long-term care facilities with the elderly in high-density housing) (1,3,8,23–37).

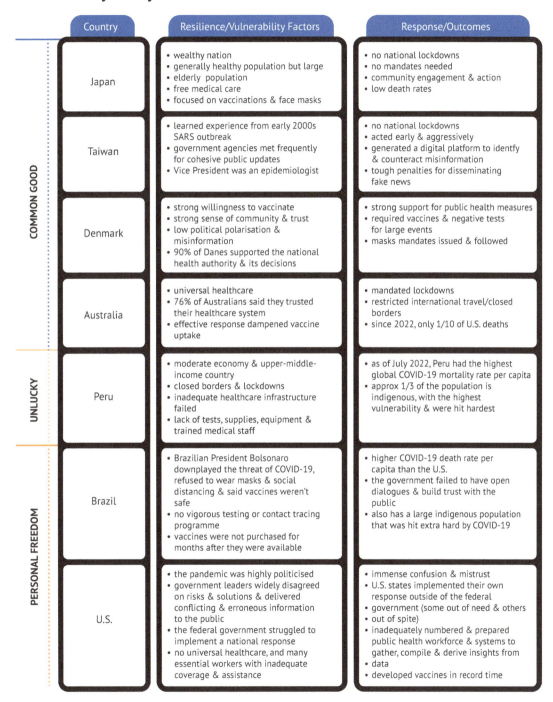

Figure 38.6: Analysis of COVID-19 response of select countries by resilience/vulnerability factors and responses/outcomes

RETHINKING MEASURES AND ELEMENTS OF PREPAREDNESS

The Global Health Security Agenda

The COVID-19 pandemic exposed profound deficiencies and disparities in pandemic response across the globe despite over a decade of focused support. The Global Health Security Agenda (GHSA) was launched in 2014 and has international and non-governmental organisations and private sector companies in more than 70 countries working to secure global health security. It is focused on capacity-building for the detection, prevention, and active responses to threats. As of 2018, the U.S. government alone had already spent almost US$ 1 billion supporting these activities (38). That same year, all parties agreed to the next phase (GHSA 2024) which encourages countries to strengthen their national global health security efforts and complete the Joint External Evaluation (JEE), achieving a score of at least four out of five in a minimum of five technical areas (39).

The deficiencies and within-country disparities were no more evident than in the U.S. In 2019, the U.S. was ranked number one in the Global Health Security Index (GHSI) on preparedness to combat a future outbreak, based on over 100 criteria (11). Much to the surprise of the global health community, the U.S. struggled with the epidemic, clocking in 17 per cent of global deaths despite comprising only 4 per cent of the world population. The inability of these indicators of preparedness to predict successful responses demonstrates the need to revisit our metrics for preparedness. However, it also highlights that responses take place in very dynamic settings and changing political contexts, both of which may be unpredictable, not to mention difficult to measure in advance. Success on metrics of preparedness may not guarantee success in response, especially if we are not measuring the right predictors of success, such as prior resiliency and political trust.

JEEs

JEEs, a key component of the International Health Regulations (IHR) Monitoring and Evaluation Framework, are a voluntary assessment of a country across 19 technical sectors to determine the country's capacity to prevent, detect, and rapidly respond to public health emergencies. The evaluation aims to find gaps and weaknesses in the country's health security so they can focus on improvement (40).

Another metric often used in global outbreak preparedness includes the World Health Organization (WHO) JEEs, which assess the progress of compliance with international requirements, rather than actual readiness and preparedness for a specific public health threat (e.g., a simulation exercise [SimEX]) or response to prior outbreaks (e.g., 7-1-7 [detect in seven days, notify in one day, and respond in seven days]) (41–42). A country could engage its resources and capacity to fulfil all 48 indicators, receive a full five out of five compliance score, and yet not be ready for the next pandemic (examples shown in **Figure 38.6**). JEEs have simply too many indicators of questionable utility (38).

> **How much can the GHSI and JEEs tell us about response?**
>
> A multiple linear regression analysis on the value of GHSI and JEE scores on predicted preparedness and actual outcomes from the COVID-19 pandemic found that they had a "lower predictive value for detection response time and mortality outcome due to COVID-19". Of the top 20 countries with the highest preparedness scores in 2020, half of them had the highest rates of deaths per million from the COVID-19 pandemic (43). The authors suggested that high-income countries could afford the necessities required to score high on the metric scale but would also have to deal with national competing (political) interests that would detract from a community-focused response during a pandemic. The revision of the JEE in 2022 (44) addressed many of these issues but as of April 2023, only two countries have used the new evaluation tool.

In the U.S., the National Health Security Preparedness Index (NHSPI) defines national health security as the state where a nation and its populace are well prepared, protected, and resilient in the face of potential health threats or incidents. This index assesses U.S. states' collective health security preparedness, providing an annual update to gauge the country's progress in readiness, prevention, and response to potential health incidents.

The NHSPI encompasses 129 measures of capabilities crucial in safeguarding individuals from the health consequences of large-scale hazards and emergencies. The responsibility for achieving these capabilities extends across public and private sector entities, including federal, state, and local public health and emergency management, as well as healthcare providers, businesses, and volunteer organisations throughout the U.S. (45).

The NHSPI provided an independent review which in hindsight was a more accurate snapshot of U.S. preparedness (46). In 2019, the NHSPI index poorly scored the U.S. with 6.8 out of 10, with the lowest scores due to poor healthcare readiness and low community engagement, both critical faults within the pandemic response (47). The 2021 index found that the U.S. scores varied considerably across the country. As expected, areas with the highest economic and social vulnerabilities had the lowest health security and preparedness levels (48).

The global health community needs to make considerable effort to improve the ways in which we currently measure preparedness to better focus attention and target resources. The COVID-19 pandemic has shown the world that most countries failed to adequately assess the impact of COVID-19 on their communities, engage these same communities, implement and evaluate public health measures, communicate with an aligned scientific and political voice, and establish a resilient healthcare system (33). The quality of health and equity in a population may be the best predictor of mortality and morbidity rates for the next pandemic. If a country cannot do routine public health, is it prepared for the next pandemic? For example, if vaccine coverage of adolescent vaccines (human papillomavirus [HPV] where available) or the second dose of the measles vaccine is not 95 per cent, this suggests the country is not prepared for the next pandemic. These countries have not solved trust and community engagement issues and the delivery of rudimentary public health and health services. Similarly, the way a health authority responds to a small outbreak (using metrics such as 7-1-7) is probably the best predictor of how it will respond to a large event. If it is unable to mobilise resources and communities for the rapid control of an epidemic, it will not be able to do the same at scale.

In this case, prior response to events in the previous years could be a powerful predictor of future response.

This approach to measuring preparedness in an even more comprehensive process is the basis for a new WHO tool called the Universal Health and Preparedness Review (UHPR). This is a voluntary mechanism of peer-to-peer review, led by Member States, that is not only meant to promote a whole-of-government approach to preparedness and greater, more effective international cooperation, but also assesses UHC health systems, population health and their contribution to preparedness, pandemic preparedness and all-hazards risk management, compliance with the IHR, health security, and ethics, equity, human rights, and gender equity in public health (49).

RETHINKING PANDEMICS AND CREATING RESILIENT, HEALTHY COMMUNITIES

The global and national responses to the COVID-19 pandemic provide a template to essentially rethink preparedness efforts that were recodified at the end of the last century, as nation-states tackled the avian influenza pandemic, bioterrorism in the U.S., and regional outbreaks such as Zika and SARS. This process continues, without resolution at time of writing, through negotiations for a new Pandemic Preparedness Treaty. To ready an effective response, preparedness core capabilities, approaches, and measures must be as attuned to public health warfare against a microbe as to information warfare against mis- and disinformation (**See Chapter 34, Infodemics**). While the intensity of emergency public health responses is distinct in scale and scope from routine public health activities, the foundation of that response is still generally centred on some national version of the twelve WHO Essential Public Health Functions (EPHFs) (See **Figure 38.7** for the U.S. version of the 10 EPHFs) (50–51). The main difference is that emergencies require a dedicated focus on medical countermeasures (e.g., COVID vaccines, mpox diagnostics, PPE, ventilators, etc.) and the assorted supply chains (**See Chapter 7, Logistics**), as well as transparent multilateral coordination and data sharing (**See Chapter 9, Surveillance**) (52).

While our reframing of preparedness (**Figure 38.8**) leans heavily on building trust to counter disinformation and change behaviour—since the science of microbial prevention is centuries old—the universal observation and inconvenient truth is that there is little new information in the litany of recommendations from the dozens of national and global post-mortems on this pandemic. Little of what we observed during this pandemic had not been identified as gaps during prior outbreaks and exercises. Gaps were often well documented not just in white papers and the media, but even expertly depicted in fictionalised movies (e.g., just substitute ivermectin for forsythia in the movie Contagion). The litany has gone from "lessons learned" to lessons relearned to lessons ignored to lessons observed. Any brilliant new exposition of how to improve preparedness must address why the hundreds of other reports over the decades failed to catalyse the necessary national changes.

We have seen modest and piecemeal implementation. The reasons are legion hinging on overlapping or missing legislative, regulatory, and other authorities, complexity, and resources—which were unavailable, inadequate, or unsustained as part of a boom-and-bust cycle targeting the disease *du jour*. A solution is a single national authority with the responsibility, budgetary authority, and accountability to drive preparedness across the whole-of-government and the private sector. This does not necessarily require that key

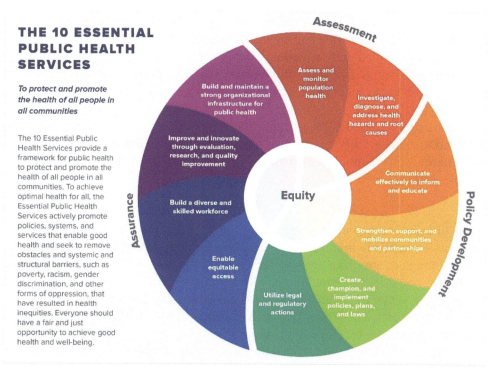

Figure 38.7: The 10 EPHFs in the U.S. (51)

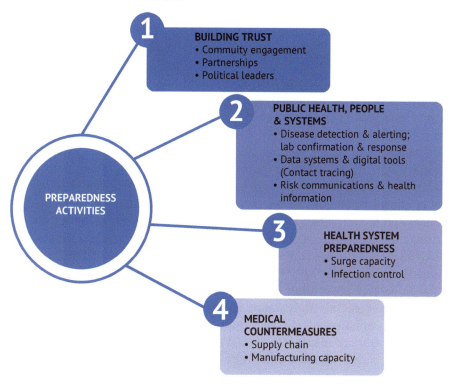

Figure 38.8: Rethinking preparedness activities at the national level

national response and preparedness entities be organisationally restructured or combined, but there needs to be an entity that has the oversight and visibility on the whole-of-enterprise. We propose this be coupled with two other changes:
- Core funding from the nation's health budget should be directed toward public health and prevention with objective evidence of adequacy based on a needs-based approach and fiscal sustainability.
- Stable funding for these health security activities with an emergency contingency fund, again tied to metrics. Only this approach will ensure the necessary resources, prioritisation of needs, and essential coordination across numerous verticals of excellence across multiple sectors.

Trust

High levels of public trust were a consistently significant source of success in handling the COVID-19 pandemic. While intangible and multifaceted (but measurable), public trust in our governments and each other is a decisive factor in a country's efforts to mobilise successfully during a public health crisis. Populations with strong trust in their governments tended to more consistently follow requirements such as mask-wearing and social distancing and had higher vaccination rates. These countries will continue to be leaders in pandemic preparedness with the most successful outcomes (14).

To have trust, the elements of excellent leadership—competency, honesty, acting with goodwill, commitment to communications and community engagement, an equity focus, and the willingness to form strong partnerships—are needed at all levels. Public health practitioners may have little ability to ensure that a populace trusts its government, has outstanding political leadership, or that the response remains non-partisan, with a unified political voice. Still, they can engage their political leaders often in exercises and workshops to educate policymakers on pandemics and proposed plans. This could build the necessary relationships so that they can become trusted advisors and should help bolster the political will to stimulate policy changes to address preparedness gaps. In contrast, public health officials have the ability and must work on their leadership and communications skills to improve and independently engender trust within their own communities. The right time for leaders to make public health more visible to their populace is when the lessons of COVID-19 are still vivid in memory—the first time a community sees its public health leader and team should not be when they are ordering some sort of mandate. Resilience comes from a population trusting the country's public health communications and policies. Science needs to be seen as non-political and factual albeit incomplete and changing. This is where public health can excel and bridge those gaps to encourage better outcomes in future pandemics.

The COVID-19 pandemic has underscored the critical need to focus on health equity and the social determinants of health (SDOH) in future pandemic planning. Major inequalities in wages, the impact of prevention measures, and housing conditions have led to a wide range of health outcomes. One study found a direct association between the number of cases, death rates, and income inequality across the U.S. (34). In some areas, simply driving 10–20 miles would reveal marked disparities in COVID-19 mortality rates. Precision public health leverages data from both traditional and innovative sources to tailor interventions to specific populations, aiming to reduce health disparities (25).

The pandemic has exacerbated the effects of SDOH, with "essential" jobs often offering low pay and high risk, disproportionately affecting marginalised groups such as racial/ethnic minorities, women, and undocumented workers. Public health experts and policymakers have a moral obligation to address these determinants equitably, especially during crises (53).

The COVID-19 pandemic highlighted existing inequities in healthcare access and outcomes. Low-income communities and people of colour faced higher risks due to crowded housing, limited healthcare access, and higher rates of underlying health conditions. Indigenous populations struggled with healthcare access due to remoteness, cultural factors, and historical mistrust. Early in the pandemic, testing and treatment resources were scarce, with marginalised communities facing greater barriers to access. The digital divide excluded those without reliable internet from telehealth services, and language barriers disadvantaged non-English speakers.

Economic factors also played a significant role. Job losses and economic insecurity affected low-wage workers, making healthcare unaffordable and preventative measures difficult. Food insecurity worsened health outcomes, and vulnerable populations like the elderly in care homes, people with disabilities, and homeless individuals faced unique challenges.

Similar disparities were observed globally. In Europe, low-income communities and ethnic minorities saw higher COVID-19 mortality rates due to crowded housing and limited healthcare access. Migrant workers in precarious jobs faced increased infection risks (**See Seasonal agricultural migrant workers**). In Latin America, large informal economies left workers without social safety nets or health insurance, while indigenous communities faced significant healthcare access challenges.

Addressing these inequities requires a coordinated effort to integrate health equity into all aspects of pandemic response and preparedness, ensuring that all communities receive the support and resources needed to protect their health.

Seasonal agricultural migrant workers in Germany

Numerous countries, like Germany, declared their seasonal migrant workers "essential" at the start of the COVID-19 pandemic. Germany brought in an additional 80,000 seasonal agricultural workers from Central and Eastern Europe. However, this status of "essential" did not correlate with increased improvements or support for these workers. Many of them did not speak German, worked and lived in poor conditions, had perpetual exposure to health risks, and by and large were excluded from Germany's health insurance or social security infrastructure (54).

Risk communication and community engagement are significant capabilities that must be built to maintain trust for an effective response (**See Chapter 33, RCCE**). We know misinformation (false or inaccurate information) and disinformation (deliberate false information to deceive for personal gain) are deadly. In May 2020, the WHO passed a resolution for member countries to target misinformation in their own countries (35). Governments must hold people, mainly social media companies, accountable for harmful misinformation while amplifying trustworthy information. Scientists, public health professionals, and journalists must also become more proficient in pre-bunking and other strategies for challenging misinformation and disinformation (55–56). This has been a significant cause of confusion and lack of confidence in the COVID-19 vaccines, which has kept vaccination rates in some populations frustratingly low. Vaccines were initially in high demand, with long lines at clinics. However, in some areas, millions of vaccine doses are being discarded due to expiration (**See Destroyed vaccine doses**) because either the country's infrastructure does not allow them to be stored in bulk or many citizens still do not want to be vaccinated (57).

> **Destroyed vaccine doses in Africa**
>
> Despite a commitment to structured, coordinated, and equitable vaccine distribution, millions of COVID-19 vaccine doses sent to African and other low- and middle-income countries were discarded due to a lack of infrastructure and organisation. Many of these discarded vaccines were short shelf-life doses delivered early in the pandemic to expedite vaccination efforts. In 2021, Malawi destroyed almost 20,000 doses, South Sudan destroyed nearly 60,000 doses, and Nigeria disposed of over one million expired doses. Some doses were reassigned to neighbouring countries in the hopes of use before expiration. Many recipient countries stopped accepting short shelf-life doses and accused donor countries of "dumping" vaccines on them (58–59).
>
> The core issue was that the recipient countries had no agency over the timing of vaccine deliveries, leaving them unprepared to receive and administer the doses. The hyper-centralised ACT-A system exacerbated the situation by sending vaccines with short shelf lives and insufficient prior notice, then unjustly blaming the recipient countries for not being ready. This approach ignored the significant logistical and political challenges involved in organising mass vaccination campaigns and failed to account for the broader context in which these countries operate.
>
> In 2022, Moderna announced a US$ 500 million investment in Kenya to produce 500 million mRNA vaccine doses annually for Africa, but by April 2024, the plan was paused due to waning demand. This is the latest in failed attempts to diversify pharmaceutical production in Africa. While regional centres could address equity and supply chain issues, they must be economically viable and sustainable. Local production often fails due to inefficiencies, poor infrastructure, and regulatory barriers. Governments and stakeholders should commit to building adaptable and profitable vaccine production facilities to meet current and future needs (60).

Health practitioners and scientists must credibly and promptly share information tailored to the community. They need to recognise that while public health authorities may have the "correct" message, they may not always be the right messengers. They must engage community members and leaders early in the information efforts, and work across the spectrum of community factions. Most critically, the role of responders is to share responsibility, so the responses are community centred. Trust is bilateral. A common misstep seen in many communities is that public health practitioners cannot trust the community to serve as advisors on the various response pillars (**Table 38.1**)—including the community engagement pillar! In a national response that can cost millions to billions of dollars, almost everyone is profiting except the patients – a situation which breeds mistrust. In the future, direct financial assistance for persons subject to isolation and quarantine should be a part of every response.

Pillar #	Public health preparedness and response area
1	Coordination, planning, financing, and monitoring
2	Risk communication, community engagement, and infodemic management
3	Surveillance, epidemiologic investigations, contact tracing, and adjustment of public health and social measures
4	Points of entry, international travel and transport, and mass gatherings
5	Laboratories and diagnostics
6	Infection prevention and control, and protection of the health workforce
7	Case management, clinical operations, and therapeutics
8	Operational support and logistics, and supply chains
9	Maintaining essential health services and systems
10	Vaccination

Table 38.1: Ten pillars of the WHO Strategic Preparedness and Response Plan for COVID-19 (as of February 2021) (61)

The WHO's strategy to combat COVID-19 is structured around ten interconnected technical and operational pillars (**Table 38.1**). These pillars guide coordinated action at national, regional, and global levels to address ongoing challenges, mitigate inequities, and navigate the pandemic. Key components of the strategy include the consistent implementation of context-appropriate public health and social measures at the local level, the introduction and deployment of new tools, and the simultaneous maintenance of essential health services and systems. Emphasising the restoration, reinforcement, and strengthening of health systems, the strategy also integrates COVID-19 surveillance and management into broader respiratory disease frameworks. The WHO's response plan is organised around these pillars, recognising their interdependence in shaping an effective and comprehensive public health response to COVID-19.

Public health systems

With the limits of its workforce and systems, every nation must be able to assess its population's health, and diagnose and address health threats. These capabilities are at the core of any response and should not be compartmentalised from health security; they are "dual-use capacities". The core functions include surveillance (**See Chapter 9, Surveillance**), laboratory testing (**See Chapter 19, Laboratory capacity**), data analytics (**See Chapter 17, Integrated outbreak analytics**), and rapid and emergency response (e.g., rapid response, incident management systems [**See Chapter 3, Leading and partnering**; **See Chapter 6, Teamwork**], financing, logistics [**See Chapter 7, Logistics**], planning, and exercises).

Surveillance systems cannot be standalone; they must integrate healthcare information, especially from social media and other sources of information. In the U.S., the idea of bringing together dataflows from disparate sources into a "fusion centre" emerged as a response to intelligence failures post-9/11. From 2008–2009, the U.S. Centers for Disease Control and Prevention (U.S. CDC) conducted a pilot programme called BioPHusion. It tested the capacity of the over 70 Fusion Centres across the U.S. to collect, analyse, and interpret information from traditional and nontraditional sources. Fusion Centres are U.S. state-operated hubs that gather and share threat-related information among state, local, tribal, and territorial (SLTT) partners, federal agencies, and the private sector. As part of the National Network of Fusion Centers, they provide a unique perspective on security threats, acting as intermediaries between frontline personnel, state, and local leaders, and the broader Homeland Security Enterprise. The National Network facilitates collaboration, representing a new standard in homeland security, by enhancing information exchange between the federal government, SLTT partners, and the private sector to prevent and respond to various threats and hazards (62). The goal of the programme was to create best practices for a nationwide network of state and local public health fusion centres (63).

All countries should invest in a national laboratory system with core technology that can be easily adapted for a new pathogen. This should also include genomic surveillance (**See Chapter 21, Genomics**). Although unknown pathogens are harder to detect and monitor, improvements in pathogen-agnostic genome-sequencing methods have created the ability to conduct open-ended searches (34).

Advances in genomics utilised during COVID-19 responses offer a promising avenue for enhanced pathogen detection in the future. This is particularly significant as the application of genomic surveillance extends beyond high-income countries. Initiatives such as the Africa Pathogen Genomics Initiative (Africa PGI), launched by Africa CDC in 2020, exemplify the potential of integrating pathogen genomics and bioinformatics into public health surveillance and outbreak investigations. Sharing information and skills between countries and collaborating with organisations such as the WHO can further amplify the benefits of these genomic advancements for global disease control and prevention.

Similar efforts have started in Latin America and the Caribbean as a result of the COVID-19 pandemic. In 2020, the COVID-19 Genomic Surveillance Regional Network (CoViGEN) was established in the Americas to enhance the sequencing capabilities of participating laboratories. The primary goal is to establish routine genomic sequencing of SARS-CoV-2 to increase the availability of genetic data globally. This data is crucial for developing diagnostic protocols, supporting vaccine development, and gaining insights into the evolution and molecular epidemiology of SARS-CoV-2. The network comprises in-country sequencing and external sequencing through eight regional sequencing laboratories. The Pan American Health Organization (PAHO) facilitates regional- and country-level training and provides support for timely SARS-CoV-2 genomic sequencing data. All countries in the Americas can participate through their National Public Health Laboratories, with encouragement to share genetic information via the GISAID platform (64).

Small countries with no previous genomics experience became empowered in sequencing and bioinformatics methods and started to actively participate in regular pathogen genomic surveillance (65). A lesson from COVID-19 and the more recent mpox pandemic is that laboratory capacity can be distributed across a country and diagnostics should not be limited to public laboratories during an emergency. Some laboratories are at academic centres or in the private sector, while others are in public health departments. During the next public health crisis, we should divide the workload amongst these competent labs which have the resources to achieve the fastest results and better outcomes and rely more heavily on rapid diagnostics (66).

Many countries have the means to collect copious data (laboratory, pharmacy, illness, healthcare utilisation, etc.). The problem is often building relationships and legal frameworks to share data and to develop rules that affect what can be shared, to whom, and for what purpose. Well-designed protocols ensure that all actors involved know what to do and with whom to share data on any outbreak that can potentially become a pandemic. The public health sector needs to develop new health intelligence capabilities that integrate social networks, law enforcement, and healthcare utilisation, and use tools like outbreak analytics, BioPHusion, and artificial intelligence to increase reaction speed and decrease death rates (67). Researchers need to determine and specify the exact data formats that are necessary for accurate information sharing. Governments must foster expertise on data sources, who to contact, and how to access it. All parties must work to protect the data to keep it secure and protect patient privacy where applicable (68).

The GISAID initiative, formally launched in May 2008 as an alternative to the public domain sharing model, has evolved into a crucial platform for the swift exchange of data. This initiative, designed by scientists for scientists, facilitates the sharing of genetic sequences and clinical and epidemiological information, aiding researchers in understanding the evolution and spread of viruses during epidemics and pandemics. GISAID addresses the barriers and restrictions that previously hindered data sharing before formal publication, ensuring open access for individuals adhering to its sharing mechanism. Users commit to acknowledging originating and submitting laboratories, fostering the fair utilisation of results. Supported by public–private partnerships and various governmental and academic institutions globally, the initiative emphasises open collaboration and respect for all rights and interests while enhancing the sharing of data (69). For example, earlier and more conclusive data would have helped scientists to determine more quickly that even asymptomatic people can spread SARS-CoV-2 through airborne transmission (34). That may have prompted the advocation for mask-wearing and extensive testing earlier in the pandemic.

Health system preparedness
A mistake from decades of preparedness is that the healthcare sector cannot be ignored in planning and response efforts. Emergency responses mirror real life; prevention takes a back seat to meeting an ill person's immediate needs. The healthcare sector should be integrated into preparedness planning and response efforts. They must anticipate surges in patients, need to implement emergency standards of care, and must address infection control.

The juice
Medical countermeasures are unique and often need to be pathogen-specific to be effective. This capacity is the most sensitive to financial resources, for example, to purchase goods, map supply chain vulnerabilities, and maintain the capacity for rapid scale-up of vaccines. Even in the U.S., in the early days of the COVID-19 pandemic, the public learned that the U.S. Strategic National Stockpile (SNS) of PPE, intensive care unit (ICU) equipment such as venti-

lators, and other critical supplies had not been replenished after the 2009 H1N1 pandemic. What remained was depleted almost immediately (70). A resilient national healthcare system must be able to respond immediately and effectively to any public health need. It should have all the financial resources it needs from the government to be self-sufficient for two to three months in case of supply line failings. Vaccines typically have the highest impact when discussing medical countermeasures because they can prevent, reduce the effects, or even stop an infectious disease pandemic (71). All nations should invest in at least one core warm-based vaccine platform, either individually or regionally, or have a number of prior agreements to assure access to these critical countermeasures. During the next pandemic, affluent countries will, again, meet their needs before sharing vaccines with others.

Bringing it all together

Routine public activities are linked to emergency response through planning and exercises for continued improvement. Nonetheless, simply having that plan, while necessary, is not enough. A plan can delineate how those capabilities and capacities will go operational during a crisis to be effective in the new health situation. A country must ensure the continuity of essential care to its population during the crisis, and that there are no major disruptions to existing programmes such as social services (**See Chapter 23, Essential services**). Once a plan has been created and implemented, it must be practised and challenged through table-top and full-scale exercises. It should also be well funded so that the resources, procedures, and infrastructure upon which the plan relies are in place before the next event happens. A plan is never complete and should be updated often to keep up with ever-changing technologies, national policies, and the health status of a population. Countries do not have the same resources or starting points. Leaders and public health experts should exchange knowledge, successes, and pitfalls within their global health societies and networks, and especially with their neighbouring countries. Infectious diseases do not stop at political borders or geographic boundaries, so it is vital to run multi-country exercises, including, among others, sharing expertise and planning for cross-deployments.

Ten steps for national preparedness

The authors have developed these ten steps for national preparedness. Many of these steps consider areas that are the subject of chapters in this book.

1. Build trust with elected leaders and citizens.
2. Establish clear top-level authority to coordinate national and subnational efforts for preparedness and response.
3. Dedicate adequate resources for a public health system, operational coordination, and developing practitioners.
4. Dedicate adequate resources for preparedness—including community resiliency—and a contingency fund for emergencies.
5. Invest in a national laboratory system with core technology to easily adapt for new pathogens.

6. Improve health intelligence with updated disease detection systems with health information from a wide variety of sources (including healthcare and social media) and new analytic tools.
7. Build the in-country legal framework for public health responses including quarantine and isolation.
8. Integrate the healthcare system into preparedness and response efforts.
9. Guarantee access to a cache of critical medical supplies and equipment across mapped supply chains.
10. Invest in warm-based vaccine manufacturing entities or agreements for access to critical medical countermeasures.

CONCLUSION

Our future preparedness plans must build upon trust and leadership, community engagement, improvements to public health communications and policy creation, data collection and disease modelling, rapid response capacity, integration of healthcare as a unified public health response, supply chain management, preparedness measurement tools, and the ability to develop therapies and vaccines (34). One must also make allowances for critical distinctions between countries with differing economies. Low- and middle-income countries will have a pared-down set of capabilities centred on core vigilance activities (scaling laboratory and health information systems, personnel, access to PPE, and stockpiles of vaccines and antivirals). They can optimise building relationships and networks across sectors and improve their leadership and community trust-building guidance.

COVID-19 was a deadly and disruptive pandemic. The next one has the potential to be even deadlier. The 14–28 million persons who would not be dead today were it not for COVID-19 would consider the global response a failure. There was a 3.4 per cent drop in global economic growth resulting in over US$ 2 trillion of lost economic output in 2020. By February 2022, schools globally had been closed because of COVID-19 for an average of 4.5 months, affecting an estimated 1.6 billion students and creating what the United Nations has called the largest disruption to education in history. Due to this interruption of education, UNESCO estimates that these students will lose US$ 17 trillion in potential lifetime earnings (72). Estimates are that roughly 10 per cent of persons who were infected with COVID-19 have long COVID symptoms.

It did not have to be this way. Some countries were able to protect their economies while maintaining a zero-to-low COVID policy, in many cases with few mandates restricting personal freedoms. Miraculously, within one year of the pandemic, there was the availability (if inequitable) of multiple safe and highly effective vaccines and therapeutics. Tackling the disinformation that led to the negative outcomes, improving inadequate public health infrastructure, and correcting public health missteps will require a new approach to trust-based preparedness. Making these foundational changes will require dedicated, sustained resources at the national level and a national authority with the responsibility, budgetary authority, and accountability to drive preparedness across the whole-of-government and private sector.

REFERENCES:

1. Bremmer I. The best global responses to the covid-19 pandemic, 1 year later. TIME; 2020 [updated 2021 Feb 23; cited 2022 Sept 25]. https://time.com/5851633/best-global-responses-covid-19/.

2. Ntoumi F, Zumla A. Advancing accurate metrics for future pandemic preparedness. Lancet. 2022 Apr;399(10334):1443–5. https://doi.org/10.1016/S0140-6736(22)00425-1 PMID:35430007.
3. Bollyky TJ, Hulland EN, Barber RM, Collins JK, Kiernan S, Moses M, et al.; COVID-19 National Preparedness Collaborators. Pandemic preparedness and COVID-19: an exploratory analysis of infection and fatality rates, and contextual factors associated with preparedness in 177 countries, from Jan 1, 2020, to Sept 30, 2021. Lancet. 2022 Apr;399(10334):1489–512. https://doi.org/10.1016/S0140-6736(22)00172-6 PMID:35120592.
4. Morens DM, Taubenberger JK, Fauci AS. A centenary tale of two pandemics: the 1918 influenza pandemic and COVID-19, Part II. Am J Public Health. 2021 Jul;111(7):1267–72. https://doi.org/10.2105/AJPH.2021.306326 PMID:34111372.
5. Kuhfeld MS, Lewis K, Morton E. The pandemic has had devastating impacts on learning. What will it take to help students catch up? Brookings; 2022. https://www.brookings.edu/articles/the-pandemic-has-had-devastating-impacts-on-learning-what-will-it-take-to-help-students-catch-up/.
6. Stone G, Witzig T, McIntosh C. The impact of COVID-19 on school-age children. Psychol Sch. 2022 Dec 1:10.1002/pits.22831. https://doi.org/10.1002/pits.22831.
7. Torbay R. Are we ready for the next pandemic? Health Aff (Millwood). 2020 Jun;39(6):1104. https://doi.org/10.1377/hlthaff.2020.00467 PMID:32479216.
8. Sachs JD, Horton R, Bagenal J, Ben Amor Y, Karadag Caman O, Lafortune G. The Lancet COVID-19 Commission. Lancet. 2020 Aug 15;396(10249):454-455. https://doi.org/10.1016/S0140-6736(20)31494-X PMID:32653081.
9. Bloomberg. The Covid resilience ranking the best and worst places to be as world enters next Covid phase 2022 [updated 2022 Jun 29; cited 2022 Sept 29]. https://www.bloomberg.com/graphics/covid-resilience-ranking/#:~:text=A%20consistently%20strong%20performer%20in,rounding%20out%20the%20top%20five.
10. Lyu S, Qian C, McIntyre A, Lee CH. One pandemic, two solutions: comparing the U.S.-China response and health priorities to COVID-19 from the perspective of "two types of control". Healthcare (Basel). 2023 Jun;11(13):1848. https://doi.org/10.3390/healthcare11131848 PMID:37444682.
11. Maxmen A, Tollefson J. Two decades of pandemic war games failed to account for Donald Trump. Nature [Internet]. 2020 Aug 4;584(7819):26–9. http://dx.doi.org/10.1038/d41586-020-02277-6.
12. Bollyky TJ, Angelino O, Wigley S, Dieleman JL. Trust made the difference for democracies in COVID-19. Lancet. 2022 Aug;400(10353):657. https://doi.org/10.1016/S0140-6736(22)01532-X PMID:36030809.
13. Abed Alah M, Abdeen S, Kehyayan V. The first few cases and fatalities of Corona Virus Disease 2019 (COVID-19) in the Eastern Mediterranean Region of the World Health Organization: a rapid review. J Infect Public Health. 2020 Oct;13(10):1367–72. https://doi.org/10.1016/j.jiph.2020.06.009 PMID:32586684.
14. Ward A. World leaders who denied the coronavirus's danger made us all less safe. Vox; 2020 [updated 2020, Mar 30; cited 2022 Oct 2]. https://www.vox.com/2020/3/30/21195469/coronavirus-usa-china-brazil-mexico-spain-italy-iran.
15. Beer T. All the times Trump compared Covid-19 to the flu, even after he knew Covid-19 was far more deadly. Forbes; 2020 [updated 2021 Jun 30; cited 2022 Oct 4]. https://www.forbes.com/sites/tommybeer/2020/09/10/all-the-times-trump-compared-covid-19-to-the-flu-even-after-he-knew-covid-19-was-far-more-deadly/?sh=589f7828f9d2.
16. Our World in Data. Coronavirus (COVID-19) Deaths 2024. https://ourworldindata.org/covid-deaths.
17. Larkin HD. COVID-19 health policies and economies in Nordic countries. JAMA. 2022 Sep;328(11):1029. https://doi.org/10.1001/jama.2022.14713 PMID:36125463.
18. Irfan FB, Minetti R, Telford B, Ahmed FS, Syed AY, Hollon N, et al. Coronavirus pandemic in the Nordic countries: health policy and economy trade-off. J Glob Health. 2022 Aug;12:05017. https://doi.org/10.7189/jogh.12.05017 PMID:35932219.
19. GAO. Operation Warp Speed: accelerated COVID-19 vaccine development status and efforts to address manufacturing challenges. U.S. Government Accountability Office; 2021 [updated 2021 Feb 11; cited 2022 Oct 1]. https://www.gao.gov/products/gao-21-319.
20. Abutaleb Y, McGinley L, Johnson CY. How the 'deep state' scientists vilified by Trump helped him deliver an unprecedented achievement. The Washington Post; 2020 [updated 2020 Dec 14; cited 2022 Oct 1]. https://www.washingtonpost.com/health/2020/12/14/trump-operation-warp-speed-vaccine/.
21. Fitzpatrick MC, Moghadas SM, Pandey A, Galvani AP. Two years of U.S. COVID-19 vaccines have prevented millions of hospitalizations and deaths. The Commonwealth Fund; 2022 [updated Dec 13, 2022. https://www.commonwealthfund.org/blog/2022/two-years-covid-vaccines-prevented-millions-deaths-hospitalizations.

22. SOGC Guideline Retirement Notice No. 2. J Obstet Gynaecol Can. 2022 Oct;44(10):1104– 1112. https://doi.org/10.1016/j.jogc.2022.08.012. PMID: 36241341.

23. Davis HE, McCorkell L, Vogel JM, Topol EJ. Long COVID: major findings, mechanisms and recommendations. Nat Rev Microbiol. 2023 Mar;21(3):133–46. https://doi.org/10.1038/s41579-022-00846-2 PMID:36639608.

24. Matsuyama K, Mayber J. How Japan achieved one of the world's lowest COVID-19 death rates. Japan Times; 2022 [updated 2022 Jun 18; cited 2022 Sept 13]. https://www.japantimes.co.jp/news/2022/06/18/national/science-health/japan-coronavirus-deaths-low/.

25. Sales C, Kim Y, Kim G, Lin B, Palaniappan L. Precision public health matters: an international assessment of communication, preparedness, and coordination for successful COVID-19 responses. Am J Public Health. 2021 Mar;111(3):392–4. https://doi.org/10.2105/AJPH.2020.306129 PMID:33566659.

26. Adler-Nissen R, Lehmann S, Roepstorff A. Denmark's hard lessons about trust and the pandemic. The New York Times; 2021 [updated 2021 Nov 14; cited 2022 Sept 13]. https://www.nytimes.com/2021/11/14/opinion/denmark-trust-covid-vaccine.html. https://www.nytimes.com/2021/11/14/opinion/denmark-trust-covid-vaccine.html.

27. Cave D. How Australia saved thousands of lives while Covid killed a million Americans. The New York Times; 2022 [updated 2022 May 17; cited 2022 Sept 13]. https://www.nytimes.com/2022/05/15/world/australia/covid-deaths.html?smid=tw-share.

28. Statista. Coronavirus (COVID-19) deaths worldwide per one million population as of July 13, 2022, by country. Statista; 2022 [updated 2022 Jul 13; cited 2022 Oct 2]. https://www.statista.com/statistics/1104709/coronavirus-deaths-worldwide-per-million-inhabitants/.

29. Malca CG, Gideon J, Romero MJ. How Peru became the country with the highest COVID-19 death rate in the world. Down to Earth; 2021 [updated 2021 17 Nov; cited 2022 Oct 2]. https://www.downtoearth.org.in/blog/health/how-peru-became-the-country-with-the-highest-covid-19-death-rate-in-the-world-80239.

30. Castaneda S. In Peru's Amazon, Indigenous COVID-19 patients get too little, too late. The New Humanitarian; 2020 [updated 2020 Sept 1; cited 2022 Oct 2]. https://www.thenewhumanitarian.org/photo-feature/2020/09/01/Peru-Amazon-Indigenous-coronavirus-health.

31. Guerin O. Covid-19 pandemic: 'Everything you should not do, Brazil has done'. BBC News; 2021 [updated 2021 Jul 9; cited 2022 Oct 2]. https://www.bbc.com/news/world-latin-america-57733540.

32. Andreoni M. Coronavirus in Brazil: what you need to know. The New York Times; 2021 [updated 2021 Oct 19; cited 2022 Oct 2]. https://www.nytimes.com/article/brazil-coronavirus-cases.html.

33. Wang Z, Duan Y, Jin Y, Zheng ZJ. Coronavirus disease 2019 (COVID-19) pandemic: how countries should build more resilient health systems for preparedness and response. Glob Health J. 2020 Dec;4(4):139–45. https://doi.org/10.1016/j.glohj.2020.12.001 PMID:33312747.

34. Maxmen A. Has COVID taught us anything about pandemic preparedness? Nature. 2021 Aug;596(7872):332–5. https://doi.org/10.1038/d41586-021-02217-y PMID:34389832.

35. Kumar P, Lurie E, Parthasarathy R. Building the US public-health workforce of the future. McKinsey & Company; 2022. https://www.mckinsey.com/industries/public-and-social-sector/our-insights/building-the-us-public-health-workforce-of-the-future.

36. Leider JP, McCullough JM, Singh SR, Sieger A, Robins M, Fisher JS, et al. Staffing up and sustaining the public health workforce. J Public Health Manag Pract. 2023 May-Jun 01;29(3):E100-E107. https://doi.org/10.1097/PHH.0000000000001614 PMID:36228097.

37. Woolhandler S, Himmelstein DU, Ahmed S, Bailey Z, Bassett MT, Bird M, et al. Public policy and health in the Trump era. Lancet. 2021 Feb;397(10275):705–53. https://doi.org/10.1016/S0140-6736(20)32545-9 PMID:33581802.

38. Asghar RJ, Kimball AM, Khan AS. Global Health Security: rethinking joint external evaluations to ensure readiness? Health Secur. 2019;17(6):504–6. https://doi.org/10.1089/hs.2019.0104 PMID:31770009.

39. Centers for Disease Control and Prevention. Global Health - CDC and the Global Health Security Agenda 2022. Updated 2022 May 20. https://www.cdc.gov/globalhealth/security/what-is-ghsa.htm.

40. World Health Organization. Joint External Evaluation (JEE). WHO; 2023 [updated 24 Mar 2023. https://extranet.who.int/sph/jee?region=All&country=341#.

41. Frieden TR, Lee CT, Bochner AF, Buissonnière M, McClelland A. 7-1-7: an organising principle, target, and accountability metric to make the world safer from pandemics. Lancet. 2021 Aug;398(10300):638-40. https://doi.org/10.1016/S0140-6736(21)01250-2 PMID:34242563.

42. Resolve to Save Lives. 7-1-7: a global target for early detection & response 2024. https://resolvetosavelives.org/prevent-epidemics/7-1-7-early-disease-detection/.
43. Haider N, Yavlinsky A, Chang YM, Hasan MN, Benfield C, Osman AY, et al. The Global Health Security Index and Joint External Evaluation score for health preparedness are not correlated with countries' COVID-19 detection response time and mortality outcome. Epidemiol Infect. 2020 Sep;148 e210:e210. https://doi.org/10.1017/S0950268820002046 PMID:32892793.
44. Global Health Security Agenda. Revisions to the Joint External Evaluation. 2022.
45. PREPARED. Measures List for 2019 Release. 2019.
46. PREPARED. National Health Security Preparedness Index [cited 2022 Sept 15]. https://nhspi.org/about/.
47. Keim ME, Lovallo AP. Validity of the National Health Security Preparedness Index as a predictor of excess COVID-19 mortality. Prehosp Disaster Med. 2021 Apr;36(2):141–4. https://doi.org/10.1017/S1049023X20001521 PMID:33397547.
48. Mays G. Health security levels in 2021 show that inequities are large, persistent but solvable. National Health Security Preparedness Index; 2021 [updated 2021 Sept 28; cited 2022 15 Sept]. https://nhspi.org/blog/health-security-levels-in-2021-show-that-inequities-are-large-persistent-but-solvable/.
49. Tedros AG. Universal Health and Preparedness Review (UHPR). 2020 Oct 21.
50. World Health Organization. Essential public health functions. https://www.who.int/teams/primary-health-care/health-systems-resilience/essential-public-health-functions.
51. 10 Essential Public Health Services Futures Initiative Task Force. The 10 Essential Public Health Services 2020 [updated Sept 9, 2020]. https://debeaumont.org/10-essential-services/.
52. Pan American Health Organization. Essential public health functions https://www.paho.org/en/topics/essential-public-health-functions.
53. Bowleg L. We're not all in this together: on COVID-19, intersectionality, and structural inequality. Am J Public Health. 2020 Jul;110(7):917. https://doi.org/10.2105/AJPH.2020.305766 PMID:32463703.
54. Bogoeski V. Continuities of exploitation: seasonal migrant workers in German agriculture during the COVID-19 pandemic. J Law Soc. 2022;49(4):681–702. https://doi.org/10.1111/jols.12389.
55. Cook J, Lewandowsky S, Ecker UK. Neutralizing misinformation through inoculation: exposing misleading argumentation techniques reduces their influence. PLoS One. 2017 May;12(5):e0175799. https://doi.org/10.1371/journal.pone.0175799 PMID:28475576.
56. Bond S. False information is everywhere. 'Pre-bunking' tries to head it off early. NPR; 2022 [updated Oct 28, 2022]. https://www.npr.org/2022/10/28/1132021770/false-information-is-everywhere-pre-bunking-tries-to-head-it-off-early.
57. Guza M, Moreland H. More than 2 million covid vaccines discarded across Pa. as doses expire. TRIB Live; 2022 [updated 2022, Jul 21; cited 2022 Sept 27]. https://triblive.com/local/regional/more-than-2-million-covid-vaccines-discarded-across-pa-as-doses-expire/.
58. Mwai P. Covid-19 vaccines: why some African states can't use their vaccines. BBC News; 2021 [updated 2021 Jun 8]. https://www.bbc.com/news/56940657.
59. Adepoju P. African countries to decline COVID-19 vaccines with short shelf lives. Devex; 2021 [updated 2021 Dec 16]. https://www.devex.com/news/african-countries-to-decline-covid-19-vaccines-with-short-shelf-lives-102324.
60. Mercurio B. Moderna cancels Kenya vaccine project due to familiar economic hurdles. Think Global Health; 2024. https://www.thinkglobalhealth.org/article/moderna-cancels-kenya-vaccine-project-due-familiar-economic-hurdles#:~:text=Moderna%20Cancels%20Kenya%20Vaccine%20Project%20Due%20to%20Familiar%20Economic%20Hurdles,-The%20cancellation%20reminds&text=On%20April%2011%2C%202024%2C%20Moderna,are%20unlikely%20to%20be%20resurrected.
61. World Health Organization. COVID-19 Strategic Preparedness and Response Plan (SPRP 2021), February 24, 2021. https://www.who.int/publications/i/item/WHO-WHE-2021.02.
62. Homeland Security. Fusion Centers 2022. https://www.dhs.gov/fusion-centers.
63. Khan AS, Fleischauer A, Casani J, Groseclose SL. The next public health revolution: public health information fusion and social networks. Am J Public Health. 2010 Jul;100(7):1237–42. https://doi.org/10.2105/AJPH.2009.180489 PMID:20530760.
64. Pan American Health Organization. COVID-19 Genomic Surveillance Regional Network 2023. https://www.paho.org/en/topics/influenza-and-other-respiratory-viruses/covid-19-genomic-surveillance-regional-network.

65. A continent-wide collaboration on genomics surveillance show the power of African science and how the majority of COVID-19 variants were introduced into Africa [press release]. 15 Sept 2022.

66. Maxmen A. Pandemic whistle-blower: we need a non-political way to track viruses. Nature. 2021 Apr;592(7852):21. https://doi.org/10.1038/d41586-021-00760-2 PMID:33742176.

67. Shakeri Hossein Abad Z, Kline A, Sultana M, Noaeen M, Nurmambetova E, Lucini F, et al. Digital public health surveillance: a systematic scoping review. NPJ Digit Med. 2021 Mar;4(1):41. https://doi.org/10.1038/s41746-021-00407-6 PMID:33658681.

68. Wanted: rules for pandemic data access that everyone can trust. Nature. 2021 Jun;594(7861):8. https://doi.org/10.1038/d41586-021-01460-7 PMID:34075248.

69. GISAID. About Us 2023 [cited 2023 16 Nov]. https://gisaid.org/.

70. Finkenstadt DJ, Handfield R, Guinto P. Why the U.S. still has a severe shortage of medical supplies: Harvard Business Review; 2020 [updated 2020, Sept 17; cited 2022 Oct 1]. https://hbr.org/2020/09/why-the-u-s-still-has-a-severe-shortage-of-medical-supplies.

71. Adalja A, Watson M, Cicero A, Inglesby T. Vaccine Platforms: state of the field and looming challenges. 2019 Apr. https://centerforhealthsecurity.org/sites/default/files/2022-12/190423-opp-platform-report.pdf.

72. Pearson H. COVID derailed learning for 1.6 billion students. Here's how schools can help them catch up. Nature. 2022 May;605(7911):608–11. https://doi.org/10.1038/d41586-022-01387-7 PMID:35614241.

CHAPTER 39

MOVING FORWARD GLOBALLY TO IMPROVE HEALTH OUTCOMES

by Thomas Frieden, Amanda McClelland, and Precious Matsoso

Inadequate preparedness contributed to the devastating consequences of the COVID-19 pandemic. Although public health measures, including vaccines, saved millions of lives, it is inevitable that another pandemic will strike in the future. It is imperative that the world moves forward by learning from the lessons of COVID-19. This chapter explores the role of public health and primary healthcare in pandemic prevention, detection, and control. We need to strengthen our public health infrastructure and implement new strategies to better prevent, detect, and respond to disease outbreaks, improve primary healthcare systems to strengthen capacities for routine care as well as response to health emergencies, and promote resilience so that individuals and communities can get and stay healthier and be better able to withstand health threats of all types.

This will require a coordinated all-of-society approach that broadly engages governments, technical agencies, diverse communities, civil society organisations, health systems, and donors. The need, tools, and effective models exist; the single most important component lacking is political commitment.

INTRODUCTION

The devastating human, economic, social, and educational costs of the COVID-19 pandemic illustrate the risks of insufficient preparedness. Countries failed to prevent millions of deaths, tens of millions of individuals experienced severe illness, hundreds of millions of students fell behind on their education, and there have been trillions of dollars in economic damage (1). Although the world has made substantial progress in response to the COVID-19 pandemic, the disease continues to cause widespread illness and death, and we remain unprepared for and unprotected from disease outbreaks; no country is fully prepared, and most have substantial work to do (2).

Increasing levels of vaccine-induced immunity and natural immunity from infection, improved treatments, better knowledge of the pathology of COVID-19, and mutations that may have made the SARS-CoV-2 coronavirus less virulent (though more transmissible) have shifted COVID-19 from a pandemic to an endemic phase. We are unlikely to experience again the high infection and death rates when COVID-19 first emerged. However, ongoing viral evolution and propagation of highly transmissible subvariants means that there will likely be ongoing spread for many years, along with flare-ups in different times and places, and the risk of a more severe, immune-escape variant is omnipresent. People will continue to die, most of them avoidably, and the long-term health impacts from infection (i.e., "long COVID") are substantial.

Moving forward

Although COVID-19 may be under better control, the next pandemic is coming. It is inevitable. We do not know where, or when, or how bad it might be, but the world needs to improve preparedness to avert its negative impacts when it does arrive. To accomplish this, we require fundamental changes in our approach to promote progress in a broad range of areas so that we keep people healthy as we prepare for the next pandemic.

The chapters in this book present the latest consensus from the outbreak response community on what we can do to improve our ability to detect infectious disease outbreaks, respond effectively to keep outbreaks from expanding into epidemics or pandemics, and prevent the emergence of pathogens. However, we also need an overarching, all-of-society strategy to improve health, including maintaining essential health services during disruptions. These essential health services include not only vaccination against communicable diseases and maternal-child health interventions, but also care for the increasing burden of hypertension, diabetes, and other non-communicable diseases.

The 3 Rs

To prevent avoidable illness and death from the next pandemic, and to improve health and productivity regardless of when the next deadly variant or microbe emerges, societies need to need get the "3 Rs" right (3). First, a *Renaissance* in public health to improve our capacity to find, stop, and prevent health threats. Second, *Robust* primary healthcare that is at the centre of healthcare systems. Third, *Resilience* so that people can get and stay healthier and live in communities where they can trust healthcare and other public services, and are thus better able to withstand and effectively respond to health threats of all types. Progress in these areas is essential not only to improve detection of and response to future health threats, but also to accelerate progress toward universal health coverage and achieving the world's Sustainable Development Goals.

RENAISSANCE IN PUBLIC HEALTH

Our public health agencies need to work in a more integrated fashion, with better alignment across local, city, state, national, and global levels. Improved coordination with political and community leaders will prioritise evidence-based action and enable multisectoral coordination. Because health is greatly affected by social determinants, we need to involve many segments of society (economic, educational, social, etc.) to maximise health protection and impact. As human populations expand into previously uninhabited areas, adoption of the multisectoral One Health approach that recognises the interconnection between people, animals, plants, and their shared environment will be essential to achieving optimal health outcomes and avoiding zoonotic spillover. Lab security is another area that can be improved, reducing the risk of an intentional or unintentional release of pathogens. There must also be sufficient and assured funding, including at local levels, which is often neglected despite its key position at the front lines of public health.

The role of the WHO

The World Health Organization (WHO) is pivotal to effective global response. The WHO is essential and necessary for data, guidance, global collaboration, and country support; as the anchor of our global health architecture, it needs stronger authorities and capacities and a larger, more flexible budget. The WHO must also be reinforced by human resource improvements, increased resources, functional partnerships with development banks and other organisations, and safeguards from inappropriate political interference (4).

Even before the COVID-19 pandemic, the WHO recognised the need for organisational reform to reduce fragmentation and compartmentalisation of programmes, increase funding to ensure sustainability, and close gaps in emergency preparedness and response (5). COVID-19 has intensified calls for agency restructuring and spurred negotiations among WHO Member States for a new pandemic preparedness treaty to accompany revisions that strengthen the International Health Regulations to improve preparedness for future pandemics and other health emergencies (6) (**See Chapter 4, Legal frameworks**).

Further improvements in the WHO are necessary, but these alone will not be sufficient to greatly improve global readiness; the scope of financial, technical, and operational support required to coordinate and respond effectively to the next pandemic is likely to remain beyond the reach of any single institution. The WHO's consensus-building approach is appropriate to most situations but would need to be further enhanced to be effective in the context of rapid action for emergency notification and response. There is a need for improved mechanisms for distribution and spending of financial resources, rapid deployment of health and public health staff, coordination at local, city, state/province, national, regional, and global levels, and collaboration across multidisciplinary pillars of preparedness and response.

At least US$ 5–10 billion a year of new funding will be required for at least a decade to substantially increase preparedness in low- and middle-income countries. In addition, substantial resources are needed to finance the zoonotic spillover prevention efforts that address the root causes of pandemics, including deforestation, the commercial wildlife trade, and inadequate agricultural biosecurity (7). More efficient financial mechanisms, stronger collaboration, and new ways of working together must recognise the reality—so vividly illustrated by the COVID-19 pandemic—of our mutual dependency and accountability.

Public health infrastructure

In addition to increased financial support, the world's public health infrastructure needs robust and intensive technical support. There must be sufficiently trained and experienced leadership, with practical experts equipped with real-time data to enable the best decisions to be made and ensure that financial resources result in improved functional capacities. Operational support is also needed to create stronger organisations with improved managerial capacity and governance. Leadership must have sufficient staff capable of implementing programmes, which will require staff who are well trained and appropriately compensated.

Incident command structures are crucial to response activities. Regular scenario planning is a useful component of the emergency planning process. Tabletop and simulation exercises can be useful as a complementary approach to the analysis of real-world responses to examine a broad range of possibilities, actions, and potential outcomes, enabling advance identification of the most effective strategies to allow for rapid and targeted response when needed.

The 7-1-7 approach

One approach to increasing accountability is to implement timeliness metrics as a means to assess and advocate for resources that improve preparedness and to accelerate progress improving preparedness. A global target of 7-1-7 for early outbreak detection, notification, and response provides a basis for accountability, to assess and improve performance, and can also be applied locally to promote equity in detection and context-appropriate response capabilities (8). The 7-1-7 target can help break the cycle of planning and more planning, using instead an approach of promptly finding and quickly fixing gaps in preparedness.

Under the 7-1-7 performance standard, every suspected outbreak is identified within seven days of emergence, is reported to public health authorities with initiation of investigation and response efforts within one day, and is effectively responded to—as defined by objective benchmarks—within seven days. This allows for the assessment of the performance of surveillance, reporting, investigation, and response systems, and is a means to assess, advocate for, and provide accountability for the efficient use of resources that improve preparedness.

The 7-1-7 target is feasible to measure and achieve, and assessment with this framework can identify areas for rapid performance improvement and help prioritise national planning. The 7-1-7 target provides a systems framework through which countries were able to assess their epidemic preparedness capabilities and complements existing preparedness measures by identifying bottlenecks and enablers of response (9–10).

Trust

It is essential to restore and rebuild the trust in public health and primary healthcare that, in many countries, became damaged during the COVID-19 pandemic, and to develop better ways of functioning in low-trust contexts while trust is being built. Trust cannot be surged during a health emergency; public health and primary healthcare systems must work together to strengthen the population's trust.

Building and maintaining community trust will strengthen the ability to detect disease outbreaks rapidly and respond effectively. Risk communication and community engagement readiness is essential to mount a rapid and effective response that will protect the public's health and save lives (11). Community engagement is core to all elements of health system resilience, but strategies must be developed with the affected communities, taking into account their specific cultural contexts and needs (12). Existing community engagement structures can support contextually specific, acceptable, and appropriate prevention and control measures, which will be particularly important to reach marginalised populations and respond in ways that support health equity (13) (**See Chapter 33, RCCE**).

Faster and more effective public health action is needed, with real-time surveillance, better communication and community engagement, and rapid response. Improved primary healthcare can address symptomatic conditions as well as the leading drivers of disability and death. Environments can be structured to make healthy choices the default choices.

ROBUST PRIMARY HEALTHCARE

One of the most important lessons from the COVID-19 pandemic is that primary healthcare should be central to healthcare systems. Population health is better in areas with more primary care physicians, people who receive care from primary care providers are healthier, and the primary care model of healthcare provision is associated with better health (14). The WHO has endorsed this approach to improve individual and population health and promote health equity (15). Strong, reliable primary healthcare systems that are accountable and provide high-quality primary care that is accessible to all are essential to improve the health of individuals and populations, and to promote community resilience against disease outbreaks and other health threats.

Despite the critical importance of primary healthcare systems, they are the most neglected component of many of the world's health systems and are often the weak link in community and national response. Most outbreaks that are stopped early were diagnosed by alert clinicians with strong connections to their local public health systems who knew to suspect an unusual disease, arrange for testing, and promptly report to public health authorities (16–17). Strengthening systems to improve healthcare provider performance and build connections with public health will therefore be essential (3).

Characteristics of high-performing primary healthcare systems

High-performing primary healthcare systems share many characteristics. Although countries will face different challenges, and solutions must be adapted to different country contexts, all countries have the potential to develop and sustain strong and reliable primary healthcare systems. Thailand and Costa Rica, both middle-income countries, have built on decades of political consensus to provide high-quality primary healthcare services available to all, with reliance on taxes and other broad financing mechanisms for funding (18). Thailand's system benefits from broad public participation, including a remarkable one million health volunteers, while Costa Rica integrates community health workers into care provision. Low-income countries will likely encounter greater challenges, particularly regarding system financing, but can steadily strengthen primary healthcare with sustained political commitment, effective governance, and appropriate financing mechanisms and choices.

Optimally, primary healthcare systems assign every person in a community to a specific primary healthcare clinician who leads a multidisciplinary team that provides culturally-competent, patient-centred care, enabling doctors and other trained healthcare workers (including nurses and community-level workers) working as part of a multidisciplinary team to use their skills where needed most to support the management of larger patient panels. Clinical encounters are at times and places convenient to patients, and out-of-pocket costs are minimised or eliminated. Continuity of care is achieved when patients receive care over the years by the same team (although its members can change) which has ready access to laboratory and other diagnostic testing, as well as priority referral for specialist care and hospitalisation when indicated.

Primary healthcare systems need sustained funding, including for staff and facilities, particularly in rural and underserved areas. Payment reforms, including well-designed performance incentives and a shift toward capitation, can improve patient outcomes by encouraging effective, quality, high-value care, and not just quantity of care (19). Ultimately, primary healthcare will have the greatest impact by doing what improves health the most and saves the most lives.

A culture of quality monitoring and continuous improvement is a consistent characteristic of the highest performing primary healthcare systems (20). Comprehensive health information management systems that integrate with electronic health records create feedback loops that facilitate continuous learning and innovation to improve value and quality of care, as well as increase patient and staff satisfaction.

An optimally functioning primary healthcare system also involves the community it serves. In this way, community members and leadership can be informed of health challenges and participate in the design and implementation of programmes to address these challenges. Furthermore, a highly functioning primary healthcare system will hold itself accountable for the health outcomes of all people assigned to its care, and each facility will be aware of its status in the delivery of effective services—as prioritised by the national government and local community—to the empanelled population.

Epidemic-ready primary healthcare

Epidemic-ready primary healthcare is central to protect communities from infectious disease outbreaks and promote community resilience (21). Primary healthcare plays an important role in preventing epidemics by detecting and managing infectious diseases, including through the rapid detection of unusual health events and reporting of these events to public health authorities, as well as through vaccination programmes and laboratory networks (22).

Many recent disease outbreaks and epidemics, including H1N1 influenza, Ebola, and coronaviruses (e.g., SARS, MERS, and likely COVID-19), were zoonotic diseases that emerged after initial spread between animals and people. Avian influenza (particularly the H5N1 strain) presents a major and ongoing risk of a pandemic among humans as well as animals. To achieve the One Health goal of balancing and optimising the health of people, animals, and the environment, and preventing spillover events, primary healthcare must integrate with public health, veterinary, and environmental sectors in a collaborative, trans-disciplinary approach to rapidly detect and reduce health threats at the human-animal-ecosystem interface. Laboratory security must also be strengthened to prevent the unintentional release of pathogens into the environment.

Epidemic-ready primary healthcare provides patients with accurate, timely, and high-quality prevention, diagnosis, and care, and bridges the gap between clinical care and public health (22). Resilient health facilities at all levels of the health system are able to maintain core services (including preventive care) during pandemics or other societal disruptions and ensure the safety of health workers and patients, who are at the highest risk of infection from disease outbreaks, with effective infection prevention and control measures (23).

Virtuous cycles

Emerging lessons point to a phenomenon of virtuous cycles in strengthening primary healthcare. High-quality primary healthcare services that are valued by communities are recognised and rewarded with increased funding and support from policymakers. As government funding for primary healthcare grows, health services are expanded and enhanced, and the services are appreciated and increasingly used by the community.

As the cycle repeats, momentum and public support for public healthcare grows, eventually achieving escape velocity by transcending partisanship and becoming recognised as a national priority and resource that is part of the fundamental social contract between the state and its citizens. The U.K., Thailand, Costa Rica, and Sri Lanka have achieved this, with primary healthcare services supported by budgets that are endorsed by nearly all political parties and governments (24).

RESILIENT INDIVIDUALS AND COMMUNITIES

One reason COVID-19 has been so deadly is that so many people were vulnerable because of their poor health status and lack of social safety nets. Many communities—defined by geography, political affiliation, race, ethnicity, and other factors—were alienated from healthcare and government services. More resilient individuals and communities are better able to withstand health threats of all types (3).

Although individuals make choices that can result in either good health or illness, many of these choices are largely determined by societal incentives and structures. Resilience is strengthened when environments are structured to make healthy behaviours the default choice and when communities are empowered to better understand and take control of their own health. Community-wide interventions that are highly effective at improving health include high and increasing taxes on tobacco, alcohol, and unhealthy food, reduced contamination of air and water, policies that reduce disparities and inequalities, land use policies that promote physical activity and safe active transportation (e.g., bicycling, walking), and food policies that encourage healthier eating, including the elimination of artificial trans fat (25). Environments structured to reduce avoidable illness, injury, disability, death, and health disparities help reduce risk and harm from future health emergencies.

Non-communicable disease prevention

In addition to providing essential public health functions, including response to epidemic diseases and other public health crises, primary healthcare is critical to preventing and coordinating life-long management of chronic conditions such as heart disease and diabetes (19). The healthier people are, the more they are able to withstand health shocks, including COVID-19 and other pandemic diseases. Healthier populations are more resilient, more productive, and have lower healthcare costs. Strengthening primary healthcare systems can shift baseline outcomes for all controllable conditions.

Cardiovascular disease presents the largest health burden globally. Hypertension is the leading preventable risk factor for heart attacks and strokes worldwide, killing more people than any other condition—more than all infectious diseases combined, and more than COVID-19 at its peak. Only about one in seven people with hypertension have controlled blood pressure (26).

Cardiovascular disease kills more than six million people aged 30–69 years worldwide each year (27). Not only are younger people having strokes and heart attacks, but disability and premature death among people in their peak wage-earning years reduce economic productivity, as does devoting time and resources to care for a parent who has had a stroke or heart attack.

Achieving high blood pressure control

Non-communicable disease programmes can achieve high blood pressure control rates, sometimes rapidly. We can learn how to do this from the world's highest performing primary healthcare systems, such as Kaiser Permanente, which controls hypertension in nearly 90 per cent of its members who have the condition (28), and countries such as Canada, which has controlled blood pressure in 60–70 per cent of all people with the condition (29).

Kaiser Permanente succeeds because its financial incentives support the effort. When failure to control hypertension leads to a preventable (and expensive) stroke or heart attack, the necessary care—both emergency and ongoing—far outweighs the cost of prevention. Kaiser Permanente saves money by focusing on effective diagnosis and treatment of hypertension, with a goal of maximising prevention. Similar reimbursement structures that reward outcomes in other healthcare systems could greatly improve efforts to control hypertension. Empanelment will be an essential function of such systems, ideally with capitation central to financing (19).

Universal health coverage

Effective hypertension management programmes both require and facilitate strong primary healthcare services and are a pathfinder for universal health coverage (**See Chapter 14, Outbreak resilience**) (30). It is important to develop population-level interventions that have the greatest potential to reduce cardiovascular disease, such as the strategic approach of the WHO HEARTS technical package (31).

There is substantial synergy between universal health coverage and improved hypertension control rates, which are a key indicator of health system achievement. Improving hypertension treatment will improve many aspects of primary care and contribute to achieving universal health coverage (32). Unless primary healthcare is greatly improved, the world is unlikely to achieve the United Nations Sustainable Development Goals for health (33).

CONCLUSION

Public health and primary healthcare systems must work together to strengthen capacities for both routine and emergency care, and need to be more fully integrated with specialty clinics and hospitals as well as with health research and development efforts. Faster and more effective public health action is needed, with real-time surveillance, better communication and community engagement, coordination, and rapid response capacity. Improved primary healthcare can address symptomatic conditions as well as the leading drivers of disability and death. Environments can be structured to make healthy choices the default choices.

There is a great deal that we can and must do. The need, tools, and effective models exist; the single most important component lacking is governmental commitment to build resilient public health systems, establish accountable, high-quality primary healthcare, and implement policies such as tobacco taxation and dietary sodium reduction that save lives and promote population resilience. This will necessitate an all-of-society approach that recognises the impact of actors beyond the health system by broadly engaging governments, technical agencies, civil society organisations, health systems, and donors.

When people have access to effective public health services, high-quality primary healthcare, and societal policies to promote health, better population health can be achieved with more equitable outcomes. This will help people live longer and healthier lives as well as increase their resilience against future pandemics and other health threats.

REFERENCES:

1. Independent Panel for Pandemic Preparedness & Response. COVID-19: make it the last pandemic. 2021. https://theindependentpanel.org/wp-content/uploads/2021/05/COVID-19-Make-it-the-Last-Pandemic_final.pdf.
2. Nuclear Threat Initiative and Johns Hopkins Center for Health Security. 2021 Global Health Security Index: advancing collective action and accountability amid global crisis. 2021. https://ghsindex.org/wp-content/uploads/2021/12/2021_GHSindexFullReport_Final.pdf.

3. Frieden TR, McClelland A. Preparing for pandemics and other health threats: societal approaches to protect and improve health. JAMA. 2022 Oct;328(16):1585–6. https://doi.org/10.1001/jama.2022.18877 PMID:36206014.

4. Frieden TR, Buissonnière M, McClelland A. The world must prepare now for the next pandemic. BMJ Glob Health. 2021 Mar;6(3):e005184. https://doi.org/10.1136/bmjgh-2021-005184 PMID:33727280.

5. WHO reform continues to confuse. Lancet. 2019 Mar;393(10176):1071. https://doi.org/10.1016/S0140-6736(19)30571-9 PMID:30894255.

6. Frieden TR, Buissonnière M. Will a global preparedness treaty help or hinder pandemic preparedness? BMJ Glob Health. 2021 May;6(5):e006297. https://doi.org/10.1136/bmjgh-2021-006297 PMID:34045186.

7. Coalition to Prevent Pandemics at the Source. Toward a comprehensive financial architecture to enable pandemic prevention. 2021. https://72d37324-5089-459c-8f70-271d19427cf2.filesusr.com/ugd/518e5d_76d8fdc18ca94b9b85fb09a6c54bf099.pdf.

8. Frieden TR, Lee CT, Bochner AF, Buissonnière M, McClelland A. 7-1-7: an organising principle, target, and accountability metric to make the world safer from pandemics. Lancet. 2021 Aug;398(10300):638–40. https://doi.org/10.1016/S0140-6736(21)01250-2 PMID:34242563.

9. Bochner AF, Makumbi I, Aderinola O, Abayneh A, Jetoh R, Yemanaberhan RL, et al. Implementation of the 7-1-7 target for detection, notification, and response to public health threats in five countries: a retrospective, observational study. Lancet Glob Health. 2023 Jun;11(6):e871–9. https://doi.org/10.1016/S2214-109X(23)00133-X PMID:37060911.

10. Mayigane LN, Vedrasco L, Chungong S. 7-1-7: the promise of tangible results through agility and accountability. Lancet Glob Health. 2023 Jun;11(6):e805–6. https://doi.org/10.1016/S2214-109X(23)00167-5 PMID:37060910.

11. World Health Organization (WHO). Risk communication and community engagement readiness and response to coronavirus disease (COVID-19): interim guidance. 2020. https://www.who.int/publications/i/item/risk-communication-and-community-engagement-readiness-and-initial-response-for-novel-coronaviruses.

12. Haldane V, De Foo C, Abdalla SM, Jung AS, Tan M, Wu S, et al. Health systems resilience in managing the COVID-19 pandemic: lessons from 28 countries. Nat Med. 2021 Jun;27(6):964–80. https://doi.org/10.1038/s41591-021-01381-y PMID:34002090.

13. Gilmore B, Ndejjo R, Tchetchia A, de Claro V, Mago E, Diallo AA, et al. Community engagement for COVID-19 prevention and control: a rapid evidence synthesis. BMJ Glob Health. 2020 Oct;5(10):e003188. https://doi.org/10.1136/bmjgh-2020-003188 PMID:33051285.

14. Starfield B, Shi L, Macinko J. Contribution of primary care to health systems and health. Milbank Q. 2005;83(3):457–502. https://doi.org/10.1111/j.1468-0009.2005.00409.x PMID:16202000.

15. World Health Organization (WHO) and the United Nations Children's Fund. (UNICEF). A vision for primary health care in the 21st century: towards universal health coverage and the Sustainable Development Goals. 2018. https://apps.who.int/iris/handle/10665/328065.

16. Centers for Disease Control and Prevention (CDC). Multistate outbreak of fungal infection associated with injection of methylprednisolone acetate solution from a single compounding pharmacy - United States, 2012. MMWR Morb Mortal Wkly Rep. 2012 Oct;61(41):839–42. PMID:23076093.

17. Olivia Li JP, Shantha J, Wong TY, Wong EY, Mehta J, Lin H, et al. Preparedness among ophthalmologists: during and beyond the COVID-19 pandemic. Ophthalmology. 2020 May;127(5):569–72. https://doi.org/10.1016/j.ophtha.2020.03.037 PMID:32327128.

18. Frieden T. The politics of primary health care: a Q&A with health leaders from Costa Rica and Thailand. New York: Council on Foreign Relations; 2021 May 20. https://www.thinkglobalhealth.org/article/politics-primary-health-care.

19. Hanson K, Brikci N, Erlangga D, Alebachew A, De Allegri M, Balabanova D, et al. The Lancet Global Health Commission on financing primary health care: putting people at the centre. Lancet Glob Health. 2022 May;10(5):e715–72. https://doi.org/10.1016/S2214-109X(22)00005-5 PMID:35390342.

20. McCarthy D, Mueller K. Kaiser Permanente: bridging the quality divide with integrated practice, group accountability, and health information technology. New York: The Commonwealth Fund; 2009 June 22. https://www.commonwealthfund.org/publications/case-study/2009/jun/kaiser-permanente-bridging-quality-divide-integrated-practice.

21. Organisation for Economic Co-operation and Development. Strengthening the frontline: how primary health care helps health systems adapt during the COVID 19 pandemic. Paris: Organisation for Economic

Co-operation and Development; 2021 February 10. https://read.oecd-ilibrary.org/view/?ref=1060_1060243-snyxeld1ii&title=Strengthening-the-frontline-How-primary-health-care-helps-health-systems-adapt-during-the-COVID-19-pandemic.

22. Frieden TR, Lee CT, Lamorde M, Nielsen M, McClelland A, Tangcharoensathien V. The road to achieving epidemic-ready primary health care. Lancet Public Health. 2023 May;8(5):e383–90. https://doi.org/10.1016/S2468-2667(23)00060-9 PMID:37120262.

23. Matenge S, Sturgiss E, Desborough J, Hall Dykgraaf S, Dut G, Kidd M. Ensuring the continuation of routine primary care during the COVID-19 pandemic: a review of the international literature. Fam Pract. 2022 Jul;39(4):747–61. https://doi.org/10.1093/fampra/cmab115 PMID:34611708.

24. Balabanova D, Mills A, Conteh L, Akkazieva B, Banteyerga H, Dash U, et al. Good health at low cost 25 years on: lessons for the future of health systems strengthening. Lancet. 2013 Jun;381(9883):2118–33. https://doi.org/10.1016/S0140-6736(12)62000-5 PMID:23574803.

25. Frieden TR. A framework for public health action: the health impact pyramid. Am J Public Health. 2010 Apr;100(4):590–5. https://doi.org/10.2105/AJPH.2009.185652 PMID:20167880.

26. Mills KT, Bundy JD, Kelly TN, Reed JE, Kearney PM, Reynolds K, et al. Global disparities of hypertension prevalence and control: a systematic analysis of population-based studies from 90 countries. Circulation. 2016 Aug;134(6):441–50. https://doi.org/10.1161/CIRCULATIONAHA.115.018912 PMID:27502908.

27. Roth GA, Mensah GA, Johnson CO, Addolorato G, Ammirati E, Baddour LM, et al.; GBD-NHLBI-JACC Global Burden of Cardiovascular Diseases Writing Group. Global burden of cardiovascular diseases and risk factors, 1990-2019: update From the GBD 2019 study. J Am Coll Cardiol. 2020 Dec;76(25):2982–3021. https://doi.org/10.1161/CIRCULATIONAHA.115.01891 PMID:33309175. Erratum information can be found at https://doi.org/10.1016/j.jacc.2021.02.039.

28. Jaffe MG, Young JD. The Kaiser Permanente Northern California story: improving hypertension control from 44% to 90% in 13 years (2000 to 2013) [Greenwich]. J Clin Hypertens (Greenwich). 2016 Apr;18(4):260–1. https://doi.org/10.1111/jch.12803 PMID:26939059.

29. Campbell NR, Sheldon T. The Canadian effort to prevent and control hypertension: can other countries adopt Canadian strategies? Curr Opin Cardiol. 2010 Jul;25(4):366–72. https://doi.org/10.1097/HCO.0b013e32833a3632 PMID:20502323.

30. Frieden TR, Varghese CV, Kishore SP, Campbell NR, Moran AE, Padwal R, et al. Scaling up effective treatment of hypertension - a pathfinder for universal health coverage. J Clin Hypertens (Greenwich). 2019 Oct;21(10):1442–9. https://doi.org/10.1111/jch.13655 PMID:31544349.

31. World Health Organization (WHO). HEARTS: technical package for cardiovascular disease management in primary health care: risk-based CVD management. Geneva: World Health Organization; 2022 July 13. https://www.who.int/publications/i/item/9789240001367.

32. Varghese C, Nongkynrih B, Onakpoya I, McCall M, Barkley S, Collins TE. Better health and wellbeing for billion more people: integrating non-communicable diseases in primary care. BMJ. 2019 Jan;364:l327. https://doi.org/10.1136/bmj.l327 PMID:30692118.

33. Frieden TR, Cobb LK, Leidig RC, Mehta S, Kass D. Reducing premature mortality from cardiovascular and other non-communicable diseases by one third: achieving Sustainable Development Goal indicator 3.4.1. Glob Heart. 2020 Jul;15(1):50. https://doi.org/10.5334/gh.531 PMID:32923344.

List of Reviewers

Colleagues from the public health and responder community very kindly assisted the Chief Editor, editorial team, and authors with anonymous peer reviews of particular chapters. With gratitude for their work and input.

Ray Arthur
Agoritsa Baka
Nahid Bhadelia
Larry Brilliant
Claire Canning
Pat Drury
Gwendolen Eamer
Paul Effler
Jennifer Garland
Thomas Hofmann
Kamal Ait-Ikhlef
Amanda McClelland
Mohannad Al Nsour
Carlos Navarro Colorado
Edmund Newman
Howard Njoo
Dariusz P. Olszyna
David Paterson
Janusz T. Paweska
Paul Michael Pronyk
Ana Rivière
Lance Rodewald
Alexander Rosewell
Daniel Salmon
Hugo Sax
Soumya Swaminathan
Teo Yik Ying
Erika Valeska Rossetto
Lothar Wieler
Stephanie Williams
Hsu Li Yang
E.K. Yeoh
Mo Yin

Index

4S's, 324–7
   100 Days Mission, 266–7

Accelerated Approval for therapeutics, 370
accessibility
   of therapeutics, 201, 295–6, 373
   of vaccines, 67, 182, 214, 305, 307, 342, 346, 371, 375, 398, 400, 403, 417, 494, 495
adapting practice into context, 474–6
advance market commitments (AMCs), 399
advance purchase agreements (APAs), 399
Advisory Group on Reform of WHO's Work in Outbreaks and Emergencies, 22
affordability of vaccines, 33, 143, 265, 371, 398, 400–3
Africa Pathogen Genomics Initiative, 41, 532
African Medicines Regulatory Harmonization (AMRH) programme, 371
African Union, 23, 100, 294, 371, 387
African Vaccine Regulatory Forum (AVAREF), 370, 387
antivirals, 41, 55, 140, 276, 290, 295, 367, 369, 371, 484
Asia Pathogen Genomics Initiative, 41

Bacterial and Viral Bioinformatics Resource Center, 283
baseline mortality, 300
basic supportive care, 317–19
best clinical care, 289, 290, 296–7
best practice guidelines, 292–3
Biomedical Advanced Research and Development Authority (BARDA), 365

causes of outbreaks
   drivers
      anthropogenic, 14
      biological, 13
         pathogens, 10–12
      environmental, 13–14
   One Health
      pathogen-host-environment interplay, 10–12
   transmission, 10–11, 13–15, 17
checklists
   coordination, 458
   early identification, 457
   for patient evaluation, 317–9
   for RCCE, 456-61
   implementation, 458
   plans and strategies, 458
   reporting, 458

child labour, 148, 307, 308
child protection, 305, 307
clinical trials, 48, 49, 54, 55, 222, 228, 291, 296, 321, 365–71, 373, 374, 380–2, 387, 389–92
Coalition for Epidemic Preparedness Innovations (CEPI), 369, 385, 386, 391, 392, 397
Coalition for Ghana's Independence Now (CGIN), 404
co-infections, 157, 317, 322–3
collaboration, 25, 30, 41, 73, 89, 101, 108, 228, 229, 262, 347, 369, 386, 414, 484, 542
   case studies
      COVID-19 pandemic
         Africa Centres for Disease Control and Response, 23
      Ebola 2014–16 outbreak, 22, 39
   evidence-based approach, 24–5
   Regional Agreements, 41
   key actors, 4
      Centres for Disease Control and Response, 23
      Global Health Security Agenda (GHSA), 108
      International Association of National Public Health Institutes (IANPHI), 25
   regional agreements
      Africa
         Africa Centres for Disease Control and Prevention (Africa CDC), 41, 49
      Asia
         Association of Southeast Asian Nations (ASEAN), 41
      Europe
         European Union Legal Framework, 41
      World Health Organization's Strategic and Technical Advisory Group on Infectious Hazards with Pandemic and Epidemic Potential, 25
   operational support
      International Health Regulations (IHR) Framework, 81
   qualities, 62–4
   types of teams, 62–9
Command, Control, and Communication (C3) system, 412, 415
communicable diseases programmes, 302
communication
   Broadened Disease Coverage and Public Health Emergency of International Concern (PHEIC) Framework, 89–94
      2009 H1N1 influenza, 91–2
      COVID-19, 90, 92–5
      Ebola 2014, 93
      Ebola 2019, 93

mpox 2022, 92, 93
wild poliovirus 2014, 91–2
Zika 2016, 93
community engagement, 4, 7, 8, 24, 30, 45, 50, 54, 91, 114, 148, 172, 186, 188, 213, 263, 309, 342, 385, 415, 439, 450–62, 471, 476, 477, 482, 525, 528–30, 543
contact tracing, 5, 17, 51, 52, 94, 119, 130–8, 141, 144, 147, 148, 162, 172, 174, 196, 199, 237, 258, 274, 280, 452, 453, 479, 504
   current challenges
      mass contact tracing, 133–4
   emerging technologies
      bluetooth, 133, 134, 136
      GPS, 134, 137
      integration of technologies, 134
      QR codes, 134
   future challenges
      data storage and use issues, 132, 134, 136, 137
      disease factors, 130, 131, 133
      population factors, 136
      technology factors, 136–7
   process, 131, 132
      Convention on Biological Diversity (CBD), 34–6, 231–2
      Coronavirus Treatment Acceleration Program (CTAP), 390
Council on Health Research for Development (COHRED), 374
COVID-19 Technology Access Pool (C-TAP), 399
critical care, 314–28
cultural and social differences, 196, 483–5
   indigenous approaches in Americas, 484–5
culture-independent diagnostic tests (CIDT), 277

data accessibility, 495
data connectivity and sharing, 244–5
data sharing, 35, 52, 103, 107, 231, 244–5, 270, 271, 282, 371, 372, 375, 526, 533
decision-making processes, 413, 415
   approach, 64–7, 430, 442, 475, 478–9
   ethics as part of, 45-58
   evidence-based, 66–9, 175, 218–9
   implementation, 68
   justifications, 170
   monitoring
      COVID-19 (SARS-CoV-2), 65, 68–9
   teams, 64–9, 218
diabetes, 173, 198, 303, 439, 498, 541, 546
diagnostic tests
   challenges and solutions
      diagnostic equity, 266
      test procurement, 261
   evaluation
      performance, 253–61
      quality assurance, 261
      reference standards, 255–7, 260

      study design, 259–60
      use case, 257–9
disabilities, 305, 306, 316, 346, 422, 434, 438, 440, 441, 466, 482, 495, 529, 543, 546
disinfection, 143, 187, 293, 340, 343, 345, 356, 358, 360, 362, 504
domestic violence, 53, 169, 175, 308–9
drug development, 174, 368–70

economic diversity, 374
ELMAOUNA, shock response programme, 308
emergency cycle, 2–4
   prepare
      ethics
         variant Creutzfeldt-Jakob disease (vCJD), 51
      key actors, 71–83
      preparedness activities, 2–4, 50–1
      see also Emergency Preparedness and Response Plan (EPREP)
   prevent, 2, 3
      ethics, 47
   recover, 2, 57–8, 489–99
      ethics
         Ebola 2014–16, 58
   respond
      ethics
         COVID-19, 49, 52–3, 55–6
      key actors, 2–4, 51–7, 111–12
      outbreak investigation, 112–27
      see also pillars of response
emergency mass vaccination, 379
Emergency Preparedness and Response Plan (EPREP), 74–7
Emergency Triage Assessment and Treatment (ETAT), 316
emergency use authorisation (EUA), 228, 264, 266, 296, 368, 389
Emergency Use Listing Procedure (EUL), 267, 389
EnteroBase, 283
essential healthcare, 296, 301
essential services, 5, 7, 53, 294, 295, 334, 428, 429, 437, 442, 477, 534
ethical principles, 370
ethics
   frameworks
      European & Developing Countries Clinical Trials Partnership (EDCTP), 49
      Universal Declaration of Human Rights (UDHR), 48
   moral concepts, 46–7
   values, 46
European Centre for Disease Prevention and Control (ECDC), 100, 112
   European Medicines Agency (EMA), 371, 380
evolution of RCCE, 457
   Ebola case study, 455
excess mortality, 295, 300, 518, 519

facility infrastructure design, 331
family planning, 301, 302, 309
Federal Interagency Working Group on Influenza, 365
flow of patients, HCWs and visitors in emergency facilities, 335–7
funding, 76, 77, 91, 107, 231, 232, 234, 238, 247, 266, 342, 366, 371–2, 385–7, 397–9, 451, 476, 491, 518, 542, 544, 545

Gavi, the Vaccine Alliance, 302, 383–5, 392, 397
genomics, 41, 122, 135, 161, 225, 230, 239, 242, 253, 270–84, 391, 494, 532
genomic sequencing, 41, 230, 239, 242, 246, 253, 280, 390, 494, 532
genotypic methods, 271
GISAID, 272, 282, 283, 372, 532, 533
global health security, xi, 31, 524
Global Health Security Index, 3, 21, 32, 524
Global Health Security Initiative (GHSI), 101
Global Influenza Surveillance and Response System (GISRS), 34, 104, 107, 282
Global Outbreak Alert and Response Network (GOARN), 170, 294, 374, 504
　　Global Public Health Intelligence Network (GPHIN), 160
Global Vaccine Action Plan (GVAP), 397
Good Laboratory Practices (GLP), 382
Good Manufacturing Practices (GMP), 382

harnessing local action
　community perspectives
　　managing Ebola in Guinea, 460
　　managing mpox, 478–9
　ethical considerations, 482
　making facilities visible to community leaders, 337
　motivating volunteers, 481–2
　needs of volunteers and communities
　　community led Ebola care, 347, 480–1
　networking local HCWs, 118
　task shifting
　　case study of Red Cross, 480
health inequalities, 17, 169, 369, 403
health screening, 304–5
health-seeking behaviour, 100, 173, 289, 495
health system preparedness
　laboratory systems as essential to, 247–8
　ten steps for national preparedness, 534–5
　　health system resilience, 168–76, 242, 246
　　"herd" immunity, see immunity
hospital-acquired infections (HAI), 142, 216, 226, 270, 273, 295, 296, 301, 302, 304, 323, 325, 354
the humanitarian system, 180–1

immunity,
　"herd" immunity, 5, 51–2, 195, 380
　passive immunity, 296
　population immunity, 141, 196, 553
　　Immunization Agenda 2030 (IA2030), 397
immunogenicity, 295, 379, 381, 382, 387, 388
Infectious Diseases Control Centre (IDCC), Tokyo Games 2020, 414
infection prevention and control (IPC), 1, 14, 63, 93, 187–8, 212, 215, 228, 320, 334, 353–63, 415, 450, 491, 504, 545
infodemic management
　communicating risk, 470
　engaging and empowering communities
　　partnerships to engage vaccine hesitancy, 471
　listening to concerns, 469–70
　promoting resilience, 470
infodemics, 171, 385, 403, 416, 451, 456, 461, 465–72, 526
　impact of, 467–8
infodemiology, 471–2
institutional review boards (IRBs), 233, 370
integrated outbreak analysis, 211–21
　approaches, 216–17
　emergence, 212–15
　evidence tracking, 212–16, 219–20
　examples, 216
　key principles, 215
intellectual property (IP), 31, 187, 244, 265, 371, 398, 399
　International Association of National Public Health Institutes (IANPHI), 25
International Centre for Diarrhoeal Disease Research, Bangladesh (icddr,b), 294
International Coalition of Medicines Regulatory Authorities (ICMRA), 389
International Covenants on Civil and Political Rights (ICCPR), 32, 36–8
International Covenants on Economic, Social and Cultural Rights (ICESCR), 32, 36
International Federation of Red Cross and Red Crescent Societies (IFRC), 6, 383, 461
International Health Regulations (IHR) Framework, 6, 21, 30–6, 81, 87–9, 99
International Monetary Fund, 387
International Nucleotide Sequence Database Collaboration, 283
International Severe Acute Respiratory and emerging Infection Consortium (ISARIC), 264, 374
International Society for Infectious Diseases (ISID), 293
investigations, 14
　Bacillus cereus outbreak, 16
　and contact tracing, 133
　during humanitarian emergencies, 180
　Ebola virus disease, DRC, 2018, 246

integrated outbreak analysis, 211–21
  role of genomics, 270–1
  tuberculosis outbreaks, 135
isolation capacity, 335, 343
isolation rooms, 142, 334, 345

Jenner, Edward, 379, 380
Joint External Evaluations (JEEs), 524–5
  measuring success of RCCE, 455
Joint Research Centre (JRC) of the European Commission, 101

laboratory capacity
  building
    surge capacity, 245–6
    sustainability, 247–8
  centralisation, 241–2
  embedding within healthcare system, 241–5
  quality management, 243–4
  role, 238–40
learning loss, 147, 305, 437
legal frameworks
  considerations for research implementation, 233–4
  International Legal Instruments, *see also* communication, Broadened Disease Coverage and Public Health Emergency of International Concern (PHEIC) Framework
    Convention on Biological Diversity (CBD), *see* Convention on Biological Diversity (CBD)
    core capacities, 89, 90
    history, 87–90
    Human Rights Treaties
      International Covenants on Civil and Political Rights (ICCPR), 32, 36–8
      International Covenants on Economic, Social and Cultural Rights (ICESCR), 32, 36
      Universal Declaration of Human Rights (UDHR), 31, 36, 48
      World Health Organization (WHO) constitution, 31–7, 40
    International Health Regulations (IHR) Framework, 6, 21, 30–6, 81, 87–9, 99
    Nagoya Protocol, *see* Nagoya Protocol
    National Legal Frameworks, 29, 30, 38–9
    Pandemic Influenza Preparedness (PIP) Framework, 34–5
    World Trade Organization Trade-Related Aspects of Intellectual Property Rights (TRIPS) Agreement, *see* Trade-Related Aspects of Intellectual Property Rights (TRIPS)
logistics
  emergency preparedness and response plan (EPREP), 74–7
  operations, 74–5
  public health logisticians, 72–3

maintaining control of infectious diseases
  data collection
    comparison of surveillance, 494–5
    transmission control, 493–4
  management
    community and inpatient, 427
    emergency, 426
  management structures
    centralised, 21–2
      Global Health Security Index, 21
      International Health Regulations, 21
    decentralised, 23
Maputo Declaration, 237, 242
mass gatherings, 141, 146, 246, 408–18, 531
Médecins Sans Frontières (MSF), 6, 181, 347, 349, 427
mental health, 5, 7, 21, 40, 58, 127, 146, 147, 175, 301, 305, 308, 420–31, 434, 438, 440, 441, 452, 459, 480, 481, 485, 499, 518
MinION, 272, 276
misinformation, 7, 17, 36, 53, 171, 184, 323, 365, 367, 385, 392, 396, 397, 401–3, 416, 421, 442, 444, 454, 457, 459, 466–7, 470–2, 498, 529
modelling, applications of, 194–5, 205
modelling parameters
  basic reproduction number, 131, 193–6
  effective reproduction number, 194, 196–7
  other, 204–5
Modelling Consortium Framework, 305
morgues, 341, 342

Nagoya Protocol, 30, 34–6, 50, 231–2, 265
National Association for the Advancement of Coloured People (NAACP), 401
National Emerging Infectious Diseases Laboratory (NEIDL), US, 342
National Health Security Preparedness Index (NHSPI), 524–5
national influenza centres (NICs), 281
National Institute of Allergy and Infectious Diseases (NIAID), 371
National Institutes of Health (NIH), 342, 369
national regulatory authorities (NRAs), 370, 382
needs-based design
  components of working outcomes
    designing SMART outcomes, 506–8
    Kirkpatrick evaluation model, 508–9
new information ecosystem
  individual experience
    assessing credible and accurate information, 451, 465, 466, 470, 471, 533
    changing of needs, 466
    discerning quality of information, 466

knowing relevancy of information, 466
    making decisions, 218, 390
  science and evidence generation during epidemics, 467
next-generation sequencing (NGS), 270–2, 275, 276, 278
non-communicable diseases, 173, 243, 302, 303, 541, 546
non-pharmaceutical interventions
  categories
    community-wide response measures, 146–8
    environmental measures, 143
    personal protective measures, 140, 142–3
    targeted response measures, 144–6
  factors influencing effectiveness, 143, 147
  implementation strategies, 140–9
  objectives, 139–42
  social and ethical considerations, 141, 142, 145–8
nosocomial infections and settings, *see* hospital-acquired infections

occupational health, 296
One Health, 40, 51, 74, 101, 108, 155–64, 240, 279, 282, 541, 545
Open Research Europe (ORE), 375
organ dysfunction, 291, 314, 315, 317, 319, 320, 322
outbreak investigation
  analysis
    descriptive, 119–22
    statistical, 122–6
  case definitions, 113, 116, 118
  data management, 116–18, 121
  evaluation, 127
  field epidemiology, 111–12
  surveillance, 116–17, 119, 127
outbreak response, 179–82
  training
    just-in-time, 502–3
    non-emergency, 502–3, 505
    pre-deployment, 502–3, 505
    real-time, 502–4
outbreaks, 223–8
  2009 H1N1 influenza, 91, 92
  anthrax, 163–4
  Bacillus cereus, 16
  cholera
    global 2023, 77–8
    in Haiti (2010), 184
    in Yemen (2016–8), 187
  COVID-19 (SARS-CoV-2), 21, 23–5, 33, 49, 52–3, 55–6, 65, 68–9, 90, 92–5, 102
  diphtheria, in Cox's Bazaar (2018), 187
  Ebola virus disease (EBOD), 8, 17, 21–2, 55, 72, 93, 183, 187, 193, 199–200, 289, 322, 328, 347
    in Congo, 49, 92, 212, 214–15, 246, 260, 314, 367, 436, 497, 504
    in Gabon, 160
    in Guinea, 105, 322, 360, 460
    in Liberia, 105, 171, 322, 359, 455
    in Nigeria, 105
    in Sierra Leone, 105, 234, 306, 322
    in Uganda, 358
    in West Africa, 39, 48, 56, 58, 73, 76, 82, 91, 148, 179, 222, 227, 248, 291, 354, 386, 387–8, 391, 435, 484
  mpox 2022–3, 92, 93, 252, 266, 367
  Nipah virus, 162
  pneumonic plague 1994, 88
  Rift Valley fever virus, 163
  variant Creutzfeldt-Jakob disease (vCJD), 51
  wild poliovirus 2014, 91, 92
  Zika 2016, 92, 93, 280
outbreak training, 357, 360

palliative care, 323
Pandemic Emergency Financing Facility (PEF), 371
Pandemic Influenza Preparedness (PIP) Framework, 30, 31, 34–35, 50, 81, 399
Pandemic Preparedness Platform for Health and Emerging Infections Response (PANTHER), 264
PANDORA-ID NET Consortium, 49
Partnership for Research on the Ebola Virus in Liberia (PREVAIL 1) trial, 372
passive immunity, 296
Pasteur, Louis, 272, 379
personal protective equipment (PPE), 3, 7, 15, 23, 55, 71, 114, 142, 172, 293, 303, 325, 334, 353, 408, 437, 459, 469, 490, 504, 518
phenotypic methods, 271
phylogenies
  phylogenetic trees, 275
physiological vulnerabilities, 423
pillars of response, 2–3, 6–8, 51–7, 117–22, 213, 450–2, 479, 530–1
planning for diversity
  local actors, 482–3
populations
  bereaved, 428
  key workers
    burdens, 428
    healthcare workers, 428–30
    support, 430
  survivors, 427–8
population immunity, 141, 196, 201
post-outbreak research, 234
preventing mental illness, 423–4
principles of recovery
  capitalisation of opportunities, 498
  considering local contexts, 498
  support for welfare, 498–9
propagation
  system weaknesses, 14–17
psychosocial support, 7, 63, 323, 420–31, 480

Index

public health systems
  CoVIGEN, 532
  GISAID initiative, 532, 533
  US BioPHusion, 532
public health emergency of international concern (PHEIC), 6, 8, 22, 72, 86–96, 99
public–private partnerships (PPP), 371, 385, 533

quality clinical care, 296

randomised controlled trial (RCT), 123, 142, 323, 372
Randomized Embedded Multifactorial Adaptive Platform for Community-acquired Pneumonia (REMAP-CAP), 367
Rapidly Emerging Antiviral Drug Development Initiative (READDI), 369
rapid response mobile laboratories (RRMLs), 276
risk communications and community engagement (RCCE), 91, 188, 215, 227, 450–61, 463
  effective RCCE, 453–6
  future of, 461
  measuring success of RCCE, 455
  quality standards, 455
  RCCE and integration, 454
  RCCE and trust, 454
    lessons from Africa, 455
  RCCE in marginalised communities
    lessons from Singapore, 453, 456–8
real-world evidence
  common good, 519
  personal freedom
    Sweden and Nordic countries, 519–22
  unlucky, 522–3
reasons
  loss of coping, 421–2
  stressors, 421
regulatory reliance, 390
renaissance in public health
  7-1-7 approach, 543
  part of the 3 Rs, 541
  public health infrastructure, 542
  role of WHO, 542
  trust, 543
research, 7, 21, 24, 48–51, 54–7, 169, 174, 222–35, 239–43, 263, 292–3, 365–75, 380–4, 492
  establishing teams, 228–30
  importance, 223, 225–8
  pre-planning, 222–3, 364–5
research and development (R&D), 21, 34, 50, 54, 174, 229, 255, 266, 365, 368, 380–4
research types, 223–8
resilient health systems
  building blocks, 169, 242, 246
  definition, 168–9
  governance, trust, scientific advice, 169–71
  investment
    in health professionals and communities, 171–3
    in systems, 173–4
  private sector involvement, 169, 174
  research and development, 174
  workforce, 324
  universal health coverage
    integration with global health security, 169, 173, 174
resilient individual/communities
  high blood pressure control, 546–7
  preventing non-communicable diseases, 546
  psychological, 426
  universal health coverage, 547
resumption of health care provision
  engagement with stakeholders, 491
  improvement of logistics
    interaction with other outbreaks, 491
  prioritisation of services, 492
  reducing risk of transmission, 492
  workforce management, 491, 492
rethinking pandemics
  10 pillars of WHO plan, 531
  essential public health services, 526–8
  public trust
    destroyed vaccines in Africa, 530
    migrant workers in Germany, 529
ring vaccination, 380, 388
risk
  assessment, 181–3
  factors, 181–3
  management
    WASH initiatives, 185
risk assessment, 4, 51, 89, 93, 104, 182–3, 281–2, 410–11
  Global Health Security Index, 3, 21, 32, 524
  WHO Emergencies Programme, 4
risk communication, 7, 53, 54, 63, 173, 186, 188, 213, 227, 385, 411, 415, 418, 450–62, 470, 529, 543
risk zones, 340
robust primary healthcare
  characteristics of high-performing systems, 544–5
  epidemic ready, 545
  virtuous cycles, 545

Sanger sequencing, 272, 275
school closures, 66, 139, 141, 146, 147, 305–8, 437, 493, 495
screening, 48, 94, 115, 156, 174, 202, 228, 239, 245, 257, 281, 295, 302–4, 316, 322, 333–5, 345, 346, 348, 349, 355, 414, 428, 480
sepsis, 317–24
social inequalities, 396, 398, 401
space strategy, 332

Special Pathogens Research Network (SPRN), 370
Special Programme for Research and Training in
    Tropical Diseases (TDR), 374, 568
spectrum of disorders, 422
Stepwise Laboratory Improvement Process
    Towards Accreditation (SLIPTA), 237
Strengthening Laboratory Management Toward
    Accreditation (SLMTA), 237
supportive care, 289–91, 314–27
supply chain
    cold chain systems, 77, 80
    forecasting
        cholera 2023 outbreak, 72, 77–8
        Essential Items Estimator Tool, 78–9
        World Health Organization COVID-19
            Essential Supplies Forecasting Tool
            (COVID-ESFT), 79
    last-mile planning
        Pakistan 2022 floods, 81
    stockpiles, 71, 79–80
supporting recovery
    Anthrax outbreak in Kenya, 485–6
surge, 7, 53, 55, 73, 79, 82, 133, 201, 215, 245–7,
    290, 293–4, 324, 331, 334, 340, 343–5, 348, 354,
    357, 358, 361–2, 400, 415, 442, 479, 491, 492,
    533, 543
surge capacity, 79, 80, 245, 326, 331, 354, 358,
    361–2, 491
surveillance, 4, 7, 30, 34, 35, 40, 41, 50–2, 55, 58,
    72–4, 87, 89, 98–108, 113–17, 119, 127, 141, 157,
    159–61, 163, 170, 171, 173, 183, 184, 200, 204,
    212, 213, 216–18, 237–44, 246–8, 252, 255, 257,
    258, 261, 267, 270–83, 346, 361, 368, 369, 382,
    383, 403, 411, 412, 417, 424, 452, 459, 479, 484,
    485, 494, 495, 497, 504, 531, 532, 543
    history, 98–108
    key actors, 102–3
        Middle East Consortium on Infectious
            Disease Surveillance (MECIDS), 103
    programmes
        disease-specific
            African Centres for Disease Control and
                Prevention (Africa CDC), 100, 104
            European Centre for Disease Prevention
                and Control (ECDC), 100
        national, 98–100, 102, 106
    technology
        challenges
            Ebola 2014-16, 105
        Epidemic Intelligence from Open Sources
            (EIOS)
            COVID-19, 101–2
    types
        event-based, 100, 101, 495
        indicator-based, 100, 495
    wastewater, 69, 184, 239, 258, 494

T0 form for outbreak data, 292
T1 form for outbreak data, 292
teenage pregnancy, 308
TEKAVOUL, 308
telehealth, 296–7, 498, 529
telemonitoring, 297
terrorism, 349, 350, 526
therapeutics, 7, 34, 54, 55, 174, 198, 201, 228, 229,
    239, 264, 274, 280, 289, 295–6, 322, 323, 328,
    365–75, 389
training, 112, 127,
    of volunteers, 501–15
training, design of
    for Ebola virus disease care, 504
    for field epidemiology, 112
    GOARN non-emergency training, 505
    logistics and supply chain management, 72–5
    training, tracking of impacts, 510
training modalities
    summary of training modalities, 509–10
travel
    border closures, 20, 92–5
    COVID-19, 90, 92–5
triage, 173, 257–9, 293, 315–17, 304, 324, 327, 335,
    337, 339, 343, 345, 348, 355
Trade-Related Aspects of Intellectual Property
    Rights (TRIPS), 29–30, 33–4, 38
trust,
    in experts and medical professionals, 25, 51,
        72, 172, 205, 224, 239, 245, 289–90, 327, 372,
        453, 468, 530, 543
    general social trust, 7, 54, 91, 92, 93, 149, 172,
        188, 442, 454–5, 476, 519, 523, 526, 528–9
    between government and marginalised
        communities, 171, 439, 442, 529
    internationally, 34, 98, 107
    networks of trust, 8, 23–4, 26
    and risk communication and community
        engagement (RCCE), 454–6, 460, 475
    role of ethics to build trust, 49, 114
    and surveillance, 106, 137
    and vaccines, 397, 401, 402–4
trust-building measures, 20, 476, 528–30

U.K.-based Randomised Evaluation of COVID-19
    therapy (RECOVERY), 369
understanding communities and barriers
    building trust, 23, 24, 25, 476
    responding to epidemics, 477
undertaking effective reviews
    future preparedness, 496–7
    types of reviews, 496
UNICEF, 79, 181, 305, 308, 383, 384, 437, 461
United Nations (UN)
    Human Rights Office, 306

Mission for Ebola Emergency Response
(UNMEER), 22
United States (U.S.)
Centers for Disease Control and Prevention
(U.S. CDC), 6, 83, 98, 112, 135, 181, 248, 293,
383, 504, 532
Department of Health and Human Services
(HHS), 83, 371
Food and Drug Administration (U.S. FDA), 255,
368, 370, 380, 387, 389–91
utilities planning, 341

vaccine access, see accessibility of vaccines
vaccine affordability, see affordability
of vaccines
vaccine equity, 396–403
vaccine hesitancy, 53, 396, 398, 401–4, 471
vaccine mandates, 404
vaccine nationalism, 56, 398, 401
vaccines, 8, 14, 17, 36, 39, 40, 46, 50, 53, 56–8, 73,
76, 80–2, 91, 107, 122, 139, 148, 174, 182, 185,
186, 188, 195, 203, 204, 222, 225, 228, 229, 239,
264, 271, 281, 295, 304, 337, 365, 369, 370, 372,
379–92, 396–403, 437, 461, 465, 476, 478, 485,
491, 494, 518, 521, 525, 526, 530, 532–4, 540
virtual ward, 297
vulnerable populations
amplifiers, 441–2
children, 437
elderly
elderly in Italy, 440
indigenous populations, 439
migrant workers, 440–2
in Germany, 529
migrant workers in Singapore, 441, 456–9
people with disabilities, 438
refugees and displaced, 438

strategies
learning from mpox, 443
roles of faith and religion, 444
women and girls, 435–7

waste management in emergencies, 127, 241, 246,
336–7, 340–1
wastewater testing, see surveillance, wastewater
Wellcome Open Research Platform, 375
Wellcome Trust, 234, 375, 386
whole genome sequencing (WGS), 270–81
World Bank Financial Intermediary Fund (FIF)
for Pandemic Prevention, Preparedness and
Response (PPR), 372
World Health Organization (WHO)
constitution of, 31–7, 40
Emerging Diseases Clinical Assessment and
Response Network (EDCARN), 294
Health Emergencies Programme, 2, 22, 558,
566, 570
HEARTS technical package, 547
R&D Blueprint, 229, 261, 388–9
WHO Listed Authority (WLA), 383

zoning systems, 293
zoonotic transmission
spillback, 156
spillover
biodiversity and, 155, 157, 158
conditions promoting spillover, 157–9
factors influencing spillover, 163
reservoir hosts, 156, 159, 160
transmission
confirming spillover, 160–1
disease amplification, 161–2
transmission dynamics, 161